REFERENCE

Atlas of
Human Anatomy

F. Netter, M.D.

Consulting Editors

Jennifer K. Brueckner, PhD
Assistant Professor
Department of Anatomy and Neurobiology
University of Kentucky College of Medicine
Lexington, Kentucky

Stephen W. Carmichael, PhD, DSc
Professor
Departments of Anatomy and Orthopedic Surgery
Mayo Clinic
Rochester, Minnesota

Thomas R. Gest, PhD
Associate Professor
Division of Anatomical Sciences and Department
   of Medical Education
University of Michigan Medical School
Ann Arbor, Michigan

Noelle A. Granger, PhD
Professor
Department of Cell and Developmental Biology
University of North Carolina School of Medicine
Chapel Hill, North Carolina

John T. Hansen, PhD
Professor of Neurobiology and Anatomy
Associate Dean for Admissions
University of Rochester School of Medicine and Dentistry
Rochester, New York

Anil H. Walji, MD, PhD
Professor and Director, Division of Anatomy
Professor of Radiology and Diagnostic Imaging
Professor of Surgery
Faculty of Medicine and Dentistry
University of Alberta
Edmonton, Alberta, Canada

Atlas of
Human Anatomy

Fourth Edition

Frank H. Netter, MD

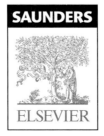

SAUNDERS

ELSEVIER

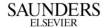

SAUNDERS
ELSEVIER

1600 John F. Kennedy Boulevard
Suite 1800
Philadelphia, Pennsylvania 19103-2899

Atlas of Human Anatomy   Edition with Student Consult Access: ISBN-13: 978-1-4160-3385-1
Fourth Edition   ISBN-10: 1-4160-3385-8

                           Professional Edition: ISBN-13: 978-1-4160-3699-9
                                                                        ISBN-10: 1-4160-3699-7

                           International Edition: ISBN-13: 978-0-8089-2384-8
                                                                        ISBN-10: 0-8089-2384-6

                           Enhanced International Edition
                           with Student Consult Access: ISBN-13: 978-0-8089-2379-4
                                                                        ISBN-10: 0-8089-2379-X

NOTICE

Neither the Publisher nor the Editors assume any responsibility for any loss or injury and/or damage to persons or property arising out of or related to any use of the material contained in this book. It is the responsibility of the treating practitioner, relying on independent expertise and knowledge of the patient, to determine the best treatment and method of application for the patient.

Previous editions copyrighted 2003, 1997, 1989.

Acquisitions Editor: Anne Lenehan
Developmental Editor: Marybeth Thiel
Publishing Services Manager: Frank Polizzano
Senior Project Manager: Cecelia Bayruns
Design Direction: Louis Forgione
Illustration Manager: Cecilia Nuyianes
Cover Design Concept: Madelene Hyde
Marketing Manager: Megan Poles

Printed in the United States of America.

Last digit is the print number: 9 8 7 6 5 4 3 2 1

To my dear wife, Vera

Foreword

The Fourth Edition of *Atlas of Human Anatomy* by Frank H. Netter, MD, has been updated by our Consulting Editor team of Jennifer K. Brueckner, Stephen W. Carmichael, Thomas R. Gest, Noelle A. Granger, John T. Hansen, and Anil H. Walji. We have each reviewed, modified, and updated a section of the *Atlas*. Throughout the book, new radiographs, computed tomographic (CT) images, CT angiograms, and magnetic resonance (MR) images have been added, which reflects the importance of diagnostic imaging in clinical anatomy and medicine. In this edition, 45 plates have been revised to show corrected anatomical relationships, 290 plates have been relabeled, and there are 17 completely new plates. Wonderful new artwork for this edition has been created by Carlos A. G. Machado, MD, who has contributed to the Netter illustrations for over ten years. Anatomical nomenclature has been brought up to date, and clinical terms and eponyms in common usage have been included parenthetically. The genius of Dr. Netter's paintings is that the anatomy is portrayed clearly, realistically, and in a clinically relatable fashion while maintaining the balance between complexity and oversimplification. We have tried to adhere to these principles in the creation of the new plates for this edition. Finally, some of the plates were rearranged as page-pairs, where appropriate, to facilitate side-by-side comparisons of commonly illustrated elements. This fourth edition owes much to the consulting editors of the earlier editions, Drs. Sharon Colacino (Oberg) (first edition), Arthur F. Dalley II (second edition), and John T. Hansen (third edition), who shepherded their editions with great skill and uncompromising professionalism, making our task significantly easier.

The head and neck is a particularly challenging area for students, residents and faculty to master, due not only to the sheer number of structures packed in this relatively small region of the human body, but also the complexity of their three-dimensional anatomical organization. The age-old aphorism that "there is more anatomy above the hyoid bone than below it" presents a unique challenge to anyone trying to portray the anatomy of this region in a simple, visually appealing, and clinically relevant manner. More than ten new plates have been added to this section. For the first time, spectacular original paintings created by Carlos Machado illustrate clinically important structures such as the uncovertebral joints of the cervical vertebrae, the vertebral veins, and the intricate vasculature of the eye, to mention a few, with artistic brilliance, anatomical precision, and visual appeal that is unsurpassed. The section includes a concise treatment of the central nervous system, including the cranial nerves and important central pathways.

In the Back section, a new plate illustrates the proper placement of a lumbar epidural anesthetic agent, as well as the location for lumbar puncture or "spinal tap." Autonomics are traditionally the bane of many students, and excellent new drawings of the autonomic nervous system by Dr. Machado will serve as a new educational resource for these difficult concepts.

The Thorax section underwent minor editorial corrections of terminology and subtle artwork modifications to more accurately reflect the most common anatomical patterns. For instance, the representation of the azygos venous system pattern was altered to reflect the most common arrangement of these highly variable veins. The inclusion of the thoracic cross-sectional images at the end of the section, rather than in the later section, reinforces the importance of knowledge of cross-sectional anatomy in the interpretation of cross-sectional MR and CT images.

The Abdomen section has had the most extensive revision for label changes and positioning of leader lines. By popular request, the plate showing the common variations in the branches of the celiac artery, which appeared in the first edition Abdomen section, has been reinstated.

The anatomy of the pelvis is a particularly difficult area to teach and, because of the depth and tight organization of the internal structures, difficult to illustrate. The Netter illustrations of pelvic anatomy are outstanding because of the clarity of their presentation and their scope of coverage. A very small number of plates were eliminated to permit the inclusion of the illustration of pelvic fascia, a parasagittal view of the broad ligament, and normal imaging (male and female radiographs, cystourethrograms, and a hysterosalpingogram). Comparative images of male and female pelvic anatomy were reorganized to allow their side-by-side comparison.

New CT angiograms have been included in the Upper Limb and Lower Limb sections. This new technology not only clearly

Foreword

demonstrates blood vessels, but vividly shows bony landmarks to which the blood vessels are related. The ligaments of the wrist have been illustrated in more detail to reflect their increased importance in arthroscopic procedures and other applications of new technology to this joint.

We hope you enjoy this new edition of the *Atlas of Human Anatomy* and that you find it useful for learning and for your career. For the standard edition and enhanced international edition of the *Atlas,* we have included access to the website www. netteranatomy.com. By registering on this website, you will be able to access supplemental material that has been organized to help you better understand anatomy and its application to the practice of clinical medicine. More information about the website, including the PIN code for access, can be found on the inside front cover of the *Atlas.*

Jennifer K. Brueckner, PhD

Stephen W. Carmichael, PhD, DSc

Thomas R. Gest, PhD

Noelle A. Granger, PhD

John T. Hansen, PhD

Anil H. Walji, MD, PhD

Acknowledgments

It has been my pleasure to work with the other members of the editorial board, Carlos Machado, MD, and the Elsevier staff. Special thanks go to John Hansen, PhD, for the opportunity to work on this editorial team. I am indebted to my family for the support and encouragement that they have provided.

—*Jennifer K. Brueckner, PhD*

I would like to thank the specialists at the Mayo Clinic who helped review the art, especially Richard A. Berger, MD, PhD, Shawn W. O'Driscoll, MD, PhD, Enrique A. Sabater, MD, and Robert J. Spinner, MD.

—*Stephen W. Carmichael, PhD, DSc*

I must thank my family and especially my daughter, Madison, and son, Taylor, for their support and understanding of my efforts on this editorial task. It was a pleasure to work with my colleagues on the editorial board and with the staff of Elsevier. It has been my sincere pleasure to work with Dr. Carlos Machado on the artwork changes for the 4th edition.

—*Thomas R. Gest, PhD*

I am deeply grateful to my colleagues at University of North Carolina School of Medicine: James Scatliff, MD, former Chair of the Department of Radiology, for his help with the imaging, and O.W. Henson, PhD, Professor Emeritus of Anatomy, for his input. I especially thank Carlos Machado, the exceptional artist whose talent made any change required in the original plates both seamless and beautiful.

—*Noelle A. Granger, PhD*

I would like to thank Marybeth Thiel, Developmental Editor, our superb medical illustrator Dr. Carlos Machado, and the entire Editorial, Production, Design, Illustration, and Marketing staff at Elsevier for shepherding this edition to completion. For all our students, past, present and future, this *Atlas* is for you. Finally, to my wife, Paula, thank you for your love and encouragement throughout the years.

—*John T. Hansen, PhD*

I would like to thank my wife, Parviz, and my daughters, Amreen and Farah, for their patience and constant support and encouragement during my involvement with this project. My special thanks go to Dr. Carlos Machado, who has my utmost admiration for his brilliant artwork and who was an absolute delight to work with. I would also like to express my sincere appreciation to all the wonderful staff at Elsevier, in particular Linda Belfus for her exemplary leadership, and Anne Lenehan, Marybeth Thiel, and Cecelia Bayruns for all of their hard work, patience, and dedication, without which this atlas would not have been possible. Finally, I would like to thank my fellow coeditors and all of my colleagues who helped with reviewing the plates, in particular Pierre Lemelin, PhD, and Daniel Livy, PhD, whose meticulous examination of the artwork has helped greatly in ensuring the accuracy of the head and neck section in this edition.

—*Anil H. Walji, MD, PhD*

Preface to the First Edition

I have often said that my career as a medical artist for almost 50 years has been a sort of "command performance" in the sense that it has grown in response to the desires and requests of the medical profession. Over these many years, I have produced almost 4,000 illustrations, mostly for *The CIBA* (now *Netter*) *Collection of Medical Illustrations* but also for *Clinical Symposia.* These pictures have been concerned with the varied subdivisions of medical knowledge such as gross anatomy, histology, embryology, physiology, pathology, diagnostic modalities, surgical and therapeutic techniques and clinical manifestations of a multitude of diseases. As the years went by, however, there were more and more requests from physicians and students for me to produce an atlas purely of gross anatomy. Thus, this atlas has come about, not through any inspiration on my part but rather, like most of my previous works, as a fulfillment of the desires of the medical profession.

It involved going back over all the illustrations I had made over so many years, selecting those pertinent to gross anatomy, classifying them and organizing them by system and region, adapting them to page size and space and arranging them in logical sequence. Anatomy of course does not change, but our understanding of anatomy and its clinical significance does change, as do anatomical terminology and nomenclature. This therefore required much updating of many of the older pictures and even revision of a number of them in order to make them more pertinent to today's ever-expanding scope of medical and surgical practice. In addition, I found that there were gaps in the portrayal of medical knowledge as pictorialized in the illustrations I had previously done, and this necessitated my making a number of new pictures that are included in this volume.

In creating an atlas such as this, it is important to achieve a happy medium between complexity and simplification. If the pictures are too complex, they may be difficult and confusing to read; if oversimplified, they may not be adequately definitive or may even be misleading. I have therefore striven for a middle course of realism without the clutter of confusing minutiae. I hope that the students and members of the medical and allied professions will find the illustrations readily understandable, yet instructive and useful.

At one point, the publisher and I thought it might be nice to include a foreword by a truly outstanding and renowned anatomist, but there are so many in that category that we could not make a choice. We did think of men like Vesalius, Leonardo da Vinci, William Hunter and Henry Gray, who of course are unfortunately unavailable, but I do wonder what their comments might have been about this atlas.

Frank H. Netter, MD
(1906–1991)

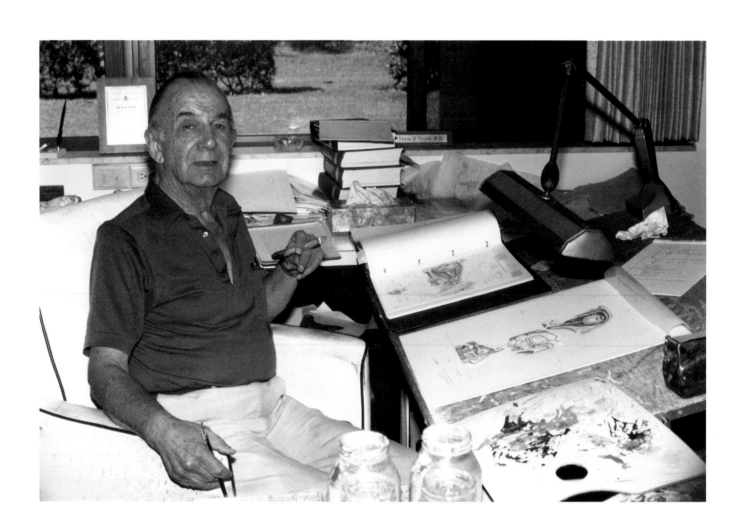

Frank H. Netter, MD

Frank H. Netter was born in New York City in 1906. He studied art at the Art Students League and the National Academy of Design before entering medical school at New York University, where he received his Doctor of Medicine degree in 1931. During his student years, Dr. Netter's notebook sketches attracted the attention of the medical faculty and other physicians, allowing him to augment his income by illustrating articles and textbooks. He continued illustrating as a sideline after establishing a surgical practice in 1933, but he ultimately opted to give up his practice in favor of a full-time commitment to art. After service in the United States Army during World War II, Dr. Netter began his long collaboration with the CIBA Pharmaceutical Company (now Novartis Pharmaceuticals). This 45-year partnership resulted in the production of the extraordinary collection of medical art so familiar to physicians and other medical professionals worldwide.

Icon Learning Systems acquired the Netter Collection in July 2000 and continued to update Dr. Netter's original paintings and to add newly commissioned paintings by artists trained in the style of Dr. Netter. In 2005, Elsevier Inc. purchased the Netter Collection and all publications from Icon Learning Systems. There are now over 50 publications featuring the art of Dr. Netter available through Elsevier Inc.

Dr. Netter's works are among the finest examples of the use of illustration in the teaching of medical concepts. The 13-book *Netter Collection of Medical Illustrations,* which includes the greater part of the more than 20,000 paintings created by Dr. Netter, became and remains one of the most famous medical works ever published. *The Netter Atlas of Human Anatomy,* first published in 1989, presents the anatomic paintings from the Netter Collection. Now translated into 16 languages, it is the anatomy atlas of choice among medical and health professions students the world over.

The Netter illustrations are appreciated not only for their aesthetic qualities, but, more importantly, for their intellectual content. As Dr. Netter wrote in 1949 "clarification of a subject is the aim and goal of illustration. No matter how beautifully painted, how delicately and subtly rendered a subject may be, it is of little value as a *medical illustration* if it does not serve to make clear some medical point." Dr. Netter's planning, conception, point of view, and approach are what inform his paintings and what make them so intellectually valuable.

Frank H. Netter, MD, physician and artist, died in 1991.

Contents

Section 1 **Head and Neck**

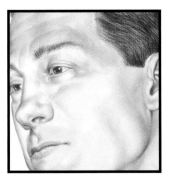
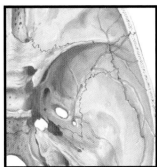
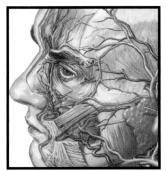
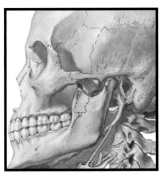

Topographic Anatomy
Plate 1

Bones and Ligaments
Plates 2–22

1 Head and Neck

Superficial Face
Plates 23–26

Neck
Plates 27–35

Nasal Region
Plates 36–50

Oral Region
Plates 51–62

Pharynx
Plates 63–73

1 Head and Neck

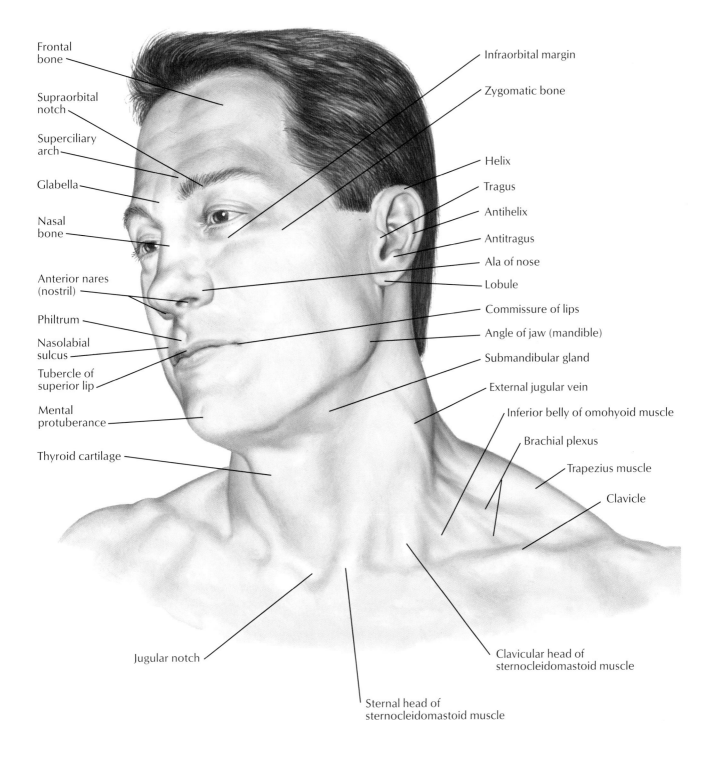

Frontal bone

Supraorbital notch

Superciliary arch

Glabella

Nasal bone

Anterior nares (nostril)

Philtrum

Nasolabial sulcus

Tubercle of superior lip

Mental protuberance

Thyroid cartilage

Jugular notch

Sternal head of sternocleidomastoid muscle

Infraorbital margin

Zygomatic bone

Helix

Tragus

Antihelix

Antitragus

Ala of nose

Lobule

Commissure of lips

Angle of jaw (mandible)

Submandibular gland

External jugular vein

Inferior belly of omohyoid muscle

Brachial plexus

Trapezius muscle

Clavicle

Clavicular head of sternocleidomastoid muscle

Topographic Anatomy

Plate 1

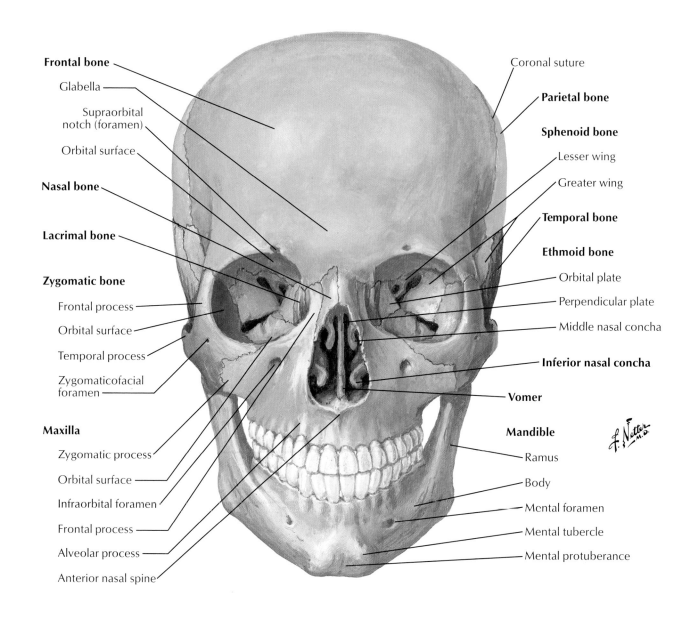

Frontal bone

Glabella

Supraorbital
notch (foramen)

Orbital surface

Nasal bone

Lacrimal bone

Zygomatic bone

Frontal process

Orbital surface

Temporal process

Zygomaticofacial
foramen

Maxilla

Zygomatic process

Orbital surface

Infraorbital foramen

Frontal process

Alveolar process

Anterior nasal spine

Coronal suture

Parietal bone

Sphenoid bone

Lesser wing

Greater wing

Temporal bone

Ethmoid bone

Orbital plate

Perpendicular plate

Middle nasal concha

Inferior nasal concha

Vomer

Mandible

Ramus

Body

Mental foramen

Mental tubercle

Mental protuberance

Right orbit: frontal and slightly lateral view

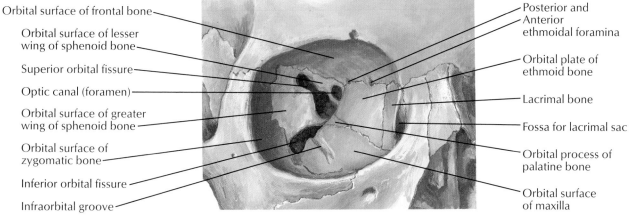

Orbital surface of frontal bone

Orbital surface of lesser
wing of sphenoid bone

Superior orbital fissure

Optic canal (foramen)

Orbital surface of greater
wing of sphenoid bone

Orbital surface of
zygomatic bone

Inferior orbital fissure

Infraorbital groove

Posterior and
Anterior
ethmoidal foramina

Orbital plate of
ethmoid bone

Lacrimal bone

Fossa for lacrimal sac

Orbital process of
palatine bone

Orbital surface
of maxilla

Plate 2

Bones and Ligaments

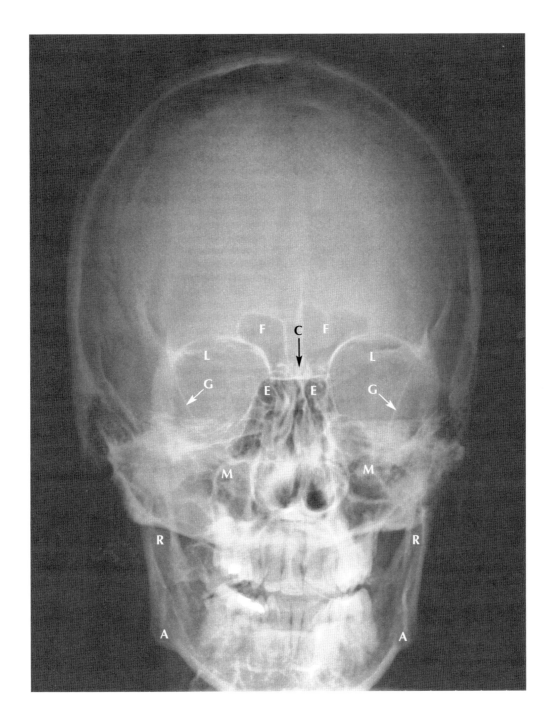

A Angle of mandible
C Crista galli
E Ethmoid air cells (sinuses)
F Frontal sinus
G Greater wing of sphenoid
L Lesser wing of sphenoid
M Maxillary sinus
R Ramus of mandible

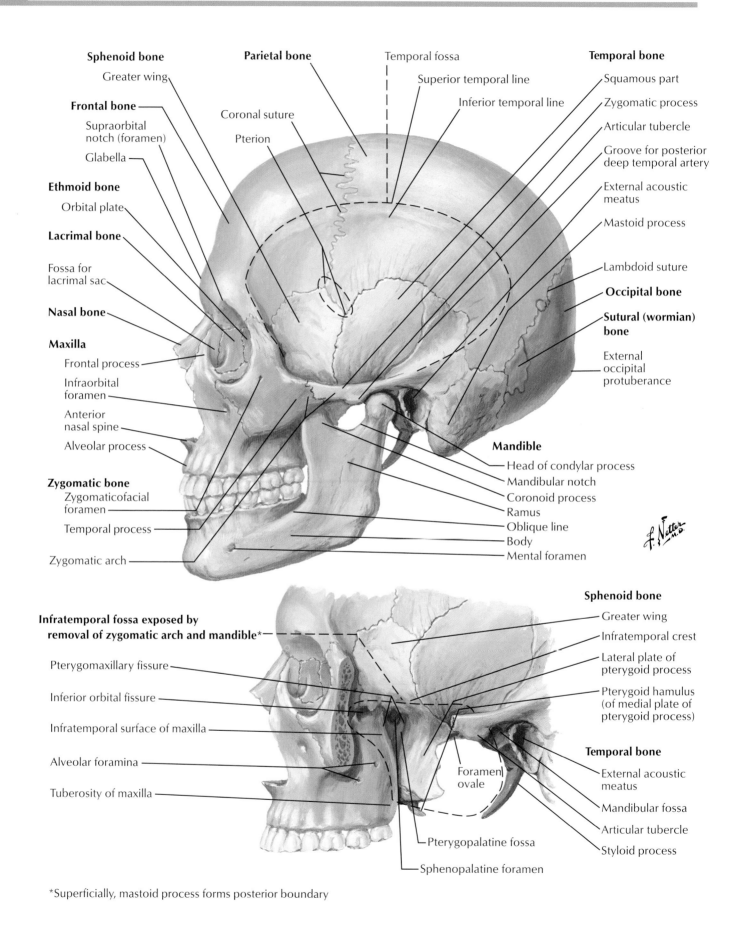

Sphenoid bone
  Greater wing

Frontal bone
  Supraorbital notch (foramen)
  Glabella

Ethmoid bone
  Orbital plate

Lacrimal bone
  Fossa for lacrimal sac

Nasal bone

Maxilla
  Frontal process
  Infraorbital foramen
  Anterior nasal spine
  Alveolar process

Zygomatic bone
  Zygomaticofacial foramen
  Temporal process
  Zygomatic arch

Parietal bone
  Coronal suture
  Pterion

Temporal fossa
  Superior temporal line
  Inferior temporal line

Temporal bone
  Squamous part
  Zygomatic process
  Articular tubercle
  Groove for posterior deep temporal artery
  External acoustic meatus
  Mastoid process
  Lambdoid suture

Occipital bone

Sutural (wormian) bone
  External occipital protuberance

Mandible
  Head of condylar process
  Mandibular notch
  Coronoid process
  Ramus
  Oblique line
  Body
  Mental foramen

Infratemporal fossa exposed by removal of zygomatic arch and mandible*

Pterygomaxillary fissure

Inferior orbital fissure

Infratemporal surface of maxilla

Alveolar foramina

Tuberosity of maxilla

Foramen ovale

Pterygopalatine fossa

Sphenopalatine foramen

Sphenoid bone
  Greater wing
  Infratemporal crest
  Lateral plate of pterygoid process
  Pterygoid hamulus (of medial plate of pterygoid process)

Temporal bone
  External acoustic meatus
  Mandibular fossa
  Articular tubercle
  Styloid process

*Superficially, mastoid process forms posterior boundary

Plate 4   **Bones and Ligaments**

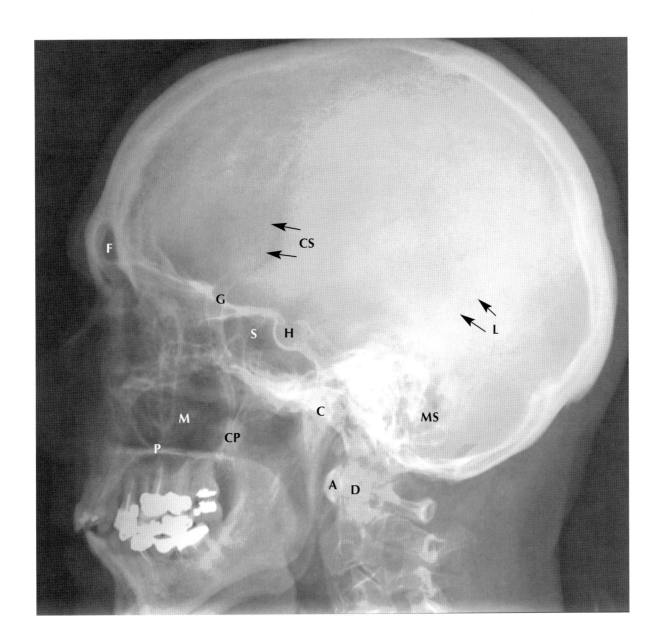

A	Anterior arch of atlas (C1 vertebra)	**G**	Greater wing of sphenoid
C	Condyle of mandible	**H**	Hypophyseal fossa (sella turcica)
CP	Coronoid process of mandible	**L**	Lambdoid suture
		M	Maxillary sinus
CS	Coronal suture	**MS**	Mastoid air cells
D	Dens of axis (C2 vertebra)	**P**	Palatine process of maxilla
F	Frontal sinus	**S**	Sphenoid sinus

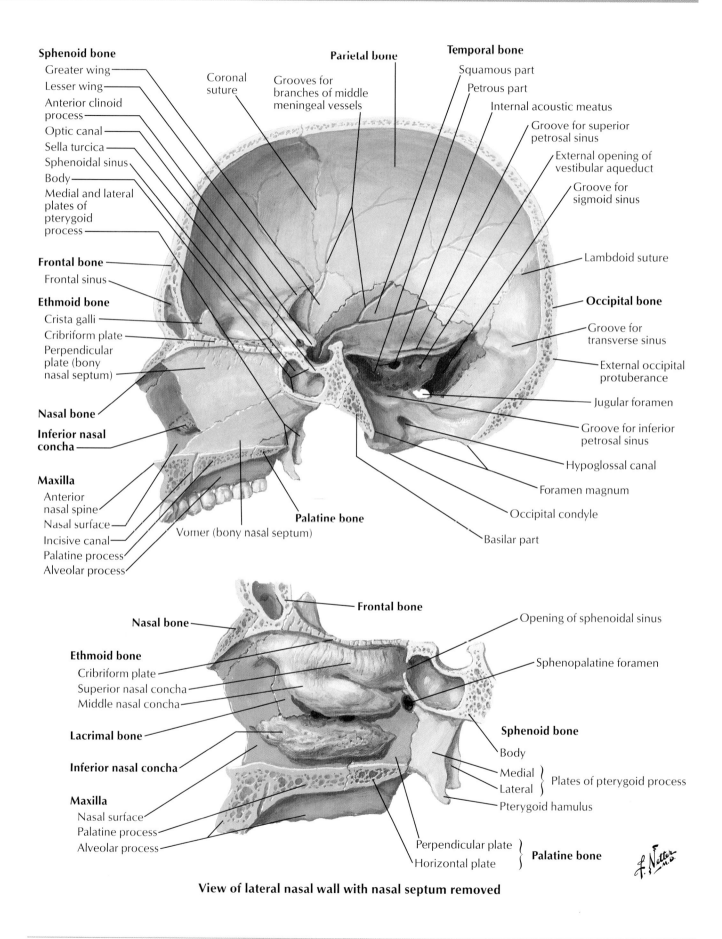

Sphenoid bone
Greater wing
Lesser wing
Anterior clinoid process
Optic canal
Sella turcica
Sphenoidal sinus
Body
Medial and lateral plates of pterygoid process

Frontal bone
Frontal sinus

Ethmoid bone
Crista galli
Cribriform plate
Perpendicular plate (bony nasal septum)

Nasal bone

Inferior nasal concha

Maxilla
Anterior nasal spine
Nasal surface
Incisive canal
Palatine process
Alveolar process

Coronal suture

Grooves for branches of middle meningeal vessels

Parietal bone

Temporal bone
Squamous part
Petrous part
Internal acoustic meatus
Groove for superior petrosal sinus
External opening of vestibular aqueduct
Groove for sigmoid sinus

Lambdoid suture

Occipital bone
Groove for transverse sinus
External occipital protuberance
Jugular foramen
Groove for inferior petrosal sinus
Hypoglossal canal
Foramen magnum
Occipital condyle
Basilar part

Vomer (bony nasal septum)

Palatine bone

Nasal bone

Ethmoid bone
Cribriform plate
Superior nasal concha
Middle nasal concha

Lacrimal bone

Inferior nasal concha

Maxilla
Nasal surface
Palatine process
Alveolar process

Frontal bone

Opening of sphenoidal sinus

Sphenopalatine foramen

Sphenoid bone
Body
Medial ⎫
Lateral ⎬ Plates of pterygoid process
Pterygoid hamulus

Perpendicular plate ⎫
Horizontal plate ⎬ **Palatine bone**

View of lateral nasal wall with nasal septum removed

Plate 6

Bones and Ligaments

Bones and Ligaments

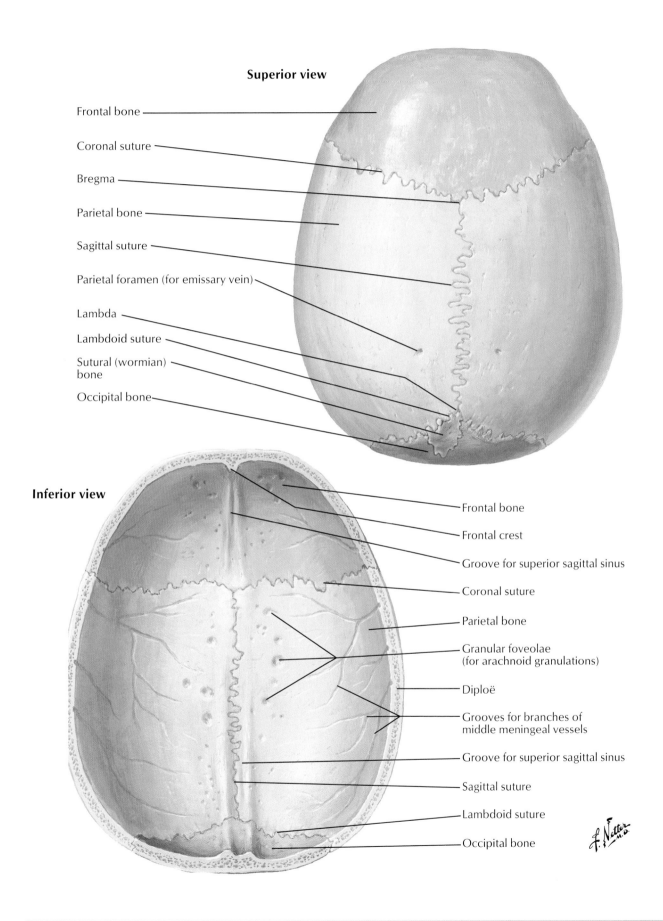

Superior view

Frontal bone

Coronal suture

Bregma

Parietal bone

Sagittal suture

Parietal foramen (for emissary vein)

Lambda

Lambdoid suture

Sutural (wormian) bone

Occipital bone

Inferior view

Frontal bone

Frontal crest

Groove for superior sagittal sinus

Coronal suture

Parietal bone

Granular foveolae (for arachnoid granulations)

Diploë

Grooves for branches of middle meningeal vessels

Groove for superior sagittal sinus

Sagittal suture

Lambdoid suture

Occipital bone

Plate 7

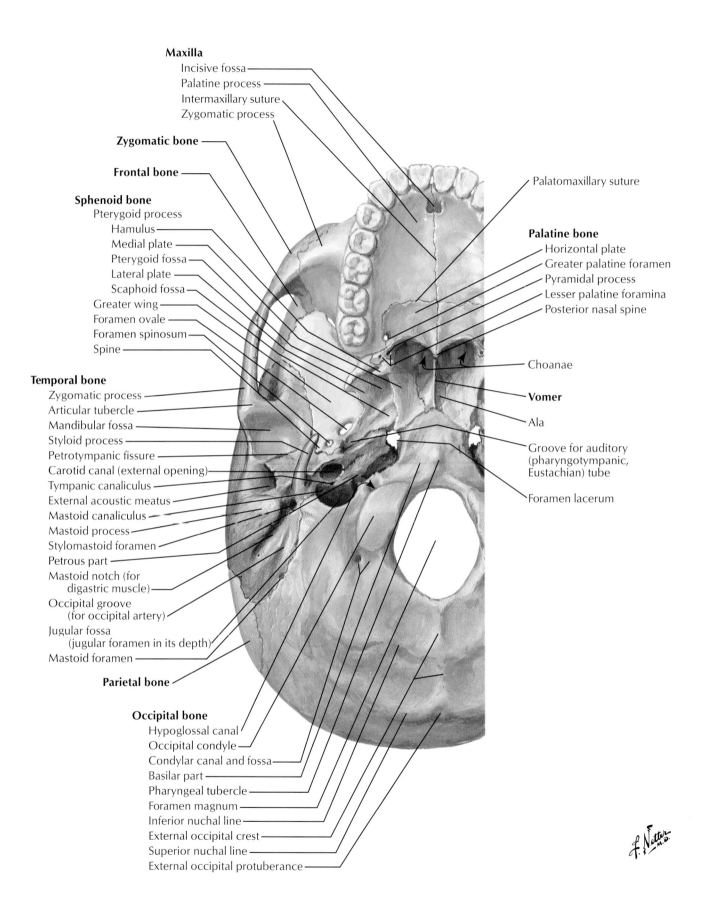

Maxilla
Incisive fossa
Palatine process
Intermaxillary suture
Zygomatic process

Zygomatic bone

Frontal bone

Sphenoid bone
Pterygoid process
Hamulus
Medial plate
Pterygoid fossa
Lateral plate
Scaphoid fossa
Greater wing
Foramen ovale
Foramen spinosum
Spine

Temporal bone
Zygomatic process
Articular tubercle
Mandibular fossa
Styloid process
Petrotympanic fissure
Carotid canal (external opening)
Tympanic canaliculus
External acoustic meatus
Mastoid canaliculus
Mastoid process
Stylomastoid foramen
Petrous part
Mastoid notch (for
 digastric muscle)
Occipital groove
 (for occipital artery)
Jugular fossa
 (jugular foramen in its depth)
Mastoid foramen

Parietal bone

Occipital bone
Hypoglossal canal
Occipital condyle
Condylar canal and fossa
Basilar part
Pharyngeal tubercle
Foramen magnum
Inferior nuchal line
External occipital crest
Superior nuchal line
External occipital protuberance

Palatomaxillary suture

Palatine bone
Horizontal plate
Greater palatine foramen
Pyramidal process
Lesser palatine foramina
Posterior nasal spine

Choanae

Vomer

Ala

Groove for auditory
(pharyngotympanic,
Eustachian) tube

Foramen lacerum

Plate 8   **Bones and Ligaments**

Frontal bone
Groove for superior sagittal sinus
Frontal crest
Groove for anterior meningeal vessels
Foramen cecum
Superior surface of orbital part

Ethmoid bone
Crista galli
Cribriform plate

Sphenoid bone
Lesser wing
Anterior clinoid process
Greater wing
Groove for middle meningeal vessels (frontal branches)
Body
Jugum
Prechiasmatic groove
Sella turcica { Tuberculum sellae
Hypophyseal fossa
Dorsum sellae
Posterior clinoid process
Carotid groove (for int. carotid a.)
Clivus

Temporal bone
Squamous part
Petrous part
Groove for lesser petrosal nerve
Groove for greater petrosal nerve
Arcuate eminence
Trigeminal impression
Groove for superior petrosal sinus
Groove for sigmoid sinus

Parietal bone
Groove for middle meningeal vessels (parietal branches)
Mastoid angle

Occipital bone
Clivus
Groove for inferior petrosal sinus
Basilar part
Groove for posterior meningeal vessels
Condyle
Groove for transverse sinus
Groove for occipital sinus
Internal occipital crest
Internal occipital protuberance
Groove for superior sagittal sinus

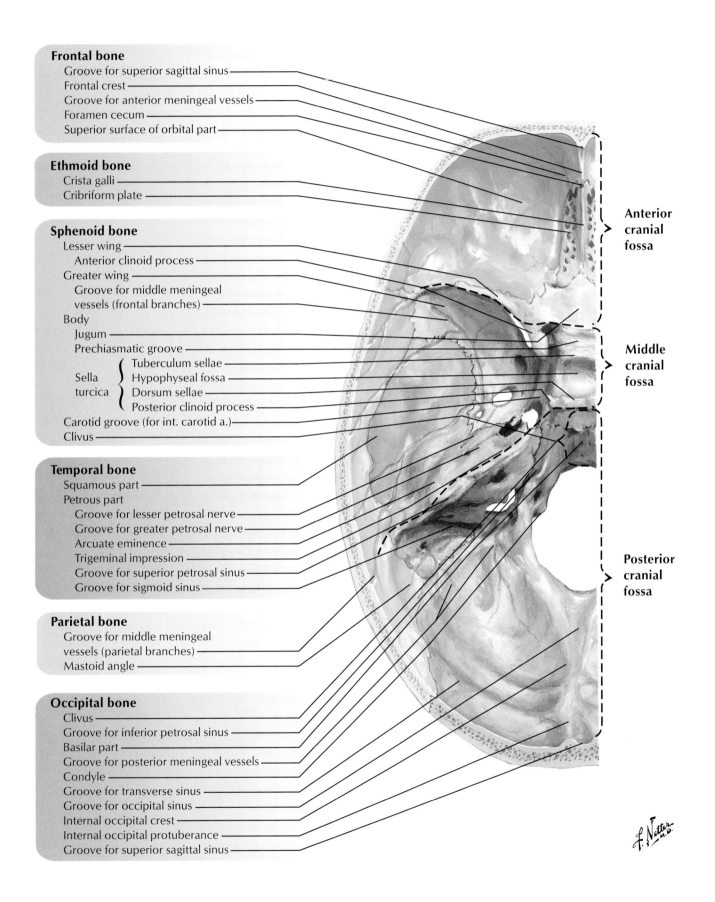

Anterior cranial fossa

Middle cranial fossa

Posterior cranial fossa

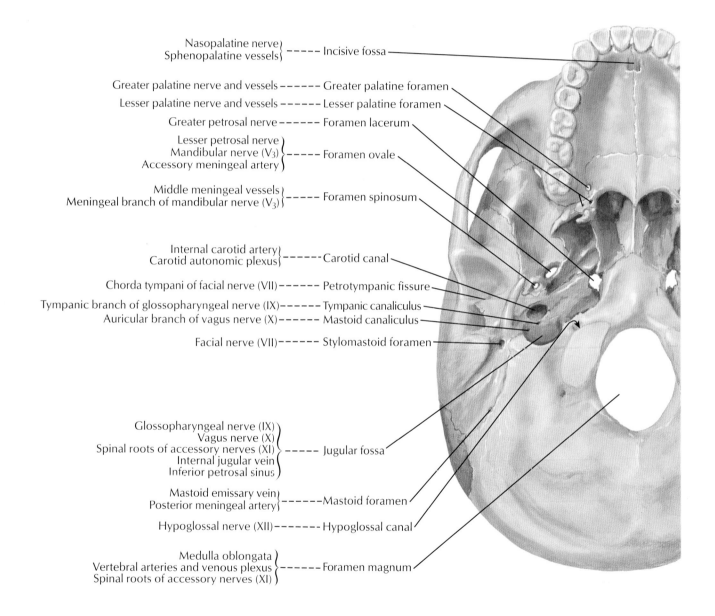

Nasopalatine nerve⎫
Sphenopalatine vessels⎭ ----- Incisive fossa

Greater palatine nerve and vessels ------ Greater palatine foramen

Lesser palatine nerve and vessels ------ Lesser palatine foramen

Greater petrosal nerve ------ Foramen lacerum

Lesser petrosal nerve⎫
Mandibular nerve (V₃)⎬----- Foramen ovale
Accessory meningeal artery⎭

Middle meningeal vessels⎫
Meningeal branch of mandibular nerve (V₃)⎭----- Foramen spinosum

Internal carotid artery⎫
Carotid autonomic plexus⎭-----Carotid canal

Chorda tympani of facial nerve (VII)----- Petrotympanic fissure

Tympanic branch of glossopharyngeal nerve (IX)----- Tympanic canaliculus

Auricular branch of vagus nerve (X)------ Mastoid canaliculus

Facial nerve (VII)------ Stylomastoid foramen

Glossopharyngeal nerve (IX)⎫
Vagus nerve (X)⎪
Spinal roots of accessory nerves (XI)⎬----- Jugular fossa
Internal jugular vein⎪
Inferior petrosal sinus⎭

Mastoid emissary vein⎫
Posterior meningeal artery⎭-----Mastoid foramen

Hypoglossal nerve (XII)------ Hypoglossal canal

Medulla oblongata⎫
Vertebral arteries and venous plexus⎬------Foramen magnum
Spinal roots of accessory nerves (XI)⎭

Plate 10   **Bones and Ligaments**

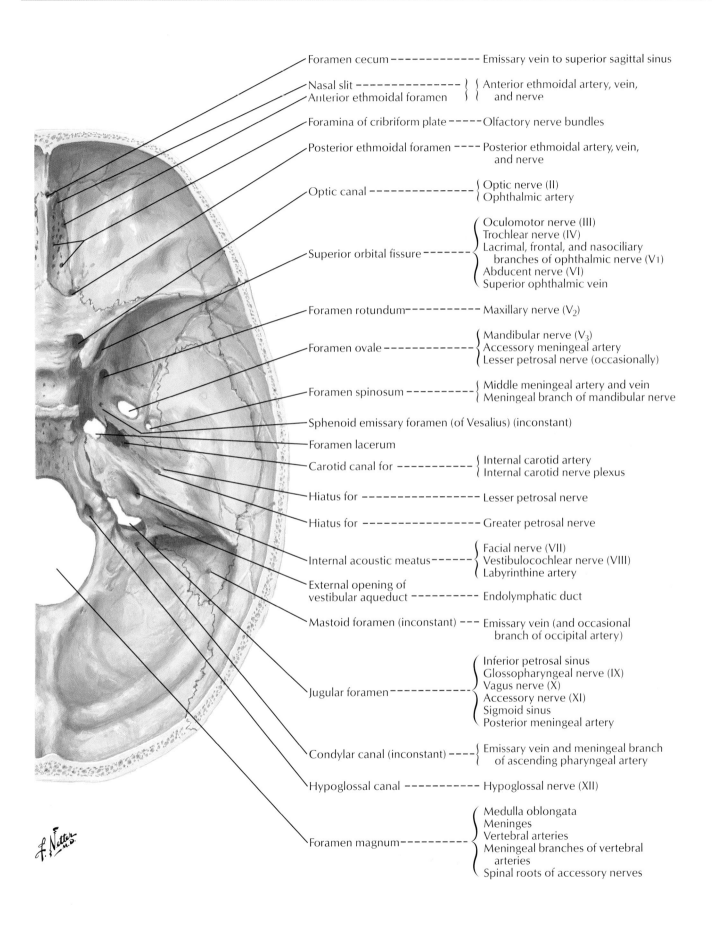

Foramen cecum ———————— Emissary vein to superior sagittal sinus

Nasal slit ————————— } { Anterior ethmoidal artery, vein,
Anterior ethmoidal foramen } {   and nerve

Foramina of cribriform plate ————Olfactory nerve bundles

Posterior ethmoidal foramen ———— Posterior ethmoidal artery, vein,
                                          and nerve

Optic canal ——————————— { Optic nerve (II)
                          { Ophthalmic artery

Superior orbital fissure ———————
{ Oculomotor nerve (III)
{ Trochlear nerve (IV)
{ Lacrimal, frontal, and nasociliary
{   branches of ophthalmic nerve (V1)
{ Abducent nerve (VI)
{ Superior ophthalmic vein

Foramen rotundum ——————————— Maxillary nerve (V₂)

Foramen ovale ————————— {
{ Mandibular nerve (V₃)
{ Accessory meningeal artery
{ Lesser petrosal nerve (occasionally)

Foramen spinosum ————————— { Middle meningeal artery and vein
                          { Meningeal branch of mandibular nerve

Sphenoid emissary foramen (of Vesalius) (inconstant)

Foramen lacerum

Carotid canal for ———————— { Internal carotid artery
                          { Internal carotid nerve plexus

Hiatus for ————————————— Lesser petrosal nerve

Hiatus for ————————————— Greater petrosal nerve

Internal acoustic meatus————— {
{ Facial nerve (VII)
{ Vestibulocochlear nerve (VIII)
{ Labyrinthine artery

External opening of
vestibular aqueduct ————————— Endolymphatic duct

Mastoid foramen (inconstant) ——— Emissary vein (and occasional
                                     branch of occipital artery)

Jugular foramen————————— {
{ Inferior petrosal sinus
{ Glossopharyngeal nerve (IX)
{ Vagus nerve (X)
{ Accessory nerve (XI)
{ Sigmoid sinus
{ Posterior meningeal artery

Condylar canal (inconstant) ———— { Emissary vein and meningeal branch
                                 {   of ascending pharyngeal artery

Hypoglossal canal ————————— Hypoglossal nerve (XII)

Foramen magnum————————— {
{ Medulla oblongata
{ Meninges
{ Vertebral arteries
{ Meningeal branches of vertebral
{   arteries
{ Spinal roots of accessory nerves

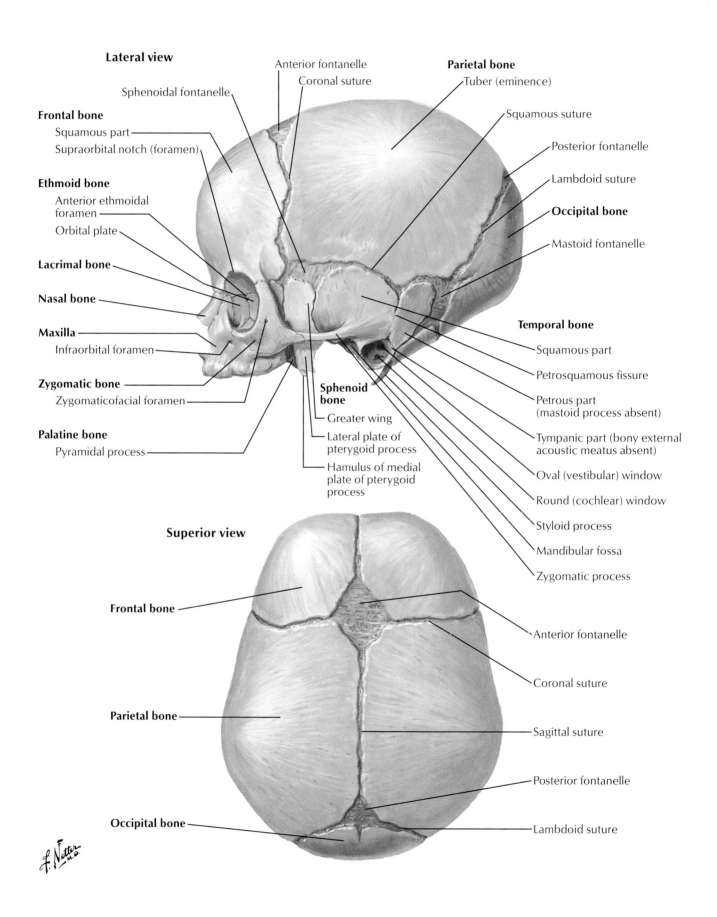

Lateral view

Frontal bone
- Squamous part
- Supraorbital notch (foramen)

Ethmoid bone
- Anterior ethmoidal foramen
- Orbital plate

Lacrimal bone

Nasal bone

Maxilla
- Infraorbital foramen

Zygomatic bone
- Zygomaticofacial foramen

Palatine bone
- Pyramidal process

Anterior fontanelle
Coronal suture
Sphenoidal fontanelle

Sphenoid bone
- Greater wing
- Lateral plate of pterygoid process
- Hamulus of medial plate of pterygoid process

Parietal bone
- Tuber (eminence)
- Squamous suture
- Posterior fontanelle
- Lambdoid suture

Occipital bone
- Mastoid fontanelle

Temporal bone
- Squamous part
- Petrosquamous fissure
- Petrous part (mastoid process absent)
- Tympanic part (bony external acoustic meatus absent)
- Oval (vestibular) window
- Round (cochlear) window
- Styloid process
- Mandibular fossa
- Zygomatic process

Superior view

Frontal bone

Parietal bone

Occipital bone

Anterior fontanelle
Coronal suture
Sagittal suture
Posterior fontanelle
Lambdoid suture

Plate 12   **Bones and Ligaments**

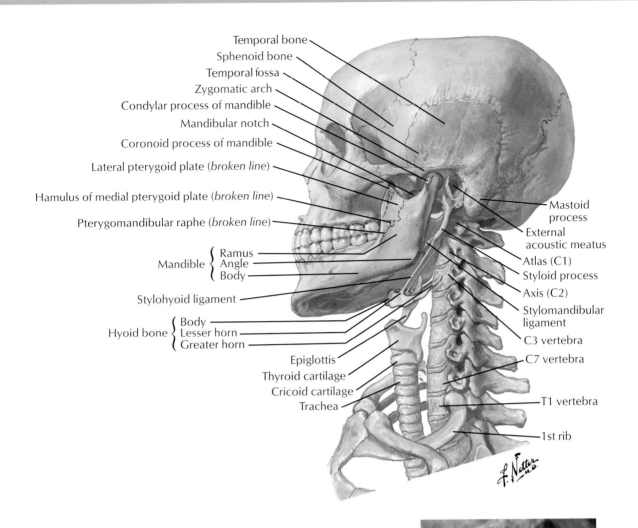

Temporal bone
Sphenoid bone
Temporal fossa
Zygomatic arch
Condylar process of mandible
Mandibular notch
Coronoid process of mandible
Lateral pterygoid plate (*broken line*)
Hamulus of medial pterygoid plate (*broken line*)
Pterygomandibular raphe (*broken line*)

Mandible { Ramus / Angle / Body
Stylohyoid ligament
Hyoid bone { Body / Lesser horn / Greater horn

Epiglottis
Thyroid cartilage
Cricoid cartilage
Trachea

Mastoid process
External acoustic meatus
Atlas (C1)
Styloid process
Axis (C2)
Stylomandibular ligament
C3 vertebra
C7 vertebra
T1 vertebra
1st rib

2nd cervical to 1st thoracic vertebrae: right lateral view

Dens
Superior articular facet
C2
Spinous processes
Foramen transversarium
C3
Intervertebral foramina for spinal nerves
C4
Articular pillar formed by articular processes and interarticular parts (pars interarticularis)
C5
Groove for spinal nerve in transverse process
C6
Zygapophyseal (facet) joints
C7
Spinous process of C7 (vertebra prominens)
T1
Costal facets (for 1st rib)

Cervical vertebrae (spine): lateral radiograph

S Spinous process (axis)
T Transverse process
VP Spinous process of C7 (vertebra prominens)
Z Zygapophyseal (facet) joint
1–7 Bodies of cervical vertebrae
··· Cervical curvature
⌐ Vertebral canal

Posterior view

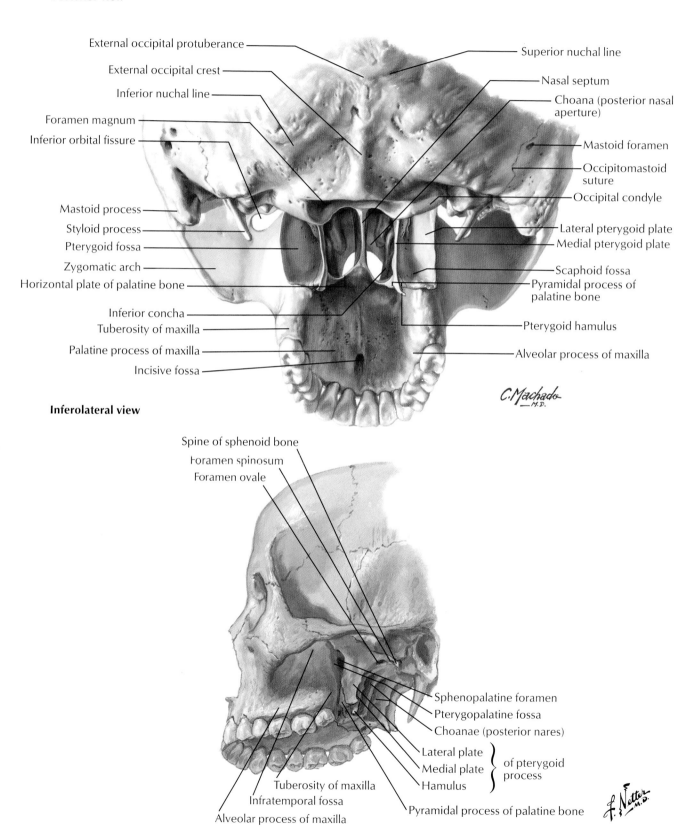

External occipital protuberance
External occipital crest
Inferior nuchal line
Foramen magnum
Inferior orbital fissure
Mastoid process
Styloid process
Pterygoid fossa
Zygomatic arch
Horizontal plate of palatine bone
Inferior concha
Tuberosity of maxilla
Palatine process of maxilla
Incisive fossa

Superior nuchal line
Nasal septum
Choana (posterior nasal aperture)
Mastoid foramen
Occipitomastoid suture
Occipital condyle
Lateral pterygoid plate
Medial pterygoid plate
Scaphoid fossa
Pyramidal process of palatine bone
Pterygoid hamulus
Alveolar process of maxilla

C. Machado —M.D.

Inferolateral view

Spine of sphenoid bone
Foramen spinosum
Foramen ovale

Sphenopalatine foramen
Pterygopalatine fossa
Choanae (posterior nares)
Lateral plate ⎫
Medial plate ⎬ of pterygoid process
Hamulus ⎭
Pyramidal process of palatine bone

Tuberosity of maxilla
Infratemporal fossa
Alveolar process of maxilla

F. Netter M.D.

Plate 14 **Bones and Ligaments**

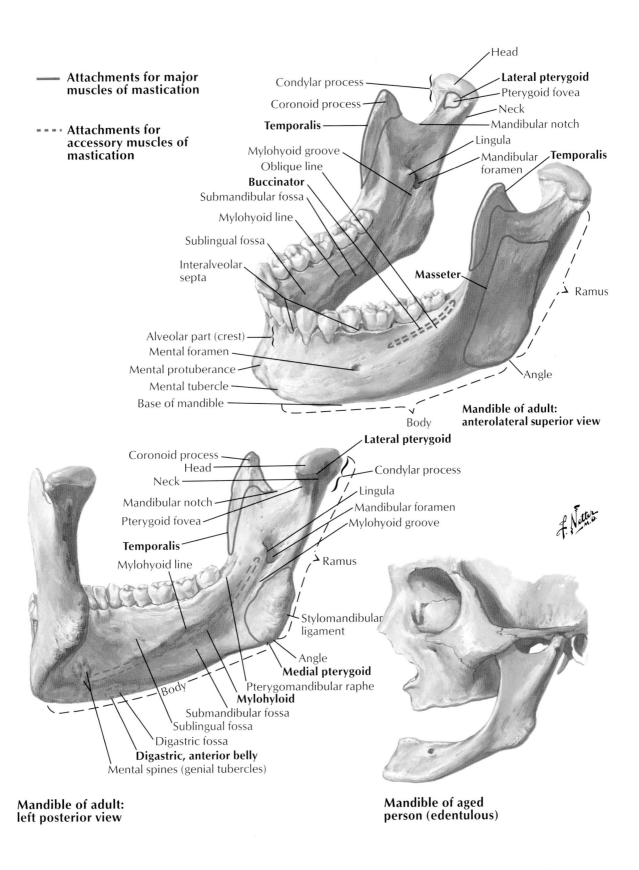

Attachments for major muscles of mastication

Attachments for accessory muscles of mastication

Head
Condylar process
Lateral pterygoid
Coronoid process
Pterygoid fovea
Temporalis
Neck
Mylohyoid groove
Mandibular notch
Oblique line
Lingula
Buccinator
Mandibular foramen
Temporalis
Submandibular fossa
Mylohyoid line
Masseter
Sublingual fossa
Interalveolar septa
Ramus
Alveolar part (crest)
Mental foramen
Mental protuberance
Mental tubercle
Angle
Base of mandible
Body
Mandible of adult: anterolateral superior view

Lateral pterygoid
Coronoid process
Head
Condylar process
Neck
Lingula
Mandibular notch
Mandibular foramen
Pterygoid fovea
Mylohyoid groove
Temporalis
Ramus
Mylohyoid line
Stylomandibular ligament
Angle
Medial pterygoid
Body
Pterygomandibular raphe
Mylohyoid
Submandibular fossa
Sublingual fossa
Digastric fossa
Digastric, anterior belly
Mental spines (genial tubercles)

Mandible of adult: left posterior view

Mandible of aged person (edentulous)

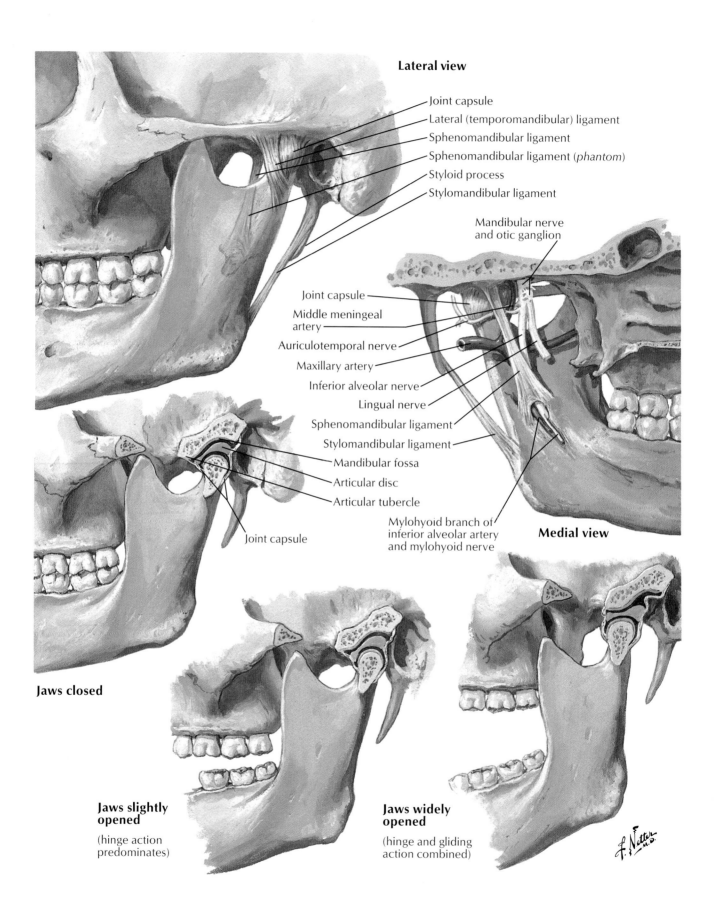

Lateral view

Joint capsule
Lateral (temporomandibular) ligament
Sphenomandibular ligament
Sphenomandibular ligament (*phantom*)
Styloid process
Stylomandibular ligament

Mandibular nerve and otic ganglion

Joint capsule
Middle meningeal artery
Auriculotemporal nerve
Maxillary artery
Inferior alveolar nerve
Lingual nerve
Sphenomandibular ligament
Stylomandibular ligament
Mandibular fossa
Articular disc
Articular tubercle
Joint capsule

Mylohyoid branch of inferior alveolar artery and mylohyoid nerve

Medial view

Jaws closed

Jaws slightly opened

(hinge action predominates)

Jaws widely opened

(hinge and gliding action combined)

Plate 16

Bones and Ligaments

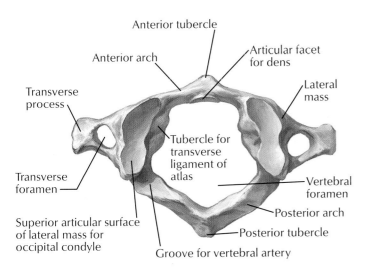

Anterior tubercle

Anterior arch

Articular facet for dens

Lateral mass

Transverse process

Tubercle for transverse ligament of atlas

Transverse foramen

Vertebral foramen

Superior articular surface of lateral mass for occipital condyle

Posterior arch

Posterior tubercle

Groove for vertebral artery

Atlas (C1): superior view

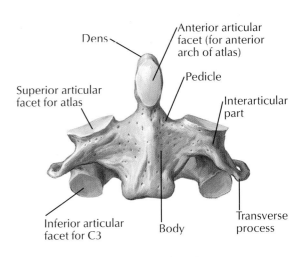

Dens

Anterior articular facet (for anterior arch of atlas)

Superior articular facet for atlas

Pedicle

Interarticular part

Inferior articular facet for C3

Body

Transverse process

Axis (C2): anterior view

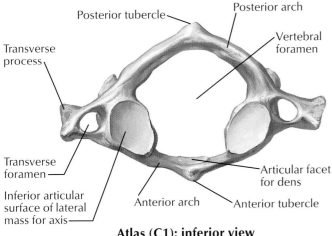

Posterior tubercle

Posterior arch

Vertebral foramen

Transverse process

Transverse foramen

Inferior articular surface of lateral mass for axis

Anterior arch

Articular facet for dens

Anterior tubercle

Atlas (C1): inferior view

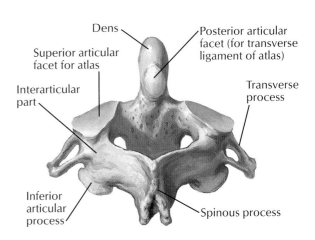

Dens

Posterior articular facet (for transverse ligament of atlas)

Superior articular facet for atlas

Interarticular part

Transverse process

Inferior articular process

Spinous process

Axis (C2): posterosuperior view

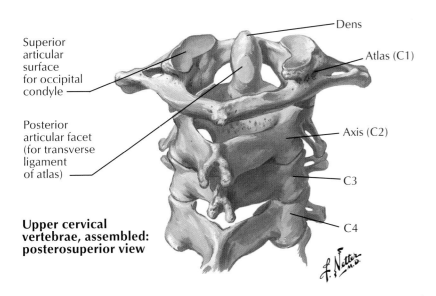

Superior articular surface for occipital condyle

Dens

Atlas (C1)

Axis (C2)

C3

C4

Posterior articular facet (for transverse ligament of atlas)

Upper cervical vertebrae, assembled: posterosuperior view

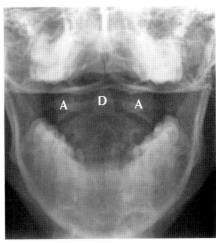

Radiograph of atlantoaxial joint (open mouth odontoid view)

A Lateral masses of atlas (C1 vertebra)

D Dens of axis (C2 vertebra)

Cervical Vertebrae (continued)

See also **Plates 13, 153**

Inferior aspect of C3 and superior aspect of C4 showing the sites of the facet and uncovertebral articulations

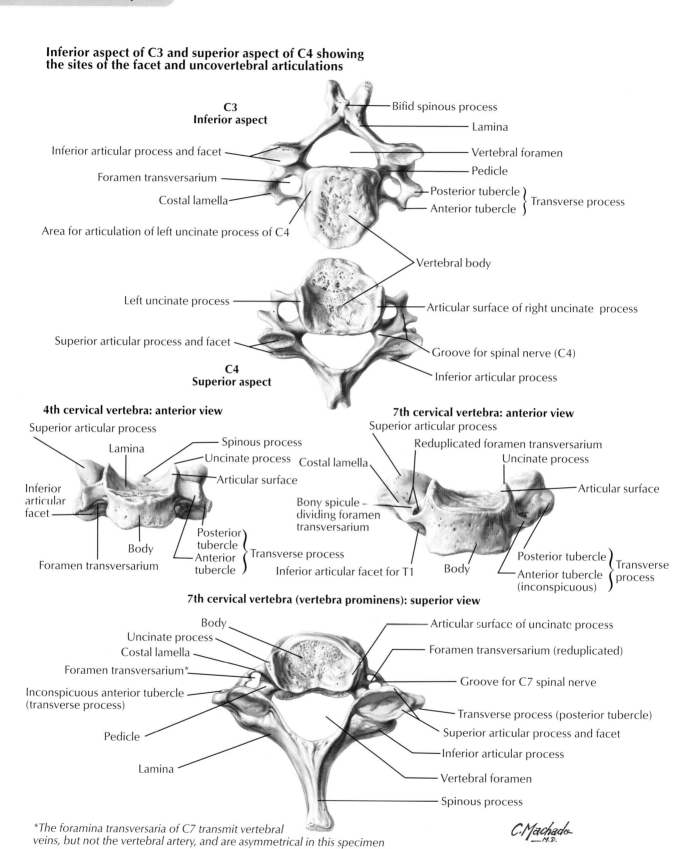

C3 Inferior aspect

Bifid spinous process

Lamina

Inferior articular process and facet

Vertebral foramen

Foramen transversarium

Pedicle

Costal lamella

Posterior tubercle

Anterior tubercle } Transverse process

Area for articulation of left uncinate process of C4

Vertebral body

Left uncinate process

Articular surface of right uncinate process

Superior articular process and facet

Groove for spinal nerve (C4)

C4 Superior aspect

Inferior articular process

4th cervical vertebra: anterior view

Superior articular process

Lamina

Spinous process

Uncinate process

Articular surface

Inferior articular facet

Body

Posterior tubercle

Anterior tubercle } Transverse process

Foramen transversarium

7th cervical vertebra: anterior view

Superior articular process

Reduplicated foramen transversarium

Uncinate process

Costal lamella

Articular surface

Bony spicule – dividing foramen transversarium

Inferior articular facet for T1

Body

Posterior tubercle

Anterior tubercle (inconspicuous) } Transverse process

7th cervical vertebra (vertebra prominens): superior view

Body

Uncinate process

Costal lamella

Foramen transversarium*

Inconspicuous anterior tubercle (transverse process)

Pedicle

Lamina

Articular surface of uncinate process

Foramen transversarium (reduplicated)

Groove for C7 spinal nerve

Transverse process (posterior tubercle)

Superior articular process and facet

Inferior articular process

Vertebral foramen

Spinous process

*The foramina transversaria of C7 transmit vertebral veins, but not the vertebral artery, and are asymmetrical in this specimen

C. Machado
_M.D.

Plate 18

Bones and Ligaments

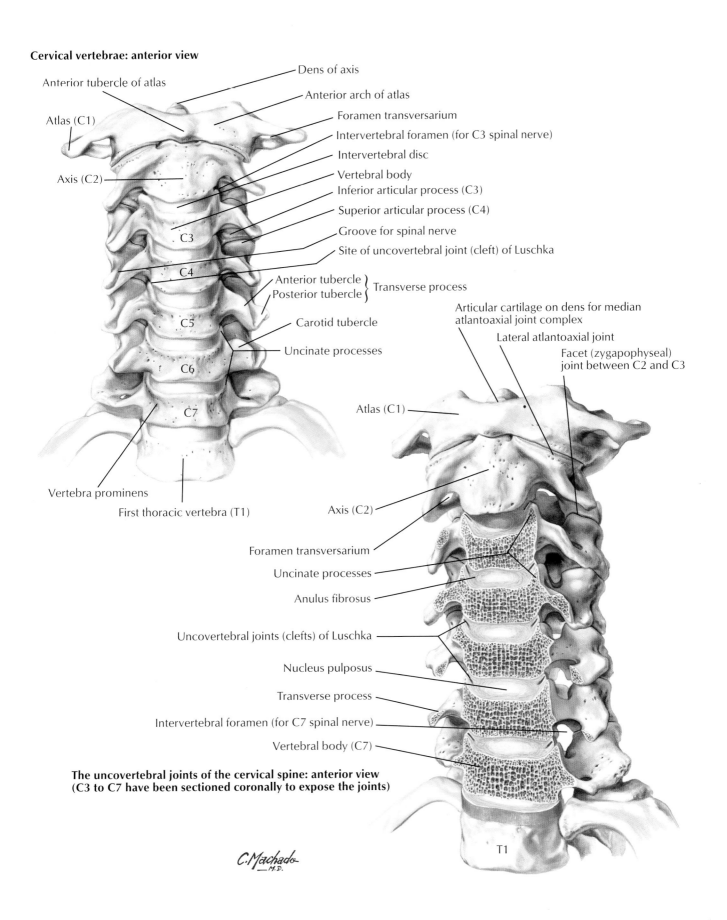

Cervical vertebrae: anterior view

Dens of axis

Anterior tubercle of atlas

Anterior arch of atlas

Atlas (C1)

Foramen transversarium

Intervertebral foramen (for C3 spinal nerve)

Intervertebral disc

Axis (C2)

Vertebral body

Inferior articular process (C3)

Superior articular process (C4)

Groove for spinal nerve

C3

Site of uncovertebral joint (cleft) of Luschka

C4

Anterior tubercle } Transverse process
Posterior tubercle }

C5

Carotid tubercle

Uncinate processes

C6

Vertebra prominens

C7

First thoracic vertebra (T1)

Articular cartilage on dens for median atlantoaxial joint complex

Lateral atlantoaxial joint

Facet (zygapophyseal) joint between C2 and C3

Atlas (C1)

Axis (C2)

Foramen transversarium

Uncinate processes

Anulus fibrosus

Uncovertebral joints (clefts) of Luschka

Nucleus pulposus

Transverse process

Intervertebral foramen (for C7 spinal nerve)

Vertebral body (C7)

**The uncovertebral joints of the cervical spine: anterior view
(C3 to C7 have been sectioned coronally to expose the joints)**

T1

C.Machado
_M.D._

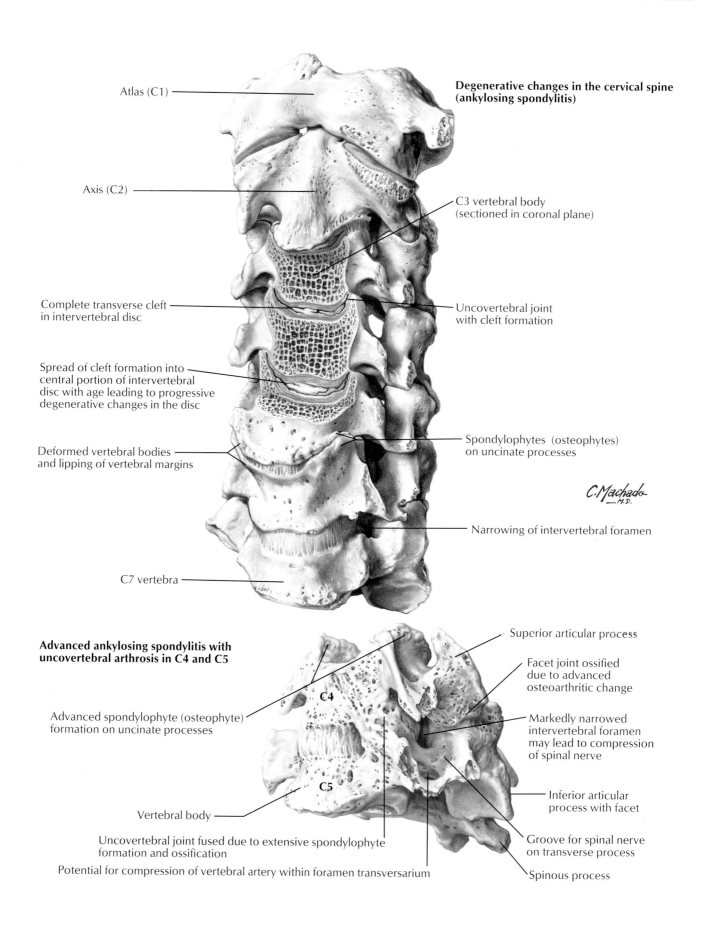

Atlas (C1)

Axis (C2)

Complete transverse cleft
in intervertebral disc

Spread of cleft formation into
central portion of intervertebral
disc with age leading to progressive
degenerative changes in the disc

Deformed vertebral bodies
and lipping of vertebral margins

C7 vertebra

**Degenerative changes in the cervical spine
(ankylosing spondylitis)**

C3 vertebral body
(sectioned in coronal plane)

Uncovertebral joint
with cleft formation

Spondylophytes (osteophytes)
on uncinate processes

Narrowing of intervertebral foramen

C. Machado
M.D.

**Advanced ankylosing spondylitis with
uncovertebral arthrosis in C4 and C5**

Advanced spondylophyte (osteophyte)
formation on uncinate processes

C4

C5

Vertebral body

Uncovertebral joint fused due to extensive spondylophyte
formation and ossification

Potential for compression of vertebral artery within foramen transversarium

Superior articular process

Facet joint ossified
due to advanced
osteoarthritic change

Markedly narrowed
intervertebral foramen
may lead to compression
of spinal nerve

Inferior articular
process with facet

Groove for spinal nerve
on transverse process

Spinous process

Plate 20   **Bones and Ligaments**

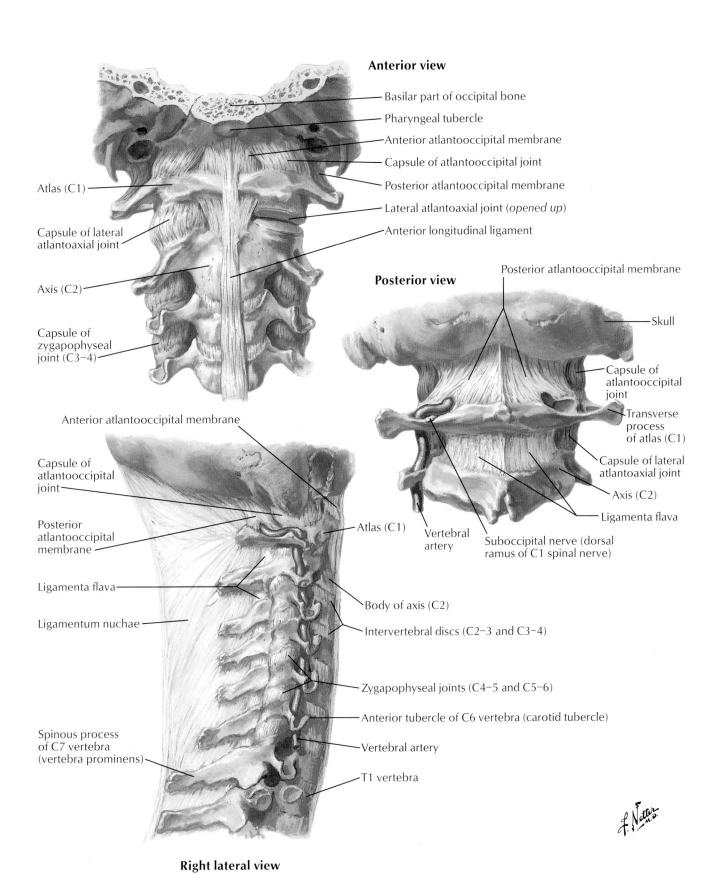

Anterior view

Basilar part of occipital bone

Pharyngeal tubercle

Anterior atlantooccipital membrane

Capsule of atlantooccipital joint

Posterior atlantooccipital membrane

Lateral atlantoaxial joint (*opened up*)

Anterior longitudinal ligament

Atlas (C1)

Capsule of lateral
atlantoaxial joint

Axis (C2)

Capsule of
zygapophyseal
joint (C3–4)

Posterior view

Posterior atlantooccipital membrane

Skull

Capsule of
atlantooccipital
joint

Transverse
process
of atlas (C1)

Capsule of lateral
atlantoaxial joint

Axis (C2)

Ligamenta flava

Vertebral
artery

Suboccipital nerve (dorsal
ramus of C1 spinal nerve)

Anterior atlantooccipital membrane

Capsule of
atlantooccipital
joint

Posterior
atlantooccipital
membrane

Ligamenta flava

Ligamentum nuchae

Atlas (C1)

Body of axis (C2)

Intervertebral discs (C2–3 and C3–4)

Zygapophyseal joints (C4–5 and C5–6)

Anterior tubercle of C6 vertebra (carotid tubercle)

Vertebral artery

T1 vertebra

Spinous process
of C7 vertebra
(vertebra prominens)

Right lateral view

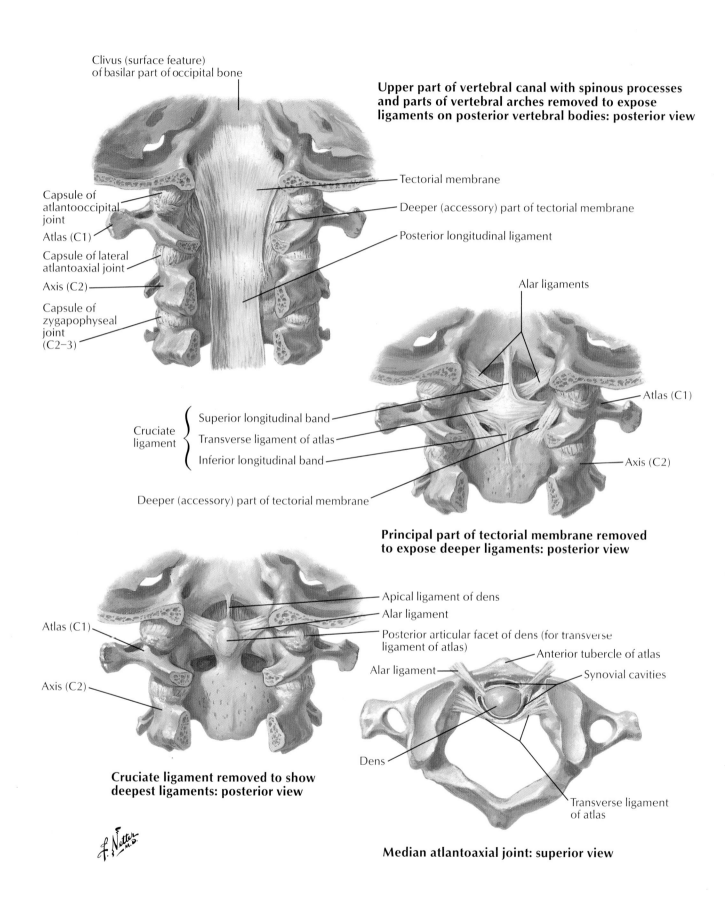

Clivus (surface feature)
of basilar part of occipital bone

**Upper part of vertebral canal with spinous processes
and parts of vertebral arches removed to expose
ligaments on posterior vertebral bodies: posterior view**

Tectorial membrane

Capsule of
atlantooccipital
joint

Deeper (accessory) part of tectorial membrane

Atlas (C1)

Posterior longitudinal ligament

Capsule of lateral
atlantoaxial joint

Axis (C2)

Capsule of
zygapophyseal
joint
(C2–3)

Alar ligaments

Atlas (C1)

Cruciate
ligament

Superior longitudinal band

Transverse ligament of atlas

Inferior longitudinal band

Axis (C2)

Deeper (accessory) part of tectorial membrane

**Principal part of tectorial membrane removed
to expose deeper ligaments: posterior view**

Apical ligament of dens

Alar ligament

Atlas (C1)

Posterior articular facet of dens (for transverse
ligament of atlas)

Anterior tubercle of atlas

Alar ligament

Synovial cavities

Axis (C2)

Dens

**Cruciate ligament removed to show
deepest ligaments: posterior view**

Transverse ligament
of atlas

Median atlantoaxial joint: superior view

Plate 22

Bones and Ligaments

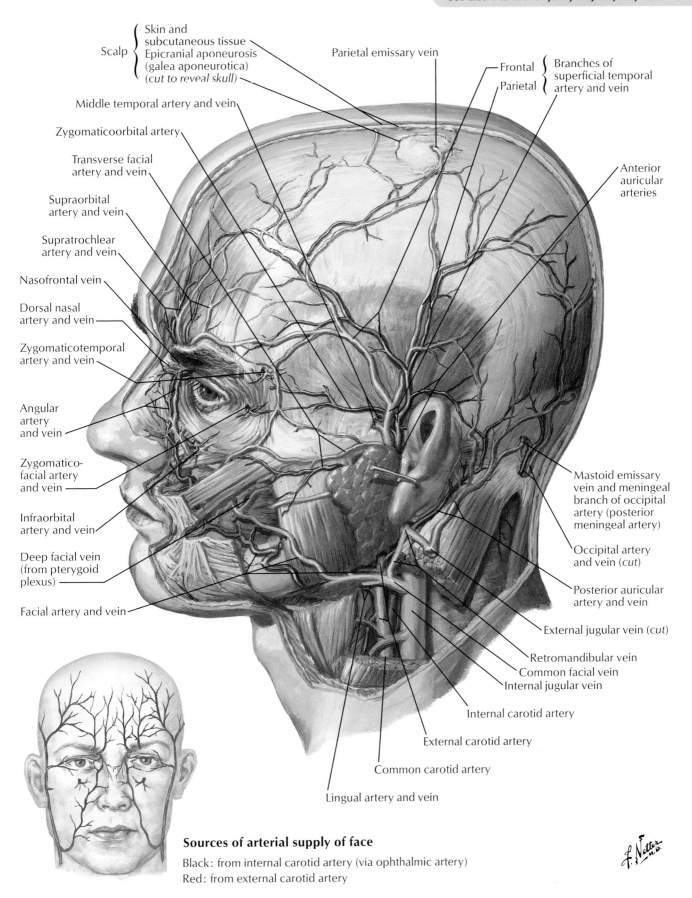

Scalp {
Skin and subcutaneous tissue
Epicranial aponeurosis (galea aponeurotica) (*cut to reveal skull*)

Middle temporal artery and vein

Zygomaticoorbital artery

Transverse facial artery and vein

Supraorbital artery and vein

Supratrochlear artery and vein

Nasofrontal vein

Dorsal nasal artery and vein

Zygomaticotemporal artery and vein

Angular artery and vein

Zygomatico-facial artery and vein

Infraorbital artery and vein

Deep facial vein (from pterygoid plexus)

Facial artery and vein

Parietal emissary vein

Frontal
Parietal
} Branches of superficial temporal artery and vein

Anterior auricular arteries

Mastoid emissary vein and meningeal branch of occipital artery (posterior meningeal artery)

Occipital artery and vein (*cut*)

Posterior auricular artery and vein

External jugular vein (*cut*)

Retromandibular vein

Common facial vein

Internal jugular vein

Internal carotid artery

External carotid artery

Common carotid artery

Lingual artery and vein

Sources of arterial supply of face

Black: from internal carotid artery (via ophthalmic artery)
Red: from external carotid artery

Superficial Face

Plate 23

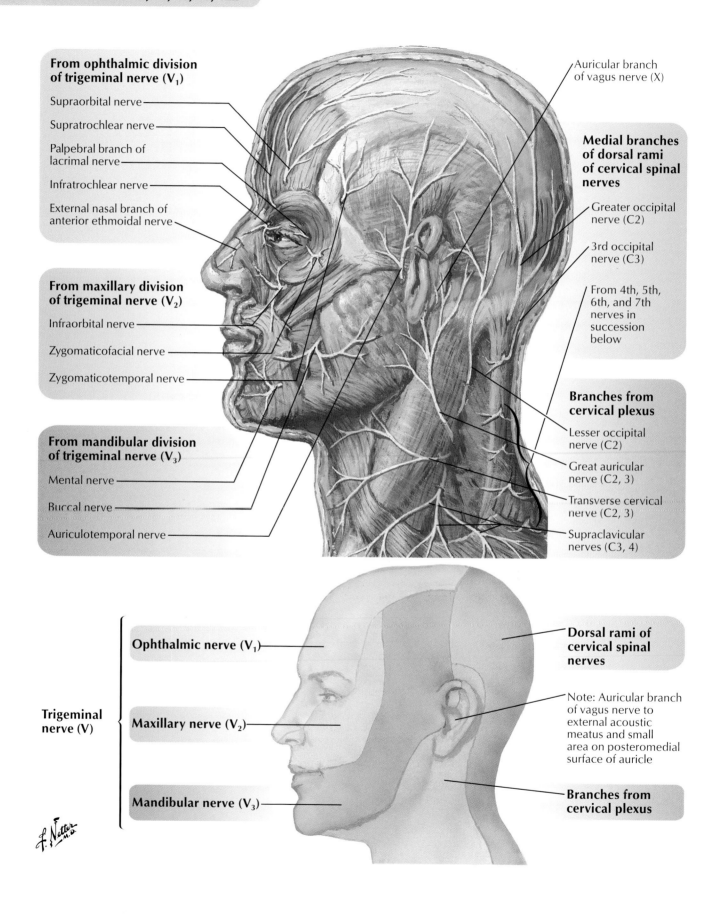

From ophthalmic division of trigeminal nerve (V₁)

Supraorbital nerve

Supratrochlear nerve

Palpebral branch of lacrimal nerve

Infratrochlear nerve

External nasal branch of anterior ethmoidal nerve

From maxillary division of trigeminal nerve (V₂)

Infraorbital nerve

Zygomaticofacial nerve

Zygomaticotemporal nerve

From mandibular division of trigeminal nerve (V₃)

Mental nerve

Buccal nerve

Auriculotemporal nerve

Auricular branch of vagus nerve (X)

Medial branches of dorsal rami of cervical spinal nerves

Greater occipital nerve (C2)

3rd occipital nerve (C3)

From 4th, 5th, 6th, and 7th nerves in succession below

Branches from cervical plexus

Lesser occipital nerve (C2)

Great auricular nerve (C2, 3)

Transverse cervical nerve (C2, 3)

Supraclavicular nerves (C3, 4)

Ophthalmic nerve (V₁)

Maxillary nerve (V₂)

Mandibular nerve (V₃)

Trigeminal nerve (V)

Dorsal rami of cervical spinal nerves

Note: Auricular branch of vagus nerve to external acoustic meatus and small area on posteromedial surface of auricle

Branches from cervical plexus

Plate 24

Superficial Face

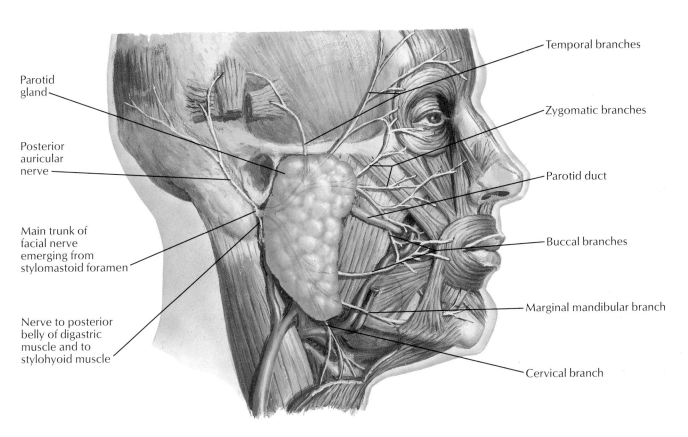

Parotid gland

Posterior auricular nerve

Main trunk of facial nerve emerging from stylomastoid foramen

Nerve to posterior belly of digastric muscle and to stylohyoid muscle

Temporal branches

Zygomatic branches

Parotid duct

Buccal branches

Marginal mandibular branch

Cervical branch

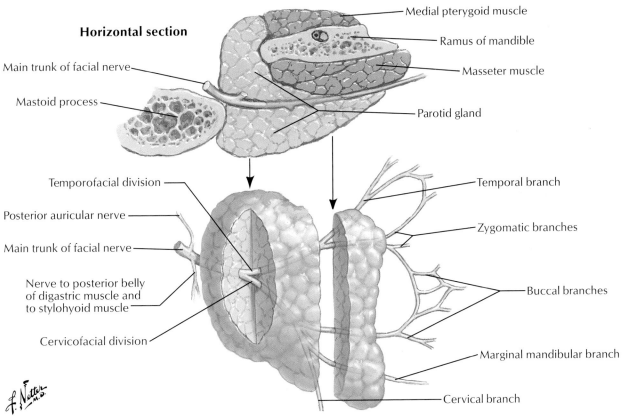

Horizontal section

Main trunk of facial nerve

Mastoid process

Medial pterygoid muscle

Ramus of mandible

Masseter muscle

Parotid gland

Temporofacial division

Posterior auricular nerve

Main trunk of facial nerve

Nerve to posterior belly of digastric muscle and to stylohyoid muscle

Cervicofacial division

Temporal branch

Zygomatic branches

Buccal branches

Marginal mandibular branch

Cervical branch

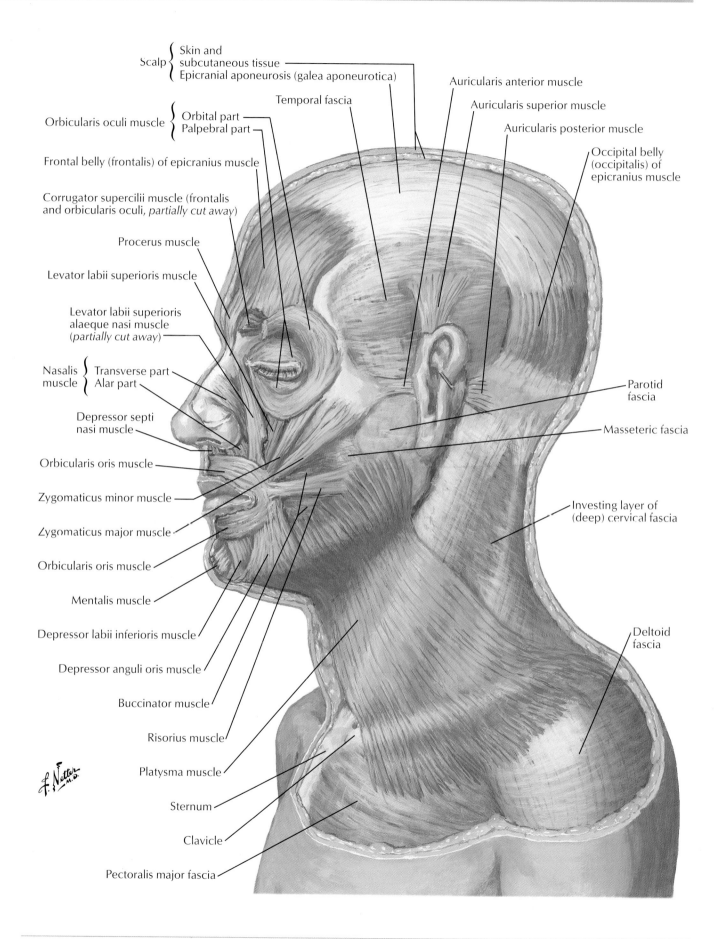

Scalp {
Skin and subcutaneous tissue
Epicranial aponeurosis (galea aponeurotica)

Temporal fascia

Auricularis anterior muscle

Auricularis superior muscle

Auricularis posterior muscle

Occipital belly (occipitalis) of epicranius muscle

Orbicularis oculi muscle {
Orbital part
Palpebral part

Frontal belly (frontalis) of epicranius muscle

Corrugator supercilii muscle (frontalis and orbicularis oculi, *partially cut away*)

Procerus muscle

Levator labii superioris muscle

Levator labii superioris alaeque nasi muscle (*partially cut away*)

Nasalis muscle {
Transverse part
Alar part

Depressor septi nasi muscle

Orbicularis oris muscle

Zygomaticus minor muscle

Zygomaticus major muscle

Orbicularis oris muscle

Mentalis muscle

Depressor labii inferioris muscle

Depressor anguli oris muscle

Buccinator muscle

Risorius muscle

Platysma muscle

Sternum

Clavicle

Pectoralis major fascia

Parotid fascia

Masseteric fascia

Investing layer of (deep) cervical fascia

Deltoid fascia

Plate 26 **Superficial Face**

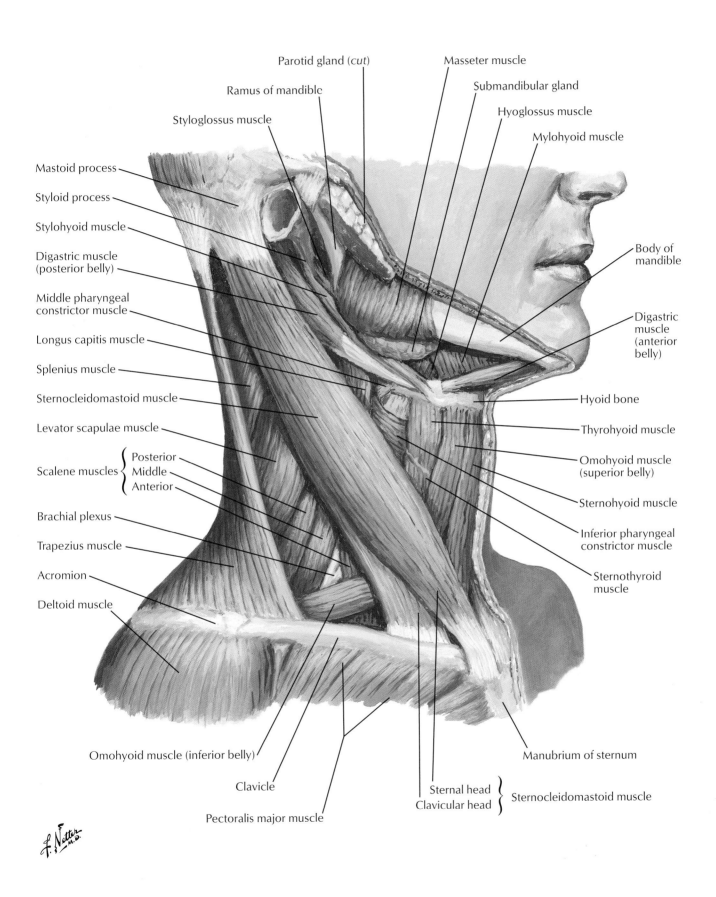

Parotid gland (*cut*)

Masseter muscle

Ramus of mandible

Submandibular gland

Styloglossus muscle

Hyoglossus muscle

Mylohyoid muscle

Mastoid process

Styloid process

Stylohyoid muscle

Body of mandible

Digastric muscle (posterior belly)

Middle pharyngeal constrictor muscle

Longus capitis muscle

Digastric muscle (anterior belly)

Splenius muscle

Sternocleidomastoid muscle

Hyoid bone

Levator scapulae muscle

Thyrohyoid muscle

Scalene muscles { Posterior Middle Anterior

Omohyoid muscle (superior belly)

Sternohyoid muscle

Brachial plexus

Trapezius muscle

Inferior pharyngeal constrictor muscle

Acromion

Sternothyroid muscle

Deltoid muscle

Omohyoid muscle (inferior belly)

Manubrium of sternum

Clavicle

Sternal head } Sternocleidomastoid muscle
Clavicular head

Pectoralis major muscle

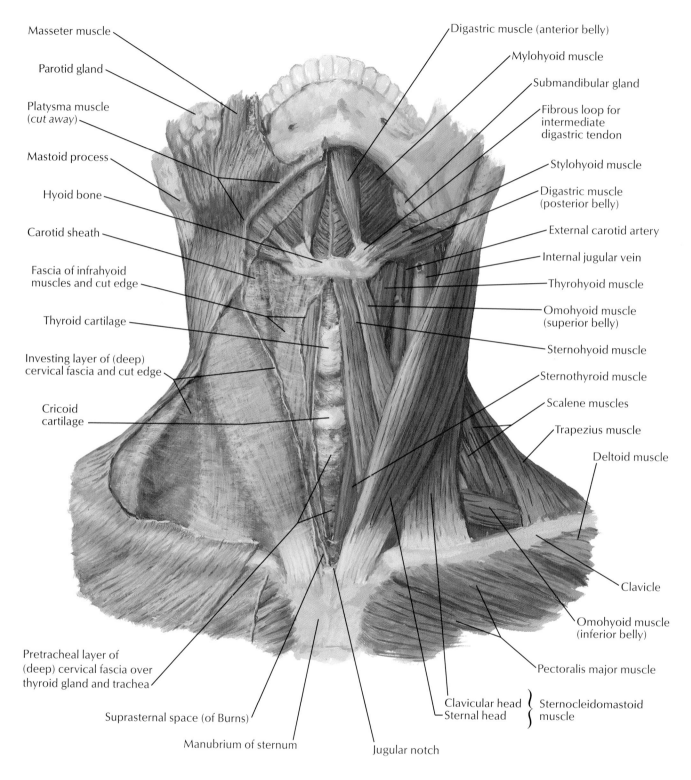

Masseter muscle

Parotid gland

Platysma muscle (*cut away*)

Mastoid process

Hyoid bone

Carotid sheath

Fascia of infrahyoid muscles and cut edge

Thyroid cartilage

Investing layer of (deep) cervical fascia and cut edge

Cricoid cartilage

Pretracheal layer of (deep) cervical fascia over thyroid gland and trachea

Suprasternal space (of Burns)

Manubrium of sternum

Digastric muscle (anterior belly)

Mylohyoid muscle

Submandibular gland

Fibrous loop for intermediate digastric tendon

Stylohyoid muscle

Digastric muscle (posterior belly)

External carotid artery

Internal jugular vein

Thyrohyoid muscle

Omohyoid muscle (superior belly)

Sternohyoid muscle

Sternothyroid muscle

Scalene muscles

Trapezius muscle

Deltoid muscle

Clavicle

Omohyoid muscle (inferior belly)

Pectoralis major muscle

Clavicular head \
Sternal head } Sternocleidomastoid muscle

Jugular notch

Plate 28

Neck

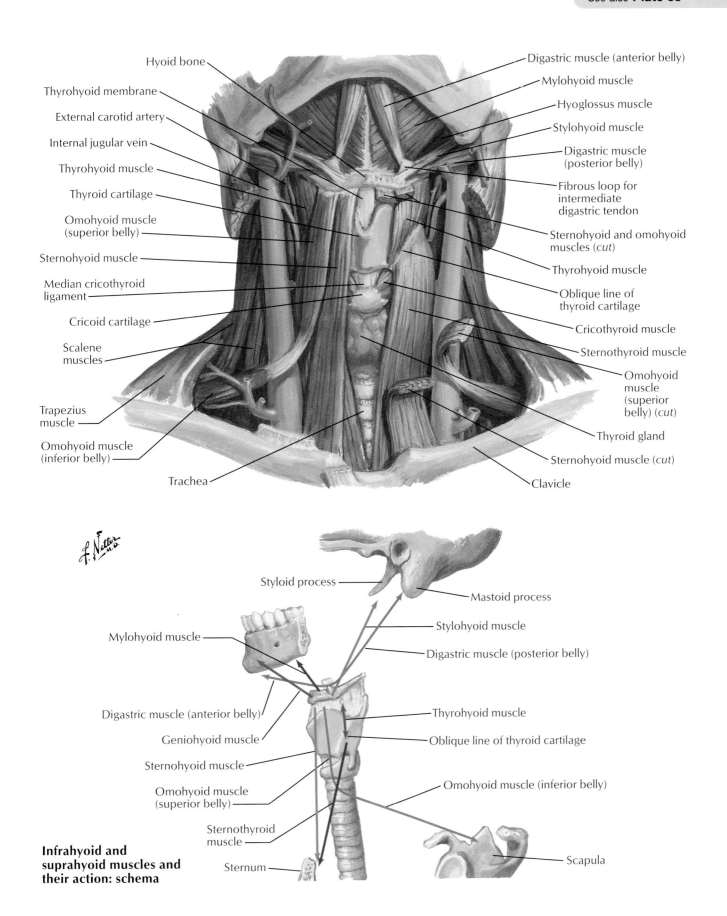

Hyoid bone

Thyrohyoid membrane

External carotid artery

Internal jugular vein

Thyrohyoid muscle

Thyroid cartilage

Omohyoid muscle (superior belly)

Sternohyoid muscle

Median cricothyroid ligament

Cricoid cartilage

Scalene muscles

Trapezius muscle

Omohyoid muscle (inferior belly)

Trachea

Digastric muscle (anterior belly)

Mylohyoid muscle

Hyoglossus muscle

Stylohyoid muscle

Digastric muscle (posterior belly)

Fibrous loop for intermediate digastric tendon

Sternohyoid and omohyoid muscles (*cut*)

Thyrohyoid muscle

Oblique line of thyroid cartilage

Cricothyroid muscle

Sternothyroid muscle

Omohyoid muscle (superior belly) (*cut*)

Thyroid gland

Sternohyoid muscle (*cut*)

Clavicle

Styloid process

Mastoid process

Stylohyoid muscle

Digastric muscle (posterior belly)

Mylohyoid muscle

Digastric muscle (anterior belly)

Geniohyoid muscle

Sternohyoid muscle

Omohyoid muscle (superior belly)

Sternothyroid muscle

Sternum

Thyrohyoid muscle

Oblique line of thyroid cartilage

Omohyoid muscle (inferior belly)

Scapula

Infrahyoid and suprahyoid muscles and their action: schema

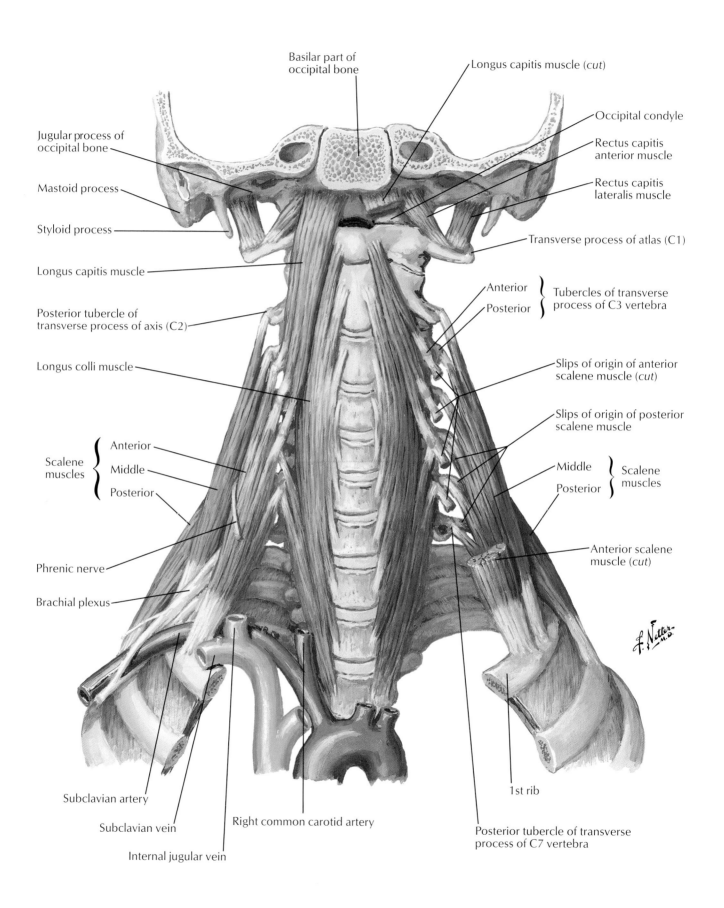

Basilar part of
occipital bone

Longus capitis muscle (*cut*)

Occipital condyle

Rectus capitis
anterior muscle

Rectus capitis
lateralis muscle

Jugular process of
occipital bone

Mastoid process

Styloid process

Transverse process of atlas (C1)

Longus capitis muscle

Anterior
Posterior

Tubercles of transverse
process of C3 vertebra

Posterior tubercle of
transverse process of axis (C2)

Slips of origin of anterior
scalene muscle (*cut*)

Longus colli muscle

Slips of origin of posterior
scalene muscle

Scalene
muscles

Anterior
Middle
Posterior

Middle
Posterior

Scalene
muscles

Anterior scalene
muscle (*cut*)

Phrenic nerve

Brachial plexus

Subclavian artery

Subclavian vein

Internal jugular vein

Right common carotid artery

1st rib

Posterior tubercle of transverse
process of C7 vertebra

Plate 30

Neck

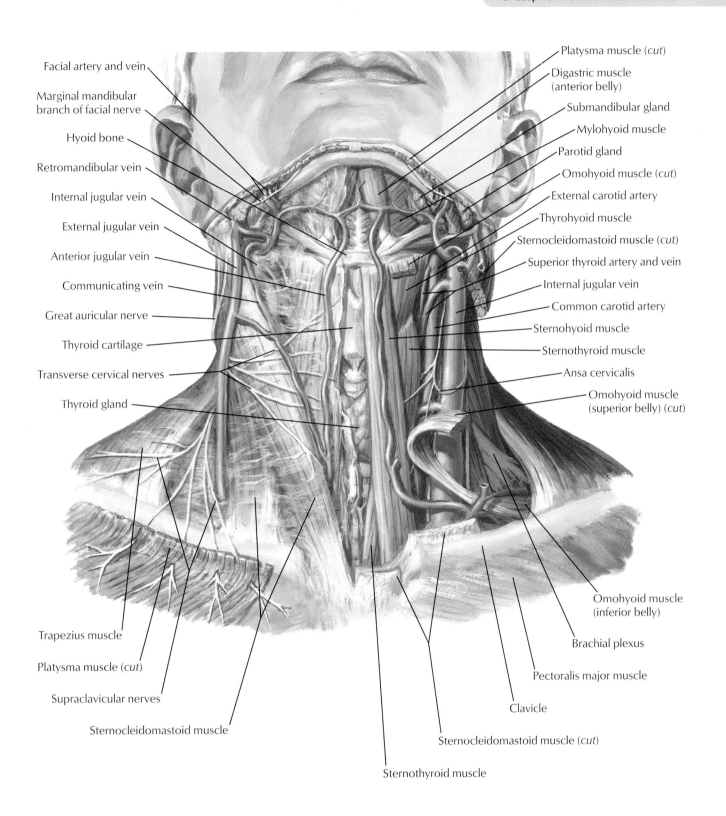

Facial artery and vein

Marginal mandibular branch of facial nerve

Hyoid bone

Retromandibular vein

Internal jugular vein

External jugular vein

Anterior jugular vein

Communicating vein

Great auricular nerve

Thyroid cartilage

Transverse cervical nerves

Thyroid gland

Trapezius muscle

Platysma muscle (*cut*)

Supraclavicular nerves

Sternocleidomastoid muscle

Sternothyroid muscle

Platysma muscle (*cut*)

Digastric muscle (anterior belly)

Submandibular gland

Mylohyoid muscle

Parotid gland

Omohyoid muscle (*cut*)

External carotid artery

Thyrohyoid muscle

Sternocleidomastoid muscle (*cut*)

Superior thyroid artery and vein

Internal jugular vein

Common carotid artery

Sternohyoid muscle

Sternothyroid muscle

Ansa cervicalis

Omohyoid muscle (superior belly) (*cut*)

Omohyoid muscle (inferior belly)

Brachial plexus

Pectoralis major muscle

Clavicle

Sternocleidomastoid muscle (*cut*)

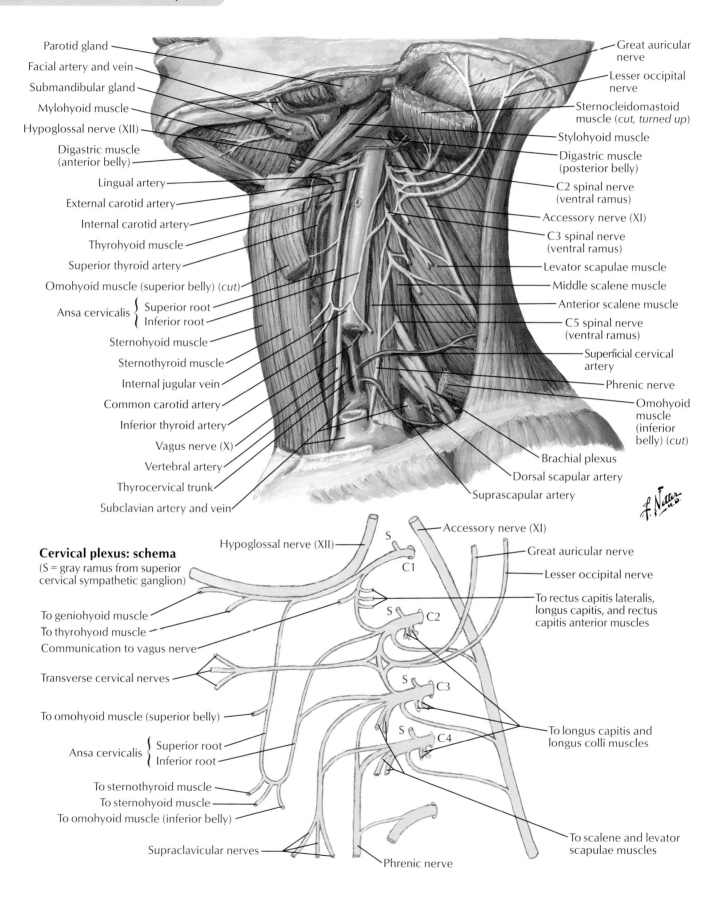

Parotid gland
Facial artery and vein
Submandibular gland
Mylohyoid muscle
Hypoglossal nerve (XII)
Digastric muscle (anterior belly)
Lingual artery
External carotid artery
Internal carotid artery
Thyrohyoid muscle
Superior thyroid artery
Omohyoid muscle (superior belly) (cut)
Ansa cervicalis { Superior root / Inferior root }
Sternohyoid muscle
Sternothyroid muscle
Internal jugular vein
Common carotid artery
Inferior thyroid artery
Vagus nerve (X)
Vertebral artery
Thyrocervical trunk
Subclavian artery and vein

Great auricular nerve
Lesser occipital nerve
Sternocleidomastoid muscle (cut, turned up)
Stylohyoid muscle
Digastric muscle (posterior belly)
C2 spinal nerve (ventral ramus)
Accessory nerve (XI)
C3 spinal nerve (ventral ramus)
Levator scapulae muscle
Middle scalene muscle
Anterior scalene muscle
C5 spinal nerve (ventral ramus)
Superficial cervical artery
Phrenic nerve
Omohyoid muscle (inferior belly) (cut)
Brachial plexus
Dorsal scapular artery
Suprascapular artery

Cervical plexus: schema
(S = gray ramus from superior cervical sympathetic ganglion)

To geniohyoid muscle
To thyrohyoid muscle
Communication to vagus nerve

Transverse cervical nerves

To omohyoid muscle (superior belly)

Ansa cervicalis { Superior root / Inferior root }

To sternothyroid muscle
To sternohyoid muscle
To omohyoid muscle (inferior belly)

Supraclavicular nerves

Hypoglossal nerve (XII)
Accessory nerve (XI)
Great auricular nerve
Lesser occipital nerve
To rectus capitis lateralis, longus capitis, and rectus capitis anterior muscles
To longus capitis and longus colli muscles
To scalene and levator scapulae muscles
Phrenic nerve

S C1
S C2
S C3
S C4

Plate 32

Neck

Right anterior dissection

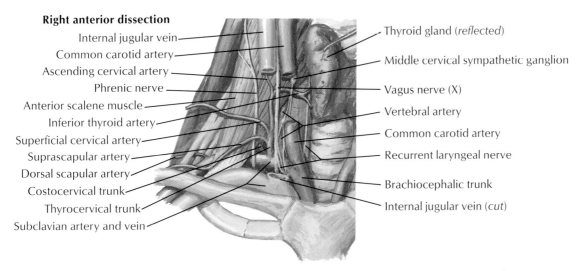

Internal jugular vein
Common carotid artery
Ascending cervical artery
Phrenic nerve
Anterior scalene muscle
Inferior thyroid artery
Superficial cervical artery
Suprascapular artery
Dorsal scapular artery
Costocervical trunk
Thyrocervical trunk
Subclavian artery and vein

Thyroid gland (*reflected*)
Middle cervical sympathetic ganglion
Vagus nerve (X)
Vertebral artery
Common carotid artery
Recurrent laryngeal nerve
Brachiocephalic trunk
Internal jugular vein (*cut*)

Common origin of superficial cervical and dorsal scapular arteries from transverse cervical artery (~30%)

Superficial branch of transverse cervical artery (superficial cervical artery)
Deep branch of transverse cervical artery (dorsal scapular artery)
Transverse cervical artery

Inferior thyroid artery
Thyrocervical trunk
Suprascapular artery

Right oblique schematic view

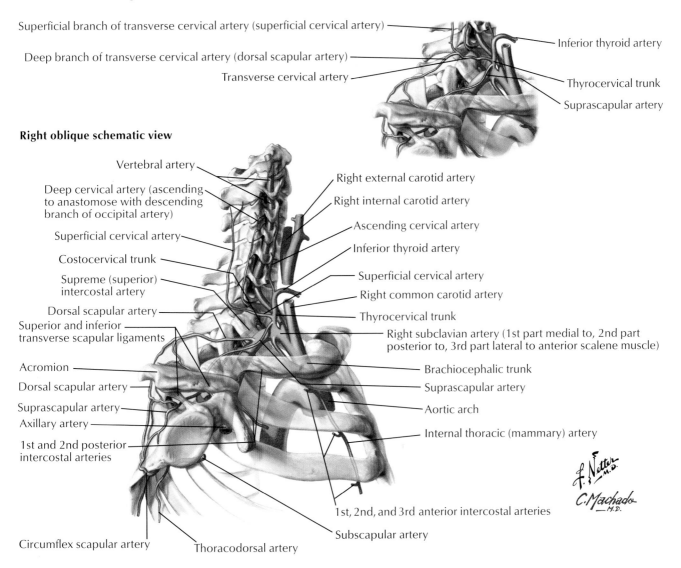

Vertebral artery
Deep cervical artery (ascending to anastomose with descending branch of occipital artery)
Superficial cervical artery
Costocervical trunk
Supreme (superior) intercostal artery
Dorsal scapular artery
Superior and inferior transverse scapular ligaments
Acromion
Dorsal scapular artery
Suprascapular artery
Axillary artery
1st and 2nd posterior intercostal arteries

Circumflex scapular artery
Thoracodorsal artery

Right external carotid artery
Right internal carotid artery
Ascending cervical artery
Inferior thyroid artery
Superficial cervical artery
Right common carotid artery
Thyrocervical trunk
Right subclavian artery (1st part medial to, 2nd part posterior to, 3rd part lateral to anterior scalene muscle)
Brachiocephalic trunk
Suprascapular artery
Aortic arch
Internal thoracic (mammary) artery

1st, 2nd, and 3rd anterior intercostal arteries
Subscapular artery

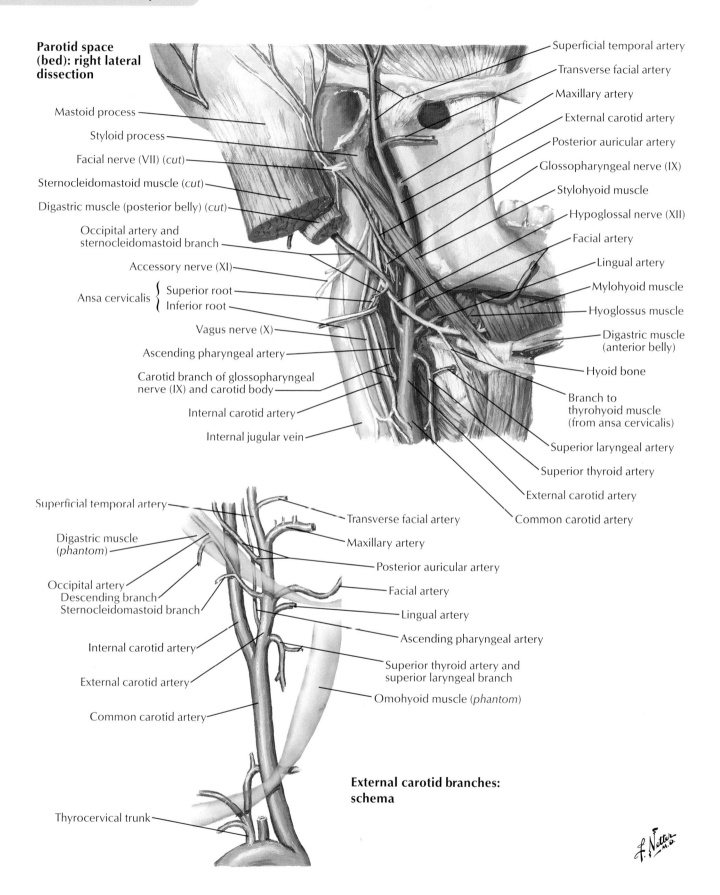

Parotid space (bed): right lateral dissection

Mastoid process

Styloid process

Facial nerve (VII) (cut)

Sternocleidomastoid muscle (cut)

Digastric muscle (posterior belly) (cut)

Occipital artery and sternocleidomastoid branch

Accessory nerve (XI)

Ansa cervicalis { Superior root / Inferior root

Vagus nerve (X)

Ascending pharyngeal artery

Carotid branch of glossopharyngeal nerve (IX) and carotid body

Internal carotid artery

Internal jugular vein

Superficial temporal artery

Transverse facial artery

Maxillary artery

External carotid artery

Posterior auricular artery

Glossopharyngeal nerve (IX)

Stylohyoid muscle

Hypoglossal nerve (XII)

Facial artery

Lingual artery

Mylohyoid muscle

Hyoglossus muscle

Digastric muscle (anterior belly)

Hyoid bone

Branch to thyrohyoid muscle (from ansa cervicalis)

Superior laryngeal artery

Superior thyroid artery

External carotid artery

Common carotid artery

Superficial temporal artery

Digastric muscle (phantom)

Occipital artery

Descending branch

Sternocleidomastoid branch

Internal carotid artery

External carotid artery

Common carotid artery

Transverse facial artery

Maxillary artery

Posterior auricular artery

Facial artery

Lingual artery

Ascending pharyngeal artery

Superior thyroid artery and superior laryngeal branch

Omohyoid muscle (phantom)

Thyrocervical trunk

External carotid branches: schema

Plate 34

Neck

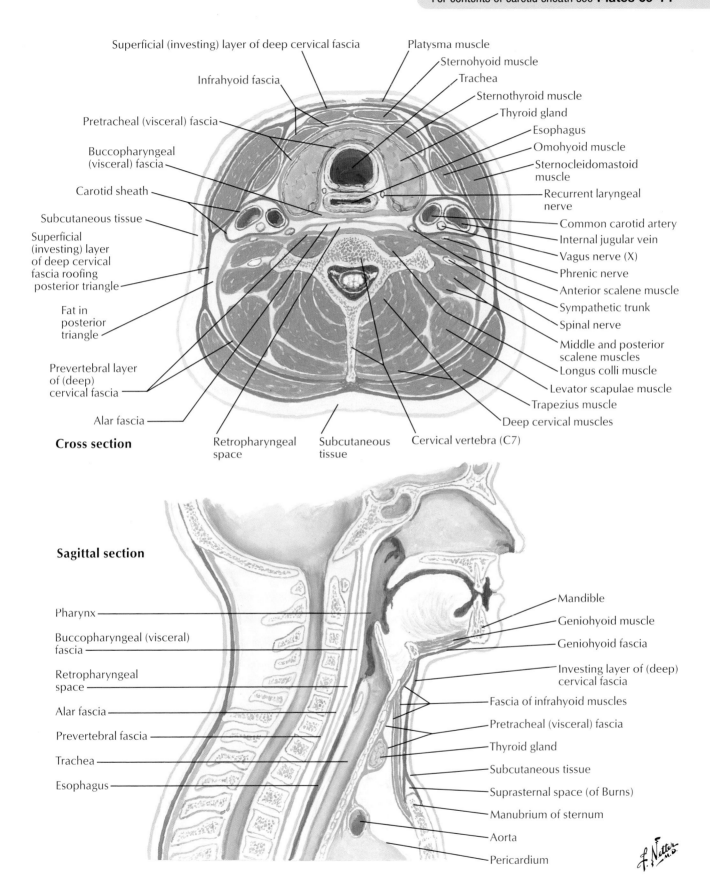

Superficial (investing) layer of deep cervical fascia

Platysma muscle

Sternohyoid muscle

Trachea

Infrahyoid fascia

Sternothyroid muscle

Thyroid gland

Pretracheal (visceral) fascia

Esophagus

Omohyoid muscle

Buccopharyngeal (visceral) fascia

Sternocleidomastoid muscle

Recurrent laryngeal nerve

Carotid sheath

Common carotid artery

Subcutaneous tissue

Internal jugular vein

Superficial (investing) layer of deep cervical fascia roofing posterior triangle

Vagus nerve (X)

Phrenic nerve

Anterior scalene muscle

Sympathetic trunk

Fat in posterior triangle

Spinal nerve

Middle and posterior scalene muscles

Prevertebral layer of (deep) cervical fascia

Longus colli muscle

Levator scapulae muscle

Trapezius muscle

Alar fascia

Deep cervical muscles

Cross section

Retropharyngeal space

Subcutaneous tissue

Cervical vertebra (C7)

Sagittal section

Pharynx

Mandible

Geniohyoid muscle

Buccopharyngeal (visceral) fascia

Geniohyoid fascia

Retropharyngeal space

Investing layer of (deep) cervical fascia

Alar fascia

Fascia of infrahyoid muscles

Prevertebral fascia

Pretracheal (visceral) fascia

Trachea

Thyroid gland

Esophagus

Subcutaneous tissue

Suprasternal space (of Burns)

Manubrium of sternum

Aorta

Pericardium

Anterolateral view

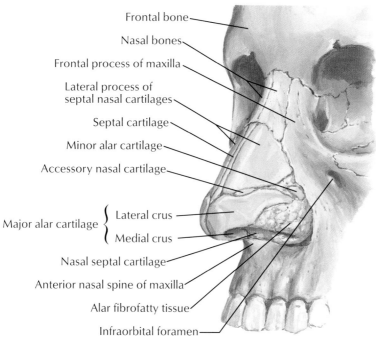

Frontal bone
Nasal bones
Frontal process of maxilla
Lateral process of septal nasal cartilages
Septal cartilage
Minor alar cartilage
Accessory nasal cartilage
Major alar cartilage { Lateral crus / Medial crus }
Nasal septal cartilage
Anterior nasal spine of maxilla
Alar fibrofatty tissue
Infraorbital foramen

Inferior view

Major alar cartilage
Lateral crus
Medial crus
Alar fibrofatty tissue
Nasal septal cartilage
Anterior nasal spine of maxilla
Intermaxillary suture

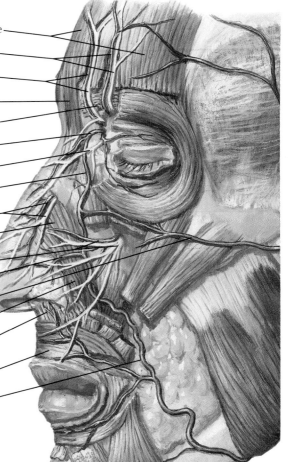

Frontalis muscle
Supraorbital artery and nerve
Supratrochlear artery and nerve
Procerus muscle
Corrugator supercilii muscle
Dorsal nasal artery
Infratrochlear nerve
Angular artery
External nasal artery and nerve
Nasalis muscle (transverse part)
Infraorbital artery and nerve
Lateral nasal artery
Transverse facial artery
Nasalis muscle (alar part)
Depressor septi nasi muscle
Orbicularis oris muscle
Facial artery

Plate 36

Nasal Region

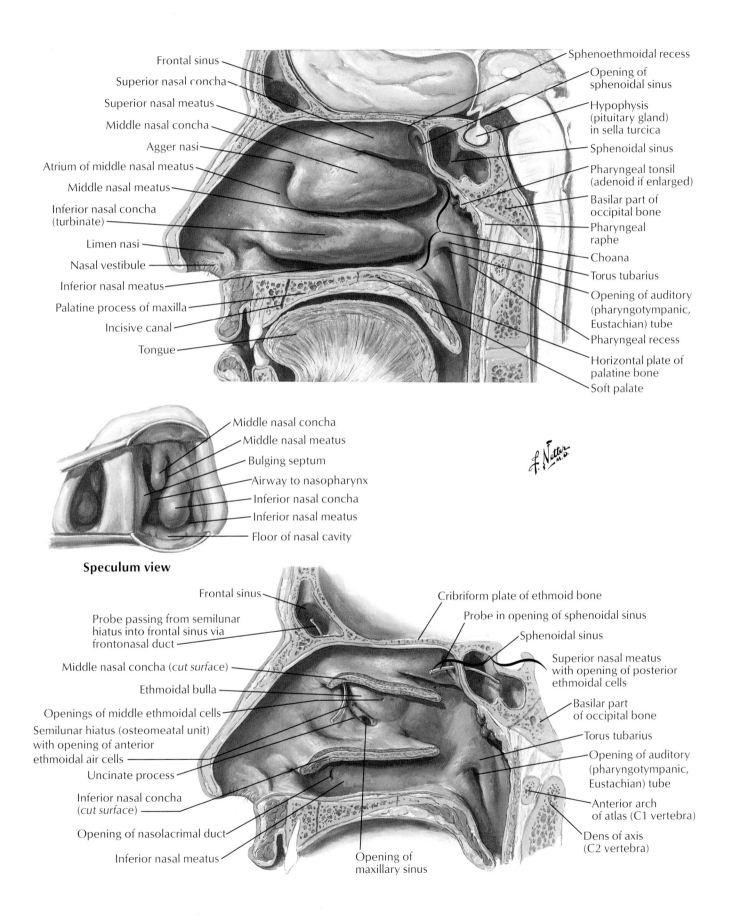

Frontal sinus

Superior nasal concha

Superior nasal meatus

Middle nasal concha

Agger nasi

Atrium of middle nasal meatus

Middle nasal meatus

Inferior nasal concha (turbinate)

Limen nasi

Nasal vestibule

Inferior nasal meatus

Palatine process of maxilla

Incisive canal

Tongue

Sphenoethmoidal recess

Opening of sphenoidal sinus

Hypophysis (pituitary gland) in sella turcica

Sphenoidal sinus

Pharyngeal tonsil (adenoid if enlarged)

Basilar part of occipital bone

Pharyngeal raphe

Choana

Torus tubarius

Opening of auditory (pharyngotympanic, Eustachian) tube

Pharyngeal recess

Horizontal plate of palatine bone

Soft palate

Middle nasal concha

Middle nasal meatus

Bulging septum

Airway to nasopharynx

Inferior nasal concha

Inferior nasal meatus

Floor of nasal cavity

Speculum view

Frontal sinus

Probe passing from semilunar hiatus into frontal sinus via frontonasal duct

Middle nasal concha (*cut surface*)

Ethmoidal bulla

Openings of middle ethmoidal cells

Semilunar hiatus (osteomeatal unit) with opening of anterior ethmoidal air cells

Uncinate process

Inferior nasal concha (*cut surface*)

Opening of nasolacrimal duct

Inferior nasal meatus

Cribriform plate of ethmoid bone

Probe in opening of sphenoidal sinus

Sphenoidal sinus

Superior nasal meatus with opening of posterior ethmoidal cells

Basilar part of occipital bone

Torus tubarius

Opening of auditory (pharyngotympanic, Eustachian) tube

Anterior arch of atlas (C1 vertebra)

Dens of axis (C2 vertebra)

Opening of maxillary sinus

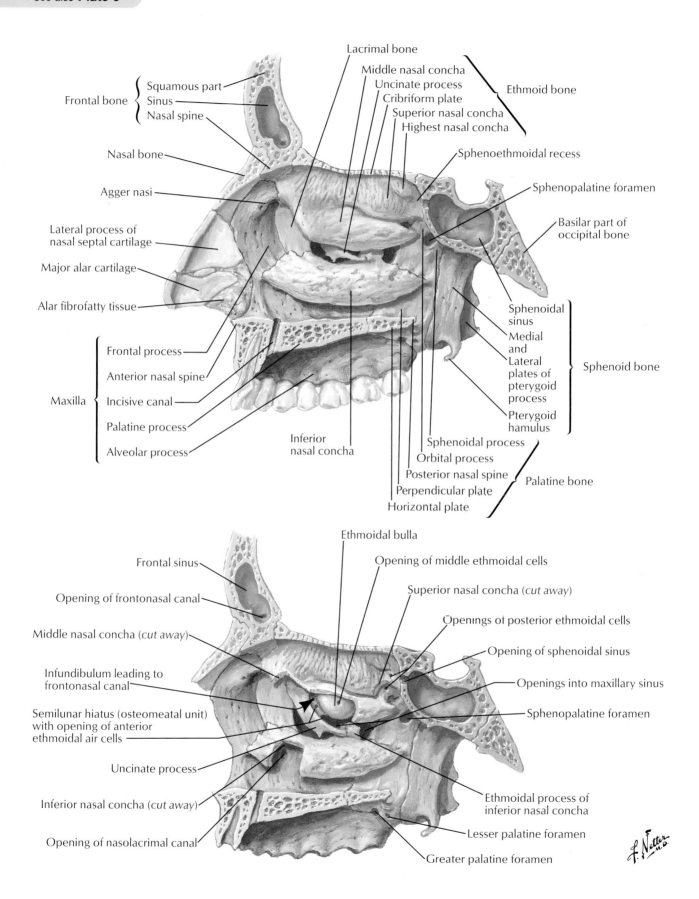

Lacrimal bone

Middle nasal concha

Uncinate process

Cribriform plate

Superior nasal concha

Highest nasal concha

Ethmoid bone

Frontal bone
- Squamous part
- Sinus
- Nasal spine

Nasal bone

Agger nasi

Lateral process of nasal septal cartilage

Major alar cartilage

Alar fibrofatty tissue

Maxilla
- Frontal process
- Anterior nasal spine
- Incisive canal
- Palatine process
- Alveolar process

Sphenoethmoidal recess

Sphenopalatine foramen

Basilar part of occipital bone

Sphenoidal sinus

Medial and Lateral plates of pterygoid process

Pterygoid hamulus

Sphenoid bone

Inferior nasal concha

Sphenoidal process

Orbital process

Posterior nasal spine

Perpendicular plate

Horizontal plate

Palatine bone

Ethmoidal bulla

Opening of middle ethmoidal cells

Superior nasal concha (cut away)

Openings of posterior ethmoidal cells

Opening of sphenoidal sinus

Openings into maxillary sinus

Sphenopalatine foramen

Frontal sinus

Opening of frontonasal canal

Middle nasal concha (cut away)

Infundibulum leading to frontonasal canal

Semilunar hiatus (osteomeatal unit) with opening of anterior ethmoidal air cells

Uncinate process

Inferior nasal concha (cut away)

Opening of nasolacrimal canal

Ethmoidal process of inferior nasal concha

Lesser palatine foramen

Greater palatine foramen

Plate 38

Nasal Region

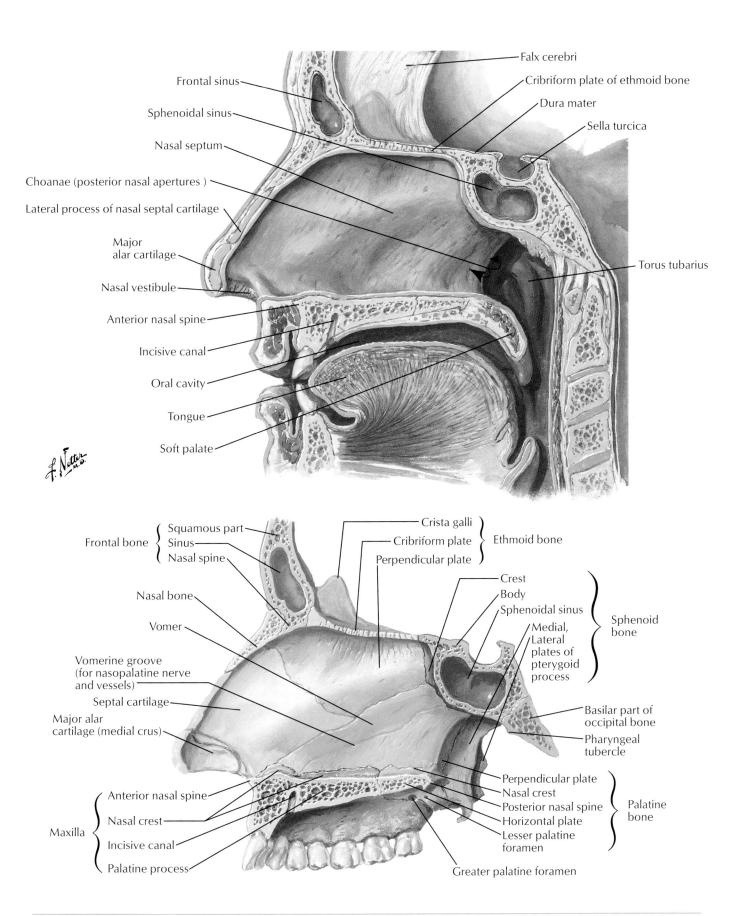

Falx cerebri

Frontal sinus

Cribriform plate of ethmoid bone

Sphenoidal sinus

Dura mater

Nasal septum

Sella turcica

Choanae (posterior nasal apertures)

Lateral process of nasal septal cartilage

Major alar cartilage

Nasal vestibule

Torus tubarius

Anterior nasal spine

Incisive canal

Oral cavity

Tongue

Soft palate

Frontal bone {
Squamous part
Sinus
Nasal spine

Crista galli
Cribriform plate
Perpendicular plate
} Ethmoid bone

Nasal bone

Crest
Body
Sphenoidal sinus

Vomer

Medial, Lateral plates of pterygoid process
} Sphenoid bone

Vomerine groove (for nasopalatine nerve and vessels)

Septal cartilage

Major alar cartilage (medial crus)

Basilar part of occipital bone

Pharyngeal tubercle

Perpendicular plate
Nasal crest
Posterior nasal spine
Horizontal plate
Lesser palatine foramen
} Palatine bone

Anterior nasal spine

Nasal crest

Maxilla {
Incisive canal

Palatine process

Greater palatine foramen

See also **Plate 34**

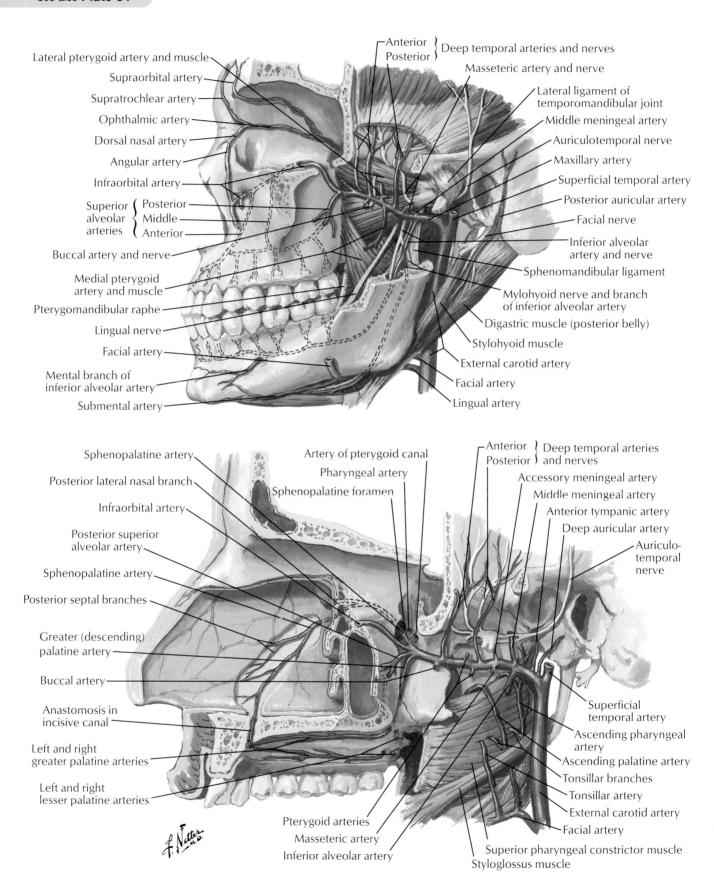

Lateral pterygoid artery and muscle

Supraorbital artery

Supratrochlear artery

Ophthalmic artery

Dorsal nasal artery

Angular artery

Infraorbital artery

Superior alveolar arteries { Posterior, Middle, Anterior

Buccal artery and nerve

Medial pterygoid artery and muscle

Pterygomandibular raphe

Lingual nerve

Facial artery

Mental branch of inferior alveolar artery

Submental artery

Anterior, Posterior } Deep temporal arteries and nerves

Masseteric artery and nerve

Lateral ligament of temporomandibular joint

Middle meningeal artery

Auriculotemporal nerve

Maxillary artery

Superficial temporal artery

Posterior auricular artery

Facial nerve

Inferior alveolar artery and nerve

Sphenomandibular ligament

Mylohyoid nerve and branch of inferior alveolar artery

Digastric muscle (posterior belly)

Stylohyoid muscle

External carotid artery

Facial artery

Lingual artery

Sphenopalatine artery

Posterior lateral nasal branch

Infraorbital artery

Posterior superior alveolar artery

Sphenopalatine artery

Posterior septal branches

Greater (descending) palatine artery

Buccal artery

Anastomosis in incisive canal

Left and right greater palatine arteries

Left and right lesser palatine arteries

Artery of pterygoid canal

Pharyngeal artery

Sphenopalatine foramen

Anterior, Posterior } Deep temporal arteries and nerves

Accessory meningeal artery

Middle meningeal artery

Anterior tympanic artery

Deep auricular artery

Auriculo-temporal nerve

Superficial temporal artery

Ascending pharyngeal artery

Ascending palatine artery

Tonsillar branches

Tonsillar artery

External carotid artery

Facial artery

Superior pharyngeal constrictor muscle

Styloglossus muscle

Pterygoid arteries

Masseteric artery

Inferior alveolar artery

Plate 40   **Nasal Region**

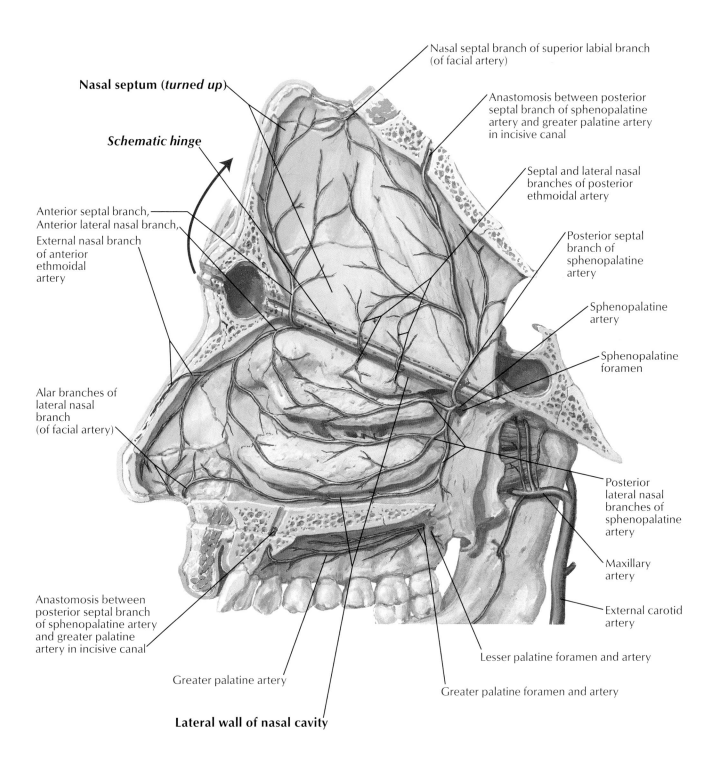

Nasal septal branch of superior labial branch (of facial artery)

Nasal septum (*turned up*)

Anastomosis between posterior septal branch of sphenopalatine artery and greater palatine artery in incisive canal

Schematic hinge

Septal and lateral nasal branches of posterior ethmoidal artery

Anterior septal branch, Anterior lateral nasal branch, External nasal branch of anterior ethmoidal artery

Posterior septal branch of sphenopalatine artery

Sphenopalatine artery

Sphenopalatine foramen

Alar branches of lateral nasal branch (of facial artery)

Posterior lateral nasal branches of sphenopalatine artery

Maxillary artery

Anastomosis between posterior septal branch of sphenopalatine artery and greater palatine artery in incisive canal

External carotid artery

Greater palatine artery

Lesser palatine foramen and artery

Lateral wall of nasal cavity

Greater palatine foramen and artery

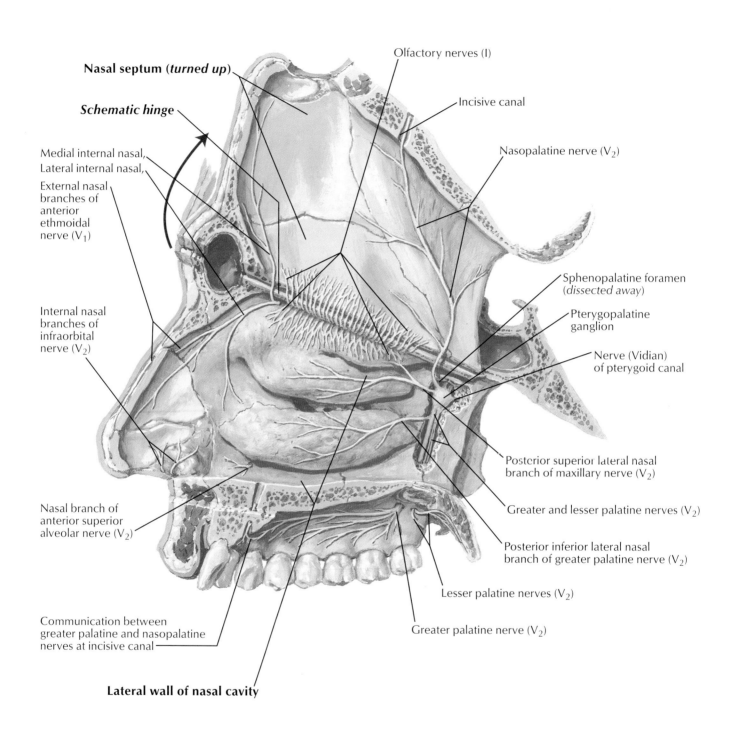

Olfactory nerves (I)

Nasal septum (*turned up*)

Incisive canal

Schematic hinge

Nasopalatine nerve (V₂)

Medial internal nasal,
Lateral internal nasal,
External nasal
branches of
anterior
ethmoidal
nerve (V₁)

Sphenopalatine foramen
(*dissected away*)

Pterygopalatine
ganglion

Internal nasal
branches of
infraorbital
nerve (V₂)

Nerve (Vidian)
of pterygoid canal

Posterior superior lateral nasal
branch of maxillary nerve (V₂)

Nasal branch of
anterior superior
alveolar nerve (V₂)

Greater and lesser palatine nerves (V₂)

Posterior inferior lateral nasal
branch of greater palatine nerve (V₂)

Lesser palatine nerves (V₂)

Communication between
greater palatine and nasopalatine
nerves at incisive canal

Greater palatine nerve (V₂)

Lateral wall of nasal cavity

Plate 42

Nasal Region

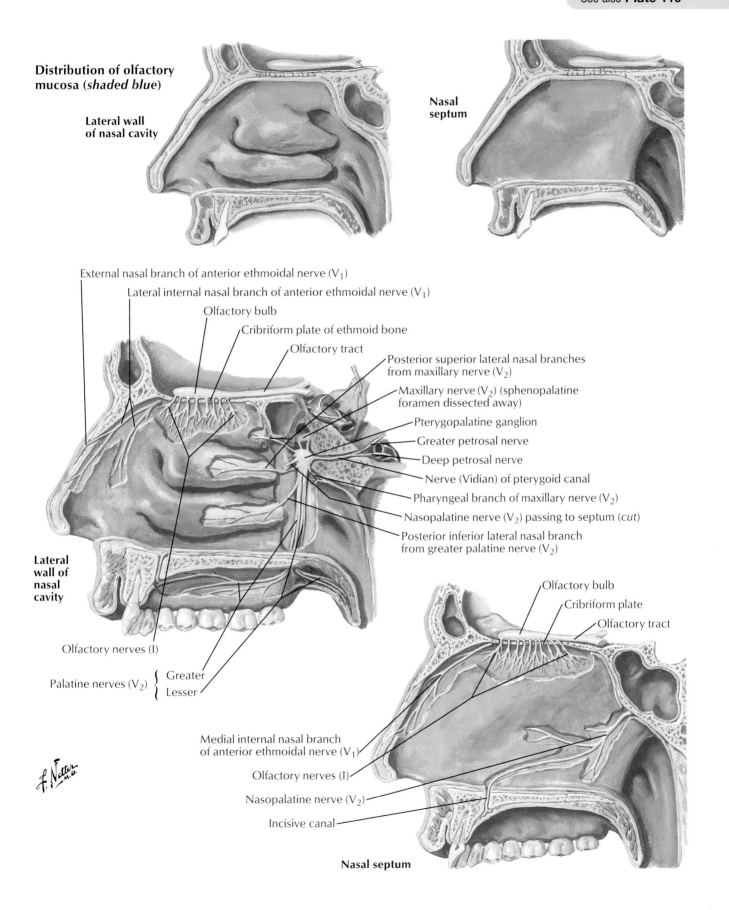

Distribution of olfactory
mucosa (*shaded blue*)

**Lateral wall
of nasal cavity**

**Nasal
septum**

External nasal branch of anterior ethmoidal nerve (V_1)

Lateral internal nasal branch of anterior ethmoidal nerve (V_1)

Olfactory bulb

Cribriform plate of ethmoid bone

Olfactory tract

Posterior superior lateral nasal branches
from maxillary nerve (V_2)

Maxillary nerve (V_2) (sphenopalatine
foramen dissected away)

Pterygopalatine ganglion

Greater petrosal nerve

Deep petrosal nerve

Nerve (Vidian) of pterygoid canal

Pharyngeal branch of maxillary nerve (V_2)

Nasopalatine nerve (V_2) passing to septum (*cut*)

Posterior inferior lateral nasal branch
from greater palatine nerve (V_2)

**Lateral
wall of
nasal
cavity**

Olfactory nerves (I)

Palatine nerves (V_2) { Greater
Lesser

Olfactory bulb

Cribriform plate

Olfactory tract

Medial internal nasal branch
of anterior ethmoidal nerve (V_1)

Olfactory nerves (I)

Nasopalatine nerve (V_2)

Incisive canal

Nasal septum

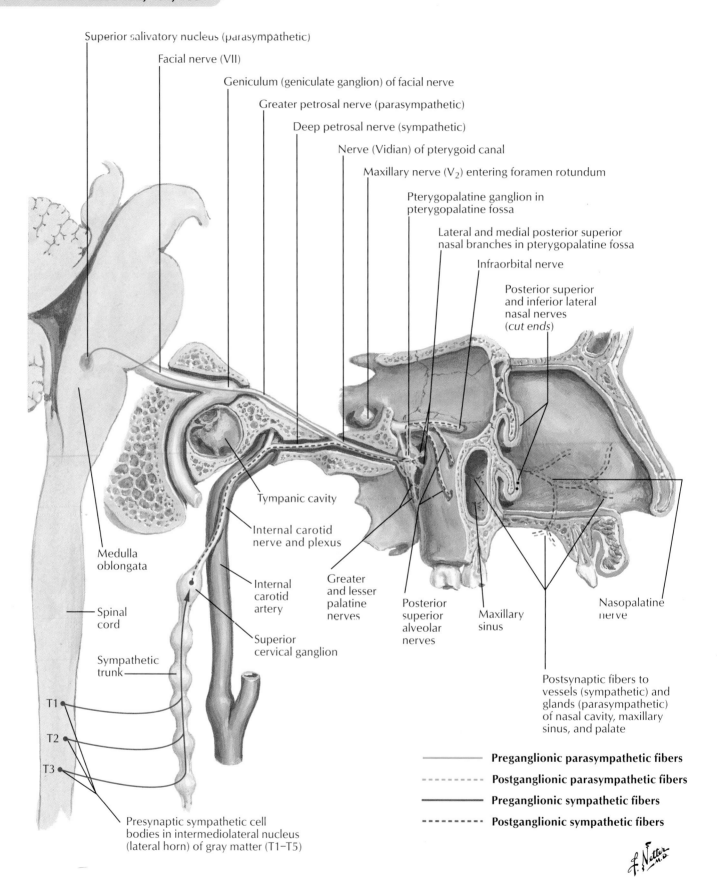

Superior salivatory nucleus (parasympathetic)

Facial nerve (VII)

Geniculum (geniculate ganglion) of facial nerve

Greater petrosal nerve (parasympathetic)

Deep petrosal nerve (sympathetic)

Nerve (Vidian) of pterygoid canal

Maxillary nerve (V_2) entering foramen rotundum

Pterygopalatine ganglion in pterygopalatine fossa

Lateral and medial posterior superior nasal branches in pterygopalatine fossa

Infraorbital nerve

Posterior superior and inferior lateral nasal nerves (*cut ends*)

Tympanic cavity

Internal carotid nerve and plexus

Medulla oblongata

Spinal cord

Internal carotid artery

Greater and lesser palatine nerves

Posterior superior alveolar nerves

Maxillary sinus

Nasopalatine nerve

Sympathetic trunk

Superior cervical ganglion

T1

T2

T3

Postsynaptic fibers to vessels (sympathetic) and glands (parasympathetic) of nasal cavity, maxillary sinus, and palate

Presynaptic sympathetic cell bodies in intermediolateral nucleus (lateral horn) of gray matter (T1–T5)

——————— **Preganglionic parasympathetic fibers**

- - - - - - - **Postganglionic parasympathetic fibers**

——————— **Preganglionic sympathetic fibers**

- - - - - - - **Postganglionic sympathetic fibers**

Plate 44

Nasal Region

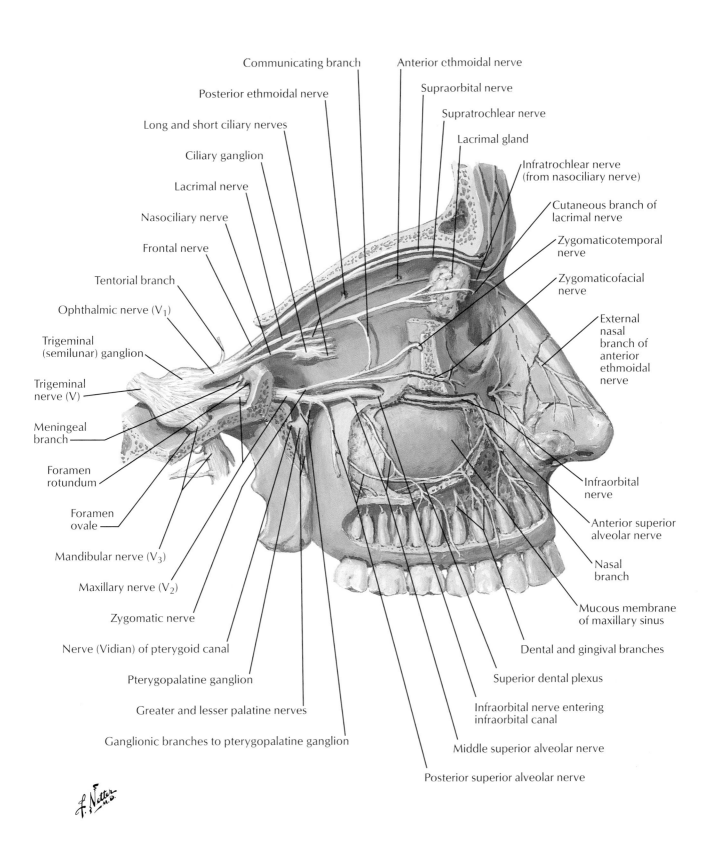

Communicating branch

Posterior ethmoidal nerve

Long and short ciliary nerves

Ciliary ganglion

Lacrimal nerve

Nasociliary nerve

Frontal nerve

Tentorial branch

Ophthalmic nerve (V₁)

Trigeminal (semilunar) ganglion

Trigeminal nerve (V)

Meningeal branch

Foramen rotundum

Foramen ovale

Mandibular nerve (V₃)

Maxillary nerve (V₂)

Zygomatic nerve

Nerve (Vidian) of pterygoid canal

Pterygopalatine ganglion

Greater and lesser palatine nerves

Ganglionic branches to pterygopalatine ganglion

Anterior ethmoidal nerve

Supraorbital nerve

Supratrochlear nerve

Lacrimal gland

Infratrochlear nerve (from nasociliary nerve)

Cutaneous branch of lacrimal nerve

Zygomaticotemporal nerve

Zygomaticofacial nerve

External nasal branch of anterior ethmoidal nerve

Infraorbital nerve

Anterior superior alveolar nerve

Nasal branch

Mucous membrane of maxillary sinus

Dental and gingival branches

Superior dental plexus

Infraorbital nerve entering infraorbital canal

Middle superior alveolar nerve

Posterior superior alveolar nerve

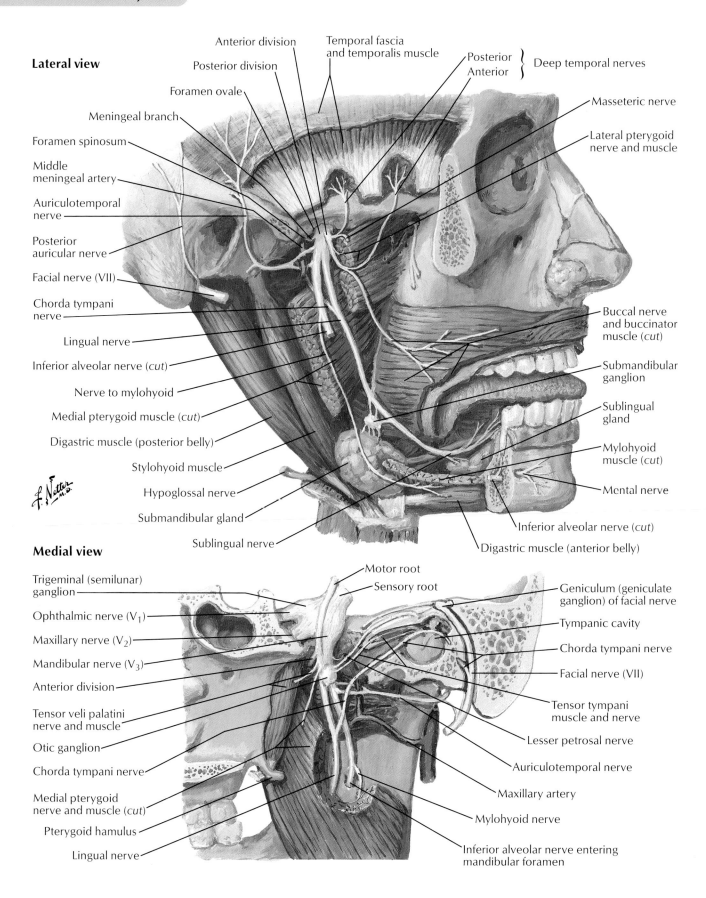

Lateral view

Anterior division

Posterior division

Temporal fascia and temporalis muscle

Posterior
Anterior } Deep temporal nerves

Foramen ovale

Meningeal branch

Masseteric nerve

Foramen spinosum

Lateral pterygoid nerve and muscle

Middle meningeal artery

Auriculotemporal nerve

Posterior auricular nerve

Facial nerve (VII)

Chorda tympani nerve

Buccal nerve and buccinator muscle (cut)

Lingual nerve

Submandibular ganglion

Inferior alveolar nerve (cut)

Sublingual gland

Nerve to mylohyoid

Medial pterygoid muscle (cut)

Mylohyoid muscle (cut)

Digastric muscle (posterior belly)

Stylohyoid muscle

Mental nerve

Hypoglossal nerve

Submandibular gland

Inferior alveolar nerve (cut)

Sublingual nerve

Digastric muscle (anterior belly)

Medial view

Motor root

Sensory root

Trigeminal (semilunar) ganglion

Geniculum (geniculate ganglion) of facial nerve

Ophthalmic nerve (V₁)

Tympanic cavity

Maxillary nerve (V₂)

Chorda tympani nerve

Mandibular nerve (V₃)

Facial nerve (VII)

Anterior division

Tensor veli palatini nerve and muscle

Tensor tympani muscle and nerve

Otic ganglion

Lesser petrosal nerve

Chorda tympani nerve

Auriculotemporal nerve

Medial pterygoid nerve and muscle (cut)

Maxillary artery

Pterygoid hamulus

Mylohyoid nerve

Lingual nerve

Inferior alveolar nerve entering mandibular foramen

Plate 46

Nasal Region

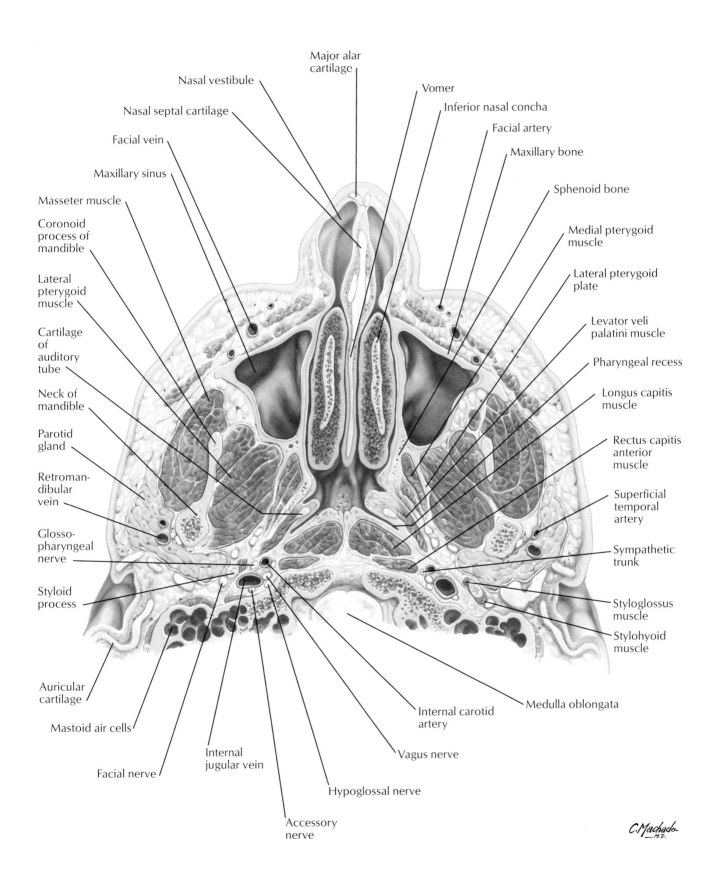

Major alar cartilage

Nasal vestibule

Nasal septal cartilage

Facial vein

Maxillary sinus

Masseter muscle

Coronoid process of mandible

Lateral pterygoid muscle

Cartilage of auditory tube

Neck of mandible

Parotid gland

Retromandibular vein

Glossopharyngeal nerve

Styloid process

Auricular cartilage

Mastoid air cells

Facial nerve

Internal jugular vein

Accessory nerve

Hypoglossal nerve

Vagus nerve

Internal carotid artery

Medulla oblongata

Stylohyoid muscle

Styloglossus muscle

Sympathetic trunk

Superficial temporal artery

Rectus capitis anterior muscle

Longus capitis muscle

Pharyngeal recess

Levator veli palatini muscle

Lateral pterygoid plate

Medial pterygoid muscle

Sphenoid bone

Maxillary bone

Facial artery

Inferior nasal concha

Vomer

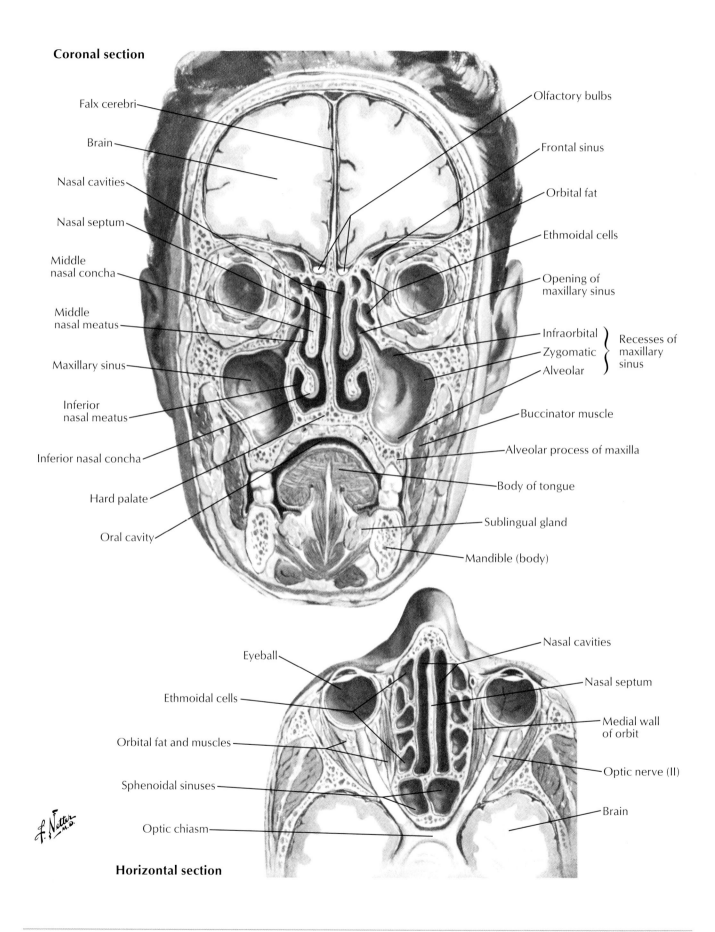

Coronal section

Falx cerebri

Brain

Nasal cavities

Nasal septum

Middle nasal concha

Middle nasal meatus

Maxillary sinus

Inferior nasal meatus

Inferior nasal concha

Hard palate

Oral cavity

Olfactory bulbs

Frontal sinus

Orbital fat

Ethmoidal cells

Opening of maxillary sinus

Infraorbital
Zygomatic
Alveolar
} Recesses of maxillary sinus

Buccinator muscle

Alveolar process of maxilla

Body of tongue

Sublingual gland

Mandible (body)

Eyeball

Ethmoidal cells

Orbital fat and muscles

Sphenoidal sinuses

Optic chiasm

Nasal cavities

Nasal septum

Medial wall of orbit

Optic nerve (II)

Brain

Horizontal section

Plate 48

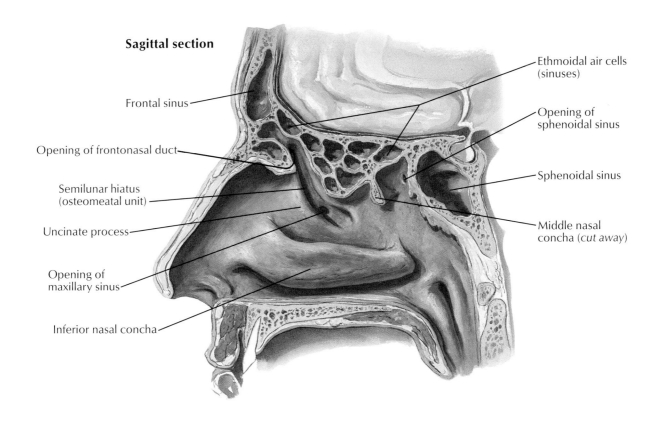

Sagittal section

Frontal sinus

Opening of frontonasal duct

Semilunar hiatus (osteomeatal unit)

Uncinate process

Opening of maxillary sinus

Inferior nasal concha

Ethmoidal air cells (sinuses)

Opening of sphenoidal sinus

Sphenoidal sinus

Middle nasal concha (*cut away*)

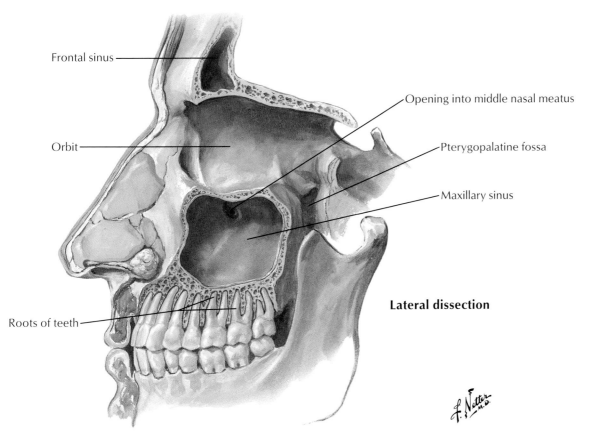

Frontal sinus

Orbit

Roots of teeth

Opening into middle nasal meatus

Pterygopalatine fossa

Maxillary sinus

Lateral dissection

Bones of nasal cavity and paranasal sinuses at birth

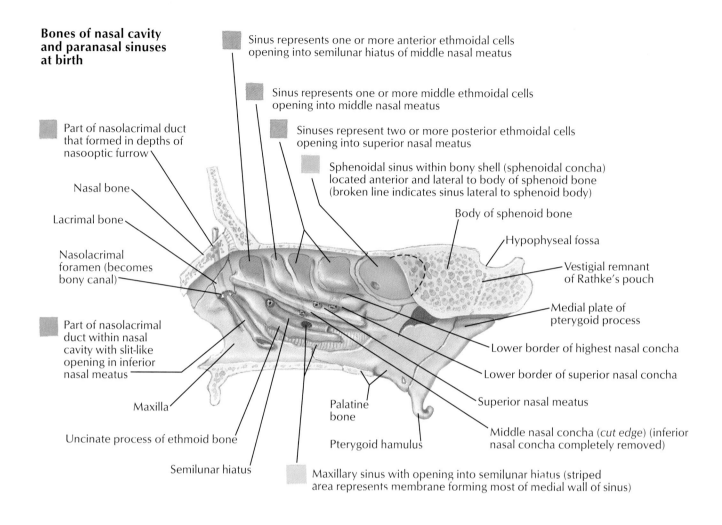

Sinus represents one or more anterior ethmoidal cells opening into semilunar hiatus of middle nasal meatus

Sinus represents one or more middle ethmoidal cells opening into middle nasal meatus

Sinuses represent two or more posterior ethmoidal cells opening into superior nasal meatus

Sphenoidal sinus within bony shell (sphenoidal concha) located anterior and lateral to body of sphenoid bone (broken line indicates sinus lateral to sphenoid body)

Part of nasolacrimal duct that formed in depths of nasooptic furrow

Nasal bone

Lacrimal bone

Nasolacrimal foramen (becomes bony canal)

Part of nasolacrimal duct within nasal cavity with slit-like opening in inferior nasal meatus

Maxilla

Uncinate process of ethmoid bone

Semilunar hiatus

Body of sphenoid bone

Hypophyseal fossa

Vestigial remnant of Rathke's pouch

Medial plate of pterygoid process

Lower border of highest nasal concha

Lower border of superior nasal concha

Superior nasal meatus

Middle nasal concha (*cut edge*) (inferior nasal concha completely removed)

Palatine bone

Pterygoid hamulus

Maxillary sinus with opening into semilunar hiatus (striped area represents membrane forming most of medial wall of sinus)

Growth of frontal and maxillary sinuses throughout life

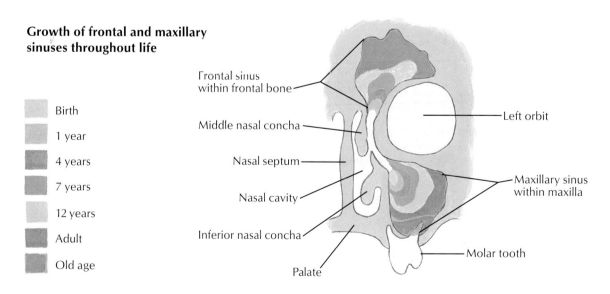

Birth

1 year

4 years

7 years

12 years

Adult

Old age

Frontal sinus within frontal bone

Middle nasal concha

Nasal septum

Nasal cavity

Inferior nasal concha

Palate

Left orbit

Maxillary sinus within maxilla

Molar tooth

Plate 50   **Nasal Region**

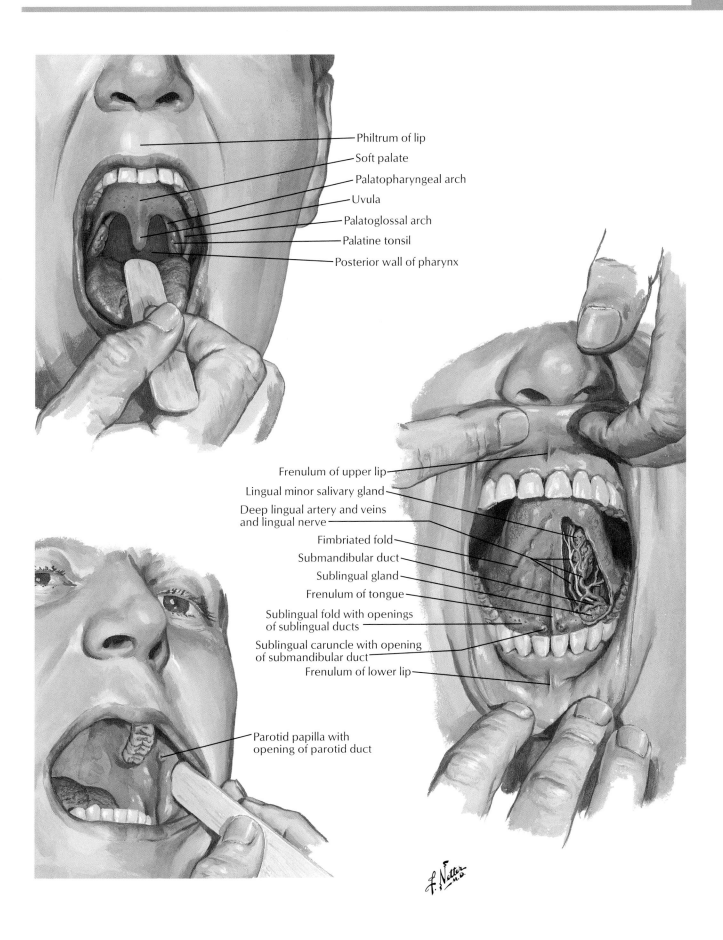

Philtrum of lip

Soft palate

Palatopharyngeal arch

Uvula

Palatoglossal arch

Palatine tonsil

Posterior wall of pharynx

Frenulum of upper lip

Lingual minor salivary gland

Deep lingual artery and veins and lingual nerve

Fimbriated fold

Submandibular duct

Sublingual gland

Frenulum of tongue

Sublingual fold with openings of sublingual ducts

Sublingual caruncle with opening of submandibular duct

Frenulum of lower lip

Parotid papilla with opening of parotid duct

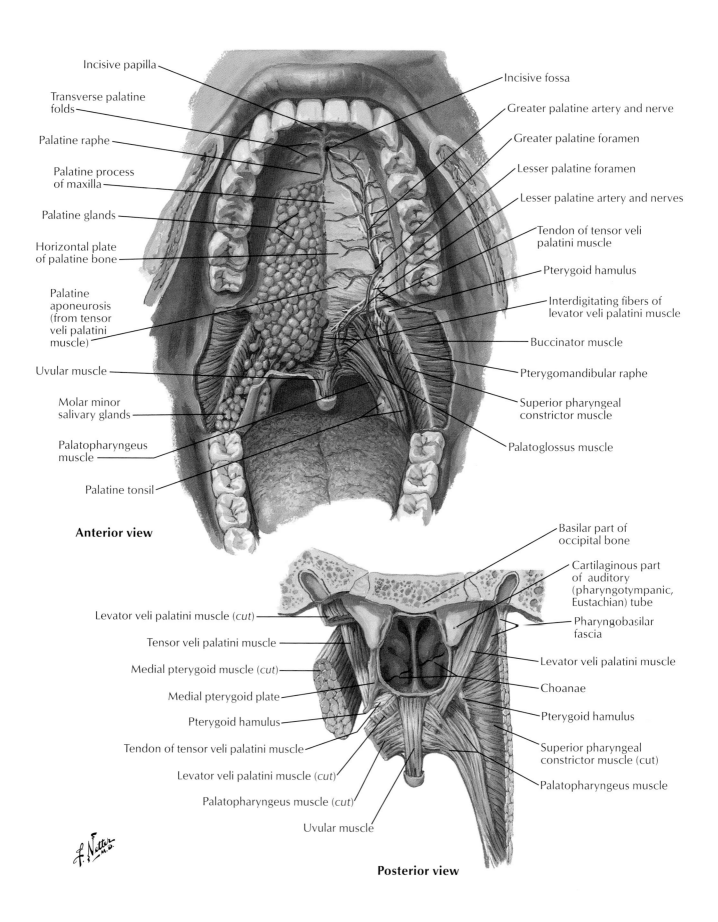

Incisive papilla

Transverse palatine folds

Palatine raphe

Palatine process of maxilla

Palatine glands

Horizontal plate of palatine bone

Palatine aponeurosis (from tensor veli palatini muscle)

Uvular muscle

Molar minor salivary glands

Palatopharyngeus muscle

Palatine tonsil

Incisive fossa

Greater palatine artery and nerve

Greater palatine foramen

Lesser palatine foramen

Lesser palatine artery and nerves

Tendon of tensor veli palatini muscle

Pterygoid hamulus

Interdigitating fibers of levator veli palatini muscle

Buccinator muscle

Pterygomandibular raphe

Superior pharyngeal constrictor muscle

Palatoglossus muscle

Anterior view

Levator veli palatini muscle (*cut*)

Tensor veli palatini muscle

Medial pterygoid muscle (*cut*)

Medial pterygoid plate

Pterygoid hamulus

Tendon of tensor veli palatini muscle

Levator veli palatini muscle (*cut*)

Palatopharyngeus muscle (*cut*)

Uvular muscle

Basilar part of occipital bone

Cartilaginous part of auditory (pharyngotympanic, Eustachian) tube

Pharyngobasilar fascia

Levator veli palatini muscle

Choanae

Pterygoid hamulus

Superior pharyngeal constrictor muscle (cut)

Palatopharyngeus muscle

Posterior view

Plate 52

Oral Region

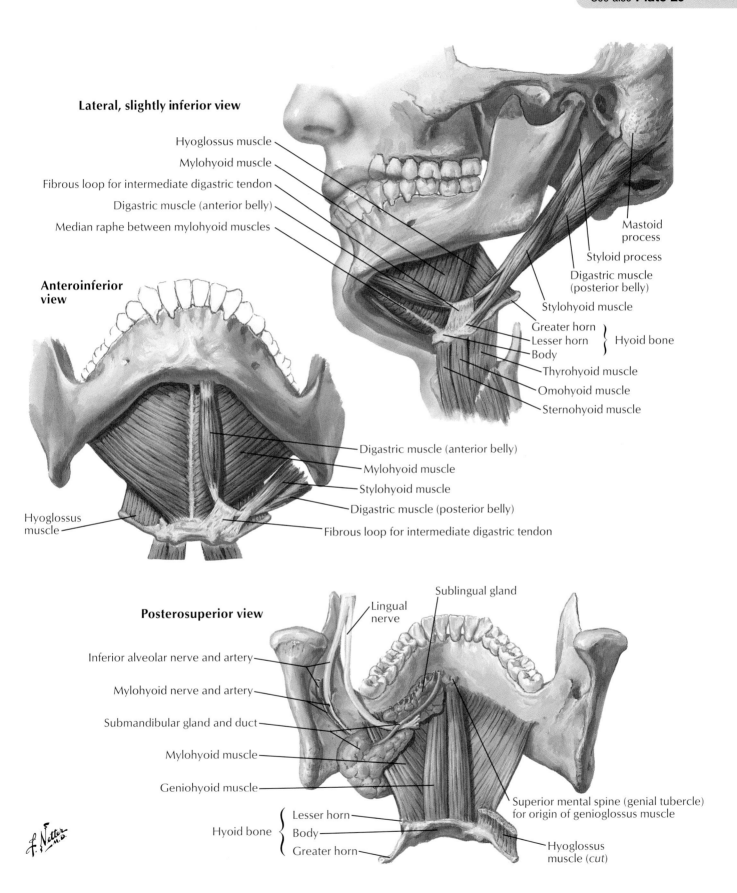

Lateral, slightly inferior view

Hyoglossus muscle

Mylohyoid muscle

Fibrous loop for intermediate digastric tendon

Digastric muscle (anterior belly)

Median raphe between mylohyoid muscles

Mastoid process

Styloid process

Digastric muscle (posterior belly)

Stylohyoid muscle

Greater horn
Lesser horn } Hyoid bone
Body

Thyrohyoid muscle

Omohyoid muscle

Sternohyoid muscle

Anteroinferior view

Digastric muscle (anterior belly)

Mylohyoid muscle

Stylohyoid muscle

Digastric muscle (posterior belly)

Fibrous loop for intermediate digastric tendon

Hyoglossus muscle

Posterosuperior view

Lingual nerve

Sublingual gland

Inferior alveolar nerve and artery

Mylohyoid nerve and artery

Submandibular gland and duct

Mylohyoid muscle

Geniohyoid muscle

Superior mental spine (genial tubercle) for origin of genioglossus muscle

Lesser horn
Hyoid bone { Body
Greater horn

Hyoglossus muscle (*cut*)

Oral Region **Plate 53**

Muscles Involved in Mastication

For facial muscles see **Plate 26**

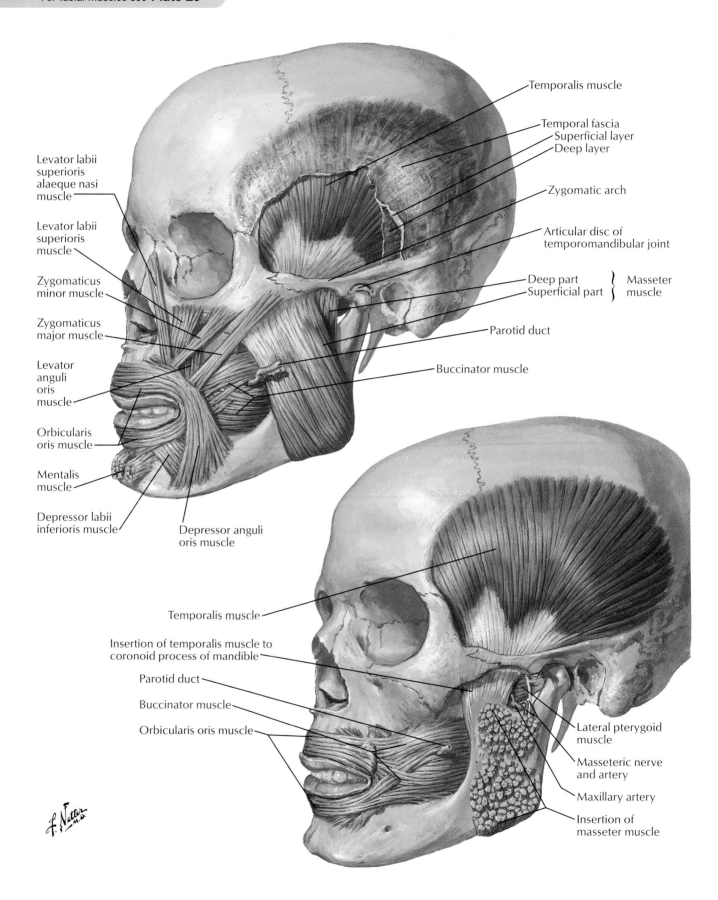

Temporalis muscle

Temporal fascia
Superficial layer
Deep layer

Zygomatic arch

Articular disc of
temporomandibular joint

Deep part } Masseter
Superficial part } muscle

Parotid duct

Buccinator muscle

Levator labii
superioris
alaeque nasi
muscle

Levator labii
superioris
muscle

Zygomaticus
minor muscle

Zygomaticus
major muscle

Levator
anguli
oris
muscle

Orbicularis
oris muscle

Mentalis
muscle

Depressor labii
inferioris muscle

Depressor anguli
oris muscle

Temporalis muscle

Insertion of temporalis muscle to
coronoid process of mandible

Parotid duct

Buccinator muscle

Orbicularis oris muscle

Lateral pterygoid
muscle

Masseteric nerve
and artery

Maxillary artery

Insertion of
masseter muscle

Plate 54

Oral Region

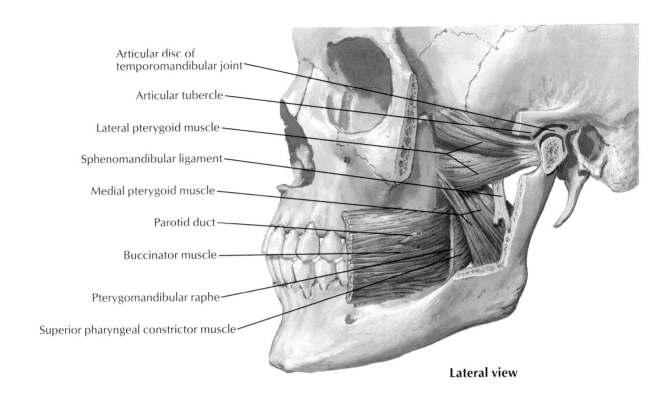

Articular disc of temporomandibular joint

Articular tubercle

Lateral pterygoid muscle

Sphenomandibular ligament

Medial pterygoid muscle

Parotid duct

Buccinator muscle

Pterygomandibular raphe

Superior pharyngeal constrictor muscle

Lateral view

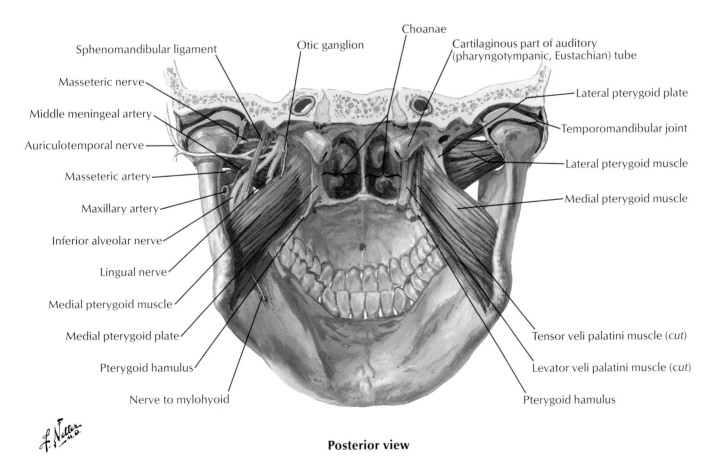

Sphenomandibular ligament

Otic ganglion

Choanae

Cartilaginous part of auditory (pharyngotympanic, Eustachian) tube

Masseteric nerve

Middle meningeal artery

Auriculotemporal nerve

Masseteric artery

Maxillary artery

Inferior alveolar nerve

Lingual nerve

Medial pterygoid muscle

Medial pterygoid plate

Pterygoid hamulus

Nerve to mylohyoid

Lateral pterygoid plate

Temporomandibular joint

Lateral pterygoid muscle

Medial pterygoid muscle

Tensor veli palatini muscle (*cut*)

Levator veli palatini muscle (*cut*)

Pterygoid hamulus

Posterior view

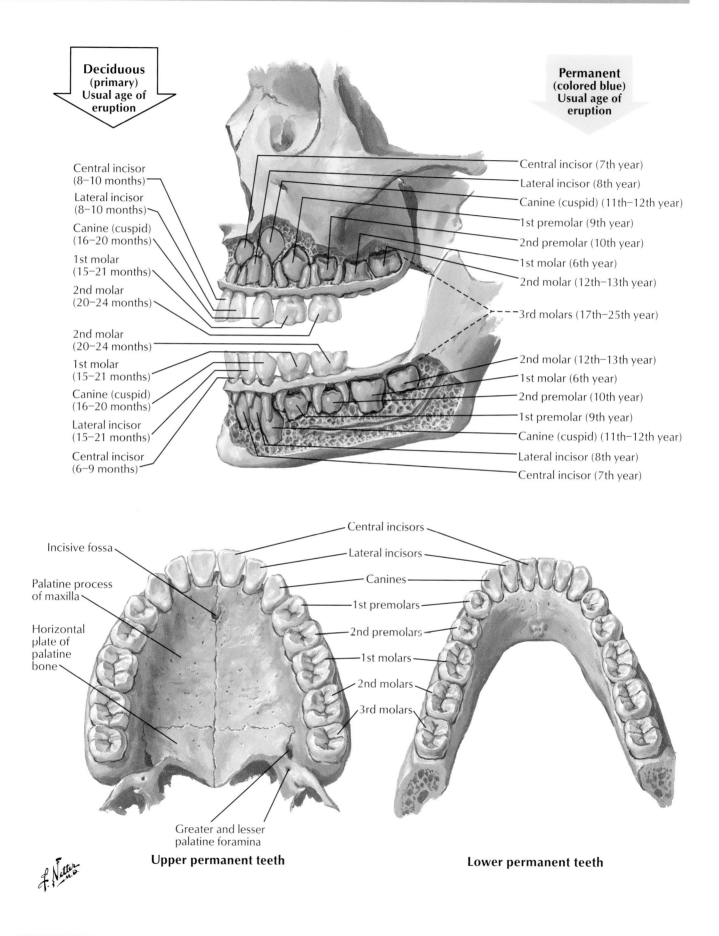

Deciduous (primary) Usual age of eruption

Central incisor (8–10 months)
Lateral incisor (8–10 months)
Canine (cuspid) (16–20 months)
1st molar (15–21 months)
2nd molar (20–24 months)

2nd molar (20–24 months)
1st molar (15–21 months)
Canine (cuspid) (16–20 months)
Lateral incisor (15–21 months)
Central incisor (6–9 months)

Permanent (colored blue) Usual age of eruption

Central incisor (7th year)
Lateral incisor (8th year)
Canine (cuspid) (11th–12th year)
1st premolar (9th year)
2nd premolar (10th year)
1st molar (6th year)
2nd molar (12th–13th year)

3rd molars (17th–25th year)

2nd molar (12th–13th year)
1st molar (6th year)
2nd premolar (10th year)
1st premolar (9th year)
Canine (cuspid) (11th–12th year)
Lateral incisor (8th year)
Central incisor (7th year)

Central incisors
Lateral incisors
Canines
1st premolars
2nd premolars
1st molars
2nd molars
3rd molars

Incisive fossa
Palatine process of maxilla
Horizontal plate of palatine bone
Greater and lesser palatine foramina

Upper permanent teeth

Lower permanent teeth

Plate 56

Oral Region

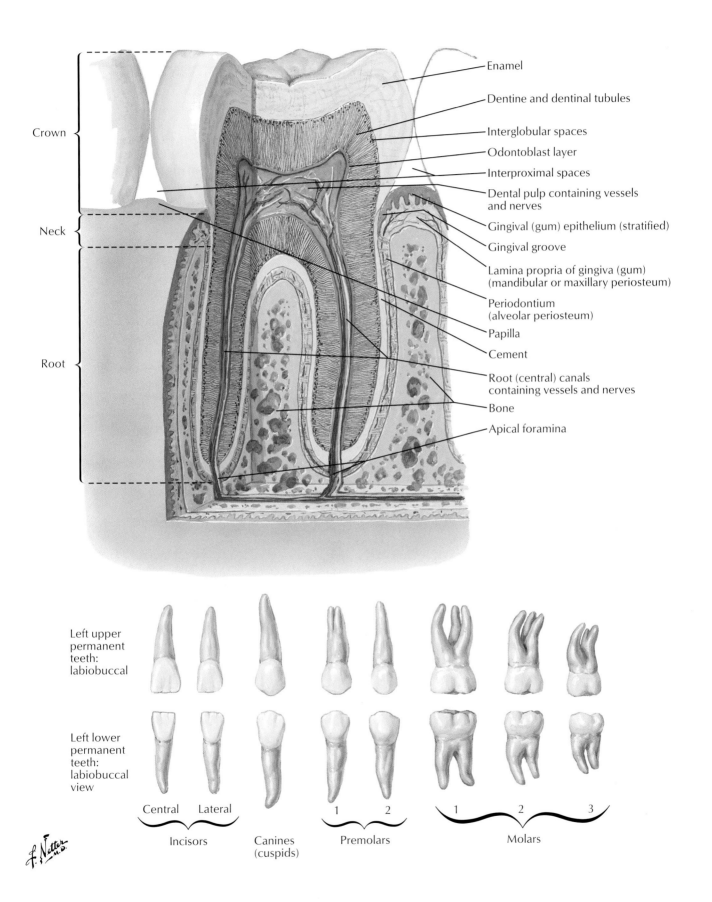

Crown

Neck

Root

Enamel

Dentine and dentinal tubules

Interglobular spaces

Odontoblast layer

Interproximal spaces

Dental pulp containing vessels and nerves

Gingival (gum) epithelium (stratified)

Gingival groove

Lamina propria of gingiva (gum) (mandibular or maxillary periosteum)

Periodontium (alveolar periosteum)

Papilla

Cement

Root (central) canals containing vessels and nerves

Bone

Apical foramina

Left upper permanent teeth: labiobuccal

Left lower permanent teeth: labiobuccal view

Central   Lateral

Incisors

Canines (cuspids)

1   2

Premolars

1   2   3

Molars

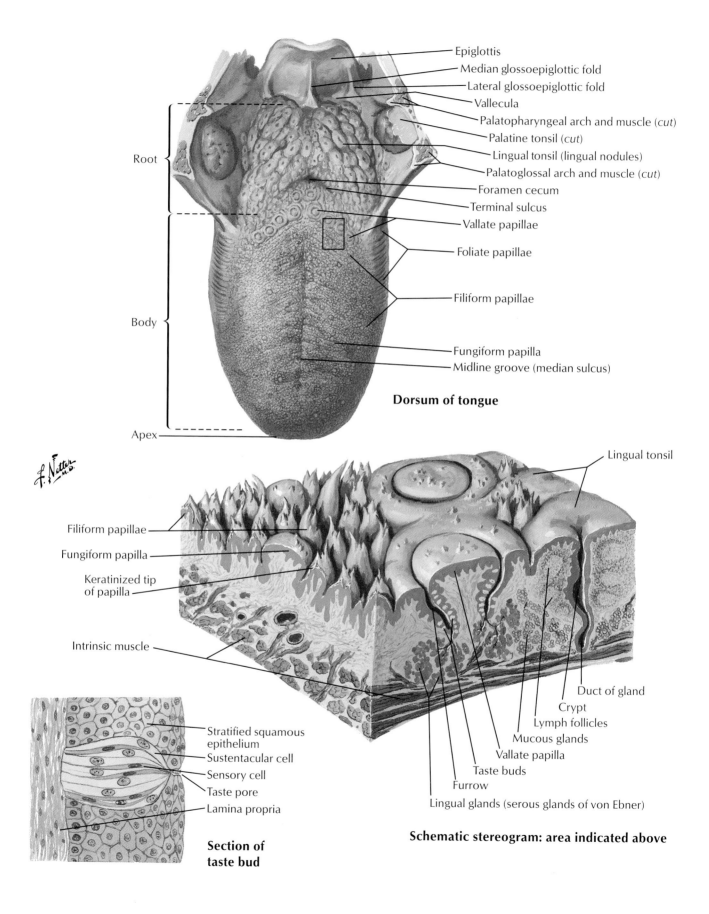

Dorsum of tongue

Epiglottis
Median glossoepiglottic fold
Lateral glossoepiglottic fold
Vallecula
Palatopharyngeal arch and muscle (*cut*)
Palatine tonsil (*cut*)
Lingual tonsil (lingual nodules)
Palatoglossal arch and muscle (*cut*)
Foramen cecum
Terminal sulcus
Vallate papillae
Foliate papillae
Filiform papillae
Fungiform papilla
Midline groove (median sulcus)

Root

Body

Apex

Lingual tonsil

Filiform papillae
Fungiform papilla
Keratinized tip of papilla
Intrinsic muscle

Duct of gland
Crypt
Lymph follicles
Mucous glands
Vallate papilla
Taste buds
Furrow
Lingual glands (serous glands of von Ebner)

Schematic stereogram: area indicated above

Stratified squamous epithelium
Sustentacular cell
Sensory cell
Taste pore
Lamina propria

Section of taste bud

Plate 58   **Oral Region**

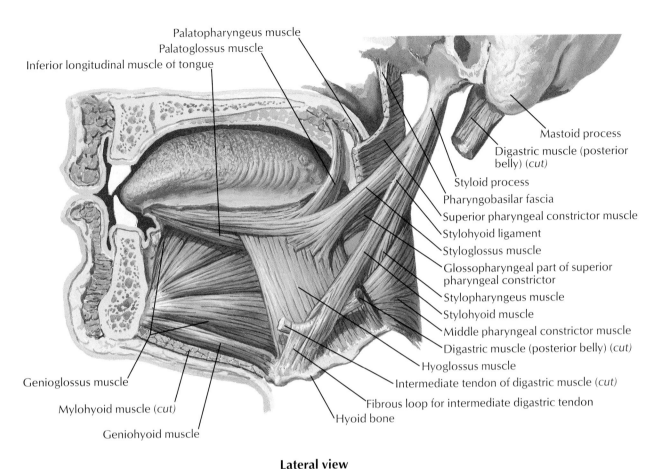

Palatopharyngeus muscle
Palatoglossus muscle
Inferior longitudinal muscle of tongue

Mastoid process
Digastric muscle (posterior belly) (*cut*)
Styloid process
Pharyngobasilar fascia
Superior pharyngeal constrictor muscle
Stylohyoid ligament
Styloglossus muscle
Glossopharyngeal part of superior pharyngeal constrictor
Stylopharyngeus muscle
Stylohyoid muscle
Middle pharyngeal constrictor muscle
Digastric muscle (posterior belly) (*cut*)
Hyoglossus muscle
Intermediate tendon of digastric muscle (*cut*)
Fibrous loop for intermediate digastric tendon

Genioglossus muscle
Mylohyoid muscle (*cut*)
Geniohyoid muscle
Hyoid bone

Lateral view

Lingual nerve
Submandibular ganglion
Deep lingual artery and venae comitantes
Artery to frenulum
Submandibular duct

Superior pharyngeal constrictor muscle
Styloglossus muscle
Palatoglossus muscle (*cut*)
Stylohyoid ligament
Stylopharyngeus muscle
Hyoglossus muscle (*cut*)
Lingual artery
External carotid artery
Internal jugular vein
Retromandibular vein
Facial vein
Common trunk for facial, retromandibular and lingual veins (common facial vein)
Lingual vein

Sublingual artery and vein
Geniohyoid muscle
Hyoid bone
Hypoglossal nerve
Dorsal lingual artery and vein
Vena comitans of hypoglossal nerve
Suprahyoid artery

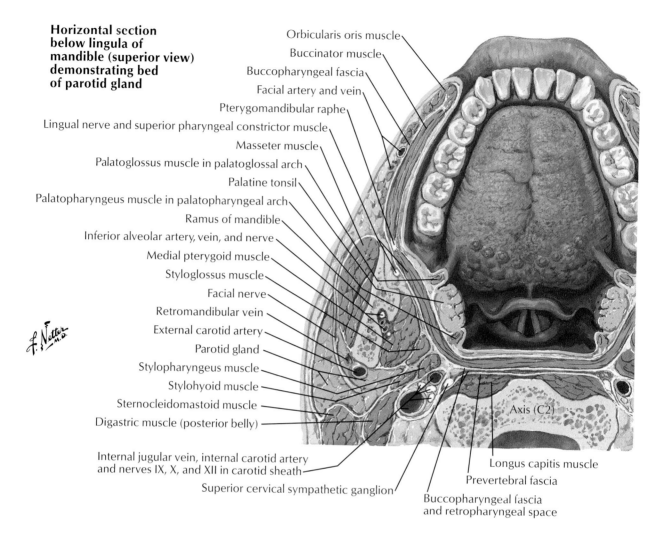

Horizontal section below lingula of mandible (superior view) demonstrating bed of parotid gland

Orbicularis oris muscle

Buccinator muscle

Buccopharyngeal fascia

Facial artery and vein

Pterygomandibular raphe

Lingual nerve and superior pharyngeal constrictor muscle

Masseter muscle

Palatoglossus muscle in palatoglossal arch

Palatine tonsil

Palatopharyngeus muscle in palatopharyngeal arch

Ramus of mandible

Inferior alveolar artery, vein, and nerve

Medial pterygoid muscle

Styloglossus muscle

Facial nerve

Retromandibular vein

External carotid artery

Parotid gland

Stylopharyngeus muscle

Stylohyoid muscle

Sternocleidomastoid muscle

Digastric muscle (posterior belly)

Internal jugular vein, internal carotid artery and nerves IX, X, and XII in carotid sheath

Superior cervical sympathetic ganglion

Axis (C2)

Longus capitis muscle

Prevertebral fascia

Buccopharyngeal fascia and retropharyngeal space

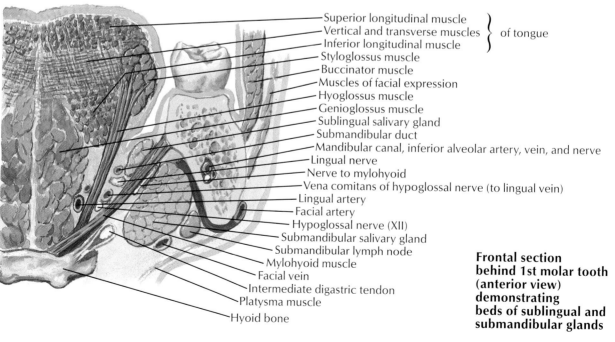

Superior longitudinal muscle

Vertical and transverse muscles ⎫ of tongue

Inferior longitudinal muscle ⎭

Styloglossus muscle

Buccinator muscle

Muscles of facial expression

Hyoglossus muscle

Genioglossus muscle

Sublingual salivary gland

Submandibular duct

Mandibular canal, inferior alveolar artery, vein, and nerve

Lingual nerve

Nerve to mylohyoid

Vena comitans of hypoglossal nerve (to lingual vein)

Lingual artery

Facial artery

Hypoglossal nerve (XII)

Submandibular salivary gland

Submandibular lymph node

Mylohyoid muscle

Facial vein

Intermediate digastric tendon

Platysma muscle

Hyoid bone

Frontal section behind 1st molar tooth (anterior view) demonstrating beds of sublingual and submandibular glands

Plate 60

Oral Region

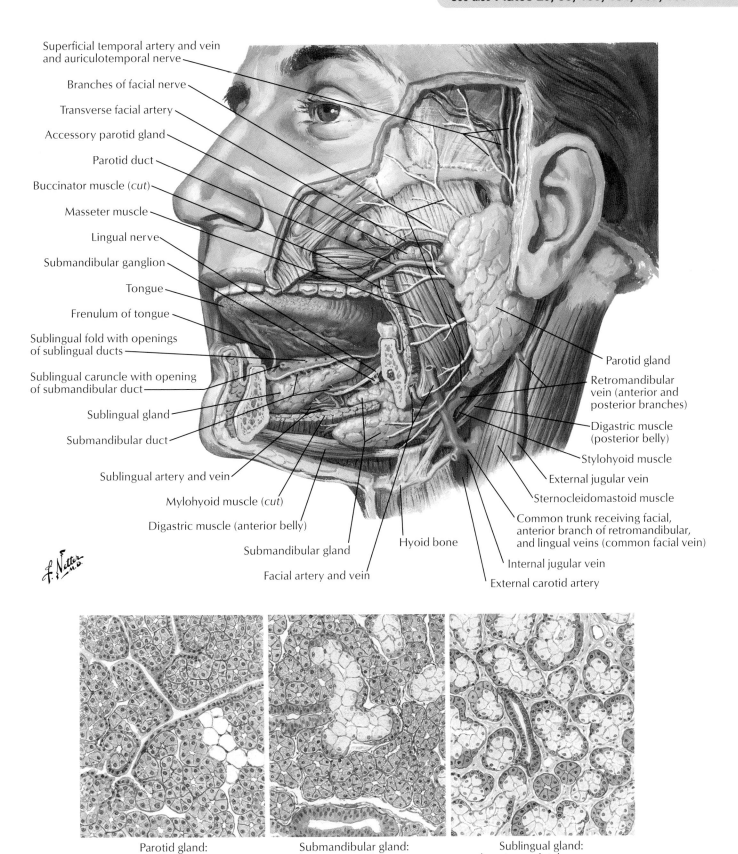

Superficial temporal artery and vein and auriculotemporal nerve

Branches of facial nerve

Transverse facial artery

Accessory parotid gland

Parotid duct

Buccinator muscle (*cut*)

Masseter muscle

Lingual nerve

Submandibular ganglion

Tongue

Frenulum of tongue

Sublingual fold with openings of sublingual ducts

Sublingual caruncle with opening of submandibular duct

Sublingual gland

Submandibular duct

Sublingual artery and vein

Mylohyoid muscle (*cut*)

Digastric muscle (anterior belly)

Submandibular gland

Facial artery and vein

Hyoid bone

Parotid gland

Retromandibular vein (anterior and posterior branches)

Digastric muscle (posterior belly)

Stylohyoid muscle

External jugular vein

Sternocleidomastoid muscle

Common trunk receiving facial, anterior branch of retromandibular, and lingual veins (common facial vein)

Internal jugular vein

External carotid artery

Parotid gland: totally serous

Submandibular gland: mostly serous, partially mucous

Sublingual gland: almost completely mucous

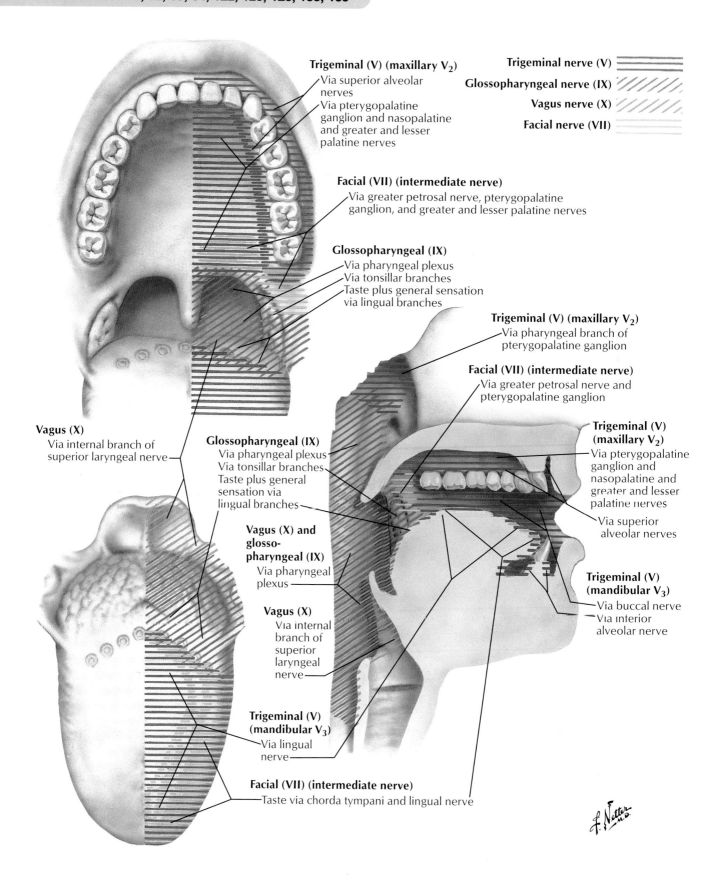

Trigeminal (V) (maxillary V$_2$)
Via superior alveolar nerves
Via pterygopalatine ganglion and nasopalatine and greater and lesser palatine nerves

Trigeminal nerve (V)
Glossopharyngeal nerve (IX)
Vagus nerve (X)
Facial nerve (VII)

Facial (VII) (intermediate nerve)
Via greater petrosal nerve, pterygopalatine ganglion, and greater and lesser palatine nerves

Glossopharyngeal (IX)
Via pharyngeal plexus
Via tonsillar branches
Taste plus general sensation via lingual branches

Trigeminal (V) (maxillary V$_2$)
Via pharyngeal branch of pterygopalatine ganglion

Facial (VII) (intermediate nerve)
Via greater petrosal nerve and pterygopalatine ganglion

Vagus (X)
Via internal branch of superior laryngeal nerve

Glossopharyngeal (IX)
Via pharyngeal plexus
Via tonsillar branches
Taste plus general sensation via lingual branches

Trigeminal (V) (maxillary V$_2$)
Via pterygopalatine ganglion and nasopalatine and greater and lesser palatine nerves
Via superior alveolar nerves

Vagus (X) and glosso-pharyngeal (IX)
Via pharyngeal plexus

Vagus (X)
Via internal branch of superior laryngeal nerve

Trigeminal (V) (mandibular V$_3$)
Via buccal nerve
Via interior alveolar nerve

Trigeminal (V) (mandibular V$_3$)
Via lingual nerve

Facial (VII) (intermediate nerve)
Taste via chorda tympani and lingual nerve

Plate 62

Oral Region

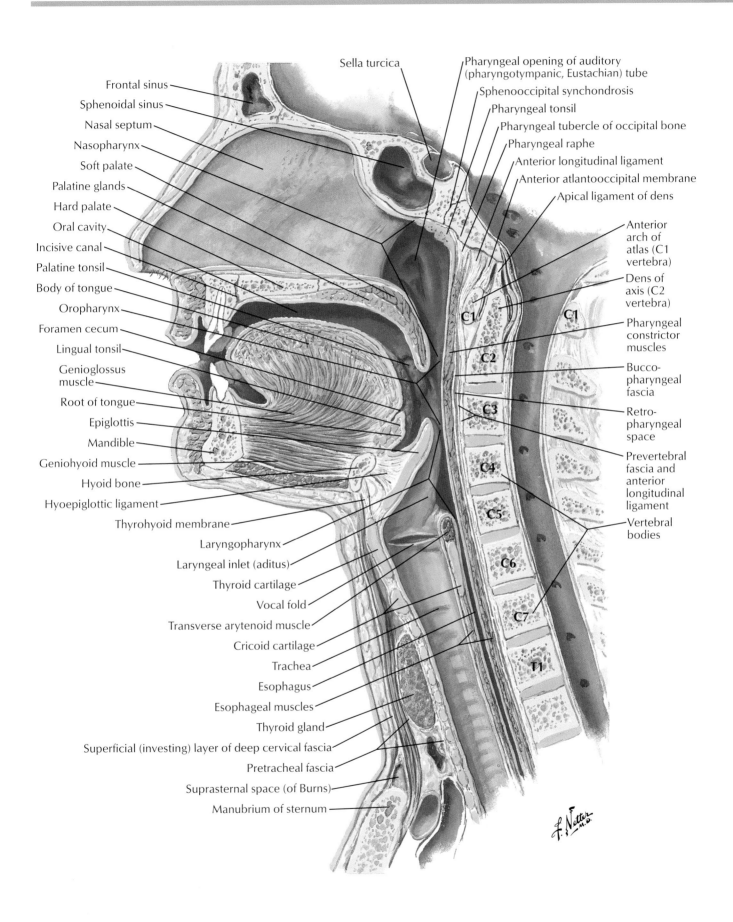

Frontal sinus
Sphenoidal sinus
Nasal septum
Nasopharynx
Soft palate
Palatine glands
Hard palate
Oral cavity
Incisive canal
Palatine tonsil
Body of tongue
Oropharynx
Foramen cecum
Lingual tonsil
Genioglossus muscle
Root of tongue
Epiglottis
Mandible
Geniohyoid muscle
Hyoid bone
Hyoepiglottic ligament
Thyrohyoid membrane
Laryngopharynx
Laryngeal inlet (aditus)
Thyroid cartilage
Vocal fold
Transverse arytenoid muscle
Cricoid cartilage
Trachea
Esophagus
Esophageal muscles
Thyroid gland
Superficial (investing) layer of deep cervical fascia
Pretracheal fascia
Suprasternal space (of Burns)
Manubrium of sternum

Sella turcica
Pharyngeal opening of auditory (pharyngotympanic, Eustachian) tube
Sphenooccipital synchondrosis
Pharyngeal tonsil
Pharyngeal tubercle of occipital bone
Pharyngeal raphe
Anterior longitudinal ligament
Anterior atlantooccipital membrane
Apical ligament of dens
Anterior arch of atlas (C1 vertebra)
Dens of axis (C2 vertebra)
Pharyngeal constrictor muscles
Bucco-pharyngeal fascia
Retro-pharyngeal space
Prevertebral fascia and anterior longitudinal ligament
Vertebral bodies

C1
C2
C3
C4
C5
C6
C7
T1

C1

Medial view
Median (sagittal) section

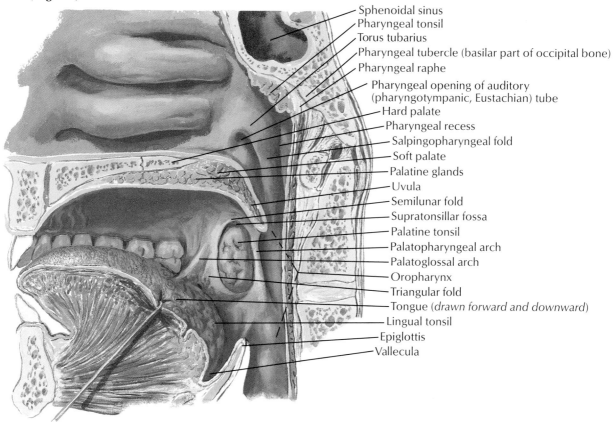

Sphenoidal sinus
Pharyngeal tonsil
Torus tubarius
Pharyngeal tubercle (basilar part of occipital bone)
Pharyngeal raphe
Pharyngeal opening of auditory (pharyngotympanic, Eustachian) tube
Hard palate
Pharyngeal recess
Salpingopharyngeal fold
Soft palate
Palatine glands
Uvula
Semilunar fold
Supratonsillar fossa
Palatine tonsil
Palatopharyngeal arch
Palatoglossal arch
Oropharynx
Triangular fold
Tongue (*drawn forward and downward*)
Lingual tonsil
Epiglottis
Vallecula

Pharyngeal mucosa removed

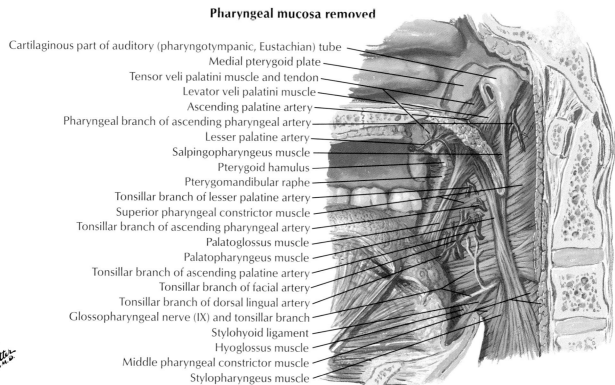

Cartilaginous part of auditory (pharyngotympanic, Eustachian) tube
Medial pterygoid plate
Tensor veli palatini muscle and tendon
Levator veli palatini muscle
Ascending palatine artery
Pharyngeal branch of ascending pharyngeal artery
Lesser palatine artery
Salpingopharyngeus muscle
Pterygoid hamulus
Pterygomandibular raphe
Tonsillar branch of lesser palatine artery
Superior pharyngeal constrictor muscle
Tonsillar branch of ascending pharyngeal artery
Palatoglossus muscle
Palatopharyngeus muscle
Tonsillar branch of ascending palatine artery
Tonsillar branch of facial artery
Tonsillar branch of dorsal lingual artery
Glossopharyngeal nerve (IX) and tonsillar branch
Stylohyoid ligament
Hyoglossus muscle
Middle pharyngeal constrictor muscle
Stylopharyngeus muscle

Plate 64   **Pharynx**

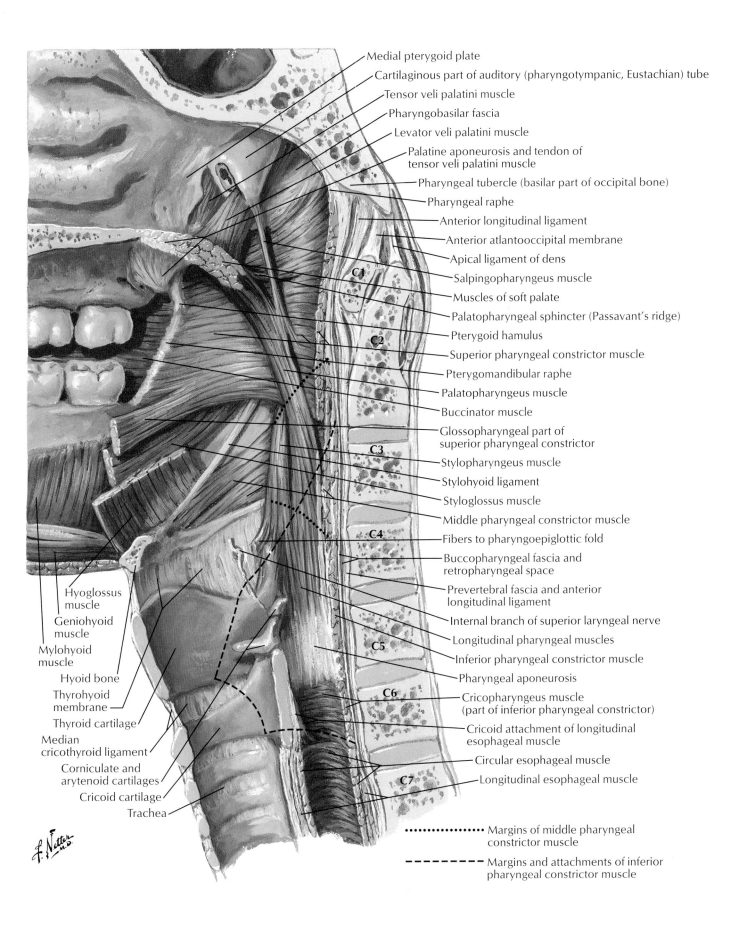

Medial pterygoid plate

Cartilaginous part of auditory (pharyngotympanic, Eustachian) tube

Tensor veli palatini muscle

Pharyngobasilar fascia

Levator veli palatini muscle

Palatine aponeurosis and tendon of tensor veli palatini muscle

Pharyngeal tubercle (basilar part of occipital bone)

Pharyngeal raphe

Anterior longitudinal ligament

Anterior atlantooccipital membrane

Apical ligament of dens

Salpingopharyngeus muscle

Muscles of soft palate

Palatopharyngeal sphincter (Passavant's ridge)

Pterygoid hamulus

Superior pharyngeal constrictor muscle

Pterygomandibular raphe

Palatopharyngeus muscle

Buccinator muscle

Glossopharyngeal part of superior pharyngeal constrictor

Stylopharyngeus muscle

Stylohyoid ligament

Styloglossus muscle

Middle pharyngeal constrictor muscle

Fibers to pharyngoepiglottic fold

Buccopharyngeal fascia and retropharyngeal space

Prevertebral fascia and anterior longitudinal ligament

Internal branch of superior laryngeal nerve

Longitudinal pharyngeal muscles

Inferior pharyngeal constrictor muscle

Pharyngeal aponeurosis

Cricopharyngeus muscle (part of inferior pharyngeal constrictor)

Cricoid attachment of longitudinal esophageal muscle

Circular esophageal muscle

Longitudinal esophageal muscle

Hyoglossus muscle

Geniohyoid muscle

Mylohyoid muscle

Hyoid bone

Thyrohyoid membrane

Thyroid cartilage

Median cricothyroid ligament

Corniculate and arytenoid cartilages

Cricoid cartilage

Trachea

C1

C2

C3

C4

C5

C6

C7

•••••••••••• Margins of middle pharyngeal constrictor muscle

– – – – – – – Margins and attachments of inferior pharyngeal constrictor muscle

f. Netter. M.D.

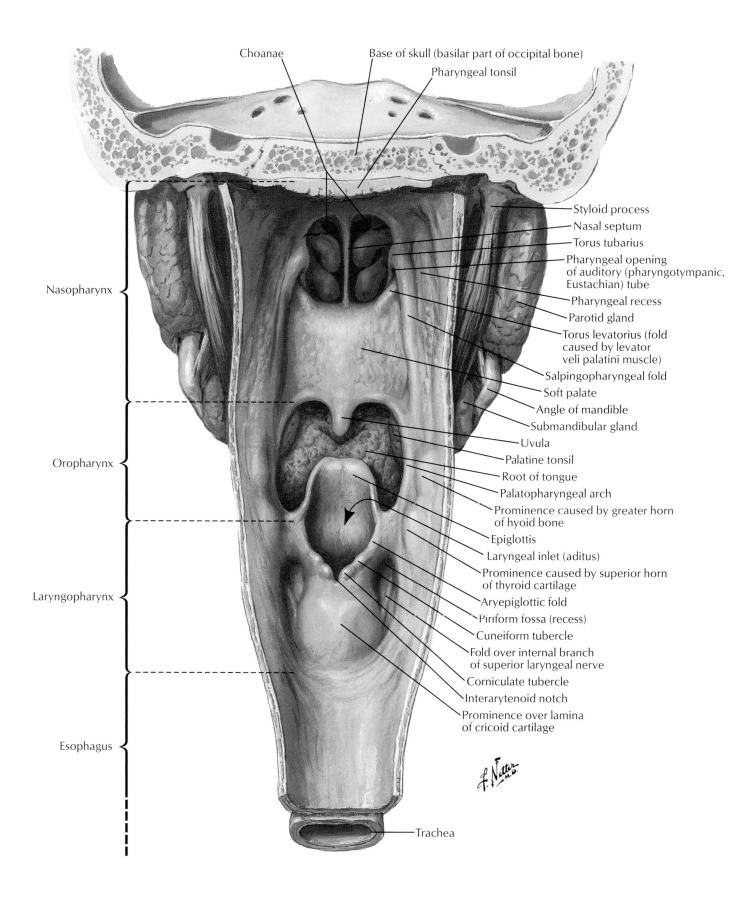

Choanae

Base of skull (basilar part of occipital bone)

Pharyngeal tonsil

Styloid process

Nasal septum

Torus tubarius

Pharyngeal opening of auditory (pharyngotympanic, Eustachian) tube

Pharyngeal recess

Parotid gland

Torus levatorius (fold caused by levator veli palatini muscle)

Salpingopharyngeal fold

Soft palate

Angle of mandible

Submandibular gland

Uvula

Palatine tonsil

Root of tongue

Palatopharyngeal arch

Prominence caused by greater horn of hyoid bone

Epiglottis

Laryngeal inlet (aditus)

Prominence caused by superior horn of thyroid cartilage

Aryepiglottic fold

Piriform fossa (recess)

Cuneiform tubercle

Fold over internal branch of superior laryngeal nerve

Corniculate tubercle

Interarytenoid notch

Prominence over lamina of cricoid cartilage

Nasopharynx

Oropharynx

Laryngopharynx

Esophagus

Trachea

Plate 66   **Pharynx**

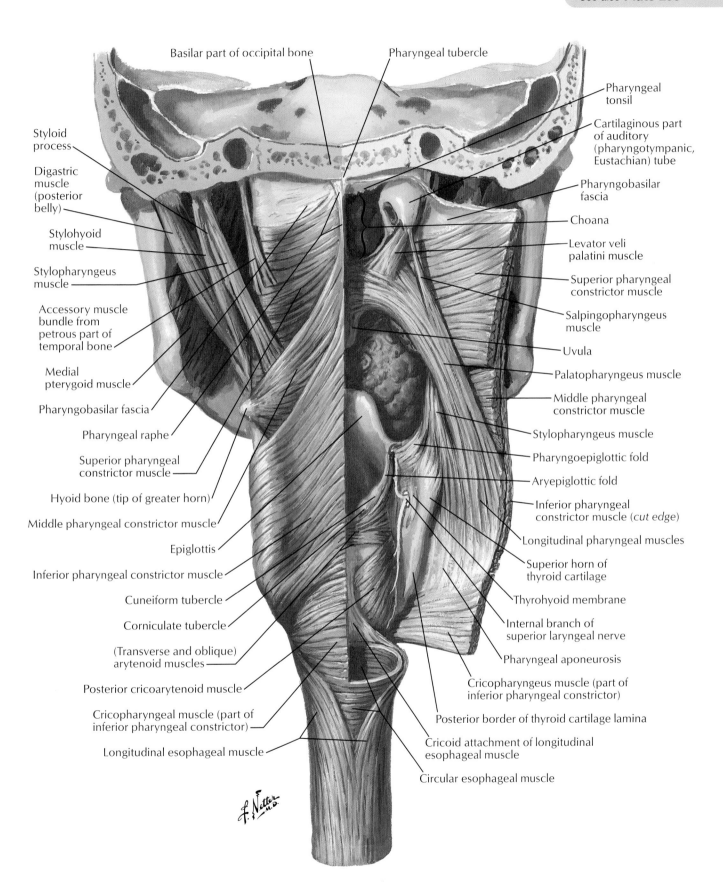

Basilar part of occipital bone

Pharyngeal tubercle

Pharyngeal tonsil

Cartilaginous part of auditory (pharyngotympanic, Eustachian) tube

Styloid process

Digastric muscle (posterior belly)

Stylohyoid muscle

Stylopharyngeus muscle

Accessory muscle bundle from petrous part of temporal bone

Medial pterygoid muscle

Pharyngobasilar fascia

Pharyngeal raphe

Superior pharyngeal constrictor muscle

Hyoid bone (tip of greater horn)

Middle pharyngeal constrictor muscle

Epiglottis

Inferior pharyngeal constrictor muscle

Cuneiform tubercle

Corniculate tubercle

(Transverse and oblique) arytenoid muscles

Posterior cricoarytenoid muscle

Cricopharyngeal muscle (part of inferior pharyngeal constrictor)

Longitudinal esophageal muscle

Pharyngobasilar fascia

Choana

Levator veli palatini muscle

Superior pharyngeal constrictor muscle

Salpingopharyngeus muscle

Uvula

Palatopharyngeus muscle

Middle pharyngeal constrictor muscle

Stylopharyngeus muscle

Pharyngoepiglottic fold

Aryepiglottic fold

Inferior pharyngeal constrictor muscle (*cut edge*)

Longitudinal pharyngeal muscles

Superior horn of thyroid cartilage

Thyrohyoid membrane

Internal branch of superior laryngeal nerve

Pharyngeal aponeurosis

Cricopharyngeus muscle (part of inferior pharyngeal constrictor)

Posterior border of thyroid cartilage lamina

Cricoid attachment of longitudinal esophageal muscle

Circular esophageal muscle

Muscles of Pharynx: Lateral View

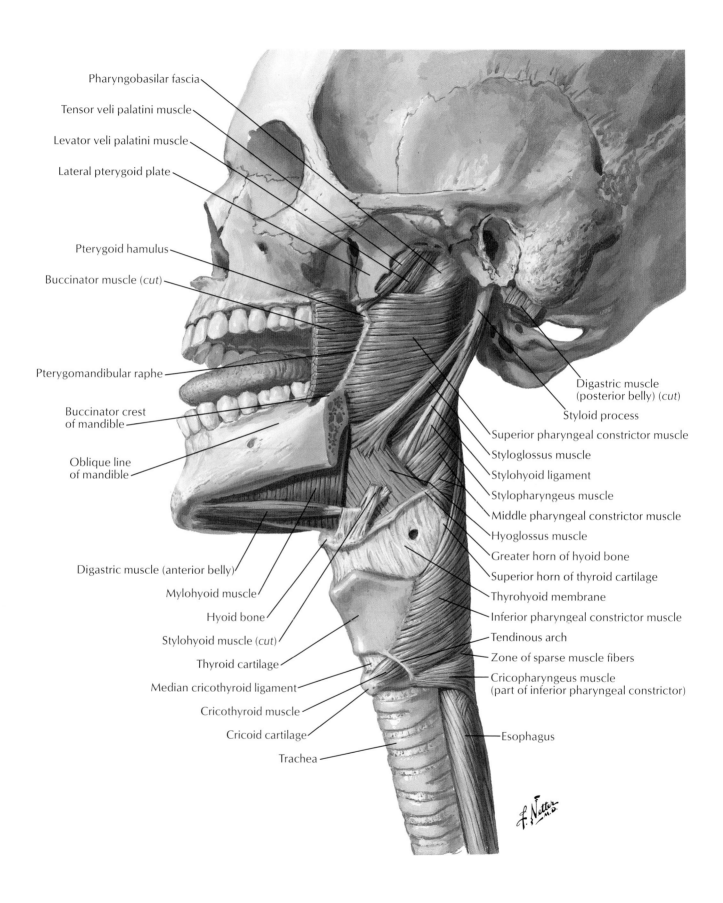

Pharyngobasilar fascia

Tensor veli palatini muscle

Levator veli palatini muscle

Lateral pterygoid plate

Pterygoid hamulus

Buccinator muscle (*cut*)

Pterygomandibular raphe

Buccinator crest of mandible

Oblique line of mandible

Digastric muscle (anterior belly)

Mylohyoid muscle

Hyoid bone

Stylohyoid muscle (*cut*)

Thyroid cartilage

Median cricothyroid ligament

Cricothyroid muscle

Cricoid cartilage

Trachea

Digastric muscle (posterior belly) (*cut*)

Styloid process

Superior pharyngeal constrictor muscle

Styloglossus muscle

Stylohyoid ligament

Stylopharyngeus muscle

Middle pharyngeal constrictor muscle

Hyoglossus muscle

Greater horn of hyoid bone

Superior horn of thyroid cartilage

Thyrohyoid membrane

Inferior pharyngeal constrictor muscle

Tendinous arch

Zone of sparse muscle fibers

Cricopharyngeus muscle (part of inferior pharyngeal constrictor)

Esophagus

Plate 68

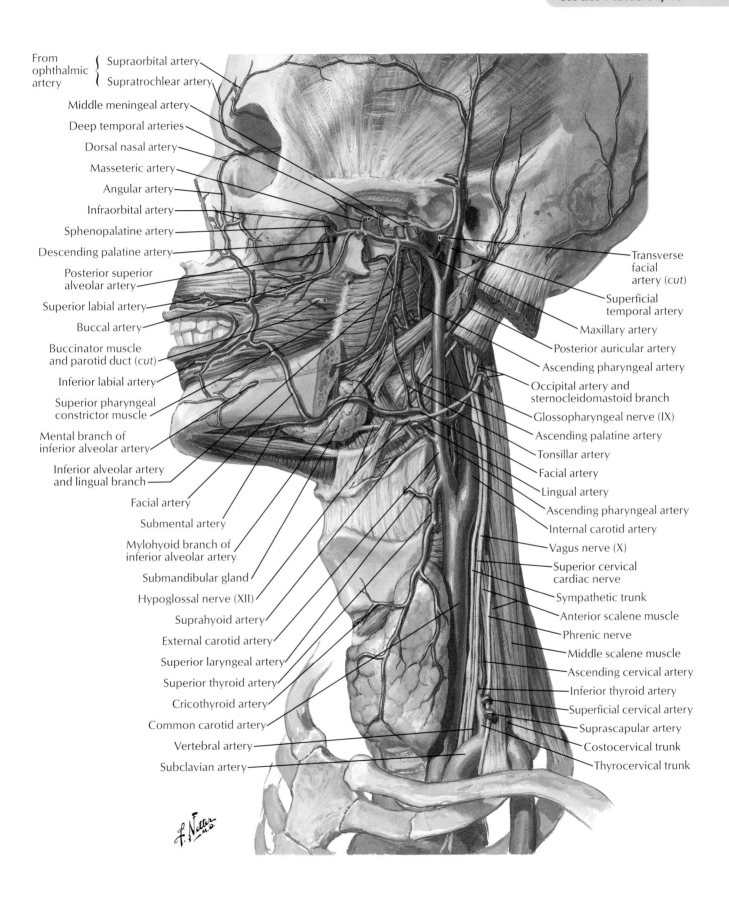

From ophthalmic artery { Supraorbital artery
Supratrochlear artery

Middle meningeal artery

Deep temporal arteries

Dorsal nasal artery

Masseteric artery

Angular artery

Infraorbital artery

Sphenopalatine artery

Descending palatine artery

Posterior superior alveolar artery

Superior labial artery

Buccal artery

Buccinator muscle and parotid duct (cut)

Inferior labial artery

Superior pharyngeal constrictor muscle

Mental branch of inferior alveolar artery

Inferior alveolar artery and lingual branch

Facial artery

Submental artery

Mylohyoid branch of inferior alveolar artery

Submandibular gland

Hypoglossal nerve (XII)

Suprahyoid artery

External carotid artery

Superior laryngeal artery

Superior thyroid artery

Cricothyroid artery

Common carotid artery

Vertebral artery

Subclavian artery

Transverse facial artery (cut)

Superficial temporal artery

Maxillary artery

Posterior auricular artery

Ascending pharyngeal artery

Occipital artery and sternocleidomastoid branch

Glossopharyngeal nerve (IX)

Ascending palatine artery

Tonsillar artery

Facial artery

Lingual artery

Ascending pharyngeal artery

Internal carotid artery

Vagus nerve (X)

Superior cervical cardiac nerve

Sympathetic trunk

Anterior scalene muscle

Phrenic nerve

Middle scalene muscle

Ascending cervical artery

Inferior thyroid artery

Superficial cervical artery

Suprascapular artery

Costocervical trunk

Thyrocervical trunk

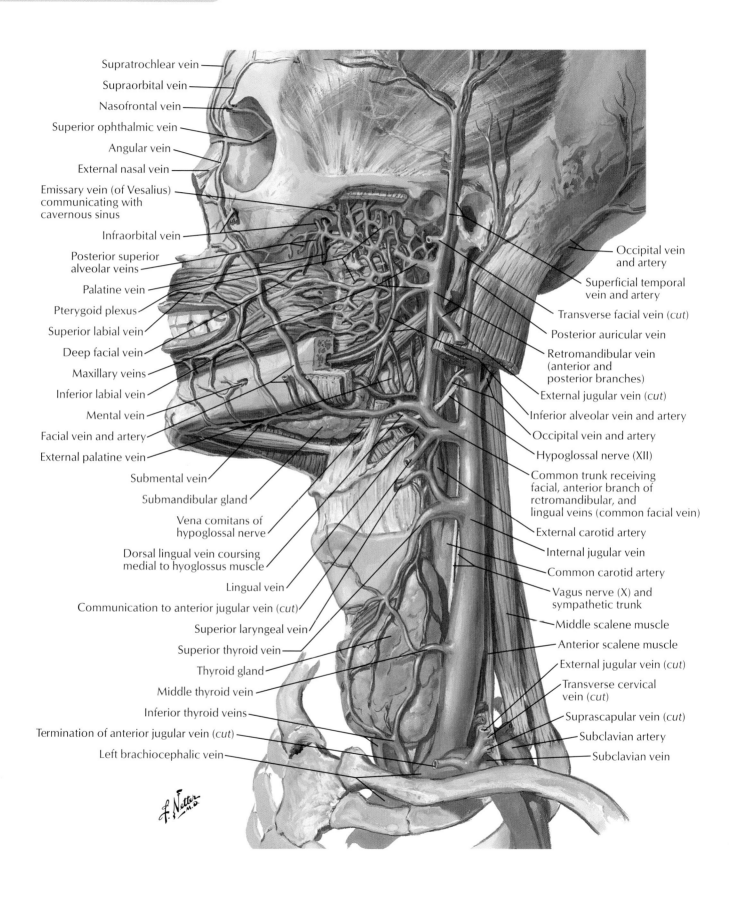

Supratrochlear vein

Supraorbital vein

Nasofrontal vein

Superior ophthalmic vein

Angular vein

External nasal vein

Emissary vein (of Vesalius) communicating with cavernous sinus

Infraorbital vein

Posterior superior alveolar veins

Palatine vein

Pterygoid plexus

Superior labial vein

Deep facial vein

Maxillary veins

Inferior labial vein

Mental vein

Facial vein and artery

External palatine vein

Submental vein

Submandibular gland

Vena comitans of hypoglossal nerve

Dorsal lingual vein coursing medial to hyoglossus muscle

Lingual vein

Communication to anterior jugular vein (cut)

Superior laryngeal vein

Superior thyroid vein

Thyroid gland

Middle thyroid vein

Inferior thyroid veins

Termination of anterior jugular vein (cut)

Left brachiocephalic vein

Occipital vein and artery

Superficial temporal vein and artery

Transverse facial vein (cut)

Posterior auricular vein

Retromandibular vein (anterior and posterior branches)

External jugular vein (cut)

Inferior alveolar vein and artery

Occipital vein and artery

Hypoglossal nerve (XII)

Common trunk receiving facial, anterior branch of retromandibular, and lingual veins (common facial vein)

External carotid artery

Internal jugular vein

Common carotid artery

Vagus nerve (X) and sympathetic trunk

Middle scalene muscle

Anterior scalene muscle

External jugular vein (cut)

Transverse cervical vein (cut)

Suprascapular vein (cut)

Subclavian artery

Subclavian vein

Plate 70

Pharynx

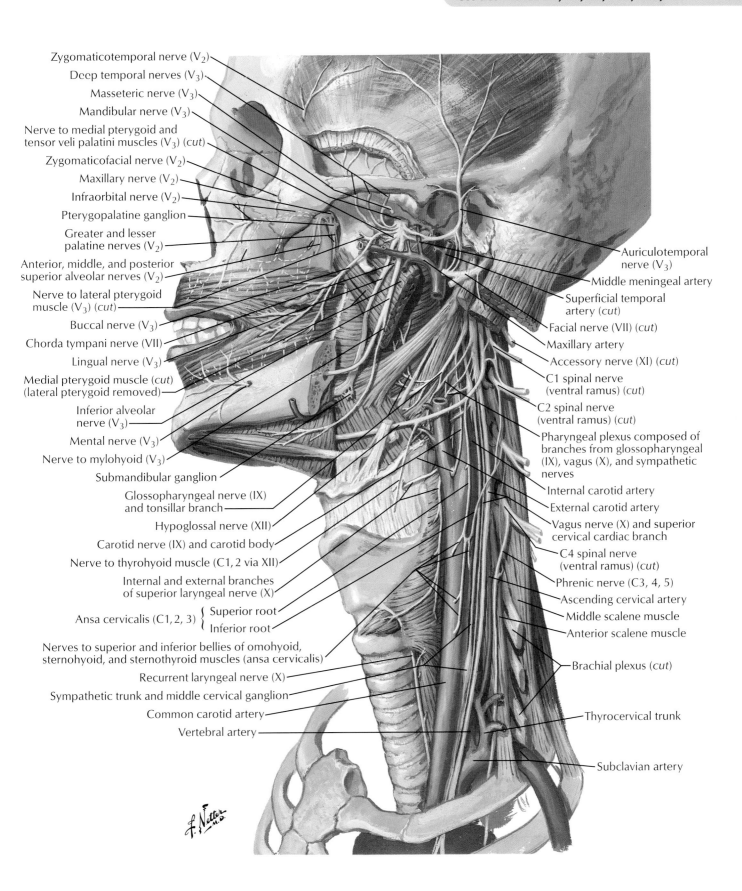

Zygomaticotemporal nerve (V₂)

Deep temporal nerves (V₃)

Masseteric nerve (V₃)

Mandibular nerve (V₃)

Nerve to medial pterygoid and tensor veli palatini muscles (V₃) (cut)

Zygomaticofacial nerve (V₂)

Maxillary nerve (V₂)

Infraorbital nerve (V₂)

Pterygopalatine ganglion

Greater and lesser palatine nerves (V₂)

Anterior, middle, and posterior superior alveolar nerves (V₂)

Nerve to lateral pterygoid muscle (V₃) (cut)

Buccal nerve (V₃)

Chorda tympani nerve (VII)

Lingual nerve (V₃)

Medial pterygoid muscle (cut) (lateral pterygoid removed)

Inferior alveolar nerve (V₃)

Mental nerve (V₃)

Nerve to mylohyoid (V₃)

Submandibular ganglion

Glossopharyngeal nerve (IX) and tonsillar branch

Hypoglossal nerve (XII)

Carotid nerve (IX) and carotid body

Nerve to thyrohyoid muscle (C1, 2 via XII)

Internal and external branches of superior laryngeal nerve (X)

Ansa cervicalis (C1, 2, 3) { Superior root / Inferior root

Nerves to superior and inferior bellies of omohyoid, sternohyoid, and sternothyroid muscles (ansa cervicalis)

Recurrent laryngeal nerve (X)

Sympathetic trunk and middle cervical ganglion

Common carotid artery

Vertebral artery

Auriculotemporal nerve (V₃)

Middle meningeal artery

Superficial temporal artery (cut)

Facial nerve (VII) (cut)

Maxillary artery

Accessory nerve (XI) (cut)

C1 spinal nerve (ventral ramus) (cut)

C2 spinal nerve (ventral ramus) (cut)

Pharyngeal plexus composed of branches from glossopharyngeal (IX), vagus (X), and sympathetic nerves

Internal carotid artery

External carotid artery

Vagus nerve (X) and superior cervical cardiac branch

C4 spinal nerve (ventral ramus) (cut)

Phrenic nerve (C3, 4, 5)

Ascending cervical artery

Middle scalene muscle

Anterior scalene muscle

Brachial plexus (cut)

Thyrocervical trunk

Subclavian artery

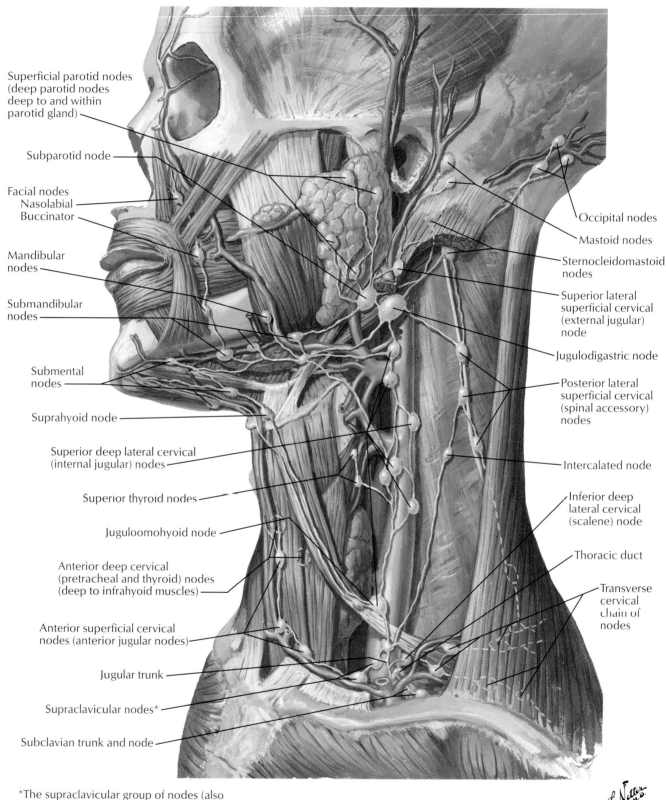

Superficial parotid nodes
(deep parotid nodes
deep to and within
parotid gland)

Subparotid node

Facial nodes
Nasolabial
Buccinator

Mandibular
nodes

Submandibular
nodes

Submental
nodes

Suprahyoid node

Superior deep lateral cervical
(internal jugular) nodes

Superior thyroid nodes

Juguloomohyoid node

Anterior deep cervical
(pretracheal and thyroid) nodes
(deep to infrahyoid muscles)

Anterior superficial cervical
nodes (anterior jugular nodes)

Jugular trunk

Supraclavicular nodes*

Subclavian trunk and node

Occipital nodes

Mastoid nodes

Sternocleidomastoid
nodes

Superior lateral
superficial cervical
(external jugular)
node

Jugulodigastric node

Posterior lateral
superficial cervical
(spinal accessory)
nodes

Intercalated node

Inferior deep
lateral cervical
(scalene) node

Thoracic duct

Transverse
cervical
chain of
nodes

*The supraclavicular group of nodes (also
known as the lower deep cervical group),
especially on the left, are also sometimes
referred to as the signal or sentinel lymph
nodes of Virchow or Troisier, especially when
sufficiently enlarged and palpable. These
nodes (or a single node) are so termed because
they may be the first recognized presumptive
evidence of malignant disease in the viscera.

Plate 72

Pharynx

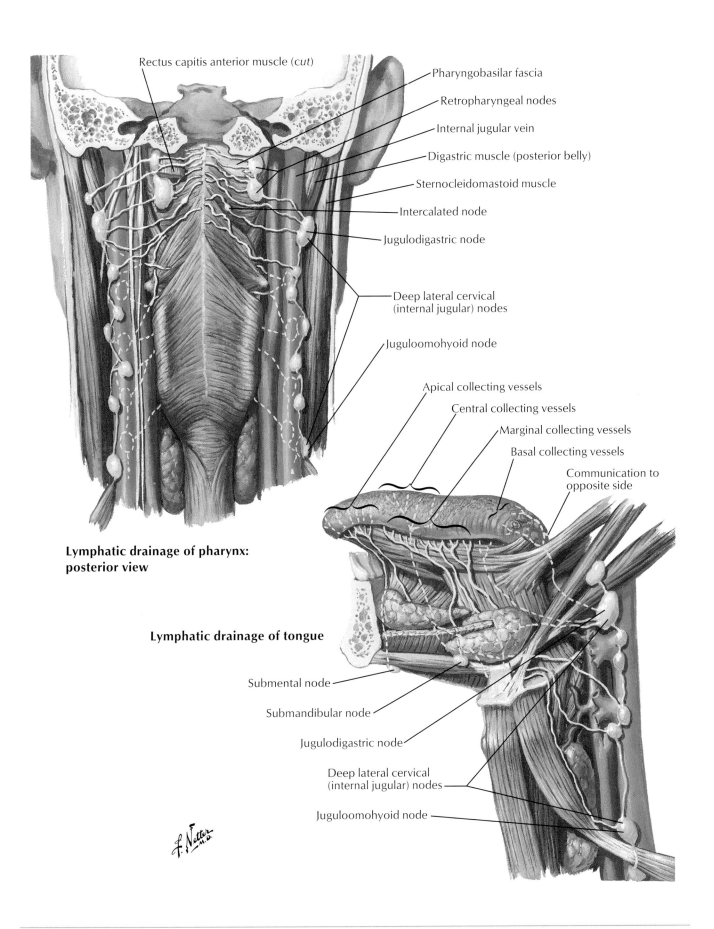

Rectus capitis anterior muscle (*cut*)

Pharyngobasilar fascia

Retropharyngeal nodes

Internal jugular vein

Digastric muscle (posterior belly)

Sternocleidomastoid muscle

Intercalated node

Jugulodigastric node

Deep lateral cervical (internal jugular) nodes

Juguloomohyoid node

Apical collecting vessels

Central collecting vessels

Marginal collecting vessels

Basal collecting vessels

Communication to opposite side

Lymphatic drainage of pharynx: posterior view

Lymphatic drainage of tongue

Submental node

Submandibular node

Jugulodigastric node

Deep lateral cervical (internal jugular) nodes

Juguloomohyoid node

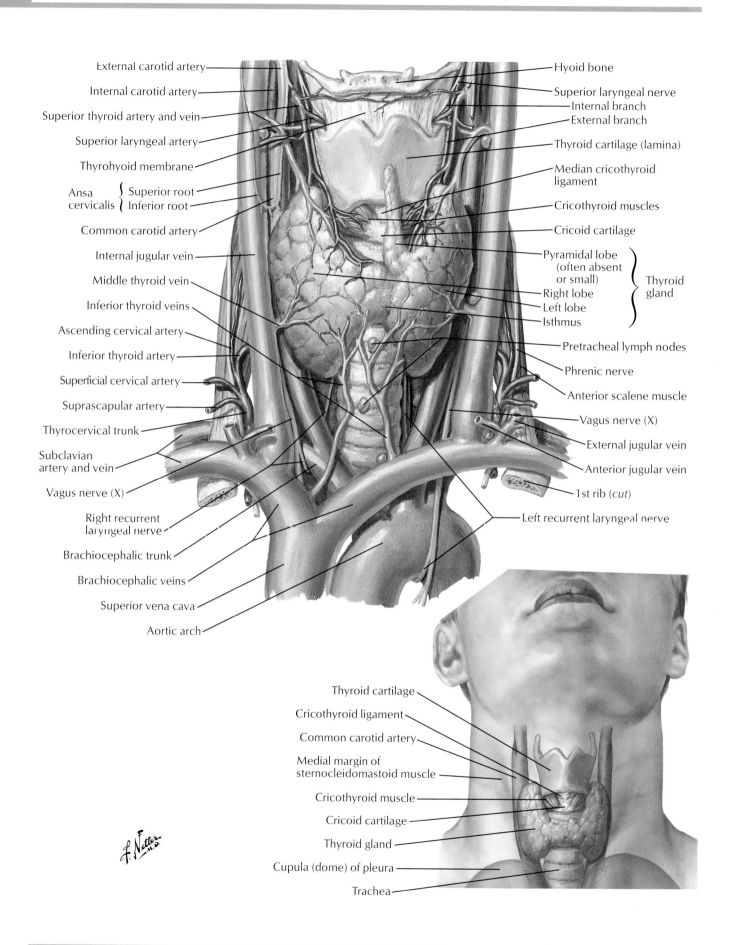

External carotid artery

Internal carotid artery

Superior thyroid artery and vein

Superior laryngeal artery

Thyrohyoid membrane

Ansa cervicalis { Superior root / Inferior root

Common carotid artery

Internal jugular vein

Middle thyroid vein

Inferior thyroid veins

Ascending cervical artery

Inferior thyroid artery

Superficial cervical artery

Suprascapular artery

Thyrocervical trunk

Subclavian artery and vein

Vagus nerve (X)

Right recurrent laryngeal nerve

Brachiocephalic trunk

Brachiocephalic veins

Superior vena cava

Aortic arch

Hyoid bone

Superior laryngeal nerve
Internal branch
External branch

Thyroid cartilage (lamina)

Median cricothyroid ligament

Cricothyroid muscles

Cricoid cartilage

Pyramidal lobe (often absent or small)
Right lobe   } Thyroid gland
Left lobe
Isthmus

Pretracheal lymph nodes

Phrenic nerve

Anterior scalene muscle

Vagus nerve (X)

External jugular vein

Anterior jugular vein

1st rib (cut)

Left recurrent laryngeal nerve

Thyroid cartilage

Cricothyroid ligament

Common carotid artery

Medial margin of sternocleidomastoid muscle

Cricothyroid muscle

Cricoid cartilage

Thyroid gland

Cupula (dome) of pleura

Trachea

Plate 74

Thyroid Gland and Larynx

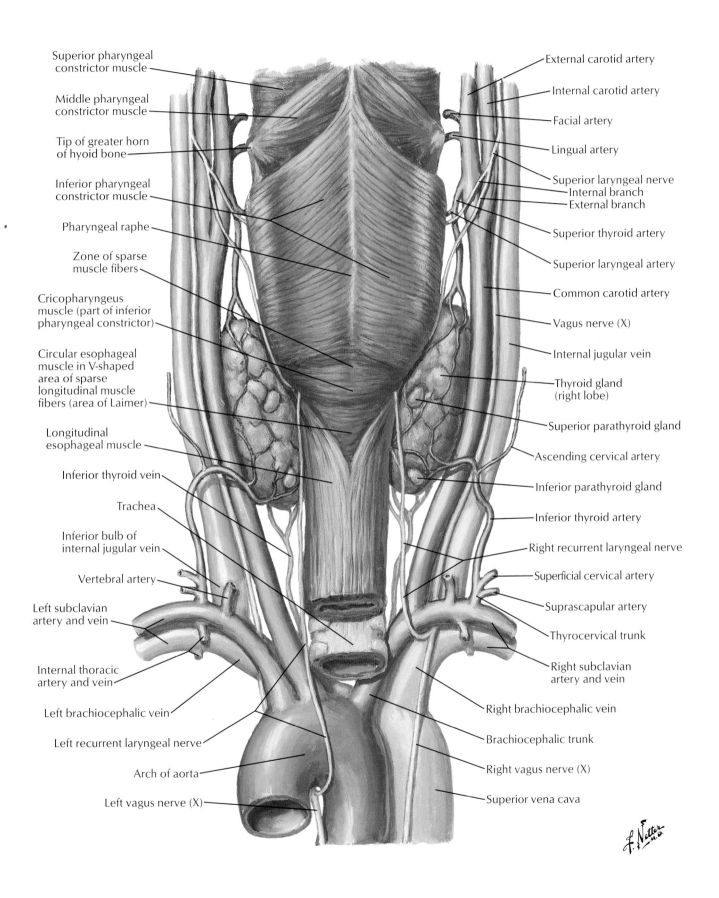

Superior pharyngeal constrictor muscle

Middle pharyngeal constrictor muscle

Tip of greater horn of hyoid bone

Inferior pharyngeal constrictor muscle

Pharyngeal raphe

Zone of sparse muscle fibers

Cricopharyngeus muscle (part of inferior pharyngeal constrictor)

Circular esophageal muscle in V-shaped area of sparse longitudinal muscle fibers (area of Laimer)

Longitudinal esophageal muscle

Inferior thyroid vein

Trachea

Inferior bulb of internal jugular vein

Vertebral artery

Left subclavian artery and vein

Internal thoracic artery and vein

Left brachiocephalic vein

Left recurrent laryngeal nerve

Arch of aorta

Left vagus nerve (X)

External carotid artery

Internal carotid artery

Facial artery

Lingual artery

Superior laryngeal nerve
Internal branch
External branch

Superior thyroid artery

Superior laryngeal artery

Common carotid artery

Vagus nerve (X)

Internal jugular vein

Thyroid gland (right lobe)

Superior parathyroid gland

Ascending cervical artery

Inferior parathyroid gland

Inferior thyroid artery

Right recurrent laryngeal nerve

Superficial cervical artery

Suprascapular artery

Thyrocervical trunk

Right subclavian artery and vein

Right brachiocephalic vein

Brachiocephalic trunk

Right vagus nerve (X)

Superior vena cava

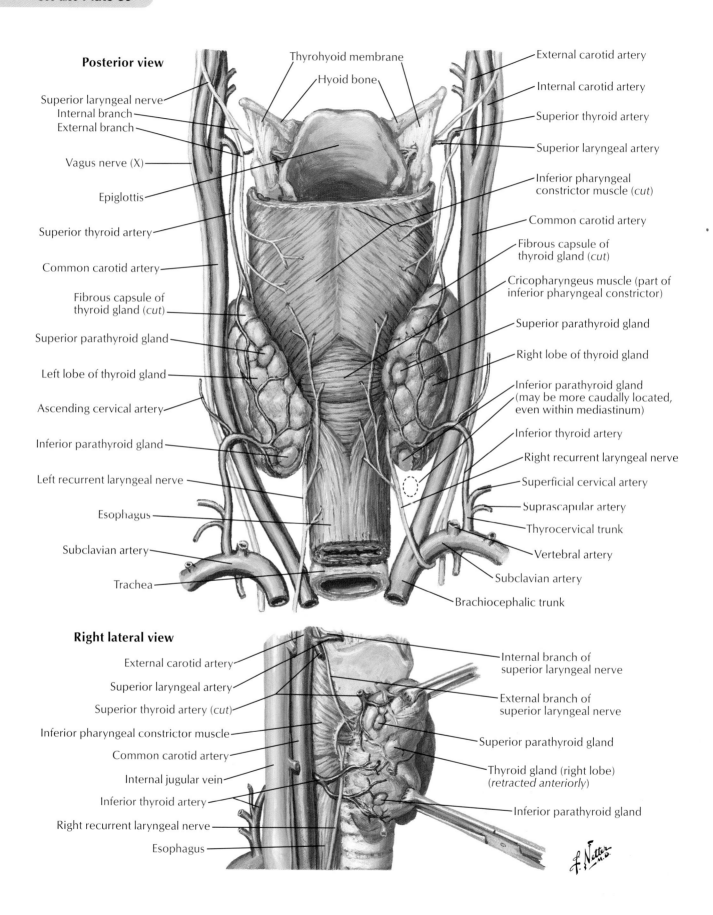

Posterior view

Superior laryngeal nerve
Internal branch
External branch

Vagus nerve (X)

Epiglottis

Superior thyroid artery

Common carotid artery

Fibrous capsule of
thyroid gland (*cut*)

Superior parathyroid gland

Left lobe of thyroid gland

Ascending cervical artery

Inferior parathyroid gland

Left recurrent laryngeal nerve

Esophagus

Subclavian artery

Trachea

Thyrohyoid membrane

Hyoid bone

External carotid artery

Internal carotid artery

Superior thyroid artery

Superior laryngeal artery

Inferior pharyngeal
constrictor muscle (*cut*)

Common carotid artery

Fibrous capsule of
thyroid gland (*cut*)

Cricopharyngeus muscle (part of
inferior pharyngeal constrictor)

Superior parathyroid gland

Right lobe of thyroid gland

Inferior parathyroid gland
(may be more caudally located,
even within mediastinum)

Inferior thyroid artery

Right recurrent laryngeal nerve

Superficial cervical artery

Suprascapular artery

Thyrocervical trunk

Vertebral artery

Subclavian artery

Brachiocephalic trunk

Right lateral view

External carotid artery

Superior laryngeal artery

Superior thyroid artery (*cut*)

Inferior pharyngeal constrictor muscle

Common carotid artery

Internal jugular vein

Inferior thyroid artery

Right recurrent laryngeal nerve

Esophagus

Internal branch of
superior laryngeal nerve

External branch of
superior laryngeal nerve

Superior parathyroid gland

Thyroid gland (right lobe)
(*retracted anteriorly*)

Inferior parathyroid gland

Plate 76

Thyroid Gland and Larynx

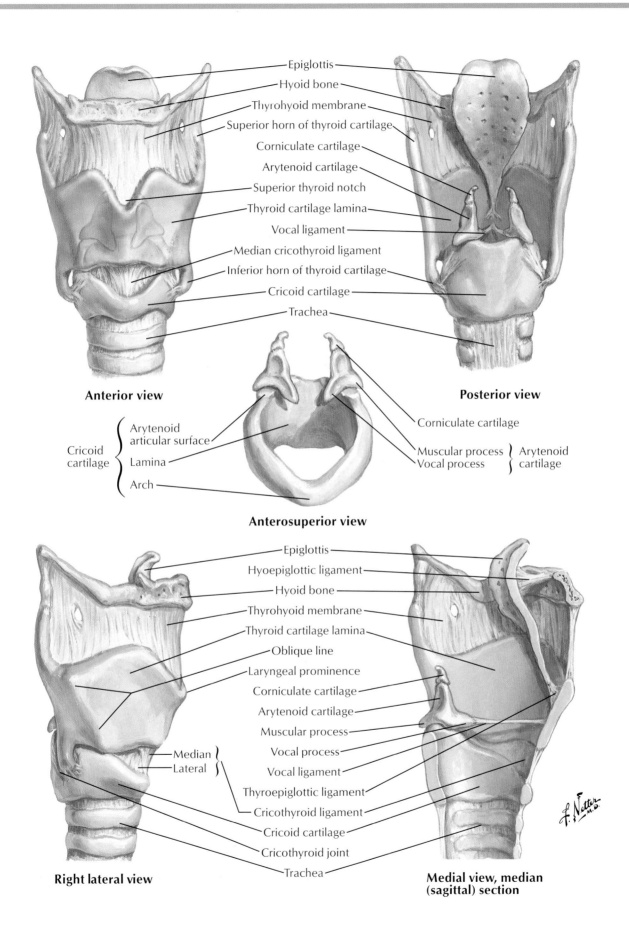

Epiglottis
Hyoid bone
Thyrohyoid membrane
Superior horn of thyroid cartilage
Corniculate cartilage
Arytenoid cartilage
Superior thyroid notch
Thyroid cartilage lamina
Vocal ligament
Median cricothyroid ligament
Inferior horn of thyroid cartilage
Cricoid cartilage
Trachea

Anterior view

Posterior view

Cricoid cartilage { Arytenoid articular surface / Lamina / Arch

Corniculate cartilage

Muscular process } Arytenoid
Vocal process } cartilage

Anterosuperior view

Epiglottis
Hyoepiglottic ligament
Hyoid bone
Thyrohyoid membrane
Thyroid cartilage lamina
Oblique line
Laryngeal prominence
Corniculate cartilage
Arytenoid cartilage
Muscular process
Vocal process
Median }
Lateral }
Vocal ligament
Thyroepiglottic ligament
Cricothyroid ligament
Cricoid cartilage
Cricothyroid joint
Trachea

Right lateral view

Medial view, median (sagittal) section

1

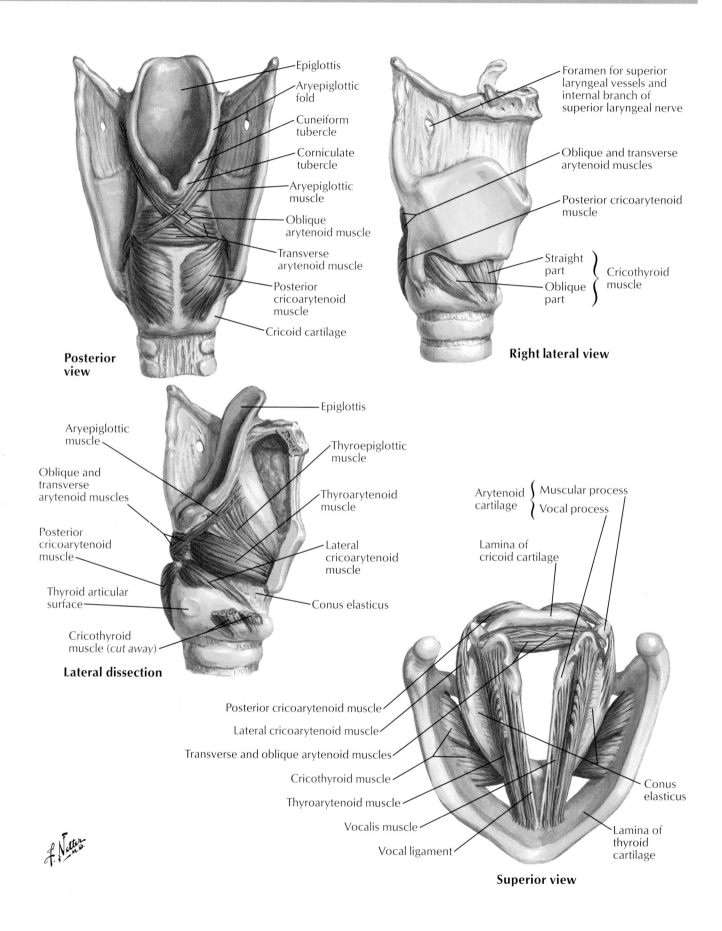

Epiglottis

Aryepiglottic fold

Cuneiform tubercle

Corniculate tubercle

Aryepiglottic muscle

Oblique arytenoid muscle

Transverse arytenoid muscle

Posterior cricoarytenoid muscle

Cricoid cartilage

Posterior view

Foramen for superior laryngeal vessels and internal branch of superior laryngeal nerve

Oblique and transverse arytenoid muscles

Posterior cricoarytenoid muscle

Straight part

Oblique part

Cricothyroid muscle

Right lateral view

Aryepiglottic muscle

Oblique and transverse arytenoid muscles

Posterior cricoarytenoid muscle

Thyroid articular surface

Cricothyroid muscle (*cut away*)

Lateral dissection

Epiglottis

Thyroepiglottic muscle

Thyroarytenoid muscle

Lateral cricoarytenoid muscle

Conus elasticus

Arytenoid cartilage

Muscular process

Vocal process

Lamina of cricoid cartilage

Posterior cricoarytenoid muscle

Lateral cricoarytenoid muscle

Transverse and oblique arytenoid muscles

Cricothyroid muscle

Thyroarytenoid muscle

Vocalis muscle

Vocal ligament

Conus elasticus

Lamina of thyroid cartilage

Superior view

Plate 78

Thyroid Gland and Larynx

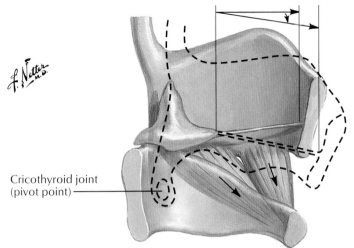

Cricothyroid joint
(pivot point)

Action of cricothyroid muscles

Lengthening (increasing tension)
of vocal ligaments

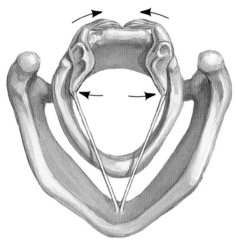

Action of posterior cricoarytenoid muscles

Abduction of vocal ligaments

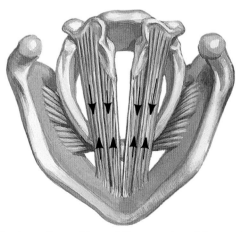

Action of lateral cricoarytenoid muscles

Adduction of vocal ligaments

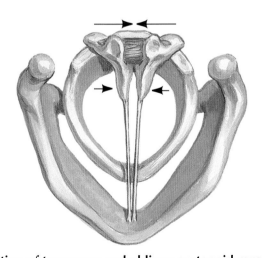

Action of transverse and oblique arytenoid muscles

Adduction of vocal ligaments

Action of vocalis and thyroarytenoid muscles

Shortening (relaxation) of vocal ligaments

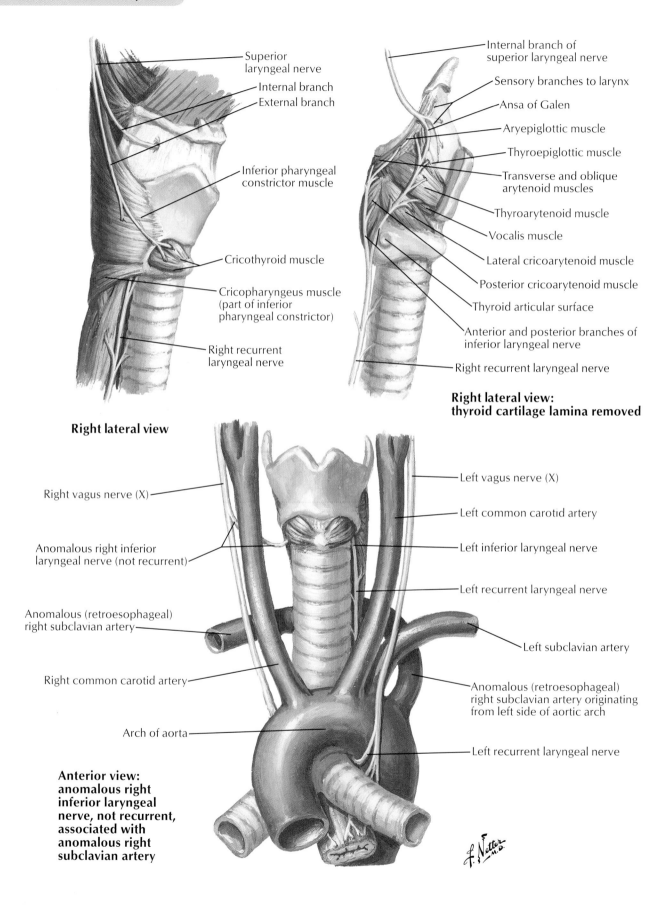

Superior
laryngeal nerve

Internal branch
External branch

Inferior pharyngeal
constrictor muscle

Cricothyroid muscle

Cricopharyngeus muscle
(part of inferior
pharyngeal constrictor)

Right recurrent
laryngeal nerve

Right lateral view

Internal branch of
superior laryngeal nerve

Sensory branches to larynx

Ansa of Galen

Aryepiglottic muscle

Thyroepiglottic muscle

Transverse and oblique
arytenoid muscles

Thyroarytenoid muscle

Vocalis muscle

Lateral cricoarytenoid muscle

Posterior cricoarytenoid muscle

Thyroid articular surface

Anterior and posterior branches of
inferior laryngeal nerve

Right recurrent laryngeal nerve

**Right lateral view:
thyroid cartilage lamina removed**

Right vagus nerve (X)

Anomalous right inferior
laryngeal nerve (not recurrent)

Anomalous (retroesophageal)
right subclavian artery

Right common carotid artery

Arch of aorta

**Anterior view:
anomalous right
inferior laryngeal
nerve, not recurrent,
associated with
anomalous right
subclavian artery**

Left vagus nerve (X)

Left common carotid artery

Left inferior laryngeal nerve

Left recurrent laryngeal nerve

Left subclavian artery

Anomalous (retroesophageal)
right subclavian artery originating
from left side of aortic arch

Left recurrent laryngeal nerve

Plate 80

Thyroid Gland and Larynx

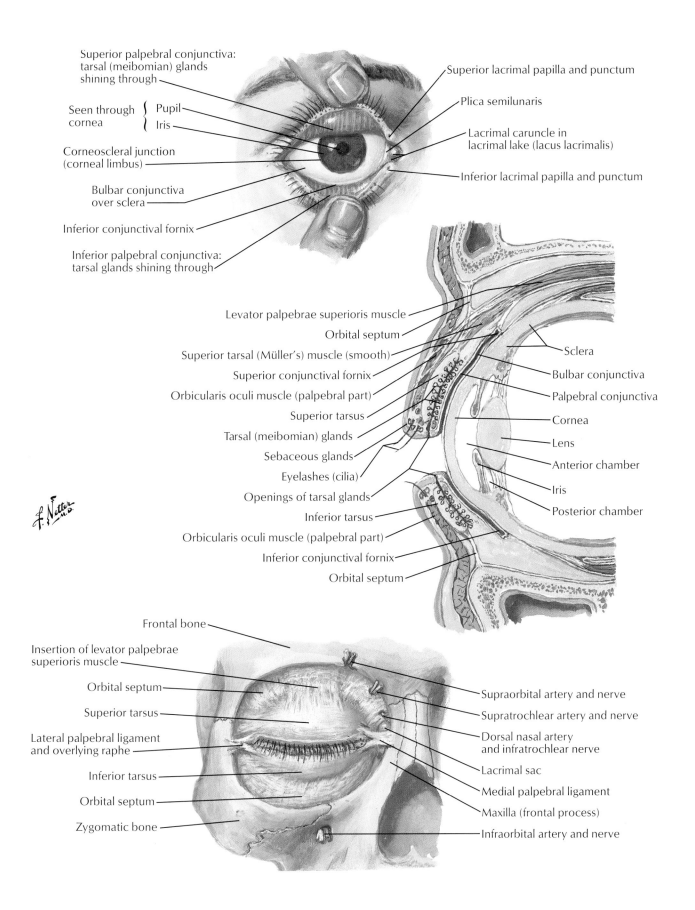

Superior palpebral conjunctiva: tarsal (meibomian) glands shining through

Seen through { Pupil
cornea { Iris

Corneoscleral junction (corneal limbus)

Bulbar conjunctiva over sclera

Inferior conjunctival fornix

Inferior palpebral conjunctiva: tarsal glands shining through

Superior lacrimal papilla and punctum

Plica semilunaris

Lacrimal caruncle in lacrimal lake (lacus lacrimalis)

Inferior lacrimal papilla and punctum

Levator palpebrae superioris muscle

Orbital septum

Superior tarsal (Müller's) muscle (smooth)

Superior conjunctival fornix

Orbicularis oculi muscle (palpebral part)

Superior tarsus

Tarsal (meibomian) glands

Sebaceous glands

Eyelashes (cilia)

Openings of tarsal glands

Inferior tarsus

Orbicularis oculi muscle (palpebral part)

Inferior conjunctival fornix

Orbital septum

Sclera

Bulbar conjunctiva

Palpebral conjunctiva

Cornea

Lens

Anterior chamber

Iris

Posterior chamber

Frontal bone

Insertion of levator palpebrae superioris muscle

Orbital septum

Superior tarsus

Lateral palpebral ligament and overlying raphe

Inferior tarsus

Orbital septum

Zygomatic bone

Supraorbital artery and nerve

Supratrochlear artery and nerve

Dorsal nasal artery and infratrochlear nerve

Lacrimal sac

Medial palpebral ligament

Maxilla (frontal process)

Infraorbital artery and nerve

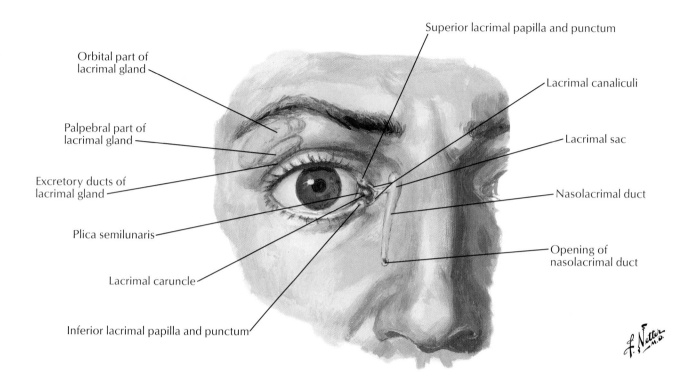

Orbital part of lacrimal gland

Palpebral part of lacrimal gland

Excretory ducts of lacrimal gland

Plica semilunaris

Lacrimal caruncle

Inferior lacrimal papilla and punctum

Superior lacrimal papilla and punctum

Lacrimal canaliculi

Lacrimal sac

Nasolacrimal duct

Opening of nasolacrimal duct

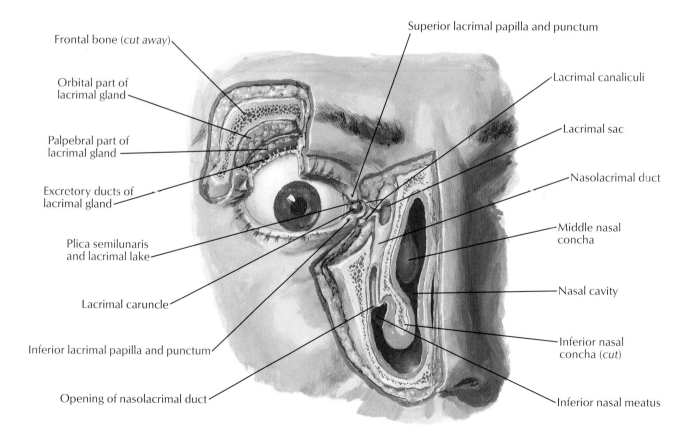

Frontal bone (*cut away*)

Orbital part of lacrimal gland

Palpebral part of lacrimal gland

Excretory ducts of lacrimal gland

Plica semilunaris and lacrimal lake

Lacrimal caruncle

Inferior lacrimal papilla and punctum

Opening of nasolacrimal duct

Superior lacrimal papilla and punctum

Lacrimal canaliculi

Lacrimal sac

Nasolacrimal duct

Middle nasal concha

Nasal cavity

Inferior nasal concha (*cut*)

Inferior nasal meatus

Plate 82

Orbit and Contents

Horizontal section

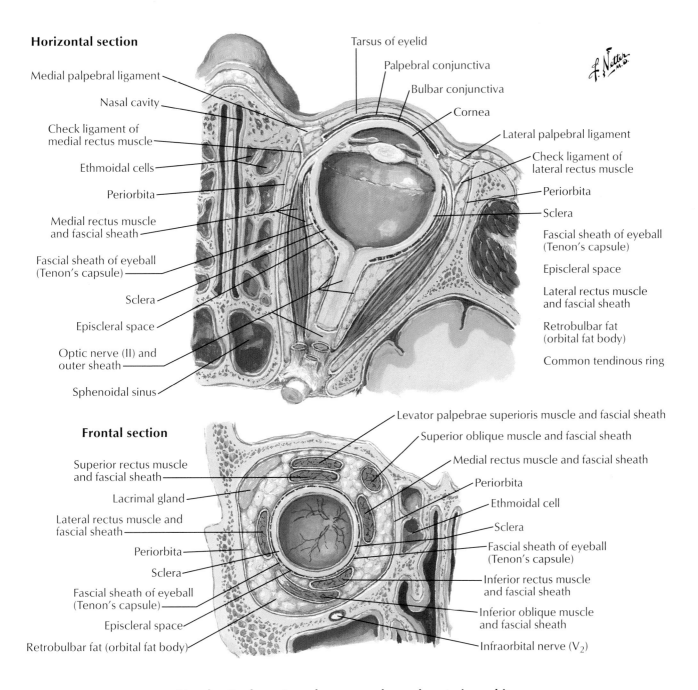

Tarsus of eyelid
Palpebral conjunctiva
Bulbar conjunctiva
Cornea
Lateral palpebral ligament
Check ligament of lateral rectus muscle
Periorbita
Sclera
Fascial sheath of eyeball (Tenon's capsule)
Episcleral space
Lateral rectus muscle and fascial sheath
Retrobulbar fat (orbital fat body)
Common tendinous ring

Medial palpebral ligament
Nasal cavity
Check ligament of medial rectus muscle
Ethmoidal cells
Periorbita
Medial rectus muscle and fascial sheath
Fascial sheath of eyeball (Tenon's capsule)
Sclera
Episcleral space
Optic nerve (II) and outer sheath
Sphenoidal sinus

Frontal section

Levator palpebrae superioris muscle and fascial sheath
Superior oblique muscle and fascial sheath
Medial rectus muscle and fascial sheath
Periorbita
Ethmoidal cell
Sclera
Fascial sheath of eyeball (Tenon's capsule)
Inferior rectus muscle and fascial sheath
Inferior oblique muscle and fascial sheath
Infraorbital nerve (V_2)

Superior rectus muscle and fascial sheath
Lacrimal gland
Lateral rectus muscle and fascial sheath
Periorbita
Sclera
Fascial sheath of eyeball (Tenon's capsule)
Episcleral space
Retrobulbar fat (orbital fat body)

Muscle attachments and nerves and vessels entering orbit

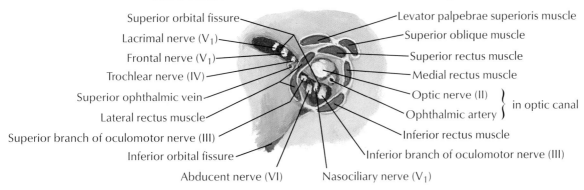

Superior orbital fissure
Lacrimal nerve (V_1)
Frontal nerve (V_1)
Trochlear nerve (IV)
Superior ophthalmic vein
Lateral rectus muscle
Superior branch of oculomotor nerve (III)
Inferior orbital fissure
Abducent nerve (VI)

Levator palpebrae superioris muscle
Superior oblique muscle
Superior rectus muscle
Medial rectus muscle
Optic nerve (II) } in optic canal
Ophthalmic artery }
Inferior rectus muscle
Inferior branch of oculomotor nerve (III)
Nasociliary nerve (V_1)

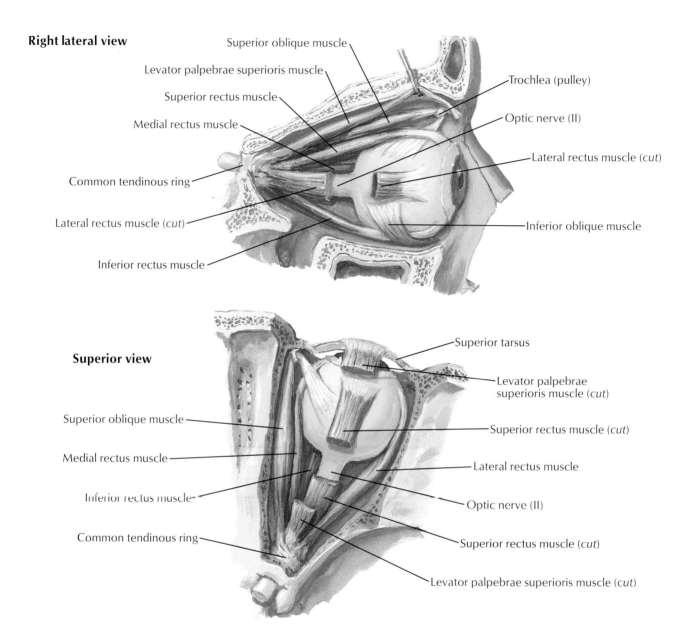

Right lateral view

Superior oblique muscle

Levator palpebrae superioris muscle

Superior rectus muscle

Medial rectus muscle

Common tendinous ring

Lateral rectus muscle (*cut*)

Inferior rectus muscle

Trochlea (pulley)

Optic nerve (II)

Lateral rectus muscle (*cut*)

Inferior oblique muscle

Superior view

Superior oblique muscle

Medial rectus muscle

Inferior rectus muscle

Common tendinous ring

Superior tarsus

Levator palpebrae superioris muscle (*cut*)

Superior rectus muscle (*cut*)

Lateral rectus muscle

Optic nerve (II)

Superior rectus muscle (*cut*)

Levator palpebrae superioris muscle (*cut*)

Innervation of extrinsic eye muscles: anterior view

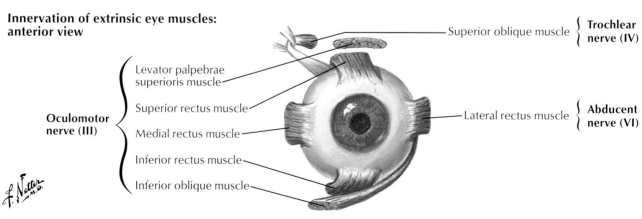

Oculomotor nerve (III)

Levator palpebrae superioris muscle

Superior rectus muscle

Medial rectus muscle

Inferior rectus muscle

Inferior oblique muscle

Superior oblique muscle — Trochlear nerve (IV)

Lateral rectus muscle — Abducent nerve (VI)

f. Netter. M.D.

Plate 84   **Orbit and Contents**

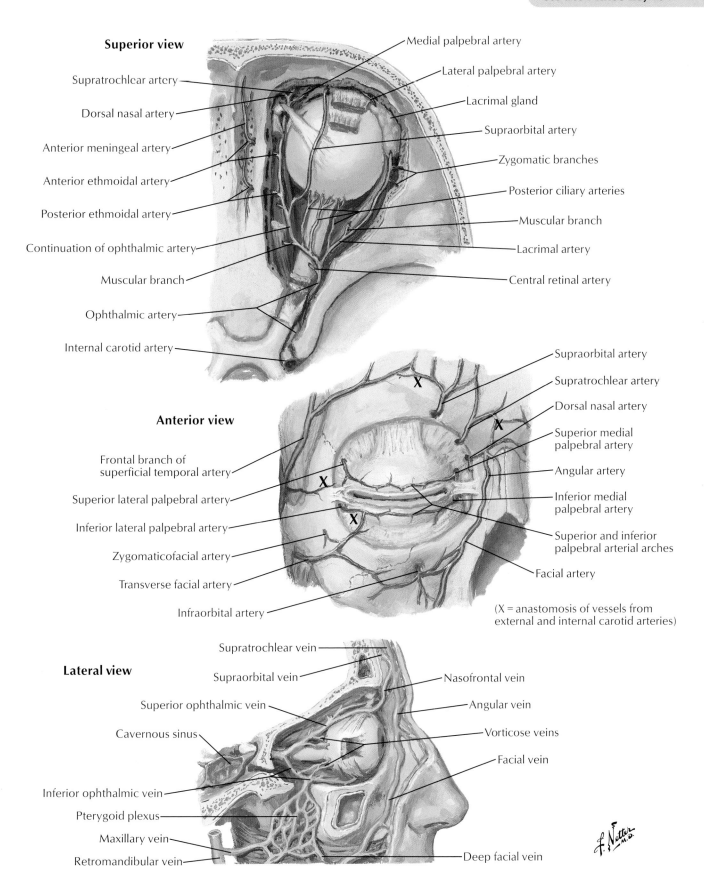

Superior view

Supratrochlear artery
Dorsal nasal artery
Anterior meningeal artery
Anterior ethmoidal artery
Posterior ethmoidal artery
Continuation of ophthalmic artery
Muscular branch
Ophthalmic artery
Internal carotid artery

Medial palpebral artery
Lateral palpebral artery
Lacrimal gland
Supraorbital artery
Zygomatic branches
Posterior ciliary arteries
Muscular branch
Lacrimal artery
Central retinal artery

Anterior view

Frontal branch of
superficial temporal artery
Superior lateral palpebral artery
Inferior lateral palpebral artery
Zygomaticofacial artery
Transverse facial artery
Infraorbital artery

Supraorbital artery
Supratrochlear artery
Dorsal nasal artery
Superior medial
palpebral artery
Angular artery
Inferior medial
palpebral artery
Superior and inferior
palpebral arterial arches
Facial artery

(X = anastomosis of vessels from
external and internal carotid arteries)

Lateral view

Supratrochlear vein
Supraorbital vein
Superior ophthalmic vein
Cavernous sinus
Inferior ophthalmic vein
Pterygoid plexus
Maxillary vein
Retromandibular vein

Nasofrontal vein
Angular vein
Vorticose veins
Facial vein
Deep facial vein

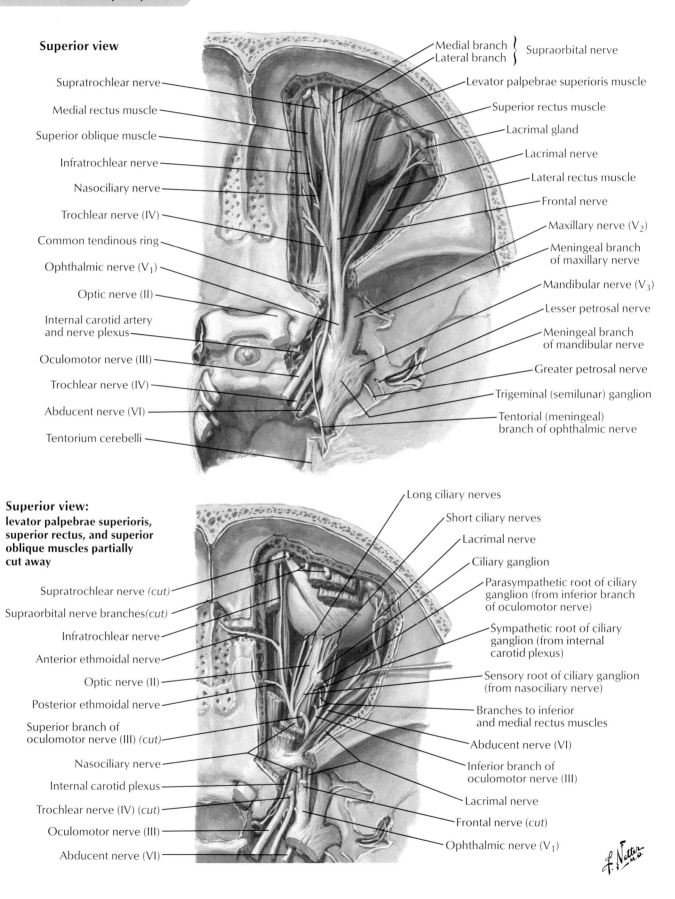

Superior view

Supratrochlear nerve

Medial rectus muscle

Superior oblique muscle

Infratrochlear nerve

Nasociliary nerve

Trochlear nerve (IV)

Common tendinous ring

Ophthalmic nerve (V₁)

Optic nerve (II)

Internal carotid artery and nerve plexus

Oculomotor nerve (III)

Trochlear nerve (IV)

Abducent nerve (VI)

Tentorium cerebelli

Medial branch } Supraorbital nerve
Lateral branch }

Levator palpebrae superioris muscle

Superior rectus muscle

Lacrimal gland

Lacrimal nerve

Lateral rectus muscle

Frontal nerve

Maxillary nerve (V₂)

Meningeal branch of maxillary nerve

Mandibular nerve (V₃)

Lesser petrosal nerve

Meningeal branch of mandibular nerve

Greater petrosal nerve

Trigeminal (semilunar) ganglion

Tentorial (meningeal) branch of ophthalmic nerve

Superior view:
levator palpebrae superioris,
superior rectus, and superior
oblique muscles partially
cut away

Supratrochlear nerve *(cut)*

Supraorbital nerve branches *(cut)*

Infratrochlear nerve

Anterior ethmoidal nerve

Optic nerve (II)

Posterior ethmoidal nerve

Superior branch of oculomotor nerve (III) *(cut)*

Nasociliary nerve

Internal carotid plexus

Trochlear nerve (IV) *(cut)*

Oculomotor nerve (III)

Abducent nerve (VI)

Long ciliary nerves

Short ciliary nerves

Lacrimal nerve

Ciliary ganglion

Parasympathetic root of ciliary ganglion (from inferior branch of oculomotor nerve)

Sympathetic root of ciliary ganglion (from internal carotid plexus)

Sensory root of ciliary ganglion (from nasociliary nerve)

Branches to inferior and medial rectus muscles

Abducent nerve (VI)

Inferior branch of oculomotor nerve (III)

Lacrimal nerve

Frontal nerve *(cut)*

Ophthalmic nerve (V₁)

Plate 86

Orbit and Contents

Horizontal section

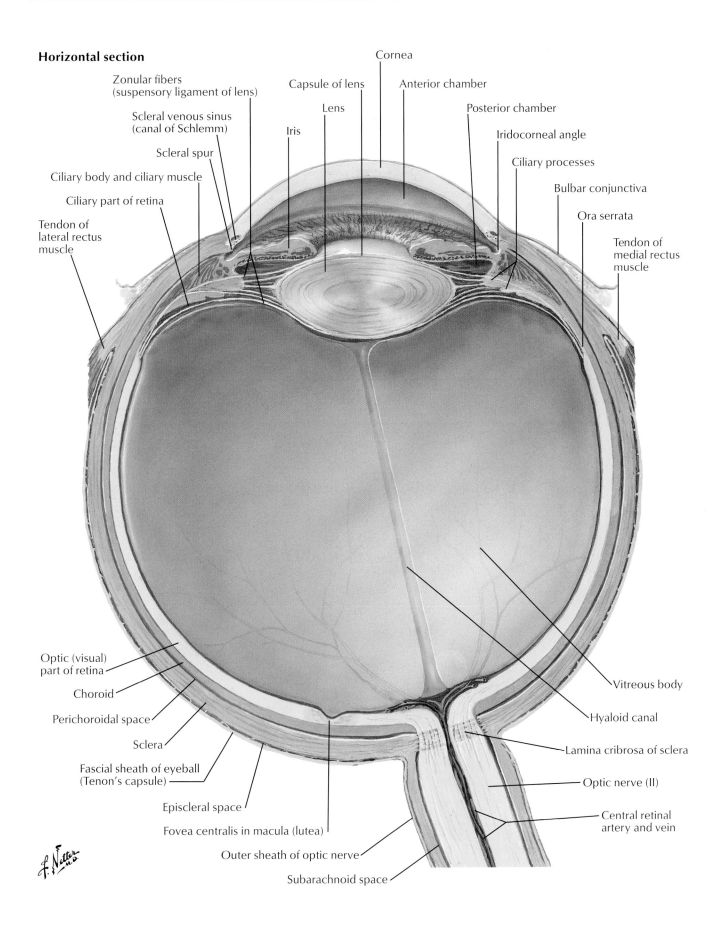

Zonular fibers
(suspensory ligament of lens)

Scleral venous sinus
(canal of Schlemm)

Scleral spur

Ciliary body and ciliary muscle

Ciliary part of retina

Tendon of
lateral rectus
muscle

Iris

Capsule of lens

Lens

Cornea

Anterior chamber

Posterior chamber

Iridocorneal angle

Ciliary processes

Bulbar conjunctiva

Ora serrata

Tendon of
medial rectus
muscle

Optic (visual)
part of retina

Choroid

Perichoroidal space

Sclera

Fascial sheath of eyeball
(Tenon's capsule)

Episcleral space

Fovea centralis in macula (lutea)

Outer sheath of optic nerve

Subarachnoid space

Vitreous body

Hyaloid canal

Lamina cribrosa of sclera

Optic nerve (II)

Central retinal
artery and vein

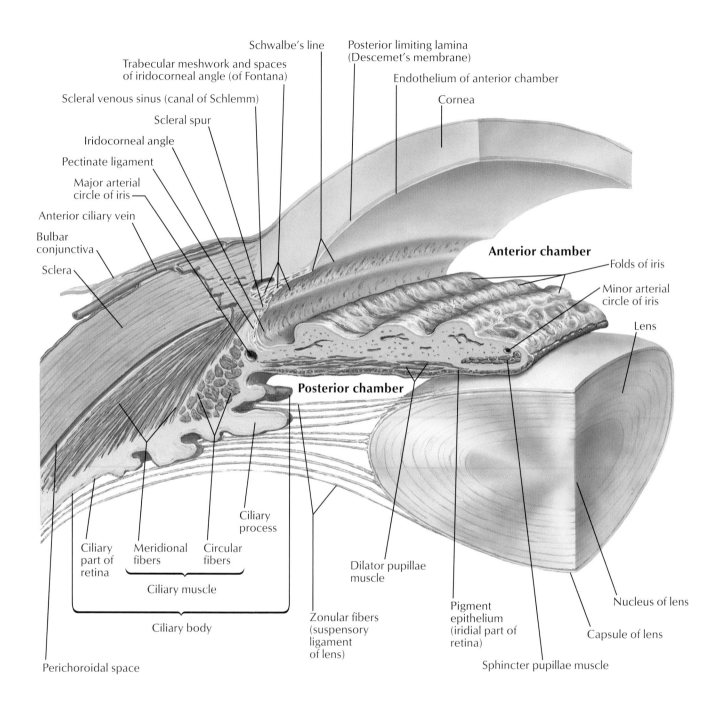

Schwalbe's line

Posterior limiting lamina
(Descemet's membrane)

Trabecular meshwork and spaces
of iridocorneal angle (of Fontana)

Endothelium of anterior chamber

Scleral venous sinus (canal of Schlemm)

Cornea

Scleral spur

Iridocorneal angle

Pectinate ligament

Major arterial
circle of iris

Anterior ciliary vein

Bulbar
conjunctiva

Sclera

Anterior chamber

Folds of iris

Minor arterial
circle of iris

Lens

Posterior chamber

Ciliary
process

Ciliary
part of
retina

Meridional
fibers

Circular
fibers

Dilator pupillae
muscle

Nucleus of lens

Pigment
epithelium
(iridial part of
retina)

Capsule of lens

Ciliary muscle

Zonular fibers
(suspensory
ligament
of lens)

Ciliary body

Sphincter pupillae muscle

Perichoroidal space

Note: For clarity, only single plane of zonular fibers shown;
actually, fibers surround entire circumference of lens.

Plate 88

Orbit and Contents

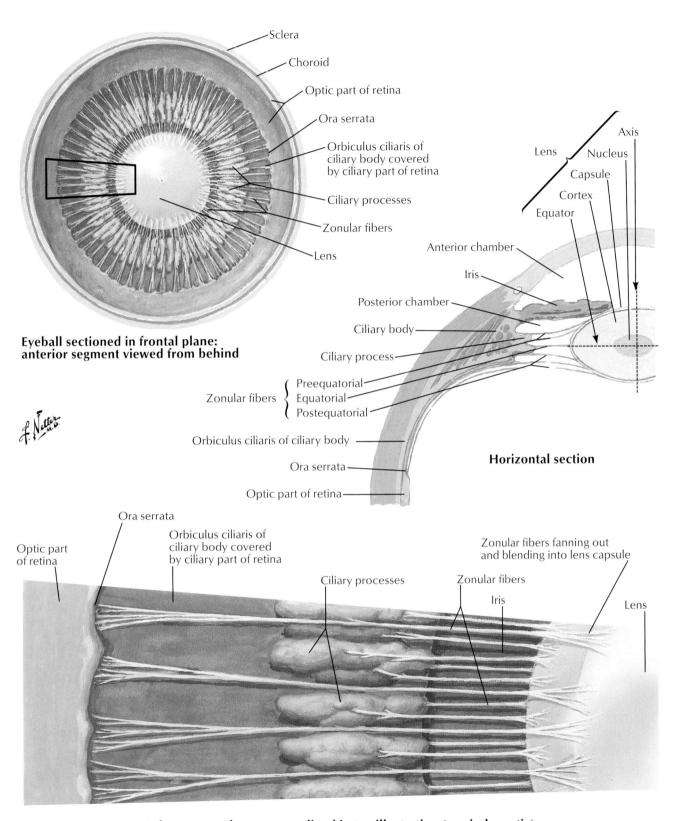

Sclera

Choroid

Optic part of retina

Ora serrata

Orbiculus ciliaris of ciliary body covered by ciliary part of retina

Ciliary processes

Zonular fibers

Lens

Eyeball sectioned in frontal plane: anterior segment viewed from behind

Axis

Lens — Nucleus

Capsule

Cortex

Equator

Anterior chamber

Iris

Posterior chamber

Ciliary body

Ciliary process

Zonular fibers { Preequatorial — Equatorial — Postequatorial

Orbiculus ciliaris of ciliary body

Ora serrata

Optic part of retina

Horizontal section

Ora serrata

Orbiculus ciliaris of ciliary body covered by ciliary part of retina

Optic part of retina

Ciliary processes

Zonular fibers fanning out and blending into lens capsule

Zonular fibers

Iris

Lens

Enlargement of segment outlined in top illustration (semischematic)

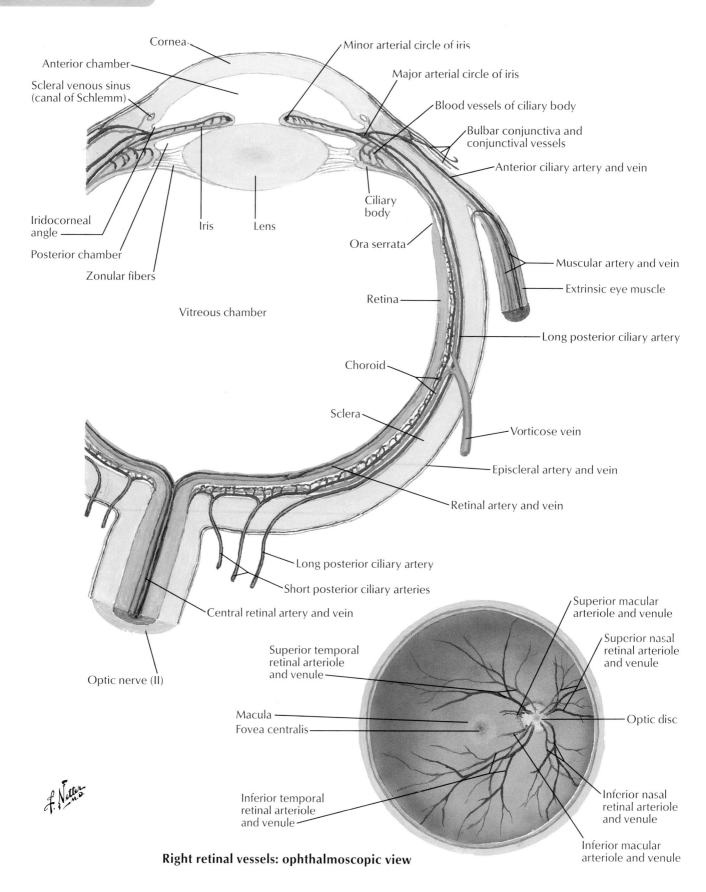

Cornea

Anterior chamber

Scleral venous sinus (canal of Schlemm)

Iridocorneal angle

Posterior chamber

Zonular fibers

Iris

Lens

Vitreous chamber

Minor arterial circle of iris

Major arterial circle of iris

Blood vessels of ciliary body

Bulbar conjunctiva and conjunctival vessels

Anterior ciliary artery and vein

Ciliary body

Ora serrata

Retina

Choroid

Sclera

Muscular artery and vein

Extrinsic eye muscle

Long posterior ciliary artery

Vorticose vein

Episcleral artery and vein

Retinal artery and vein

Long posterior ciliary artery

Short posterior ciliary arteries

Central retinal artery and vein

Optic nerve (II)

Superior temporal retinal arteriole and venule

Macula

Fovea centralis

Inferior temporal retinal arteriole and venule

Superior macular arteriole and venule

Superior nasal retinal arteriole and venule

Optic disc

Inferior nasal retinal arteriole and venule

Inferior macular arteriole and venule

Right retinal vessels: ophthalmoscopic view

Plate 90

Orbit and Contents

Vascular arrangements within the choroid (vascular tunic) of the eyeball

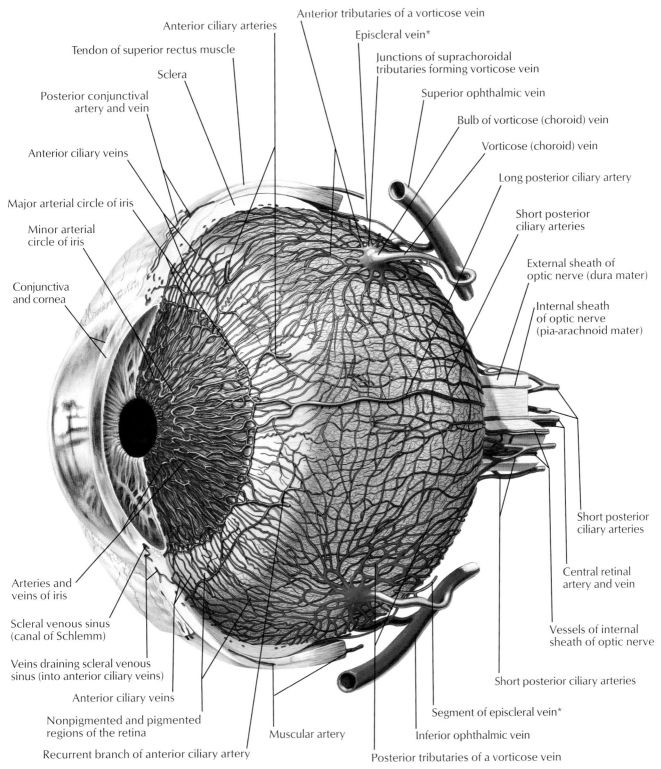

Anterior tributaries of a vorticose vein

Anterior ciliary arteries

Episcleral vein*

Tendon of superior rectus muscle

Junctions of suprachoroidal tributaries forming vorticose vein

Sclera

Superior ophthalmic vein

Posterior conjunctival artery and vein

Bulb of vorticose (choroid) vein

Vorticose (choroid) vein

Anterior ciliary veins

Long posterior ciliary artery

Major arterial circle of iris

Short posterior ciliary arteries

Minor arterial circle of iris

External sheath of optic nerve (dura mater)

Conjunctiva and cornea

Internal sheath of optic nerve (pia-arachnoid mater)

Short posterior ciliary arteries

Central retinal artery and vein

Arteries and veins of iris

Vessels of internal sheath of optic nerve

Scleral venous sinus (canal of Schlemm)

Veins draining scleral venous sinus (into anterior ciliary veins)

Short posterior ciliary arteries

Anterior ciliary veins

Segment of episcleral vein*

Nonpigmented and pigmented regions of the retina

Inferior ophthalmic vein

Muscular artery

Recurrent branch of anterior ciliary artery

Posterior tributaries of a vorticose vein

The episcleral veins are shown here anastomosing with the vorticose veins, which they do; however they also drain into the anterior ciliary veins.

C. Machado
—M.D.

Frontal section

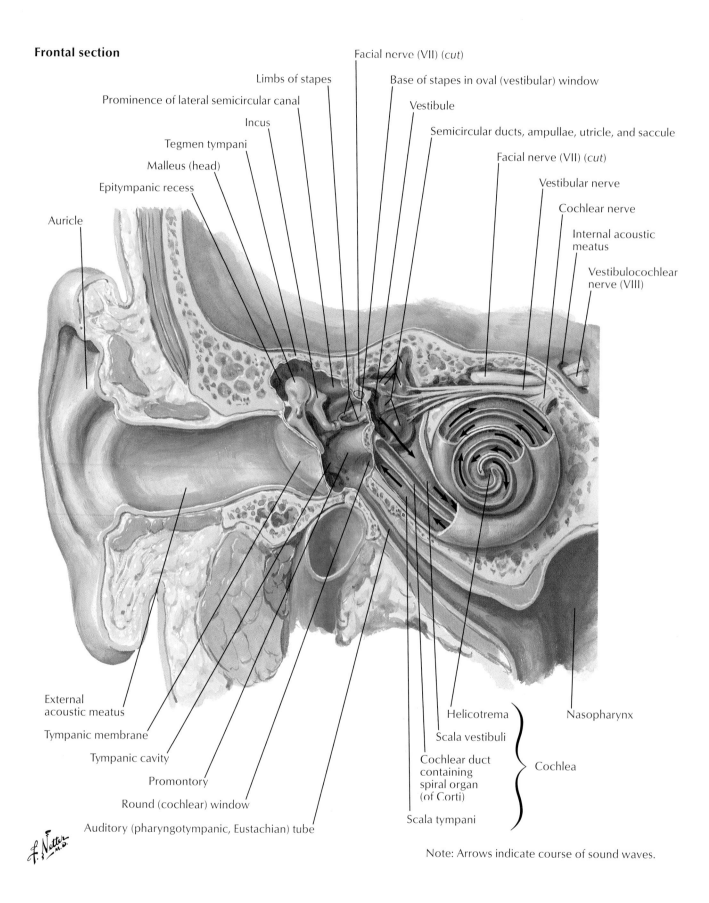

Facial nerve (VII) *(cut)*

Limbs of stapes

Base of stapes in oval (vestibular) window

Prominence of lateral semicircular canal

Vestibule

Incus

Semicircular ducts, ampullae, utricle, and saccule

Tegmen tympani

Facial nerve (VII) *(cut)*

Malleus (head)

Vestibular nerve

Epitympanic recess

Cochlear nerve

Internal acoustic meatus

Auricle

Vestibulocochlear nerve (VIII)

External acoustic meatus

Tympanic membrane

Tympanic cavity

Promontory

Round (cochlear) window

Auditory (pharyngotympanic, Eustachian) tube

Helicotrema

Scala vestibuli

Cochlear duct containing spiral organ (of Corti)

Scala tympani

Nasopharynx

Cochlea

Note: Arrows indicate course of sound waves.

Plate 92

Ear

Right auricle (pinna)

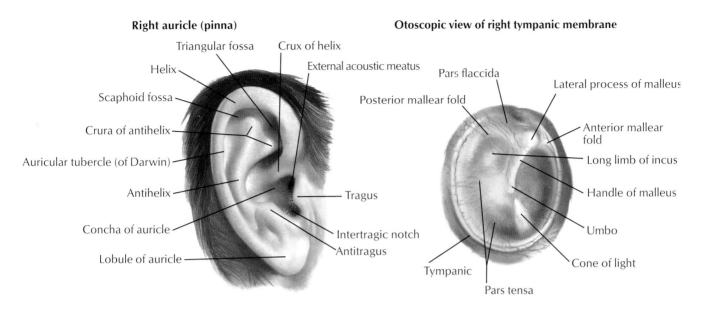

Triangular fossa

Crux of helix

Helix

External acoustic meatus

Scaphoid fossa

Posterior mallear fold

Crura of antihelix

Auricular tubercle (of Darwin)

Antihelix

Concha of auricle

Tragus

Lobule of auricle

Intertragic notch

Antitragus

Otoscopic view of right tympanic membrane

Pars flaccida

Lateral process of malleus

Anterior mallear fold

Long limb of incus

Handle of malleus

Umbo

Tympanic

Cone of light

Pars tensa

Coronal oblique section of external acoustic meatus and middle ear (tympanic cavity)

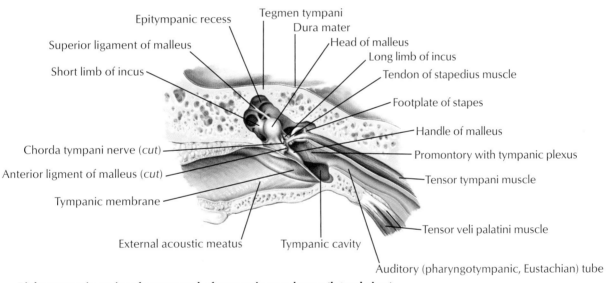

Epitympanic recess

Tegmen tympani

Dura mater

Superior ligament of malleus

Head of malleus

Short limb of incus

Long limb of incus

Tendon of stapedius muscle

Footplate of stapes

Handle of malleus

Chorda tympani nerve (cut)

Promontory with tympanic plexus

Anterior ligment of malleus (cut)

Tensor tympani muscle

Tympanic membrane

Tensor veli palatini muscle

External acoustic meatus

Tympanic cavity

Auditory (pharyngotympanic, Eustachian) tube

Right tympanic cavity after removal of tympanic membrane (lateral view)

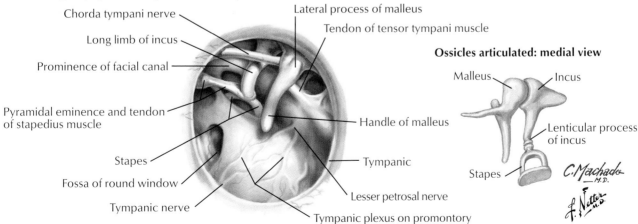

Chorda tympani nerve

Lateral process of malleus

Long limb of incus

Tendon of tensor tympani muscle

Prominence of facial canal

Ossicles articulated: medial view

Malleus

Incus

Pyramidal eminence and tendon of stapedius muscle

Handle of malleus

Lenticular process of incus

Stapes

Tympanic

Stapes

Fossa of round window

Lesser petrosal nerve

Tympanic nerve

Tympanic plexus on promontory

C. Machado —M.D.

F. Netter M.D.

Tympanic Cavity

See also **Plates 46, 123, 124, 135**

Lateral wall of tympanic cavity: medial (internal) view

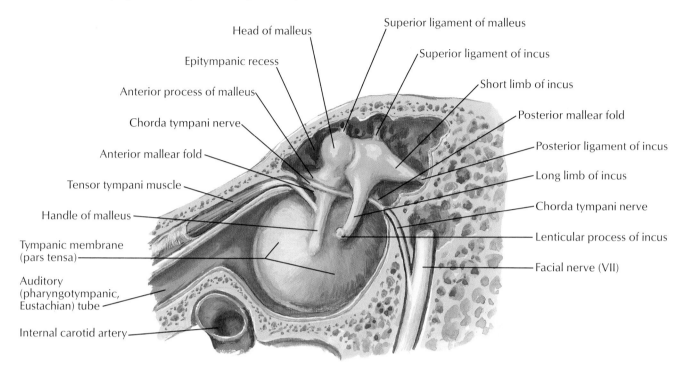

Head of malleus
Superior ligament of malleus
Superior ligament of incus
Epitympanic recess
Short limb of incus
Anterior process of malleus
Posterior mallear fold
Chorda tympani nerve
Posterior ligament of incus
Anterior mallear fold
Long limb of incus
Tensor tympani muscle
Chorda tympani nerve
Handle of malleus
Lenticular process of incus
Tympanic membrane (pars tensa)
Facial nerve (VII)
Auditory (pharyngotympanic, Eustachian) tube
Internal carotid artery

Medial wall of tympanic cavity: lateral view

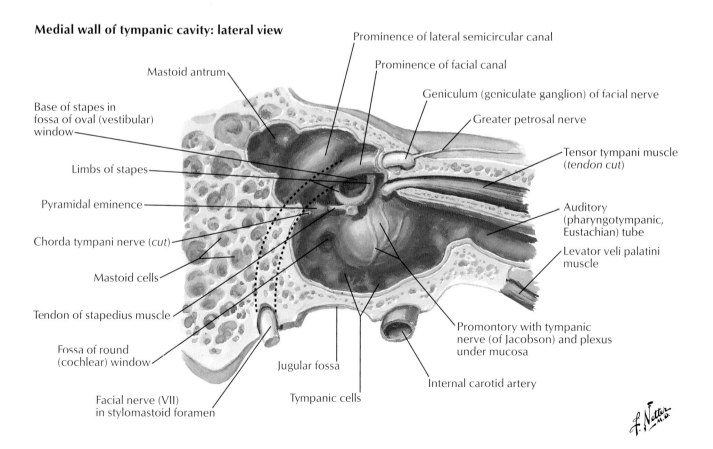

Prominence of lateral semicircular canal
Prominence of facial canal
Mastoid antrum
Geniculum (geniculate ganglion) of facial nerve
Base of stapes in fossa of oval (vestibular) window
Greater petrosal nerve
Tensor tympani muscle (tendon cut)
Limbs of stapes
Auditory (pharyngotympanic, Eustachian) tube
Pyramidal eminence
Levator veli palatini muscle
Chorda tympani nerve (cut)
Mastoid cells
Tendon of stapedius muscle
Promontory with tympanic nerve (of Jacobson) and plexus under mucosa
Fossa of round (cochlear) window
Jugular fossa
Facial nerve (VII) in stylomastoid foramen
Tympanic cells
Internal carotid artery

Plate 94

Ear

Right bony labyrinth (otic capsule), anterolateral view: surrounding cancellous bone removed

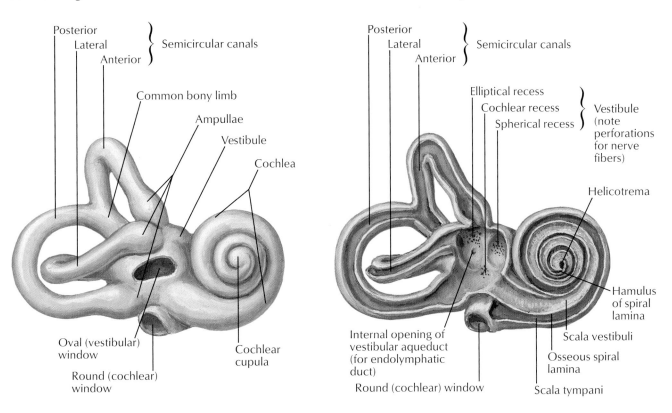

Posterior
Lateral · Semicircular canals
Anterior
Common bony limb
Ampullae
Vestibule
Cochlea

Oval (vestibular) window
Round (cochlear) window
Cochlear cupula

Dissected right bony labyrinth (otic capsule): membranous labyrinth removed

Posterior
Lateral · Semicircular canals
Anterior

Elliptical recess
Cochlear recess · Vestibule (note perforations for nerve fibers)
Spherical recess

Helicotrema

Internal opening of vestibular aqueduct (for endolymphatic duct)
Round (cochlear) window

Hamulus of spiral lamina
Scala vestibuli
Osseous spiral lamina
Scala tympani

Right membranous labyrinth with nerves: posteromedial view

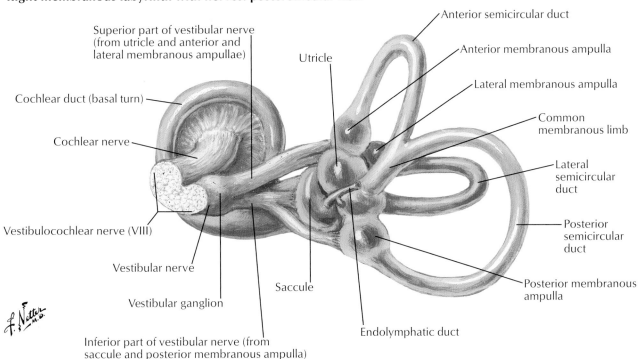

Superior part of vestibular nerve (from utricle and anterior and lateral membranous ampullae)
Cochlear duct (basal turn)
Cochlear nerve
Vestibulocochlear nerve (VIII)
Vestibular nerve
Vestibular ganglion
Inferior part of vestibular nerve (from saccule and posterior membranous ampulla)
Saccule
Utricle
Anterior semicircular duct
Anterior membranous ampulla
Lateral membranous ampulla
Common membranous limb
Lateral semicircular duct
Posterior semicircular duct
Posterior membranous ampulla
Endolymphatic duct

F. Netter, M.D.

Bony and membranous labyrinths: schema

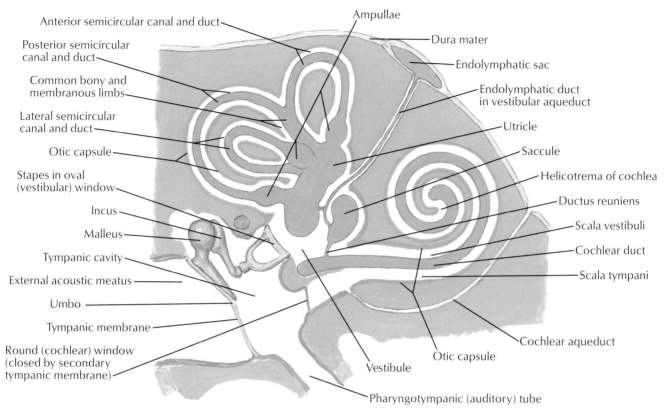

Anterior semicircular canal and duct

Posterior semicircular canal and duct

Common bony and membranous limbs

Lateral semicircular canal and duct

Otic capsule

Stapes in oval (vestibular) window

Incus

Malleus

Tympanic cavity

External acoustic meatus

Umbo

Tympanic membrane

Round (cochlear) window (closed by secondary tympanic membrane)

Ampullae

Dura mater

Endolymphatic sac

Endolymphatic duct in vestibular aqueduct

Utricle

Saccule

Helicotrema of cochlea

Ductus reuniens

Scala vestibuli

Cochlear duct

Scala tympani

Cochlear aqueduct

Otic capsule

Vestibule

Pharyngotympanic (auditory) tube

Section through turn of cochlea

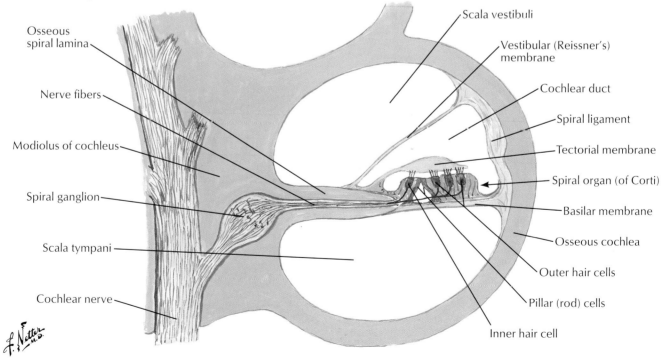

Osseous spiral lamina

Nerve fibers

Modiolus of cochleus

Spiral ganglion

Scala tympani

Cochlear nerve

Scala vestibuli

Vestibular (Reissner's) membrane

Cochlear duct

Spiral ligament

Tectorial membrane

Spiral organ (of Corti)

Basilar membrane

Osseous cochlea

Outer hair cells

Pillar (rod) cells

Inner hair cell

Plate 96

Ear

Superior projection of right bony labyrinth on floor of skull

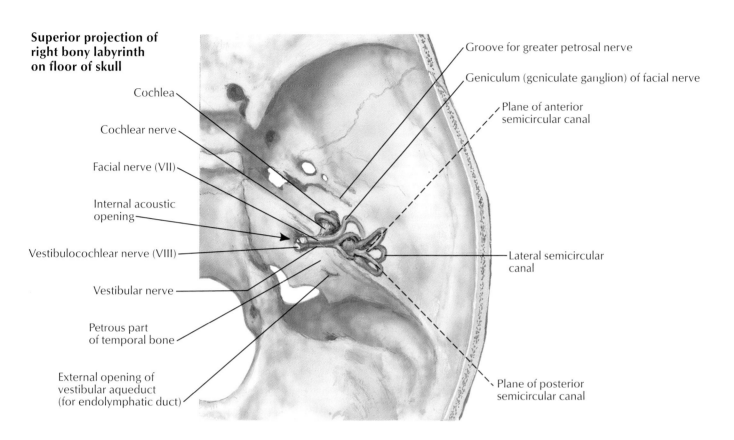

Cochlea

Cochlear nerve

Facial nerve (VII)

Internal acoustic opening

Vestibulocochlear nerve (VIII)

Vestibular nerve

Petrous part of temporal bone

External opening of vestibular aqueduct (for endolymphatic duct)

Groove for greater petrosal nerve

Geniculum (geniculate ganglion) of facial nerve

Plane of anterior semicircular canal

Lateral semicircular canal

Plane of posterior semicircular canal

Lateral projection of right membranous labyrinth

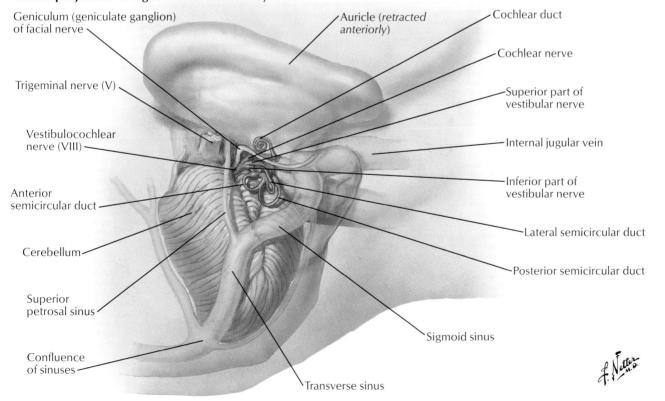

Geniculum (geniculate ganglion) of facial nerve

Trigeminal nerve (V)

Vestibulocochlear nerve (VIII)

Anterior semicircular duct

Cerebellum

Superior petrosal sinus

Confluence of sinuses

Auricle (*retracted anteriorly*)

Cochlear duct

Cochlear nerve

Superior part of vestibular nerve

Internal jugular vein

Inferior part of vestibular nerve

Lateral semicircular duct

Posterior semicircular duct

Sigmoid sinus

Transverse sinus

Auditory (Pharyngotympanic, Eustachian) Tube

See also **Plates 52, 55, 65**

Cartilaginous part of auditory (pharyngotympanic, Eustachian) tube at base of skull: inferior view

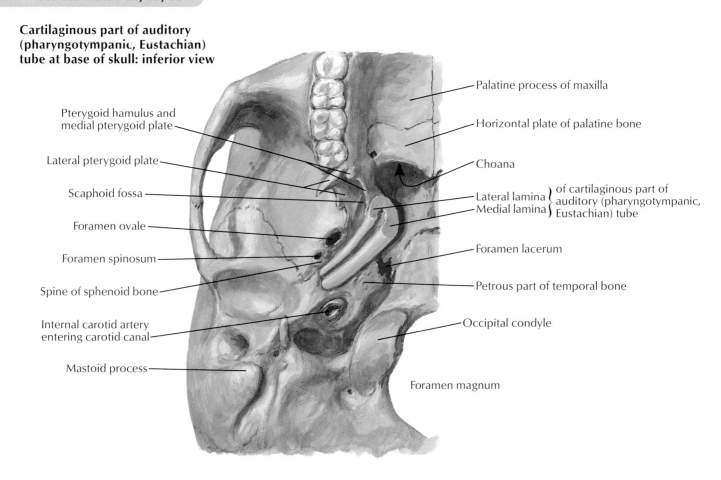

Pterygoid hamulus and medial pterygoid plate

Lateral pterygoid plate

Scaphoid fossa

Foramen ovale

Foramen spinosum

Spine of sphenoid bone

Internal carotid artery entering carotid canal

Mastoid process

Palatine process of maxilla

Horizontal plate of palatine bone

Choana

Lateral lamina } of cartilaginous part of
Medial lamina } auditory (pharyngotympanic, Eustachian) tube

Foramen lacerum

Petrous part of temporal bone

Occipital condyle

Foramen magnum

Section through cartilaginous part of auditory (pharyngotympanic, Eustachian) tube, with tube closed

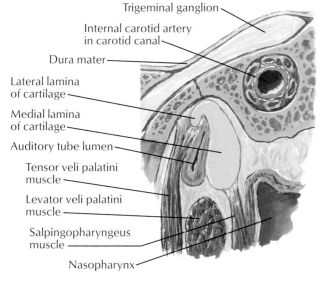

Trigeminal ganglion

Internal carotid artery in carotid canal

Dura mater

Lateral lamina of cartilage

Medial lamina of cartilage

Auditory tube lumen

Tensor veli palatini muscle

Levator veli palatini muscle

Salpingopharyngeus muscle

Nasopharynx

Auditory (pharyngotympanic, Eustachian) tube closed by elastic recoil of cartilage, tissue turgidity, and tension of salpingopharyngeus muscles

Section through cartilaginous part of auditory (pharyngotympanic, Eustachian) tube, with tube open

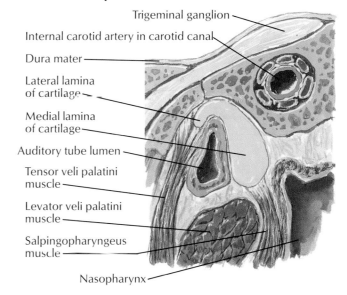

Trigeminal ganglion

Internal carotid artery in carotid canal

Dura mater

Lateral lamina of cartilage

Medial lamina of cartilage

Auditory tube lumen

Tensor veli palatini muscle

Levator veli palatini muscle

Salpingopharyngeus muscle

Nasopharynx

Lumen opened chiefly when attachment of tensor veli palatini muscle pulls wall of tube laterally during swallowing

Plate 98

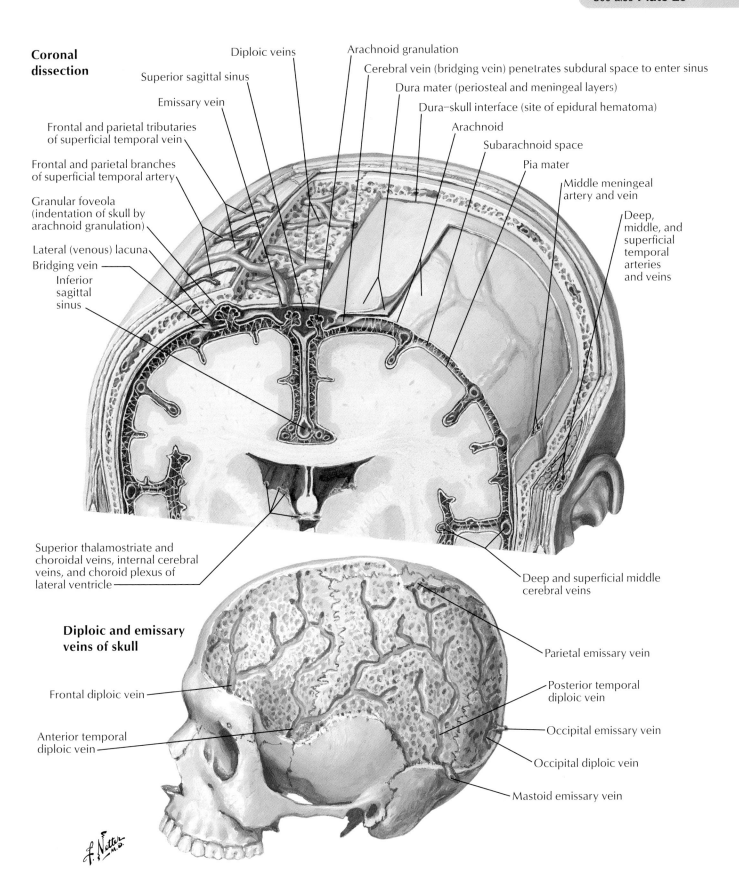

Coronal dissection

Diploic veins

Superior sagittal sinus

Emissary vein

Frontal and parietal tributaries of superficial temporal vein

Frontal and parietal branches of superficial temporal artery

Granular foveola (indentation of skull by arachnoid granulation)

Lateral (venous) lacuna

Bridging vein

Inferior sagittal sinus

Arachnoid granulation

Cerebral vein (bridging vein) penetrates subdural space to enter sinus

Dura mater (periosteal and meningeal layers)

Dura–skull interface (site of epidural hematoma)

Arachnoid

Subarachnoid space

Pia mater

Middle meningeal artery and vein

Deep, middle, and superficial temporal arteries and veins

Superior thalamostriate and choroidal veins, internal cerebral veins, and choroid plexus of lateral ventricle

Deep and superficial middle cerebral veins

Diploic and emissary veins of skull

Frontal diploic vein

Anterior temporal diploic vein

Parietal emissary vein

Posterior temporal diploic vein

Occipital emissary vein

Occipital diploic vein

Mastoid emissary vein

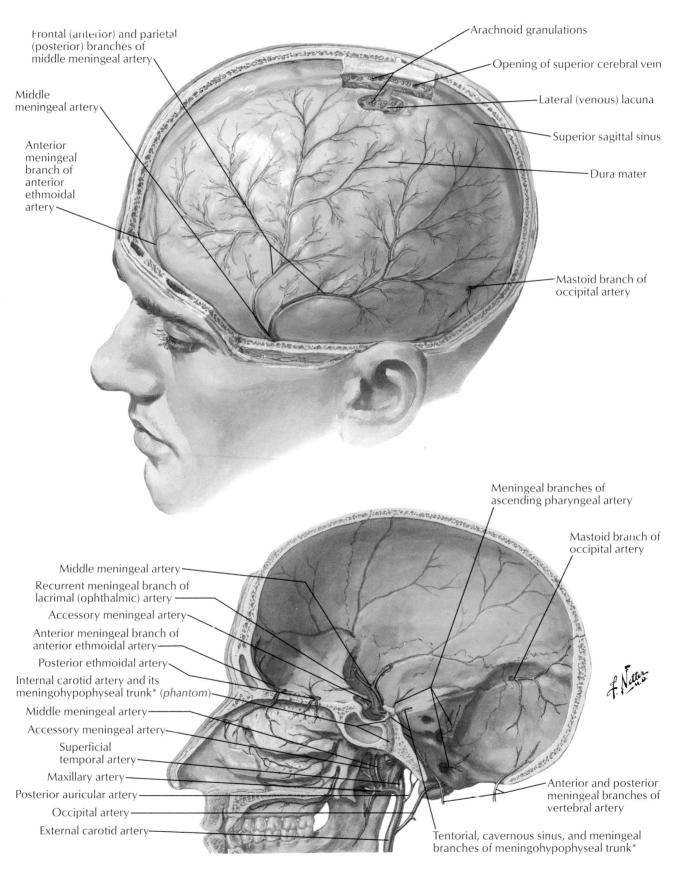

Frontal (anterior) and parietal (posterior) branches of middle meningeal artery

Middle meningeal artery

Anterior meningeal branch of anterior ethmoidal artery

Arachnoid granulations

Opening of superior cerebral vein

Lateral (venous) lacuna

Superior sagittal sinus

Dura mater

Mastoid branch of occipital artery

Meningeal branches of ascending pharyngeal artery

Mastoid branch of occipital artery

Middle meningeal artery

Recurrent meningeal branch of lacrimal (ophthalmic) artery

Accessory meningeal artery

Anterior meningeal branch of anterior ethmoidal artery

Posterior ethmoidal artery

Internal carotid artery and its meningohypophyseal trunk* (phantom)

Middle meningeal artery

Accessory meningeal artery

Superficial temporal artery

Maxillary artery

Posterior auricular artery

Occipital artery

External carotid artery

Anterior and posterior meningeal branches of vertebral artery

Tentorial, cavernous sinus, and meningeal branches of meningohypophyseal trunk*

*Variant; most commonly, these branches arise directly from internal carotid artery.

Plate 100   **Meninges and Brain**

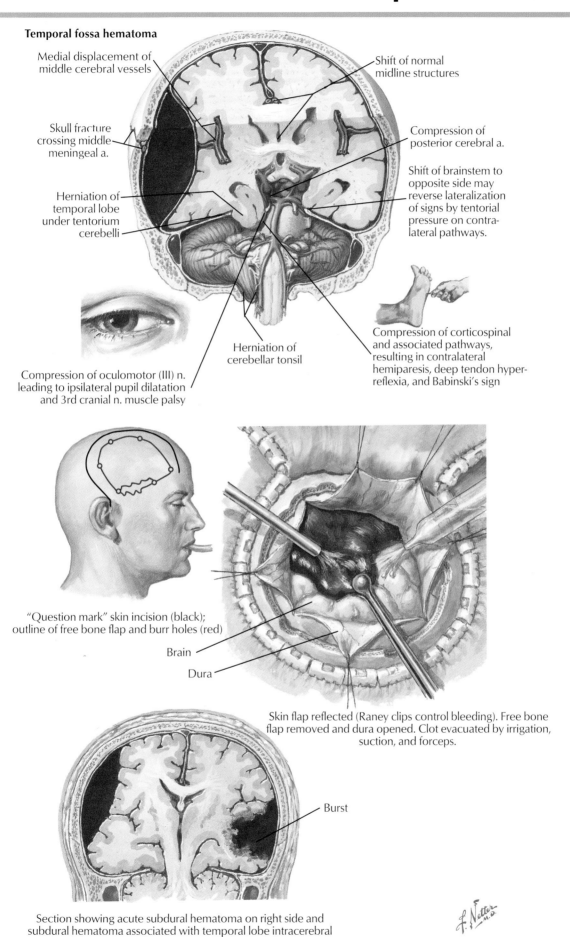

Temporal fossa hematoma

Medial displacement of middle cerebral vessels

Shift of normal midline structures

Skull fracture crossing middle meningeal a.

Compression of posterior cerebral a.

Shift of brainstem to opposite side may reverse lateralization of signs by tentorial pressure on contra-lateral pathways.

Herniation of temporal lobe under tentorium cerebelli

Herniation of cerebellar tonsil

Compression of corticospinal and associated pathways, resulting in contralateral hemiparesis, deep tendon hyper-reflexia, and Babinski's sign

Compression of oculomotor (III) n. leading to ipsilateral pupil dilatation and 3rd cranial n. muscle palsy

"Question mark" skin incision (black); outline of free bone flap and burr holes (red)

Brain

Dura

Skin flap reflected (Raney clips control bleeding). Free bone flap removed and dura opened. Clot evacuated by irrigation, suction, and forceps.

Burst

Section showing acute subdural hematoma on right side and subdural hematoma associated with temporal lobe intracerebral hematoma ("burst" temporal lobe) on left

Meninges and Brain   **Plate 101**

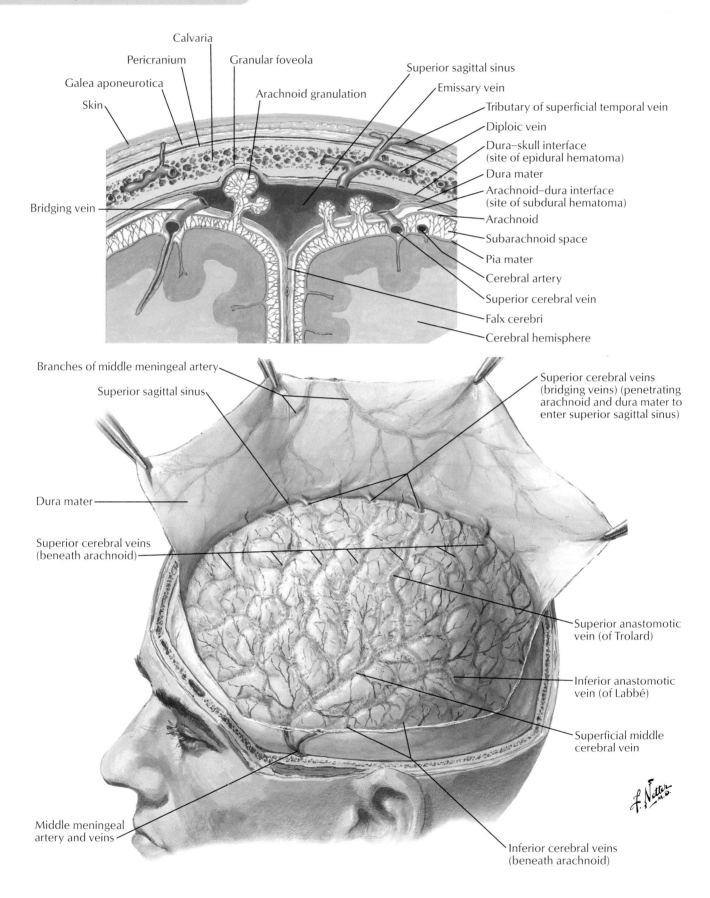

Calvaria

Pericranium

Granular foveola

Galea aponeurotica

Arachnoid granulation

Skin

Superior sagittal sinus

Emissary vein

Tributary of superficial temporal vein

Diploic vein

Dura–skull interface
(site of epidural hematoma)

Dura mater

Arachnoid–dura interface
(site of subdural hematoma)

Bridging vein

Arachnoid

Subarachnoid space

Pia mater

Cerebral artery

Superior cerebral vein

Falx cerebri

Cerebral hemisphere

Branches of middle meningeal artery

Superior sagittal sinus

Superior cerebral veins
(bridging veins) (penetrating
arachnoid and dura mater to
enter superior sagittal sinus)

Dura mater

Superior cerebral veins
(beneath arachnoid)

Superior anastomotic
vein (of Trolard)

Inferior anastomotic
vein (of Labbé)

Superficial middle
cerebral vein

Middle meningeal
artery and veins

Inferior cerebral veins
(beneath arachnoid)

Plate 102   **Meninges and Brain**

Sagittal section

Superior sagittal sinus

Straight sinus

Great cerebral vein (of Galen)

Tentorium cerebelli

Superior sagittal sinus

Falx cerebri

Inferior sagittal sinus

Sphenoparietal sinus

Anterior and posterior
intercavernous sinuses

Superior
petrosal sinus

Basilar
venous plexus

Inferior
petrosal sinus

To jugular
foramen

Sigmoid sinus

Transverse sinus

Occipital sinus

Falx cerebelli

Confluence of sinuses

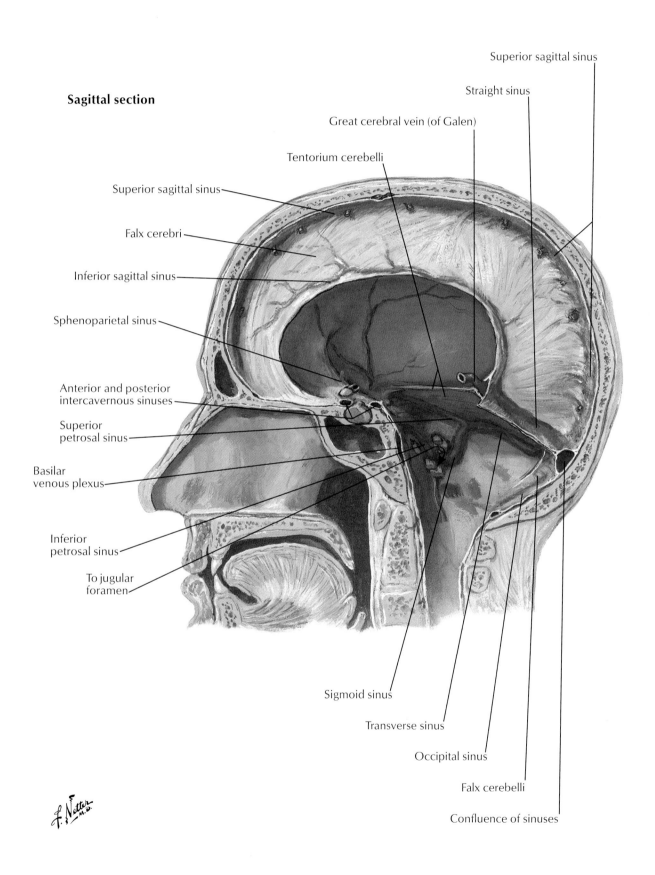

Dural Venous Sinuses (continued)

See also **Plate 85**

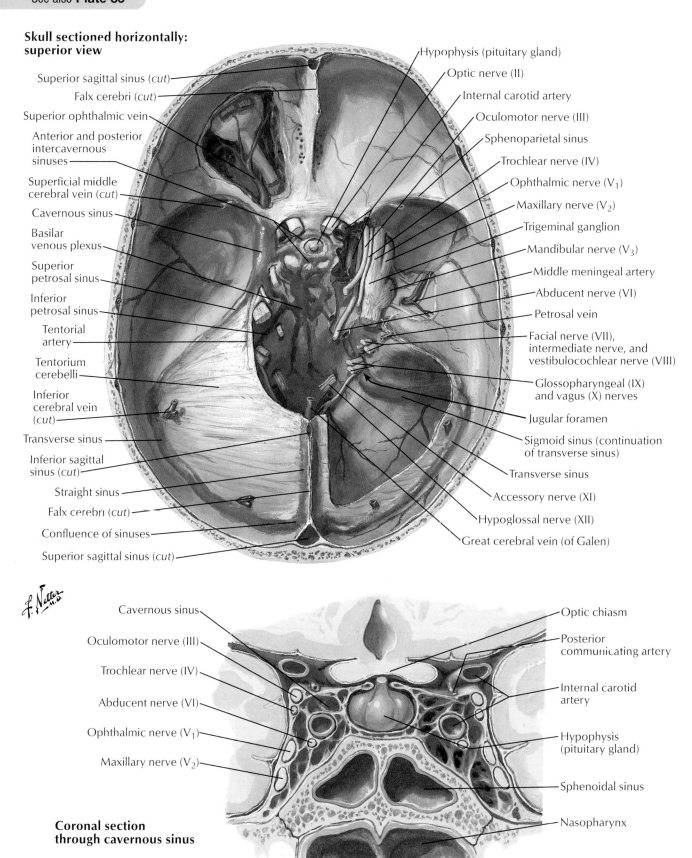

Skull sectioned horizontally: superior view

- Superior sagittal sinus (*cut*)
- Falx cerebri (*cut*)
- Superior ophthalmic vein
- Anterior and posterior intercavernous sinuses
- Superficial middle cerebral vein (*cut*)
- Cavernous sinus
- Basilar venous plexus
- Superior petrosal sinus
- Inferior petrosal sinus
- Tentorial artery
- Tentorium cerebelli
- Inferior cerebral vein (*cut*)
- Transverse sinus
- Inferior sagittal sinus (*cut*)
- Straight sinus
- Falx cerebri (*cut*)
- Confluence of sinuses
- Superior sagittal sinus (*cut*)

- Hypophysis (pituitary gland)
- Optic nerve (II)
- Internal carotid artery
- Oculomotor nerve (III)
- Sphenoparietal sinus
- Trochlear nerve (IV)
- Ophthalmic nerve (V_1)
- Maxillary nerve (V_2)
- Trigeminal ganglion
- Mandibular nerve (V_3)
- Middle meningeal artery
- Abducent nerve (VI)
- Petrosal vein
- Facial nerve (VII), intermediate nerve, and vestibulocochlear nerve (VIII)
- Glossopharyngeal (IX) and vagus (X) nerves
- Jugular foramen
- Sigmoid sinus (continuation of transverse sinus)
- Transverse sinus
- Accessory nerve (XI)
- Hypoglossal nerve (XII)
- Great cerebral vein (of Galen)

- Cavernous sinus
- Oculomotor nerve (III)
- Trochlear nerve (IV)
- Abducent nerve (VI)
- Ophthalmic nerve (V_1)
- Maxillary nerve (V_2)

- Optic chiasm
- Posterior communicating artery
- Internal carotid artery
- Hypophysis (pituitary gland)
- Sphenoidal sinus
- Nasopharynx

Coronal section through cavernous sinus

Plate 104   **Meninges and Brain**

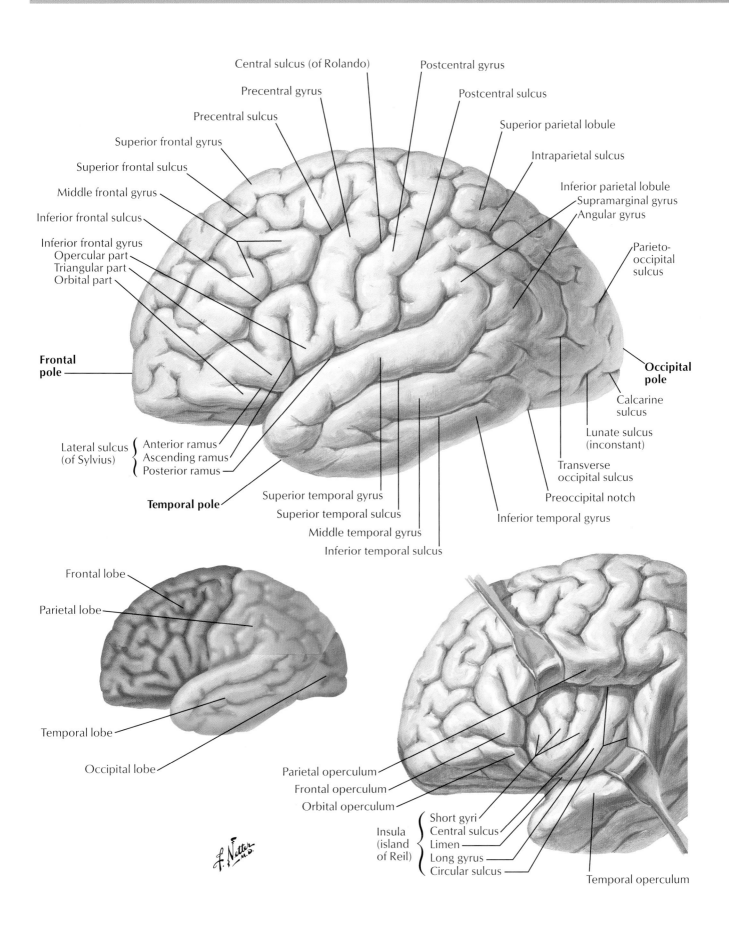

Central sulcus (of Rolando)
Precentral gyrus
Precentral sulcus
Superior frontal gyrus
Superior frontal sulcus
Middle frontal gyrus
Inferior frontal sulcus
Inferior frontal gyrus
Opercular part
Triangular part
Orbital part

Frontal pole

Lateral sulcus (of Sylvius) { Anterior ramus
Ascending ramus
Posterior ramus

Temporal pole

Postcentral gyrus
Postcentral sulcus
Superior parietal lobule
Intraparietal sulcus
Inferior parietal lobule
Supramarginal gyrus
Angular gyrus
Parieto-occipital sulcus

Occipital pole

Calcarine sulcus
Lunate sulcus (inconstant)
Transverse occipital sulcus
Preoccipital notch
Inferior temporal gyrus

Superior temporal gyrus
Superior temporal sulcus
Middle temporal gyrus
Inferior temporal sulcus

Frontal lobe
Parietal lobe
Temporal lobe
Occipital lobe

Parietal operculum
Frontal operculum
Orbital operculum

Insula (island of Reil) { Short gyri
Central sulcus
Limen
Long gyrus
Circular sulcus

Temporal operculum

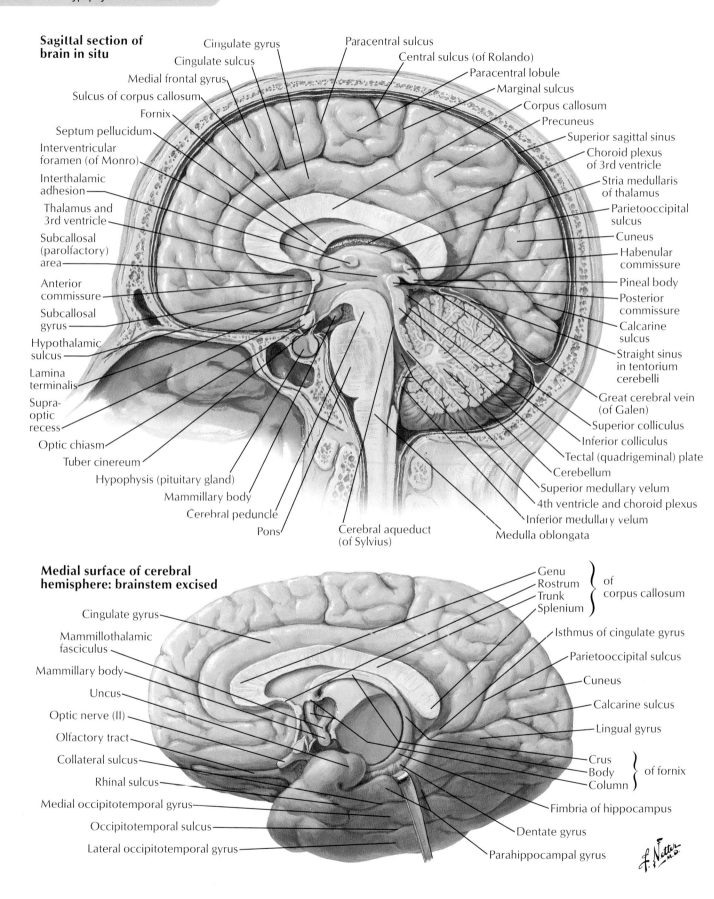

Sagittal section of brain in situ

Cingulate gyrus
Cingulate sulcus
Medial frontal gyrus
Sulcus of corpus callosum
Fornix
Septum pellucidum
Interventricular foramen (of Monro)
Interthalamic adhesion
Thalamus and 3rd ventricle
Subcallosal (parolfactory) area
Anterior commissure
Subcallosal gyrus
Hypothalamic sulcus
Lamina terminalis
Supra-optic recess
Optic chiasm
Tuber cinereum
Hypophysis (pituitary gland)
Mammillary body
Cerebral peduncle
Pons
Cerebral aqueduct (of Sylvius)

Paracentral sulcus
Central sulcus (of Rolando)
Paracentral lobule
Marginal sulcus
Corpus callosum
Precuneus
Superior sagittal sinus
Choroid plexus of 3rd ventricle
Stria medullaris of thalamus
Parietooccipital sulcus
Cuneus
Habenular commissure
Pineal body
Posterior commissure
Calcarine sulcus
Straight sinus in tentorium cerebelli
Great cerebral vein (of Galen)
Superior colliculus
Inferior colliculus
Tectal (quadrigeminal) plate
Cerebellum
Superior medullary velum
4th ventricle and choroid plexus
Inferior medullary velum
Medulla oblongata

Medial surface of cerebral hemisphere: brainstem excised

Cingulate gyrus
Mammillothalamic fasciculus
Mammillary body
Uncus
Optic nerve (II)
Olfactory tract
Collateral sulcus
Rhinal sulcus
Medial occipitotemporal gyrus
Occipitotemporal sulcus
Lateral occipitotemporal gyrus

Genu
Rostrum
Trunk
Splenium
} of corpus callosum

Isthmus of cingulate gyrus
Parietooccipital sulcus
Cuneus
Calcarine sulcus
Lingual gyrus
Crus
Body
Column
} of fornix
Fimbria of hippocampus
Dentate gyrus
Parahippocampal gyrus

Plate 106

Meninges and Brain

For hypophysis see **Plate 147**

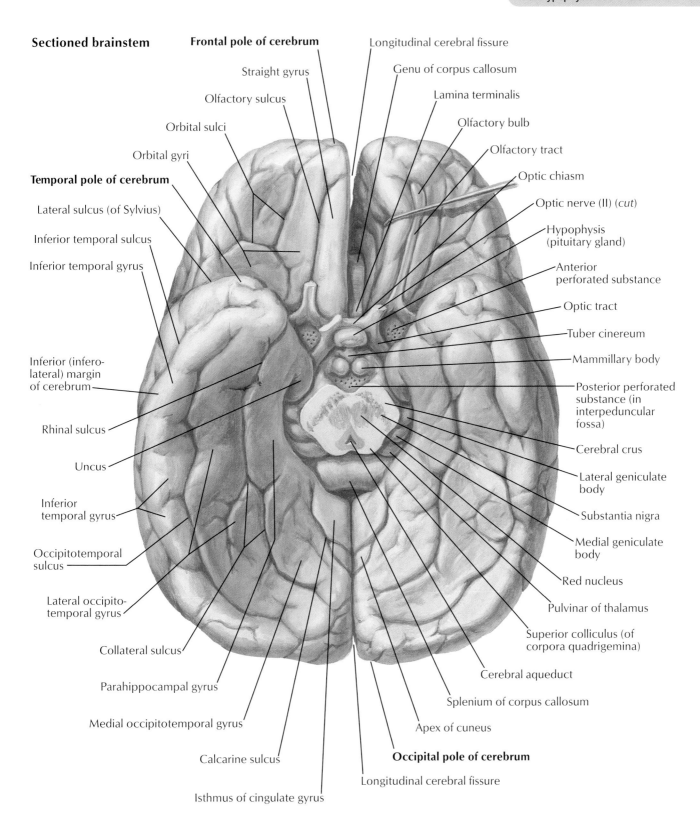

Sectioned brainstem

Frontal pole of cerebrum

Straight gyrus

Olfactory sulcus

Orbital sulci

Orbital gyri

Temporal pole of cerebrum

Lateral sulcus (of Sylvius)

Inferior temporal sulcus

Inferior temporal gyrus

Inferior (infero-lateral) margin of cerebrum

Rhinal sulcus

Uncus

Inferior temporal gyrus

Occipitotemporal sulcus

Lateral occipito-temporal gyrus

Collateral sulcus

Parahippocampal gyrus

Medial occipitotemporal gyrus

Calcarine sulcus

Isthmus of cingulate gyrus

Longitudinal cerebral fissure

Genu of corpus callosum

Lamina terminalis

Olfactory bulb

Olfactory tract

Optic chiasm

Optic nerve (II) (cut)

Hypophysis (pituitary gland)

Anterior perforated substance

Optic tract

Tuber cinereum

Mammillary body

Posterior perforated substance (in interpeduncular fossa)

Cerebral crus

Lateral geniculate body

Substantia nigra

Medial geniculate body

Red nucleus

Pulvinar of thalamus

Superior colliculus (of corpora quadrigemina)

Cerebral aqueduct

Splenium of corpus callosum

Apex of cuneus

Occipital pole of cerebrum

Longitudinal cerebral fissure

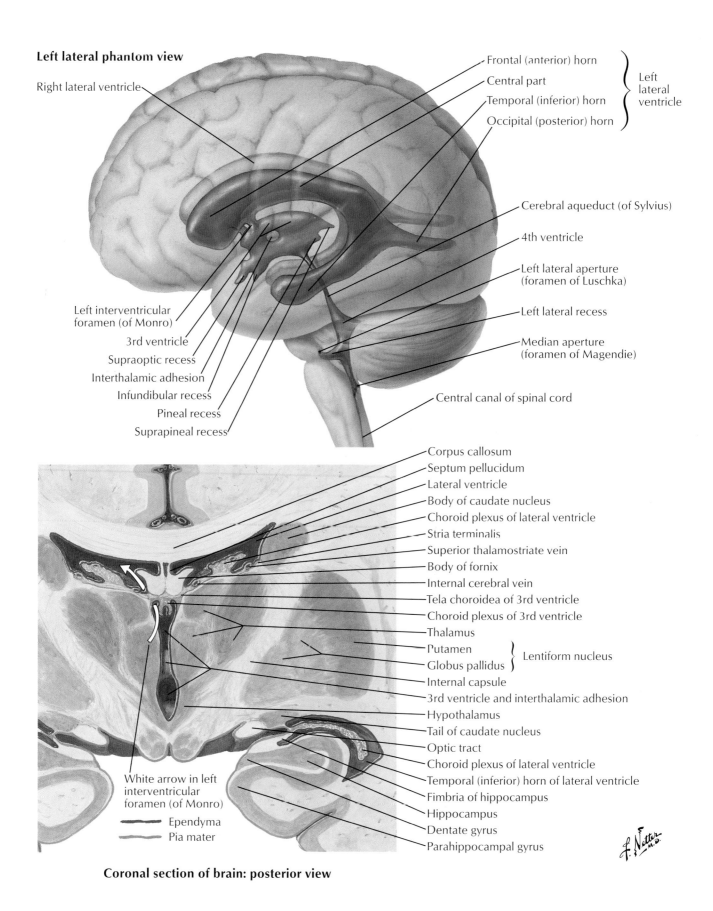

Left lateral phantom view

Right lateral ventricle

Frontal (anterior) horn

Central part

Temporal (inferior) horn

Occipital (posterior) horn

Left lateral ventricle

Cerebral aqueduct (of Sylvius)

4th ventricle

Left lateral aperture (foramen of Luschka)

Left lateral recess

Median aperture (foramen of Magendie)

Left interventricular foramen (of Monro)

3rd ventricle

Supraoptic recess

Interthalamic adhesion

Infundibular recess

Pineal recess

Suprapineal recess

Central canal of spinal cord

Corpus callosum

Septum pellucidum

Lateral ventricle

Body of caudate nucleus

Choroid plexus of lateral ventricle

Stria terminalis

Superior thalamostriate vein

Body of fornix

Internal cerebral vein

Tela choroidea of 3rd ventricle

Choroid plexus of 3rd ventricle

Thalamus

Putamen

Globus pallidus

Lentiform nucleus

Internal capsule

3rd ventricle and interthalamic adhesion

Hypothalamus

Tail of caudate nucleus

Optic tract

Choroid plexus of lateral ventricle

Temporal (inferior) horn of lateral ventricle

Fimbria of hippocampus

Hippocampus

Dentate gyrus

Parahippocampal gyrus

White arrow in left interventricular foramen (of Monro)

Ependyma

Pia mater

Coronal section of brain: posterior view

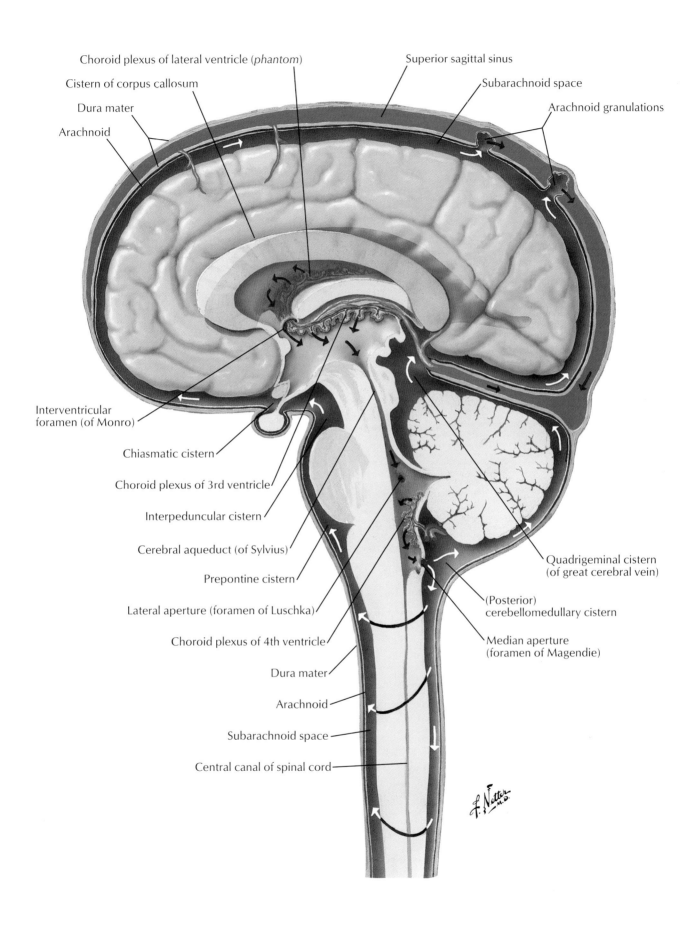

Choroid plexus of lateral ventricle (*phantom*)

Cistern of corpus callosum

Dura mater

Arachnoid

Superior sagittal sinus

Subarachnoid space

Arachnoid granulations

Interventricular foramen (of Monro)

Chiasmatic cistern

Choroid plexus of 3rd ventricle

Interpeduncular cistern

Cerebral aqueduct (of Sylvius)

Prepontine cistern

Lateral aperture (foramen of Luschka)

Choroid plexus of 4th ventricle

Dura mater

Arachnoid

Subarachnoid space

Central canal of spinal cord

Quadrigeminal cistern (of great cerebral vein)

(Posterior) cerebellomedullary cistern

Median aperture (foramen of Magendie)

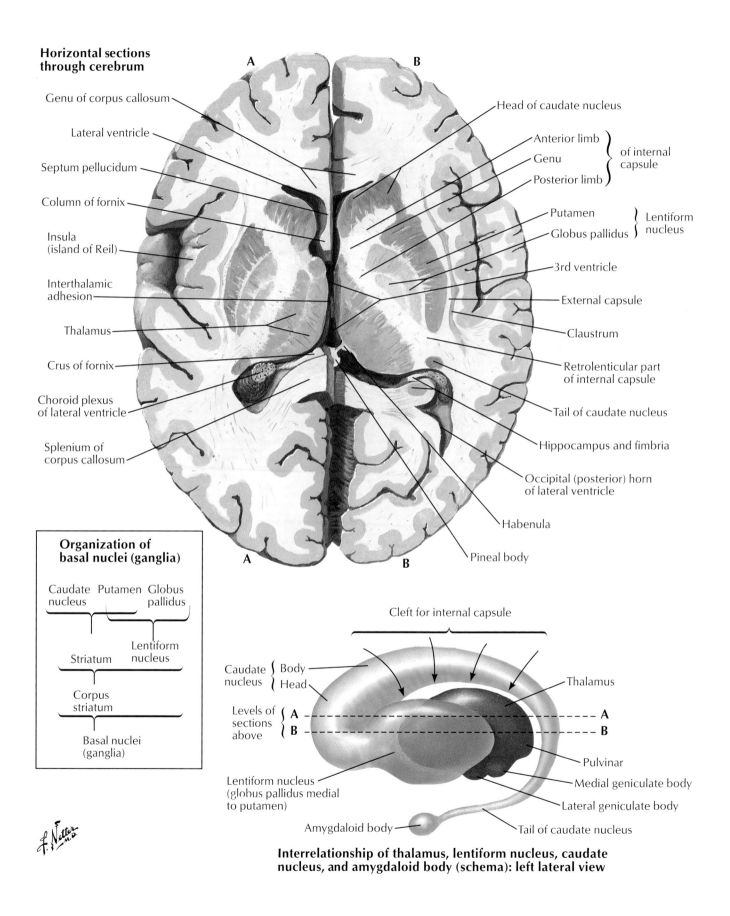

Horizontal sections through cerebrum

A   B

Genu of corpus callosum

Lateral ventricle

Septum pellucidum

Column of fornix

Insula (island of Reil)

Interthalamic adhesion

Thalamus

Crus of fornix

Choroid plexus of lateral ventricle

Splenium of corpus callosum

Head of caudate nucleus

Anterior limb
Genu
Posterior limb
} of internal capsule

Putamen
Globus pallidus
} Lentiform nucleus

3rd ventricle

External capsule

Claustrum

Retrolenticular part of internal capsule

Tail of caudate nucleus

Hippocampus and fimbria

Occipital (posterior) horn of lateral ventricle

Habenula

Pineal body

A   B

Organization of basal nuclei (ganglia)

Caudate nucleus   Putamen   Globus pallidus

Lentiform nucleus

Striatum

Corpus striatum

Basal nuclei (ganglia)

Cleft for internal capsule

Caudate nucleus { Body
{ Head

Levels of sections above { A
{ B

Lentiform nucleus (globus pallidus medial to putamen)

Amygdaloid body

Thalamus

A

B

Pulvinar

Medial geniculate body

Lateral geniculate body

Tail of caudate nucleus

Interrelationship of thalamus, lentiform nucleus, caudate nucleus, and amygdaloid body (schema): left lateral view

Plate 110　　　　　　　　　　　　**Meninges and Brain**

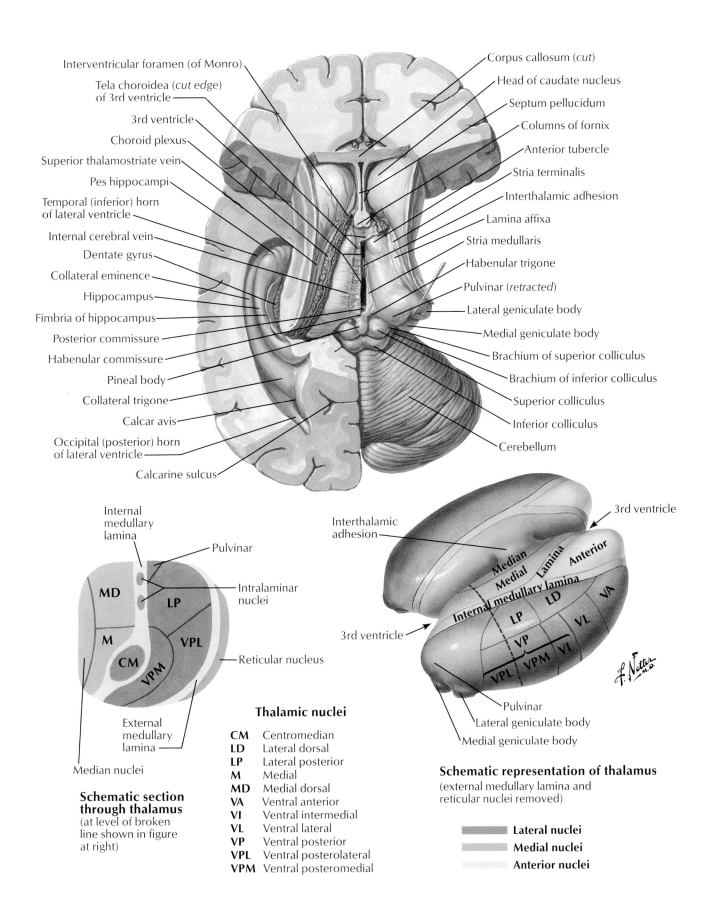

Interventricular foramen (of Monro)

Tela choroidea (*cut edge*) of 3rd ventricle

3rd ventricle

Choroid plexus

Superior thalamostriate vein

Pes hippocampi

Temporal (inferior) horn of lateral ventricle

Internal cerebral vein

Dentate gyrus

Collateral eminence

Hippocampus

Fimbria of hippocampus

Posterior commissure

Habenular commissure

Pineal body

Collateral trigone

Calcar avis

Occipital (posterior) horn of lateral ventricle

Calcarine sulcus

Corpus callosum (*cut*)

Head of caudate nucleus

Septum pellucidum

Columns of fornix

Anterior tubercle

Stria terminalis

Interthalamic adhesion

Lamina affixa

Stria medullaris

Habenular trigone

Pulvinar (*retracted*)

Lateral geniculate body

Medial geniculate body

Brachium of superior colliculus

Brachium of inferior colliculus

Superior colliculus

Inferior colliculus

Cerebellum

Internal medullary lamina

Pulvinar

Intralaminar nuclei

Reticular nucleus

MD

LP

M

VPL

CM

VPM

External medullary lamina

Median nuclei

Schematic section through thalamus (at level of broken line shown in figure at right)

Thalamic nuclei

CM	Centromedian
LD	Lateral dorsal
LP	Lateral posterior
M	Medial
MD	Medial dorsal
VA	Ventral anterior
VI	Ventral intermedial
VL	Ventral lateral
VP	Ventral posterior
VPL	Ventral posterolateral
VPM	Ventral posteromedial

Interthalamic adhesion

3rd ventricle

3rd ventricle

Median

Medial

Anterior

Lamina

Internal medullary lamina

LP

LD

VA

VP

VL

VPL

VPM

VI

Pulvinar

Lateral geniculate body

Medial geniculate body

Schematic representation of thalamus (external medullary lamina and reticular nuclei removed)

Lateral nuclei

Medial nuclei

Anterior nuclei

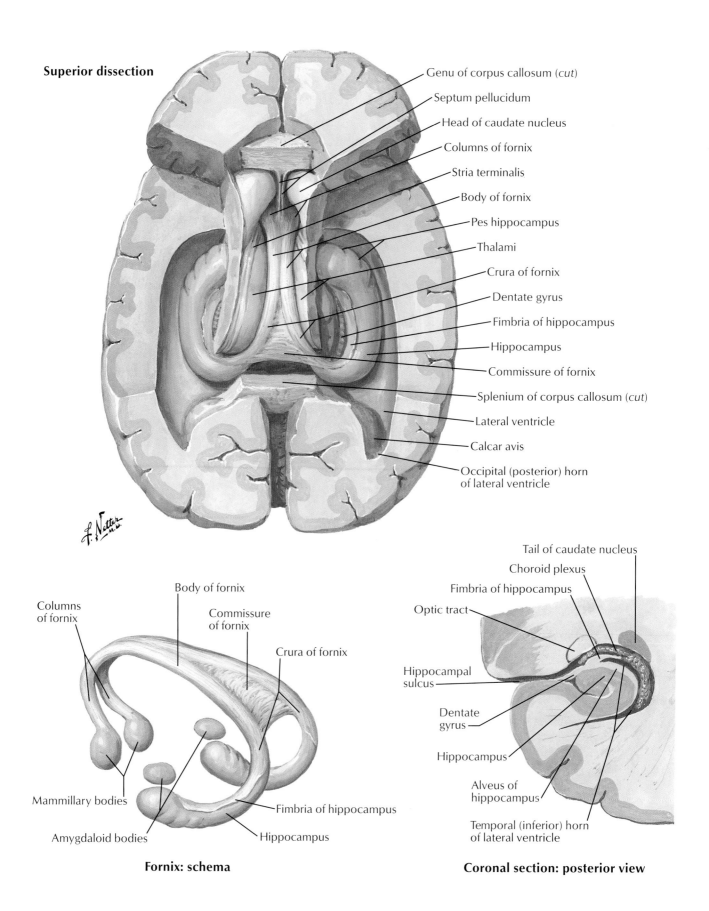

Superior dissection

Genu of corpus callosum (*cut*)

Septum pellucidum

Head of caudate nucleus

Columns of fornix

Stria terminalis

Body of fornix

Pes hippocampus

Thalami

Crura of fornix

Dentate gyrus

Fimbria of hippocampus

Hippocampus

Commissure of fornix

Splenium of corpus callosum (*cut*)

Lateral ventricle

Calcar avis

Occipital (posterior) horn of lateral ventricle

Columns of fornix

Body of fornix

Commissure of fornix

Crura of fornix

Mammillary bodies

Amygdaloid bodies

Fimbria of hippocampus

Hippocampus

Fornix: schema

Tail of caudate nucleus

Choroid plexus

Fimbria of hippocampus

Optic tract

Hippocampal sulcus

Dentate gyrus

Hippocampus

Alveus of hippocampus

Temporal (inferior) horn of lateral ventricle

Coronal section: posterior view

Plate 112   **Meninges and Brain**

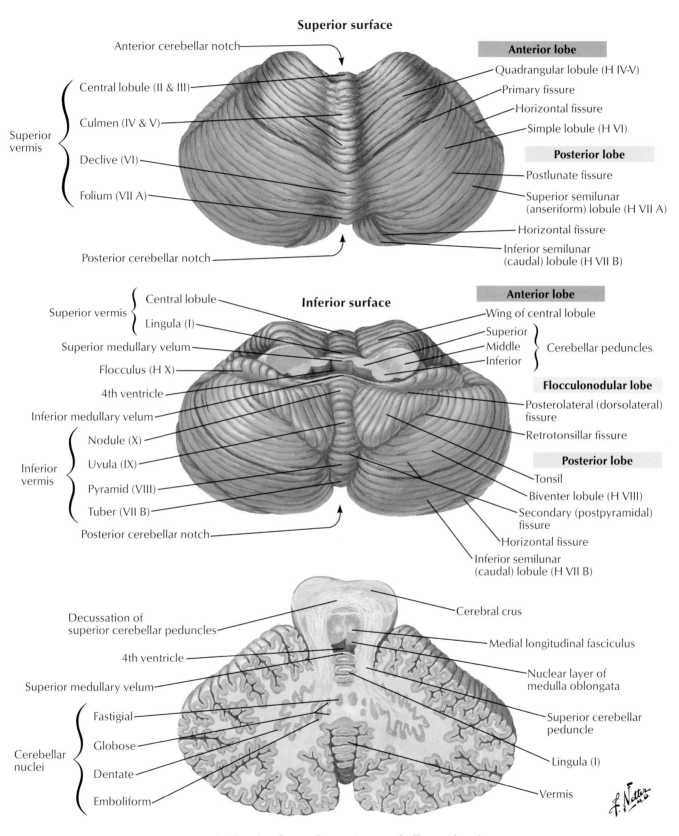

Superior surface

Anterior cerebellar notch

Anterior lobe

Central lobule (II & III)

Culmen (IV & V)

Declive (VI)

Folium (VII A)

Superior vermis

Quadrangular lobule (H IV-V)

Primary fissure

Horizontal fissure

Simple lobule (H VI)

Posterior lobe

Postlunate fissure

Superior semilunar (anseriform) lobule (H VII A)

Horizontal fissure

Inferior semilunar (caudal) lobule (H VII B)

Posterior cerebellar notch

Inferior surface

Superior vermis

Central lobule

Lingula (I)

Superior medullary velum

Flocculus (H X)

4th ventricle

Inferior medullary velum

Inferior vermis

Nodule (X)

Uvula (IX)

Pyramid (VIII)

Tuber (VII B)

Posterior cerebellar notch

Anterior lobe

Wing of central lobule

Superior

Middle

Inferior

Cerebellar peduncles

Flocculonodular lobe

Posterolateral (dorsolateral) fissure

Retrotonsillar fissure

Posterior lobe

Tonsil

Biventer lobule (H VIII)

Secondary (postpyramidal) fissure

Horizontal fissure

Inferior semilunar (caudal) lobule (H VII B)

Decussation of superior cerebellar peduncles

4th ventricle

Superior medullary velum

Cerebellar nuclei

Fastigial

Globose

Dentate

Emboliform

Cerebral crus

Medial longitudinal fasciculus

Nuclear layer of medulla oblongata

Superior cerebellar peduncle

Lingula (I)

Vermis

Section in plane of superior cerebellar peduncle

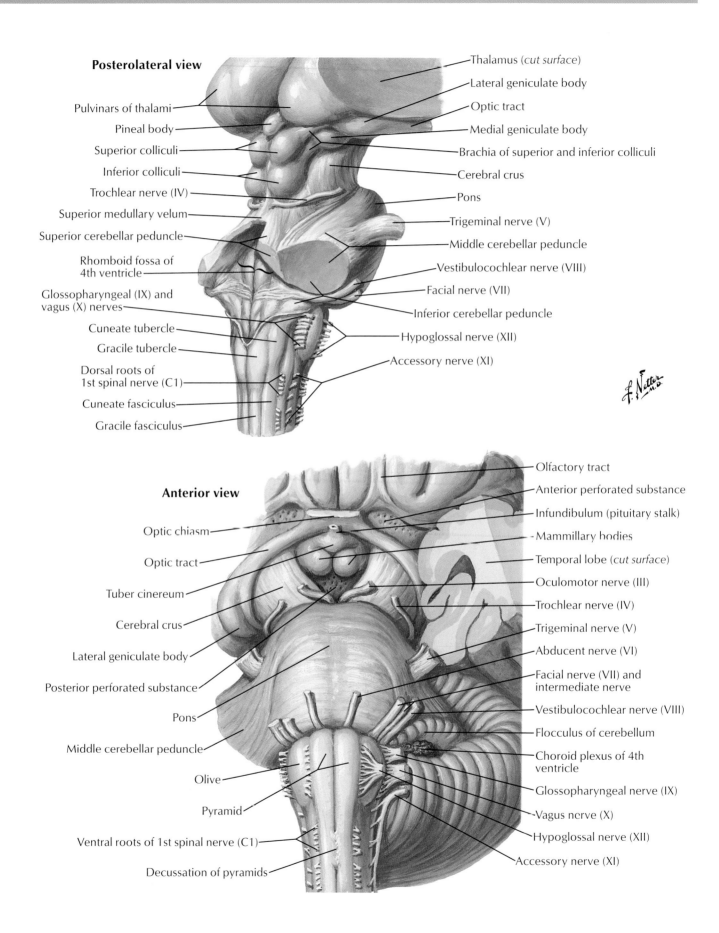

Posterolateral view

Thalamus (*cut surface*)

Pulvinars of thalami

Lateral geniculate body

Pineal body

Optic tract

Superior colliculi

Medial geniculate body

Inferior colliculi

Brachia of superior and inferior colliculi

Trochlear nerve (IV)

Cerebral crus

Superior medullary velum

Pons

Superior cerebellar peduncle

Trigeminal nerve (V)

Rhomboid fossa of 4th ventricle

Middle cerebellar peduncle

Glossopharyngeal (IX) and vagus (X) nerves

Vestibulocochlear nerve (VIII)

Facial nerve (VII)

Cuneate tubercle

Inferior cerebellar peduncle

Gracile tubercle

Hypoglossal nerve (XII)

Dorsal roots of 1st spinal nerve (C1)

Accessory nerve (XI)

Cuneate fasciculus

Gracile fasciculus

Anterior view

Olfactory tract

Anterior perforated substance

Infundibulum (pituitary stalk)

Optic chiasm

Mammillary bodies

Optic tract

Temporal lobe (*cut surface*)

Tuber cinereum

Oculomotor nerve (III)

Cerebral crus

Trochlear nerve (IV)

Trigeminal nerve (V)

Lateral geniculate body

Abducent nerve (VI)

Posterior perforated substance

Facial nerve (VII) and intermediate nerve

Pons

Vestibulocochlear nerve (VIII)

Middle cerebellar peduncle

Flocculus of cerebellum

Olive

Choroid plexus of 4th ventricle

Pyramid

Glossopharyngeal nerve (IX)

Ventral roots of 1st spinal nerve (C1)

Vagus nerve (X)

Hypoglossal nerve (XII)

Decussation of pyramids

Accessory nerve (XI)

Plate 114   **Meninges and Brain**

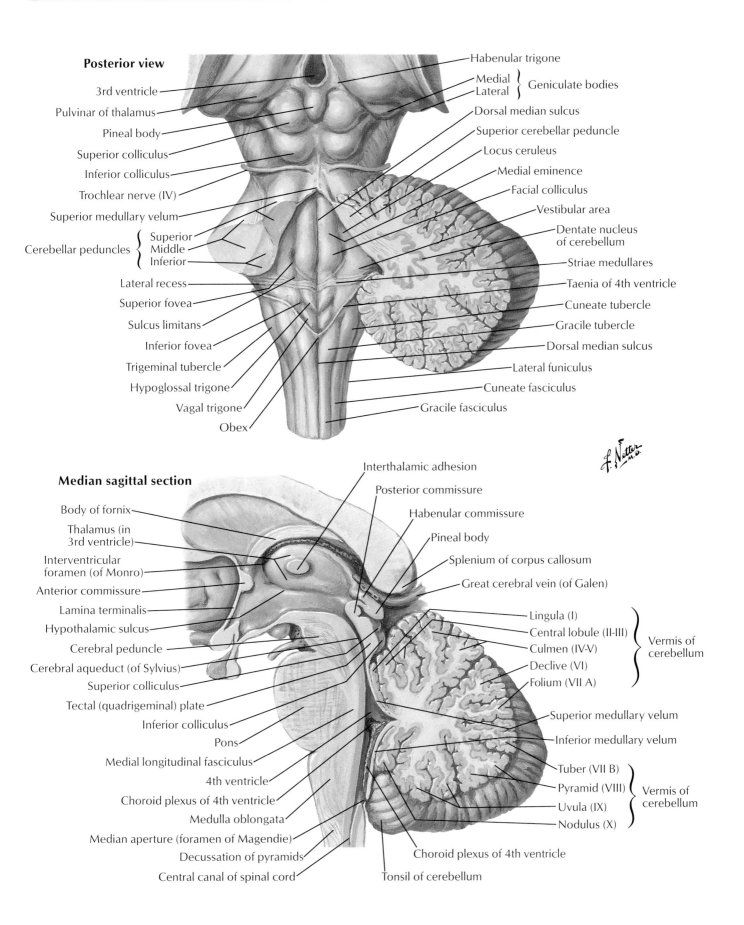

Posterior view

3rd ventricle
Pulvinar of thalamus
Pineal body
Superior colliculus
Inferior colliculus
Trochlear nerve (IV)
Superior medullary velum
Cerebellar peduncles { Superior
Middle
Inferior
Lateral recess
Superior fovea
Sulcus limitans
Inferior fovea
Trigeminal tubercle
Hypoglossal trigone
Vagal trigone
Obex

Habenular trigone
Medial } Geniculate bodies
Lateral
Dorsal median sulcus
Superior cerebellar peduncle
Locus ceruleus
Medial eminence
Facial colliculus
Vestibular area
Dentate nucleus of cerebellum
Striae medullares
Taenia of 4th ventricle
Cuneate tubercle
Gracile tubercle
Dorsal median sulcus
Lateral funiculus
Cuneate fasciculus
Gracile fasciculus

Median sagittal section

Body of fornix
Thalamus (in 3rd ventricle)
Interventricular foramen (of Monro)
Anterior commissure
Lamina terminalis
Hypothalamic sulcus
Cerebral peduncle
Cerebral aqueduct (of Sylvius)
Superior colliculus
Tectal (quadrigeminal) plate
Inferior colliculus
Pons
Medial longitudinal fasciculus
4th ventricle
Choroid plexus of 4th ventricle
Medulla oblongata
Median aperture (foramen of Magendie)
Decussation of pyramids
Central canal of spinal cord

Interthalamic adhesion
Posterior commissure
Habenular commissure
Pineal body
Splenium of corpus callosum
Great cerebral vein (of Galen)
Lingula (I)
Central lobule (II-III) } Vermis of cerebellum
Culmen (IV-V)
Declive (VI)
Folium (VII A)
Superior medullary velum
Inferior medullary velum
Tuber (VII B)
Pyramid (VIII) } Vermis of cerebellum
Uvula (IX)
Nodulus (X)
Choroid plexus of 4th ventricle
Tonsil of cerebellum

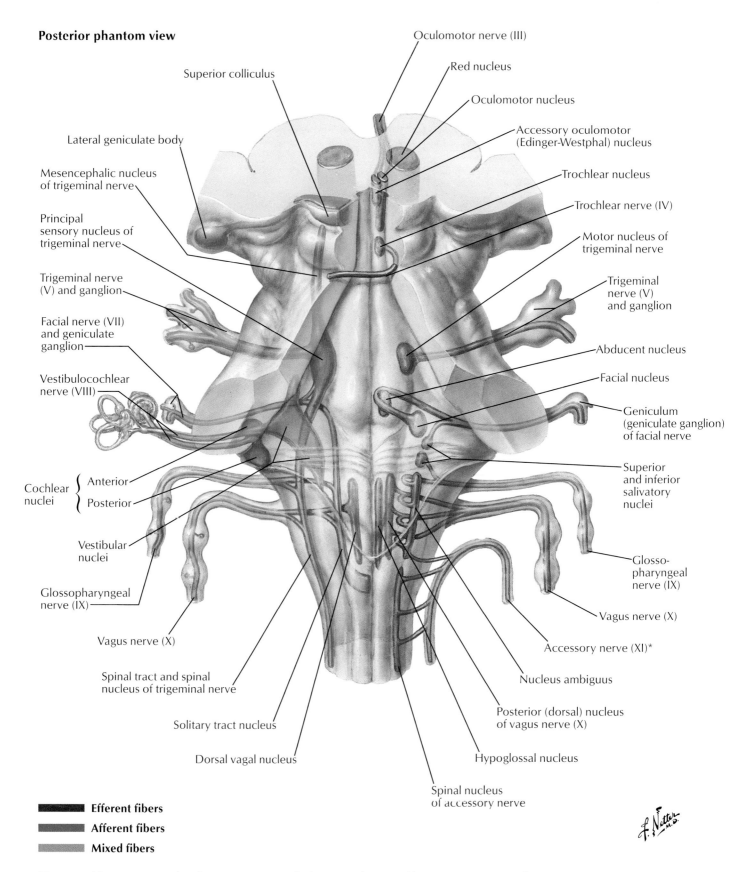

Posterior phantom view

Oculomotor nerve (III)

Superior colliculus

Red nucleus

Oculomotor nucleus

Lateral geniculate body

Accessory oculomotor (Edinger-Westphal) nucleus

Mesencephalic nucleus of trigeminal nerve

Trochlear nucleus

Principal sensory nucleus of trigeminal nerve

Trochlear nerve (IV)

Motor nucleus of trigeminal nerve

Trigeminal nerve (V) and ganglion

Trigeminal nerve (V) and ganglion

Facial nerve (VII) and geniculate ganglion

Abducent nucleus

Facial nucleus

Vestibulocochlear nerve (VIII)

Geniculum (geniculate ganglion) of facial nerve

Cochlear nuclei { Anterior / Posterior

Superior and inferior salivatory nuclei

Vestibular nuclei

Glosso-pharyngeal nerve (IX)

Glossopharyngeal nerve (IX)

Vagus nerve (X)

Vagus nerve (X)

Accessory nerve (XI)*

Spinal tract and spinal nucleus of trigeminal nerve

Nucleus ambiguus

Posterior (dorsal) nucleus of vagus nerve (X)

Solitary tract nucleus

Dorsal vagal nucleus

Hypoglossal nucleus

Spinal nucleus of accessory nerve

▬▬▬ **Efferent fibers**

▬▬▬ **Afferent fibers**

▬▬▬ **Mixed fibers**

*Recent evidence suggests that the accessory nerve lacks a cranial root and has no connection to the vagus nerve. Verification of this finding awaits further investigation.

Plate 116   **Cranial and Cervical Nerves**

Medial dissection

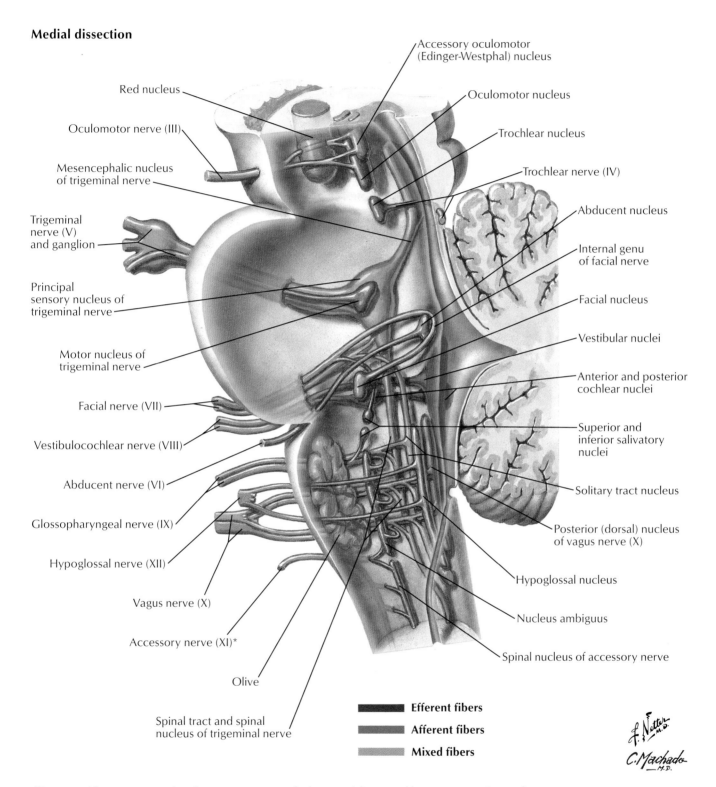

Accessory oculomotor (Edinger-Westphal) nucleus

Oculomotor nucleus

Trochlear nucleus

Red nucleus

Oculomotor nerve (III)

Mesencephalic nucleus of trigeminal nerve

Trochlear nerve (IV)

Abducent nucleus

Trigeminal nerve (V) and ganglion

Internal genu of facial nerve

Principal sensory nucleus of trigeminal nerve

Facial nucleus

Vestibular nuclei

Motor nucleus of trigeminal nerve

Anterior and posterior cochlear nuclei

Facial nerve (VII)

Vestibulocochlear nerve (VIII)

Superior and inferior salivatory nuclei

Abducent nerve (VI)

Solitary tract nucleus

Glossopharyngeal nerve (IX)

Posterior (dorsal) nucleus of vagus nerve (X)

Hypoglossal nerve (XII)

Hypoglossal nucleus

Vagus nerve (X)

Nucleus ambiguus

Accessory nerve (XI)*

Spinal nucleus of accessory nerve

Olive

Spinal tract and spinal nucleus of trigeminal nerve

▬▬ **Efferent fibers**
▬▬ **Afferent fibers**
▬▬ **Mixed fibers**

*Recent evidence suggests that the accessory nerve lacks a cranial root and has no connection to the vagus nerve. Verification of this finding awaits further investigation.

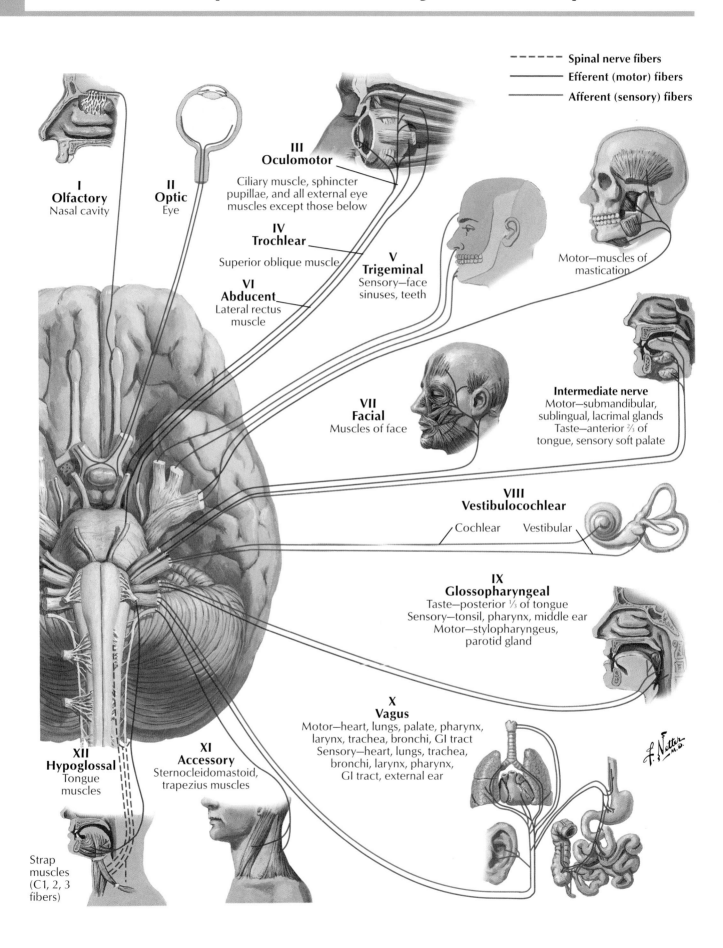

Spinal nerve fibers
Efferent (motor) fibers
Afferent (sensory) fibers

I Olfactory
Nasal cavity

II Optic
Eye

III Oculomotor
Ciliary muscle, sphincter pupillae, and all external eye muscles except those below

IV Trochlear
Superior oblique muscle

V Trigeminal
Sensory—face sinuses, teeth

VI Abducent
Lateral rectus muscle

Motor—muscles of mastication

VII Facial
Muscles of face

Intermediate nerve
Motor—submandibular, sublingual, lacrimal glands
Taste—anterior ⅔ of tongue, sensory soft palate

VIII Vestibulocochlear
Cochlear   Vestibular

IX Glossopharyngeal
Taste—posterior ⅓ of tongue
Sensory—tonsil, pharynx, middle ear
Motor—stylopharyngeus, parotid gland

X Vagus
Motor—heart, lungs, palate, pharynx, larynx, trachea, bronchi, GI tract
Sensory—heart, lungs, trachea, bronchi, larynx, pharynx, GI tract, external ear

XII Hypoglossal
Tongue muscles

XI Accessory
Sternocleidomastoid, trapezius muscles

Strap muscles (C1, 2, 3 fibers)

F. Netter M.D.

Plate 118   **Cranial and Cervical Nerves**

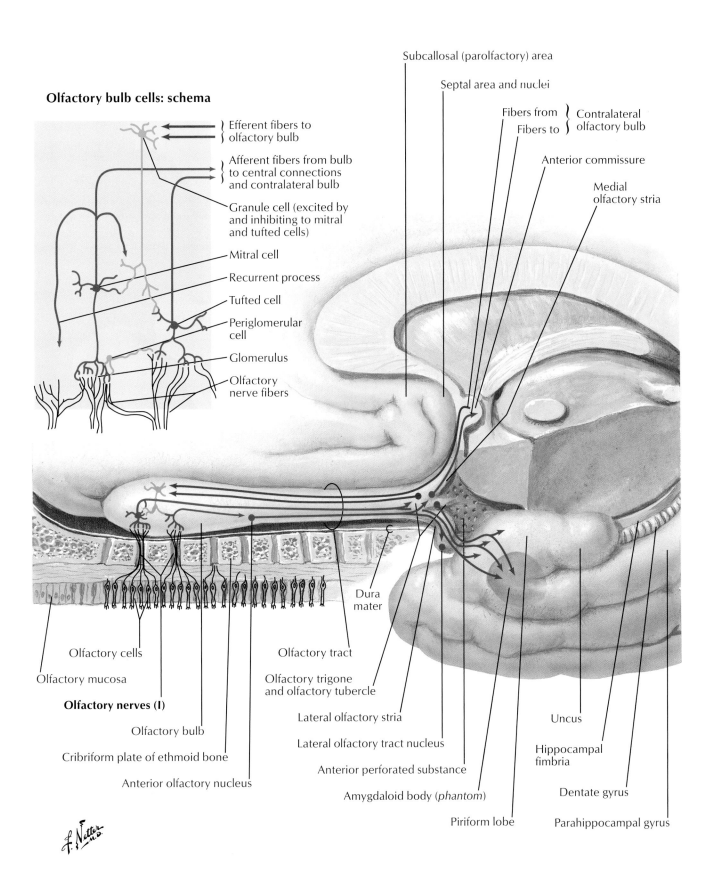

Olfactory bulb cells: schema

} Efferent fibers to olfactory bulb

} Afferent fibers from bulb to central connections and contralateral bulb

Granule cell (excited by and inhibiting to mitral and tufted cells)

Mitral cell

Recurrent process

Tufted cell

Periglomerular cell

Glomerulus

Olfactory nerve fibers

Subcallosal (parolfactory) area

Septal area and nuclei

Fibers from } Contralateral
Fibers to } olfactory bulb

Anterior commissure

Medial olfactory stria

Dura mater

Olfactory cells

Olfactory mucosa

Olfactory nerves (I)

Olfactory bulb

Cribriform plate of ethmoid bone

Anterior olfactory nucleus

Olfactory tract

Olfactory trigone and olfactory tubercle

Lateral olfactory stria

Lateral olfactory tract nucleus

Anterior perforated substance

Amygdaloid body (*phantom*)

Piriform lobe

Uncus

Hippocampal fimbria

Dentate gyrus

Parahippocampal gyrus

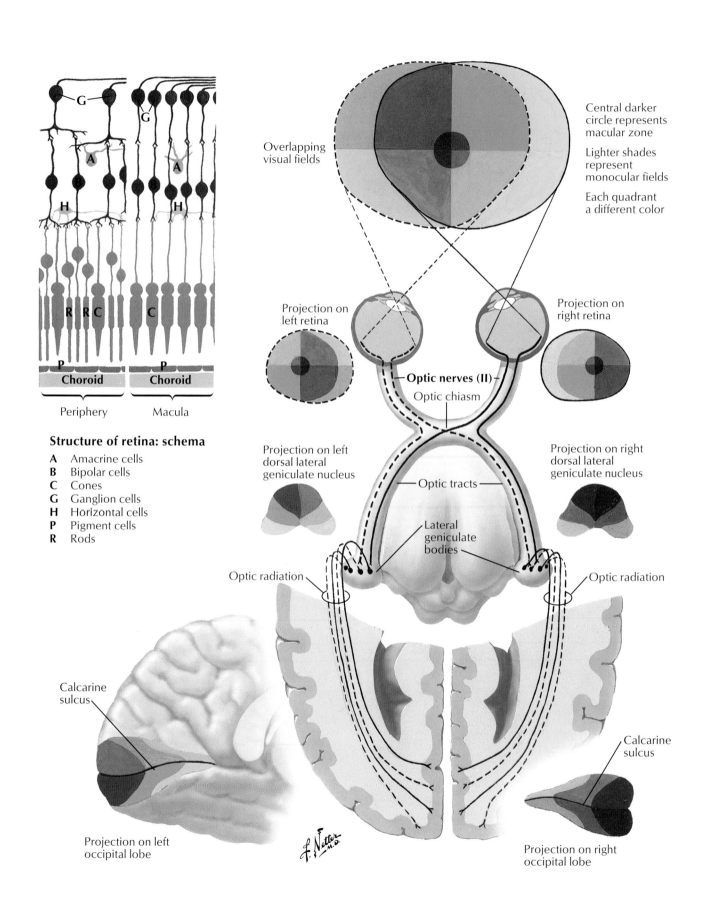

Structure of retina: schema

A Amacrine cells
B Bipolar cells
C Cones
G Ganglion cells
H Horizontal cells
P Pigment cells
R Rods

Periphery   Macula

Overlapping visual fields

Central darker circle represents macular zone

Lighter shades represent monocular fields

Each quadrant a different color

Projection on left retina

Projection on right retina

Optic nerves (II)
Optic chiasm

Projection on left dorsal lateral geniculate nucleus

Projection on right dorsal lateral geniculate nucleus

Optic tracts

Lateral geniculate bodies

Optic radiation

Optic radiation

Calcarine sulcus

Calcarine sulcus

Projection on left occipital lobe

Projection on right occipital lobe

Plate 120   **Cranial and Cervical Nerves**

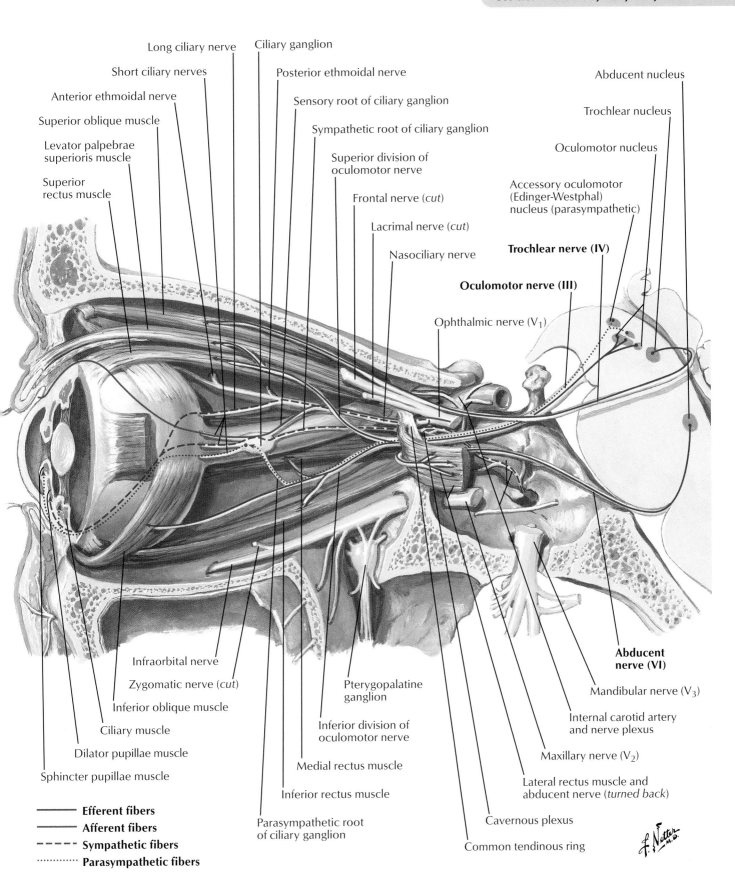

Long ciliary nerve
Short ciliary nerves
Anterior ethmoidal nerve
Superior oblique muscle
Levator palpebrae superioris muscle
Superior rectus muscle
Ciliary ganglion
Posterior ethmoidal nerve
Sensory root of ciliary ganglion
Sympathetic root of ciliary ganglion
Superior division of oculomotor nerve
Frontal nerve (cut)
Lacrimal nerve (cut)
Nasociliary nerve
Abducent nucleus
Trochlear nucleus
Oculomotor nucleus
Accessory oculomotor (Edinger-Westphal) nucleus (parasympathetic)
Trochlear nerve (IV)
Oculomotor nerve (III)
Ophthalmic nerve (V$_1$)

Infraorbital nerve
Zygomatic nerve (cut)
Inferior oblique muscle
Ciliary muscle
Dilator pupillae muscle
Sphincter pupillae muscle
Pterygopalatine ganglion
Inferior division of oculomotor nerve
Medial rectus muscle
Inferior rectus muscle
Parasympathetic root of ciliary ganglion
Abducent nerve (VI)
Mandibular nerve (V$_3$)
Internal carotid artery and nerve plexus
Maxillary nerve (V$_2$)
Lateral rectus muscle and abducent nerve (turned back)
Cavernous plexus
Common tendinous ring

———— **Efferent fibers**
———— **Afferent fibers**
– – – – **Sympathetic fibers**
·········· **Parasympathetic fibers**

Trigeminal Nerve (V): Schema

See also **Plates 24, 42, 43, 45, 46, 167, 168**

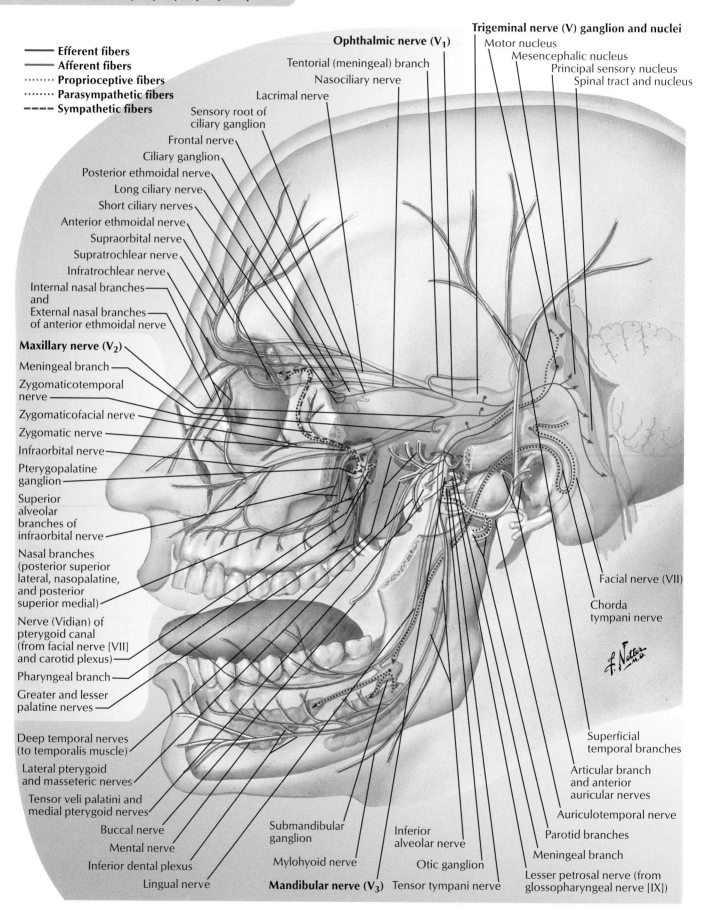

—— **Efferent fibers**
—— **Afferent fibers**
······· **Proprioceptive fibers**
········ **Parasympathetic fibers**
---- **Sympathetic fibers**

Trigeminal nerve (V) ganglion and nuclei
Motor nucleus
Mesencephalic nucleus
Principal sensory nucleus
Spinal tract and nucleus

Ophthalmic nerve (V₁)
Tentorial (meningeal) branch
Nasociliary nerve
Lacrimal nerve

Sensory root of ciliary ganglion
Frontal nerve
Ciliary ganglion
Posterior ethmoidal nerve
Long ciliary nerve
Short ciliary nerves
Anterior ethmoidal nerve
Supraorbital nerve
Supratrochlear nerve
Infratrochlear nerve
Internal nasal branches and
External nasal branches of anterior ethmoidal nerve

Maxillary nerve (V₂)
Meningeal branch
Zygomaticotemporal nerve
Zygomaticofacial nerve
Zygomatic nerve
Infraorbital nerve
Pterygopalatine ganglion
Superior alveolar branches of infraorbital nerve
Nasal branches (posterior superior lateral, nasopalatine, and posterior superior medial)
Nerve (Vidian) of pterygoid canal (from facial nerve [VII] and carotid plexus)
Pharyngeal branch
Greater and lesser palatine nerves

Deep temporal nerves (to temporalis muscle)
Lateral pterygoid and masseteric nerves
Tensor veli palatini and medial pterygoid nerves
Buccal nerve
Mental nerve
Inferior dental plexus
Lingual nerve

Submandibular ganglion
Mylohyoid nerve
Mandibular nerve (V₃)

Inferior alveolar nerve
Otic ganglion
Tensor tympani nerve

Facial nerve (VII)
Chorda tympani nerve

Superficial temporal branches
Articular branch and anterior auricular nerves
Auriculotemporal nerve
Parotid branches
Meningeal branch
Lesser petrosal nerve (from glossopharyngeal nerve [IX])

F. Netter M.D.

Plate 122

Cranial and Cervical Nerves

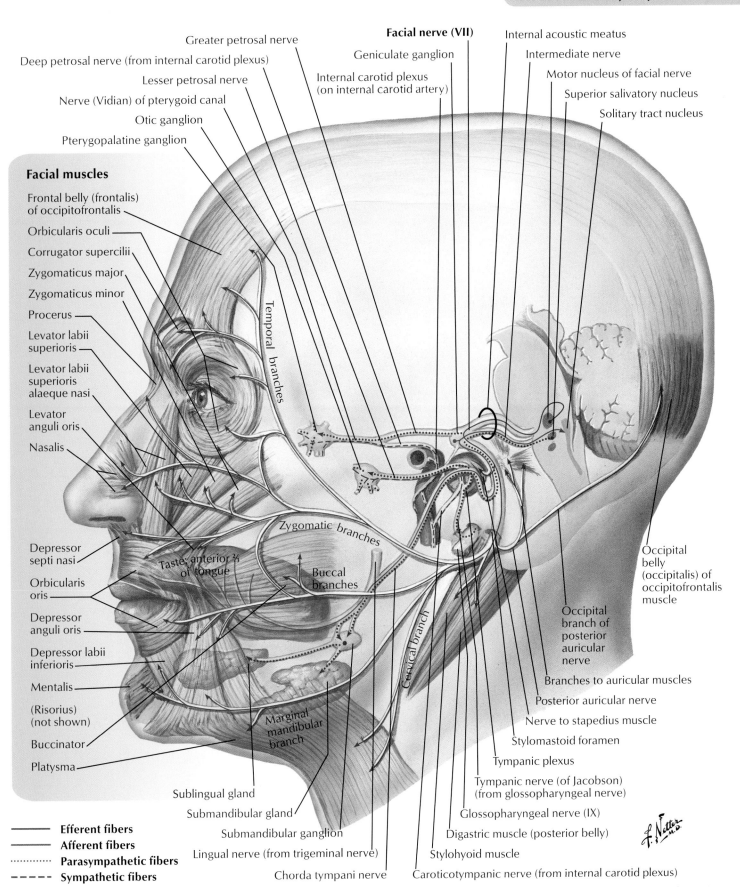

Greater petrosal nerve

Deep petrosal nerve (from internal carotid plexus)

Lesser petrosal nerve

Nerve (Vidian) of pterygoid canal

Otic ganglion

Pterygopalatine ganglion

Facial nerve (VII)

Geniculate ganglion

Internal carotid plexus (on internal carotid artery)

Internal acoustic meatus

Intermediate nerve

Motor nucleus of facial nerve

Superior salivatory nucleus

Solitary tract nucleus

Facial muscles

Frontal belly (frontalis) of occipitofrontalis

Orbicularis oculi

Corrugator supercilii

Zygomaticus major

Zygomaticus minor

Procerus

Levator labii superioris

Levator labii superioris alaeque nasi

Levator anguli oris

Nasalis

Depressor septi nasi

Orbicularis oris

Depressor anguli oris

Depressor labii inferioris

Mentalis

(Risorius) (not shown)

Buccinator

Platysma

Temporal branches

Zygomatic branches

Taste: anterior ⅔ of tongue

Buccal branches

Cervical branch

Marginal mandibular branch

Sublingual gland

Submandibular gland

Submandibular ganglion

Lingual nerve (from trigeminal nerve)

Chorda tympani nerve

Occipital belly (occipitalis) of occipitofrontalis muscle

Occipital branch of posterior auricular nerve

Branches to auricular muscles

Posterior auricular nerve

Nerve to stapedius muscle

Stylomastoid foramen

Tympanic plexus

Tympanic nerve (of Jacobson) (from glossopharyngeal nerve)

Glossopharyngeal nerve (IX)

Digastric muscle (posterior belly)

Stylohyoid muscle

Caroticotympanic nerve (from internal carotid plexus)

—— **Efferent fibers**

—— **Afferent fibers**

·········· **Parasympathetic fibers**

----- **Sympathetic fibers**

Vestibulocochlear Nerve (VIII): Schema

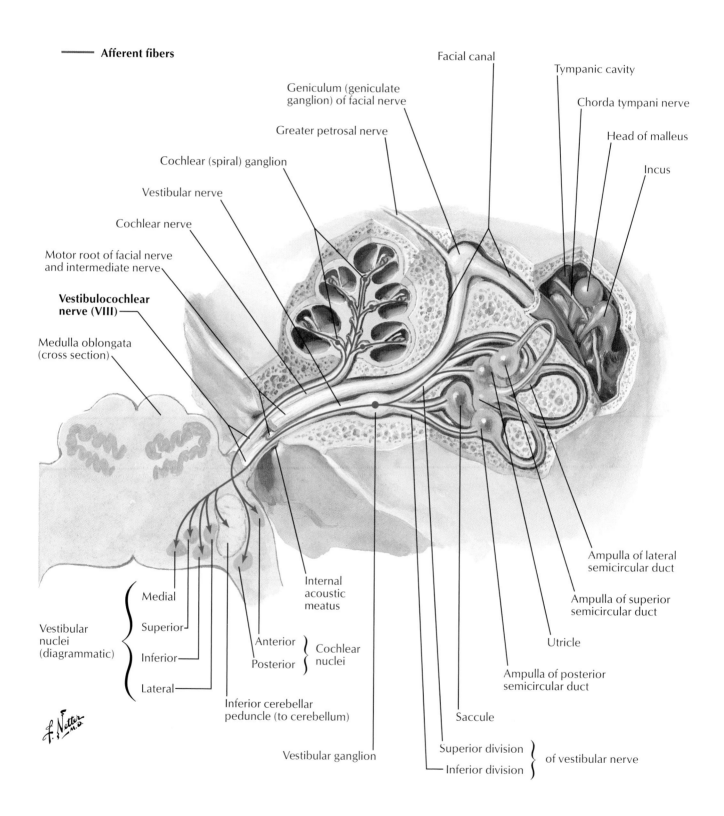

—— Afferent fibers

Facial canal

Tympanic cavity

Geniculum (geniculate ganglion) of facial nerve

Chorda tympani nerve

Greater petrosal nerve

Head of malleus

Cochlear (spiral) ganglion

Incus

Vestibular nerve

Cochlear nerve

Motor root of facial nerve and intermediate nerve

Vestibulocochlear nerve (VIII)

Medulla oblongata (cross section)

Ampulla of lateral semicircular duct

Ampulla of superior semicircular duct

Medial

Utricle

Superior

Vestibular nuclei (diagrammatic)

Internal acoustic meatus

Anterior

Inferior

Cochlear nuclei

Posterior

Ampulla of posterior semicircular duct

Lateral

Inferior cerebellar peduncle (to cerebellum)

Saccule

Vestibular ganglion

Superior division

of vestibular nerve

Inferior division

Plate 124

Cranial and Cervical Nerves

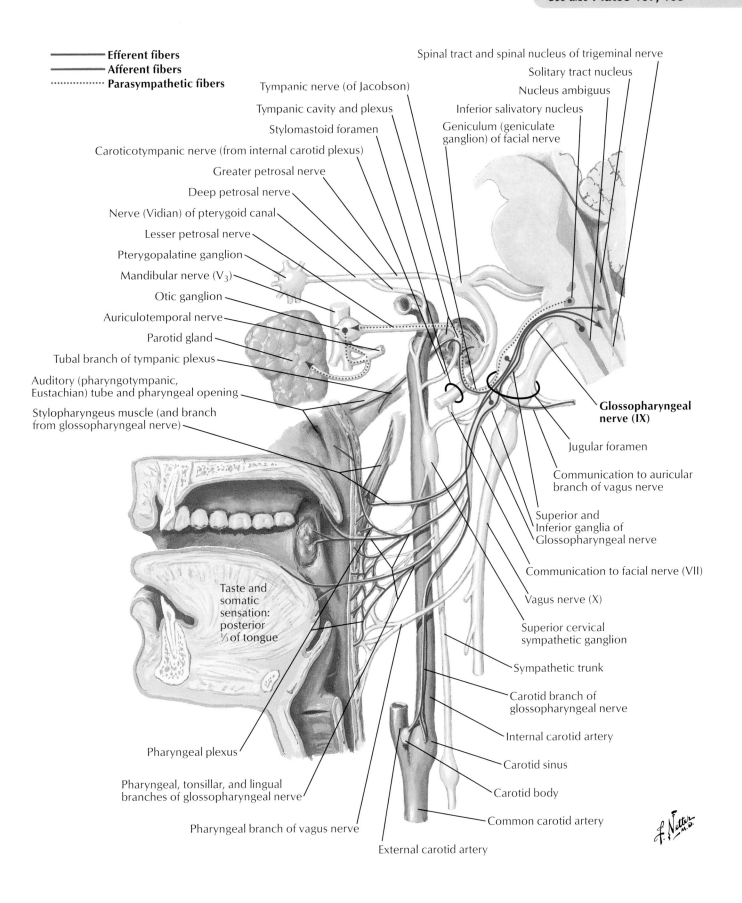

——— Efferent fibers
——— Afferent fibers
············ Parasympathetic fibers

Spinal tract and spinal nucleus of trigeminal nerve

Tympanic nerve (of Jacobson)

Tympanic cavity and plexus

Stylomastoid foramen

Solitary tract nucleus

Nucleus ambiguus

Inferior salivatory nucleus

Caroticotympanic nerve (from internal carotid plexus)

Greater petrosal nerve

Geniculum (geniculate ganglion) of facial nerve

Deep petrosal nerve

Nerve (Vidian) of pterygoid canal

Lesser petrosal nerve

Pterygopalatine ganglion

Mandibular nerve (V₃)

Otic ganglion

Auriculotemporal nerve

Parotid gland

Tubal branch of tympanic plexus

Auditory (pharyngotympanic, Eustachian) tube and pharyngeal opening

Stylopharyngeus muscle (and branch from glossopharyngeal nerve)

Glossopharyngeal nerve (IX)

Jugular foramen

Communication to auricular branch of vagus nerve

Superior and Inferior ganglia of Glossopharyngeal nerve

Communication to facial nerve (VII)

Vagus nerve (X)

Superior cervical sympathetic ganglion

Sympathetic trunk

Carotid branch of glossopharyngeal nerve

Internal carotid artery

Carotid sinus

Carotid body

Common carotid artery

Taste and somatic sensation: posterior ⅓ of tongue

Pharyngeal plexus

Pharyngeal, tonsillar, and lingual branches of glossopharyngeal nerve

Pharyngeal branch of vagus nerve

External carotid artery

Vagus Nerve (X): Schema

See also **Plates 167, 168**

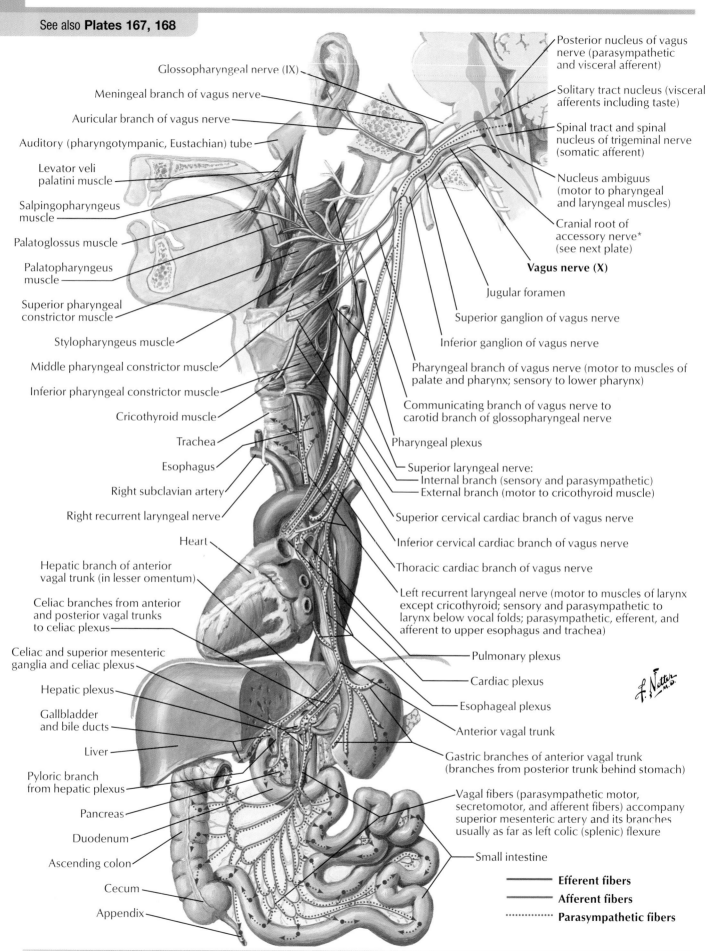

Glossopharyngeal nerve (IX)

Meningeal branch of vagus nerve

Auricular branch of vagus nerve

Auditory (pharyngotympanic, Eustachian) tube

Levator veli palatini muscle

Salpingopharyngeus muscle

Palatoglossus muscle

Palatopharyngeus muscle

Superior pharyngeal constrictor muscle

Stylopharyngeus muscle

Middle pharyngeal constrictor muscle

Inferior pharyngeal constrictor muscle

Cricothyroid muscle

Trachea

Esophagus

Right subclavian artery

Right recurrent laryngeal nerve

Heart

Hepatic branch of anterior vagal trunk (in lesser omentum)

Celiac branches from anterior and posterior vagal trunks to celiac plexus

Celiac and superior mesenteric ganglia and celiac plexus

Hepatic plexus

Gallbladder and bile ducts

Liver

Pyloric branch from hepatic plexus

Pancreas

Duodenum

Ascending colon

Cecum

Appendix

Posterior nucleus of vagus nerve (parasympathetic and visceral afferent)

Solitary tract nucleus (visceral afferents including taste)

Spinal tract and spinal nucleus of trigeminal nerve (somatic afferent)

Nucleus ambiguus (motor to pharyngeal and laryngeal muscles)

Cranial root of accessory nerve* (see next plate)

Vagus nerve (X)

Jugular foramen

Superior ganglion of vagus nerve

Inferior ganglion of vagus nerve

Pharyngeal branch of vagus nerve (motor to muscles of palate and pharynx; sensory to lower pharynx)

Communicating branch of vagus nerve to carotid branch of glossopharyngeal nerve

Pharyngeal plexus

Superior laryngeal nerve:
Internal branch (sensory and parasympathetic)
External branch (motor to cricothyroid muscle)

Superior cervical cardiac branch of vagus nerve

Inferior cervical cardiac branch of vagus nerve

Thoracic cardiac branch of vagus nerve

Left recurrent laryngeal nerve (motor to muscles of larynx except cricothyroid; sensory and parasympathetic to larynx below vocal folds; parasympathetic, efferent, and afferent to upper esophagus and trachea)

Pulmonary plexus

Cardiac plexus

Esophageal plexus

Anterior vagal trunk

Gastric branches of anterior vagal trunk (branches from posterior trunk behind stomach)

Vagal fibers (parasympathetic motor, secretomotor, and afferent fibers) accompany superior mesenteric artery and its branches usually as far as left colic (splenic) flexure

Small intestine

_____ **Efferent fibers**
_____ **Afferent fibers**
·············· **Parasympathetic fibers**

Plate 126

Cranial and Cervical Nerves

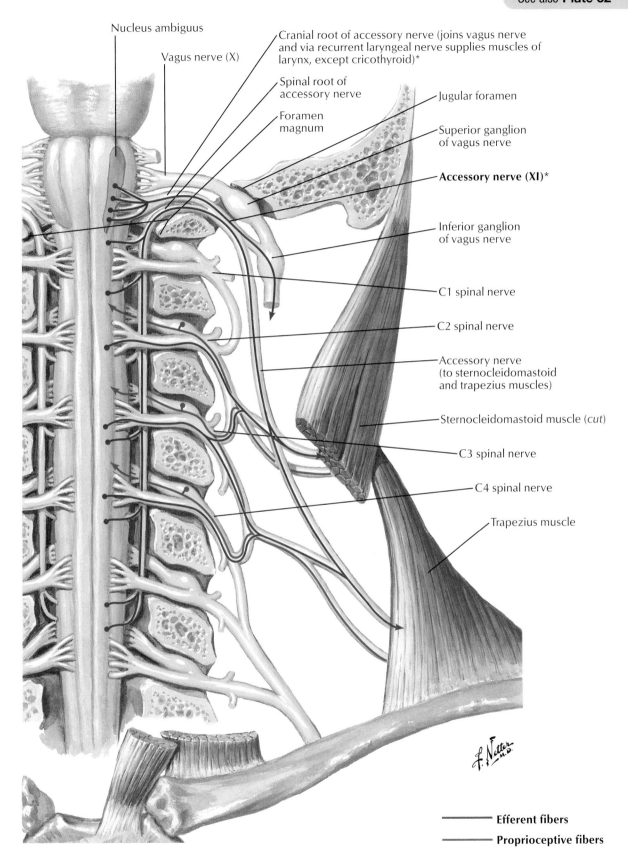

Nucleus ambiguus

Vagus nerve (X)

Cranial root of accessory nerve (joins vagus nerve and via recurrent laryngeal nerve supplies muscles of larynx, except cricothyroid)*

Spinal root of accessory nerve

Foramen magnum

Jugular foramen

Superior ganglion of vagus nerve

Accessory nerve (XI)*

Inferior ganglion of vagus nerve

C1 spinal nerve

C2 spinal nerve

Accessory nerve (to sternocleidomastoid and trapezius muscles)

Sternocleidomastoid muscle (*cut*)

C3 spinal nerve

C4 spinal nerve

Trapezius muscle

——— **Efferent fibers**

——— **Proprioceptive fibers**

*Recent evidence suggests that the accessory nerve lacks a cranial root and has no connection to the vagus nerve. Verification of this finding awaits further investigation.

Hypoglossal Nerve (XII): Schema

See also **Plate 32**

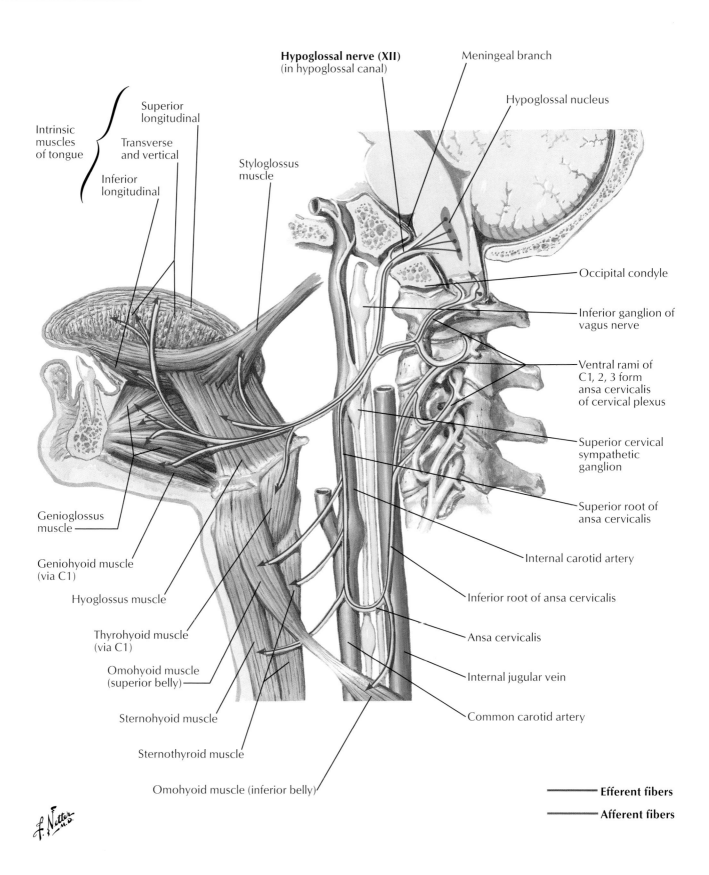

Hypoglossal nerve (XII) (in hypoglossal canal)

Meningeal branch

Hypoglossal nucleus

Intrinsic muscles of tongue
- Superior longitudinal
- Transverse and vertical
- Inferior longitudinal

Styloglossus muscle

Occipital condyle

Inferior ganglion of vagus nerve

Ventral rami of C1, 2, 3 form ansa cervicalis of cervical plexus

Superior cervical sympathetic ganglion

Superior root of ansa cervicalis

Internal carotid artery

Inferior root of ansa cervicalis

Ansa cervicalis

Internal jugular vein

Common carotid artery

Genioglossus muscle

Geniohyoid muscle (via C1)

Hyoglossus muscle

Thyrohyoid muscle (via C1)

Omohyoid muscle (superior belly)

Sternohyoid muscle

Sternothyroid muscle

Omohyoid muscle (inferior belly)

Efferent fibers

Afferent fibers

Plate 128

Cranial and Cervical Nerves

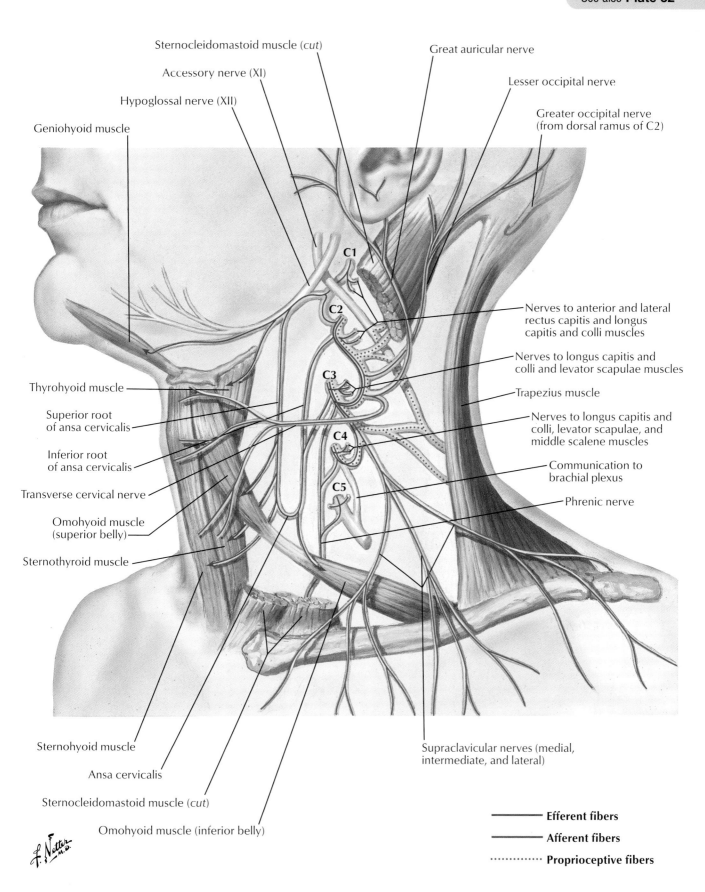

Sternocleidomastoid muscle (*cut*)

Accessory nerve (XI)

Hypoglossal nerve (XII)

Geniohyoid muscle

Great auricular nerve

Lesser occipital nerve

Greater occipital nerve
(from dorsal ramus of C2)

C1

C2

C3

C4

C5

Nerves to anterior and lateral
rectus capitis and longus
capitis and colli muscles

Nerves to longus capitis and
colli and levator scapulae muscles

Trapezius muscle

Nerves to longus capitis and
colli, levator scapulae, and
middle scalene muscles

Communication to
brachial plexus

Phrenic nerve

Thyrohyoid muscle

Superior root
of ansa cervicalis

Inferior root
of ansa cervicalis

Transverse cervical nerve

Omohyoid muscle
(superior belly)

Sternothyroid muscle

Sternohyoid muscle

Ansa cervicalis

Sternocleidomastoid muscle (*cut*)

Omohyoid muscle (inferior belly)

Supraclavicular nerves (medial,
intermediate, and lateral)

―――― **Efferent fibers**

―――― **Afferent fibers**

··········· **Proprioceptive fibers**

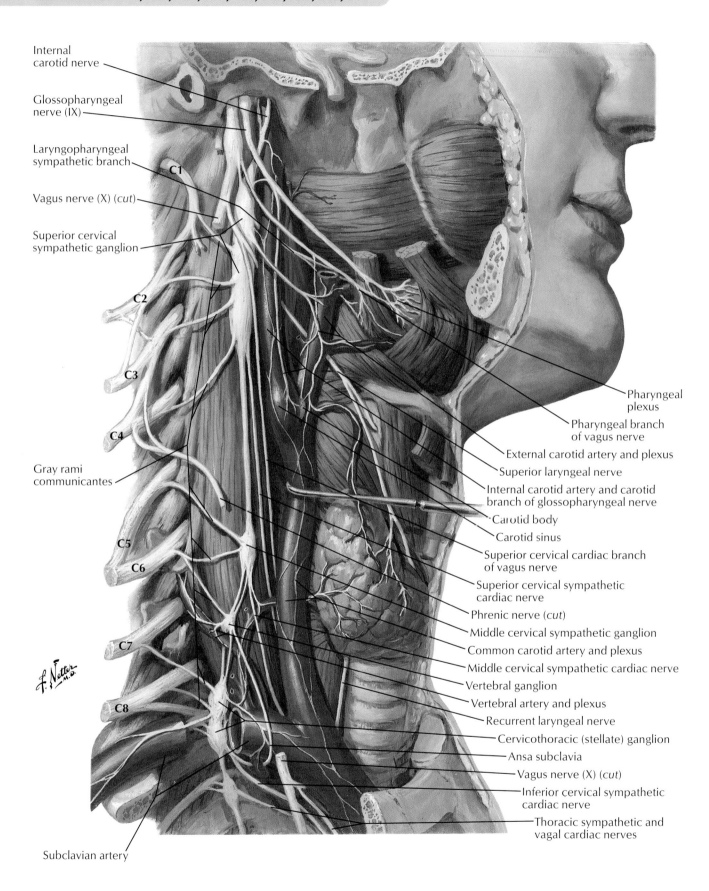

Internal carotid nerve

Glossopharyngeal nerve (IX)

Laryngopharyngeal sympathetic branch

Vagus nerve (X) (*cut*)

Superior cervical sympathetic ganglion

C1

C2

C3

C4

Gray rami communicantes

C5

C6

C7

C8

Subclavian artery

Pharyngeal plexus

Pharyngeal branch of vagus nerve

External carotid artery and plexus

Superior laryngeal nerve

Internal carotid artery and carotid branch of glossopharyngeal nerve

Carotid body

Carotid sinus

Superior cervical cardiac branch of vagus nerve

Superior cervical sympathetic cardiac nerve

Phrenic nerve (*cut*)

Middle cervical sympathetic ganglion

Common carotid artery and plexus

Middle cervical sympathetic cardiac nerve

Vertebral ganglion

Vertebral artery and plexus

Recurrent laryngeal nerve

Cervicothoracic (stellate) ganglion

Ansa subclavia

Vagus nerve (X) (*cut*)

Inferior cervical sympathetic cardiac nerve

Thoracic sympathetic and vagal cardiac nerves

Plate 130

Cranial and Cervical Nerves

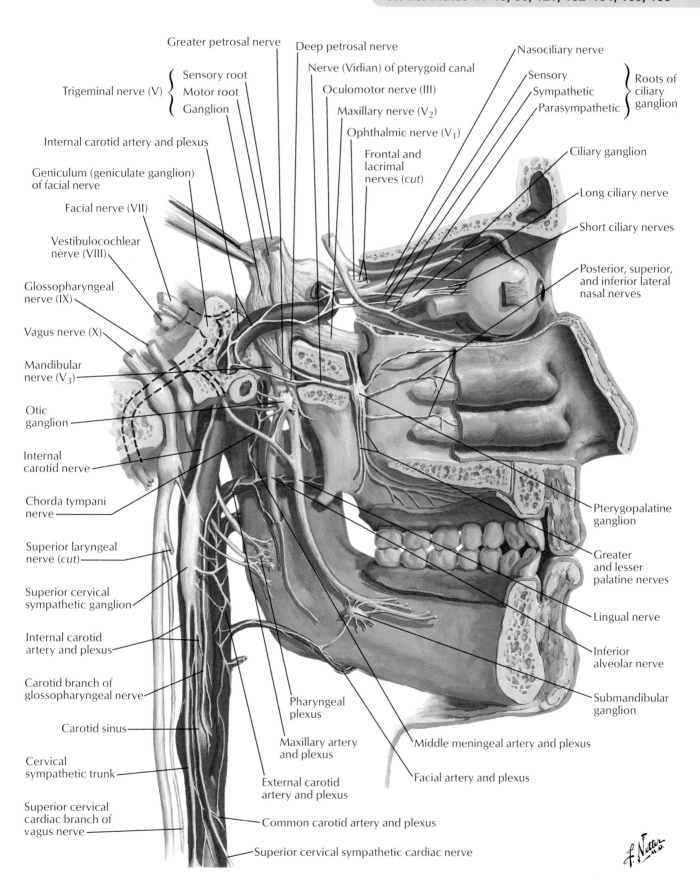

Greater petrosal nerve

Deep petrosal nerve

Nasociliary nerve

Trigeminal nerve (V) { Sensory root, Motor root, Ganglion

Nerve (Vidian) of pterygoid canal

Sensory
Sympathetic
Parasympathetic } Roots of ciliary ganglion

Oculomotor nerve (III)

Maxillary nerve (V₂)

Ophthalmic nerve (V₁)

Internal carotid artery and plexus

Frontal and lacrimal nerves (*cut*)

Ciliary ganglion

Geniculum (geniculate ganglion) of facial nerve

Long ciliary nerve

Facial nerve (VII)

Short ciliary nerves

Vestibulocochlear nerve (VIII)

Posterior, superior, and inferior lateral nasal nerves

Glossopharyngeal nerve (IX)

Vagus nerve (X)

Mandibular nerve (V₃)

Otic ganglion

Internal carotid nerve

Pterygopalatine ganglion

Chorda tympani nerve

Greater and lesser palatine nerves

Superior laryngeal nerve (*cut*)

Lingual nerve

Superior cervical sympathetic ganglion

Internal carotid artery and plexus

Inferior alveolar nerve

Carotid branch of glossopharyngeal nerve

Submandibular ganglion

Pharyngeal plexus

Carotid sinus

Maxillary artery and plexus

Middle meningeal artery and plexus

Cervical sympathetic trunk

Facial artery and plexus

Superior cervical cardiac branch of vagus nerve

External carotid artery and plexus

Common carotid artery and plexus

Superior cervical sympathetic cardiac nerve

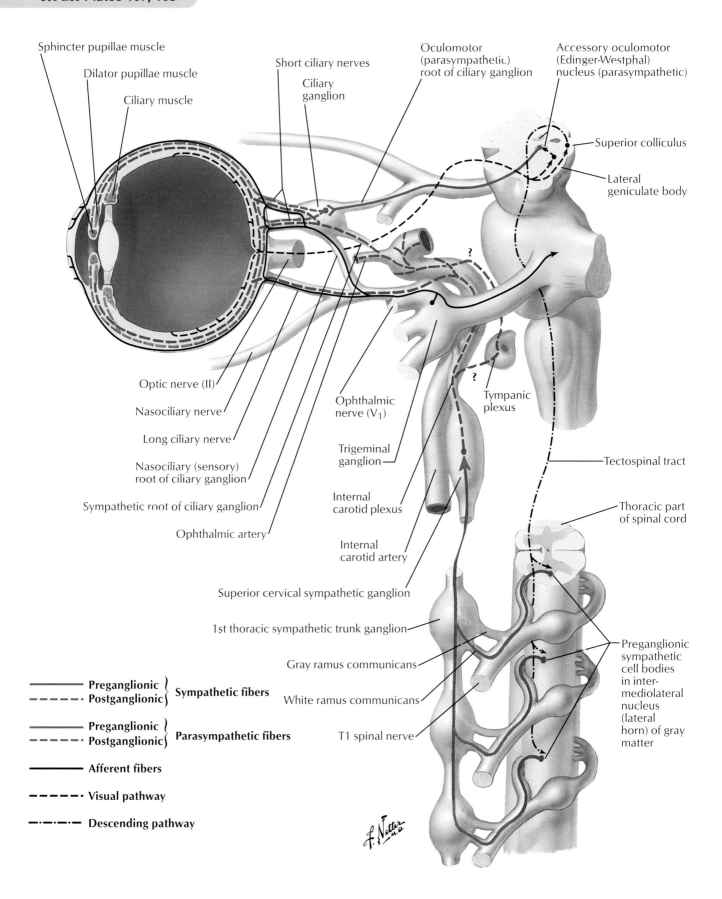

Sphincter pupillae muscle

Dilator pupillae muscle

Ciliary muscle

Short ciliary nerves

Ciliary ganglion

Oculomotor (parasympathetic) root of ciliary ganglion

Accessory oculomotor (Edinger-Westphal) nucleus (parasympathetic)

Superior colliculus

Lateral geniculate body

Optic nerve (II)

Nasociliary nerve

Long ciliary nerve

Nasociliary (sensory) root of ciliary ganglion

Sympathetic root of ciliary ganglion

Ophthalmic artery

Ophthalmic nerve (V₁)

Trigeminal ganglion

Internal carotid plexus

Internal carotid artery

Tympanic plexus

Tectospinal tract

Thoracic part of spinal cord

Superior cervical sympathetic ganglion

1st thoracic sympathetic trunk ganglion

Gray ramus communicans

White ramus communicans

T1 spinal nerve

Preganglionic sympathetic cell bodies in inter-mediolateral nucleus (lateral horn) of gray matter

—————— **Preganglionic** ⎫ **Sympathetic fibers**
– – – – – **Postganglionic** ⎭

—————— **Preganglionic** ⎫ **Parasympathetic fibers**
– – – – – **Postganglionic** ⎭

—————— **Afferent fibers**

– – – – – **Visual pathway**

–·–·–·– **Descending pathway**

Plate 132

Cranial and Cervical Nerves

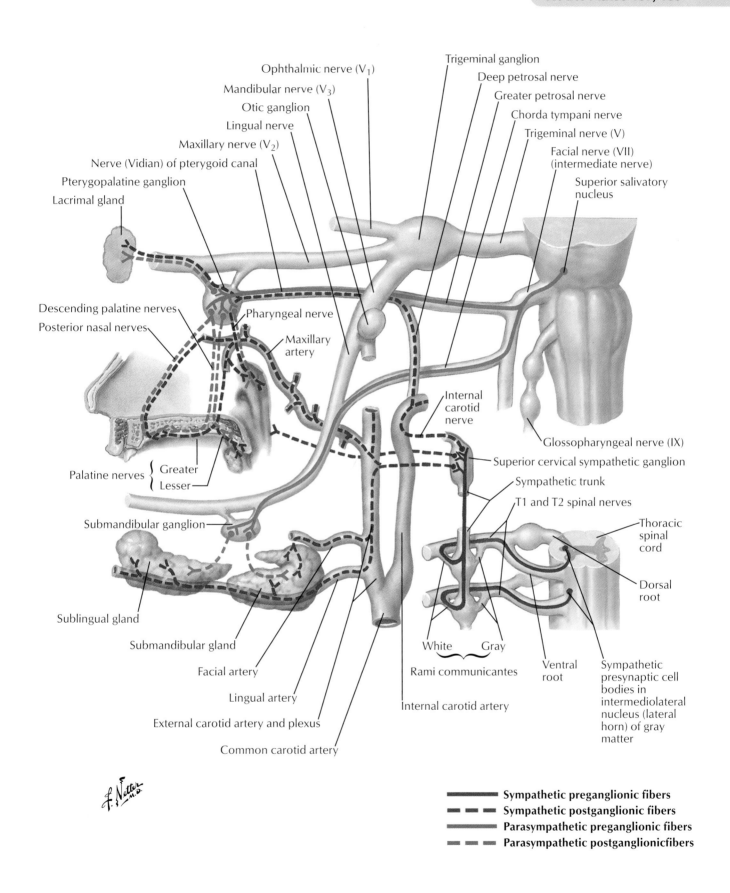

Ophthalmic nerve (V₁)

Mandibular nerve (V₃)

Otic ganglion

Lingual nerve

Maxillary nerve (V₂)

Nerve (Vidian) of pterygoid canal

Pterygopalatine ganglion

Lacrimal gland

Trigeminal ganglion

Deep petrosal nerve

Greater petrosal nerve

Chorda tympani nerve

Trigeminal nerve (V)

Facial nerve (VII) (intermediate nerve)

Superior salivatory nucleus

Descending palatine nerves

Posterior nasal nerves

Pharyngeal nerve

Maxillary artery

Internal carotid nerve

Glossopharyngeal nerve (IX)

Superior cervical sympathetic ganglion

Sympathetic trunk

T1 and T2 spinal nerves

Thoracic spinal cord

Dorsal root

Palatine nerves { Greater / Lesser

Submandibular ganglion

Sublingual gland

Submandibular gland

Facial artery

Lingual artery

External carotid artery and plexus

Common carotid artery

White   Gray

Rami communicantes

Ventral root

Internal carotid artery

Sympathetic presynaptic cell bodies in intermediolateral nucleus (lateral horn) of gray matter

═══ **Sympathetic preganglionic fibers**

─ ─ ─ **Sympathetic postganglionic fibers**

═══ **Parasympathetic preganglionic fibers**

─ ─ ─ **Parasympathetic postganglionicfibers**

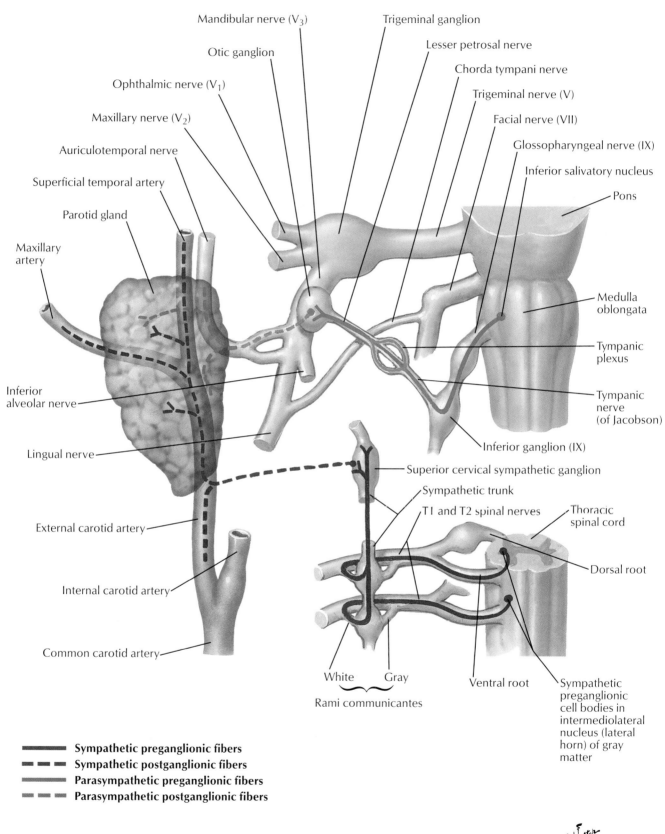

Mandibular nerve (V₃)

Otic ganglion

Ophthalmic nerve (V₁)

Maxillary nerve (V₂)

Auriculotemporal nerve

Superficial temporal artery

Parotid gland

Maxillary artery

Inferior alveolar nerve

Lingual nerve

External carotid artery

Internal carotid artery

Common carotid artery

Trigeminal ganglion

Lesser petrosal nerve

Chorda tympani nerve

Trigeminal nerve (V)

Facial nerve (VII)

Glossopharyngeal nerve (IX)

Inferior salivatory nucleus

Pons

Medulla oblongata

Tympanic plexus

Tympanic nerve (of Jacobson)

Inferior ganglion (IX)

Superior cervical sympathetic ganglion

Sympathetic trunk

T1 and T2 spinal nerves

Thoracic spinal cord

Dorsal root

Ventral root

Sympathetic preganglionic cell bodies in intermediolateral nucleus (lateral horn) of gray matter

White   Gray

Rami communicantes

━━━━━ **Sympathetic preganglionic fibers**
━ ━ ━ **Sympathetic postganglionic fibers**
━━━━━ **Parasympathetic preganglionic fibers**
━ ━ ━ **Parasympathetic postganglionic fibers**

f. Netter
M.D.

Plate 134

Cranial and Cervical Nerves

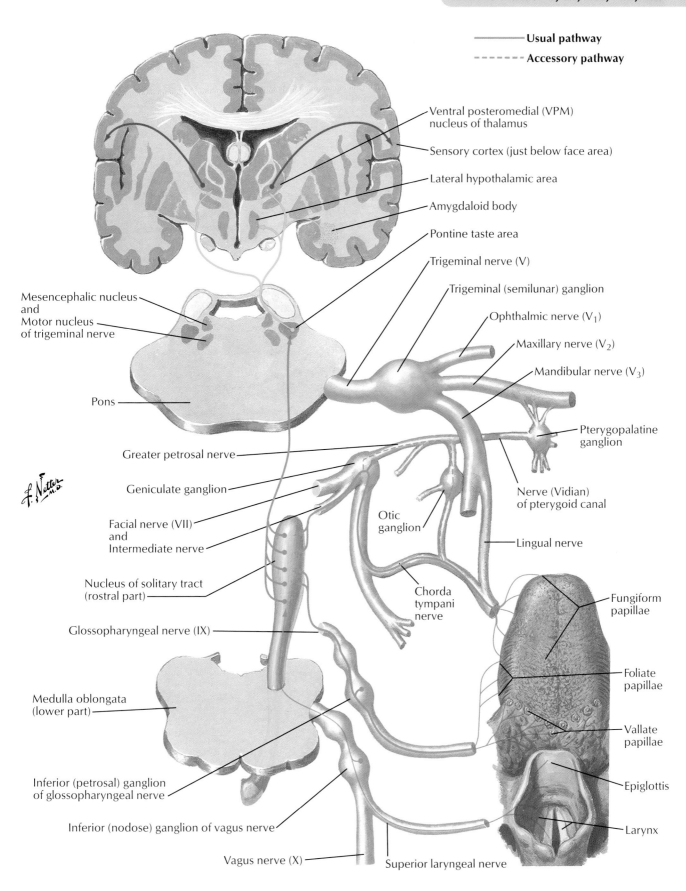

——— Usual pathway

------- Accessory pathway

Ventral posteromedial (VPM) nucleus of thalamus

Sensory cortex (just below face area)

Lateral hypothalamic area

Amygdaloid body

Pontine taste area

Trigeminal nerve (V)

Trigeminal (semilunar) ganglion

Ophthalmic nerve (V₁)

Maxillary nerve (V₂)

Mandibular nerve (V₃)

Pterygopalatine ganglion

Nerve (Vidian) of pterygoid canal

Lingual nerve

Fungiform papillae

Foliate papillae

Vallate papillae

Epiglottis

Larynx

Mesencephalic nucleus and Motor nucleus of trigeminal nerve

Pons

Greater petrosal nerve

Geniculate ganglion

Facial nerve (VII) and Intermediate nerve

Nucleus of solitary tract (rostral part)

Glossopharyngeal nerve (IX)

Medulla oblongata (lower part)

Inferior (petrosal) ganglion of glossopharyngeal nerve

Inferior (nodose) ganglion of vagus nerve

Vagus nerve (X)

Superior laryngeal nerve

Otic ganglion

Chorda tympani nerve

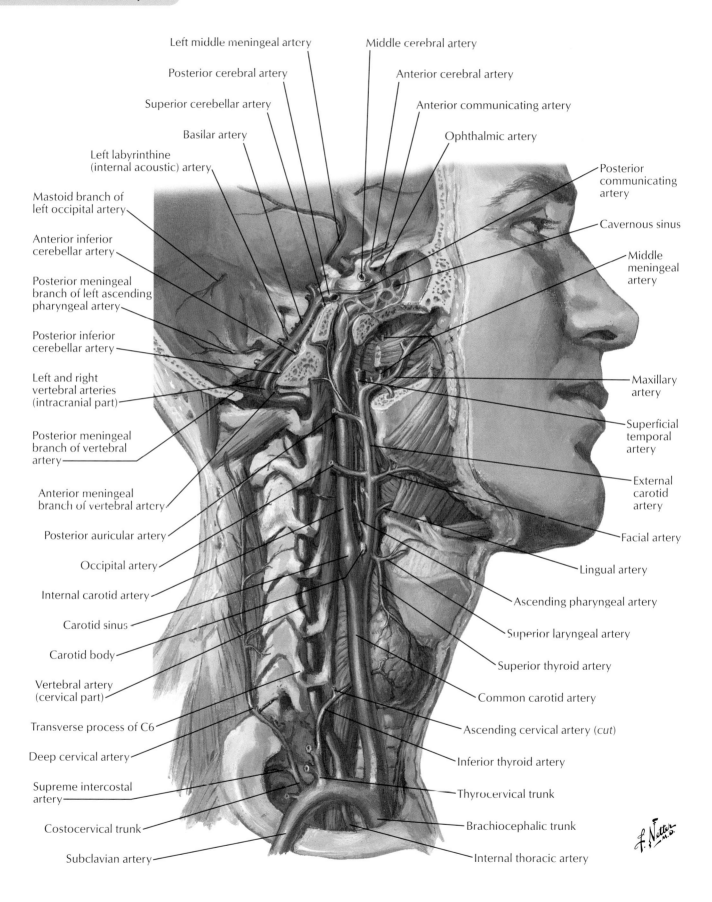

Left middle meningeal artery

Posterior cerebral artery

Superior cerebellar artery

Basilar artery

Left labyrinthine (internal acoustic) artery

Mastoid branch of left occipital artery

Anterior inferior cerebellar artery

Posterior meningeal branch of left ascending pharyngeal artery

Posterior inferior cerebellar artery

Left and right vertebral arteries (intracranial part)

Posterior meningeal branch of vertebral artery

Anterior meningeal branch of vertebral artery

Posterior auricular artery

Occipital artery

Internal carotid artery

Carotid sinus

Carotid body

Vertebral artery (cervical part)

Transverse process of C6

Deep cervical artery

Supreme intercostal artery

Costocervical trunk

Subclavian artery

Middle cerebral artery

Anterior cerebral artery

Anterior communicating artery

Ophthalmic artery

Posterior communicating artery

Cavernous sinus

Middle meningeal artery

Maxillary artery

Superficial temporal artery

External carotid artery

Facial artery

Lingual artery

Ascending pharyngeal artery

Superior laryngeal artery

Superior thyroid artery

Common carotid artery

Ascending cervical artery (*cut*)

Inferior thyroid artery

Thyrocervical trunk

Brachiocephalic trunk

Internal thoracic artery

Plate 136

Cerebral Vasculature

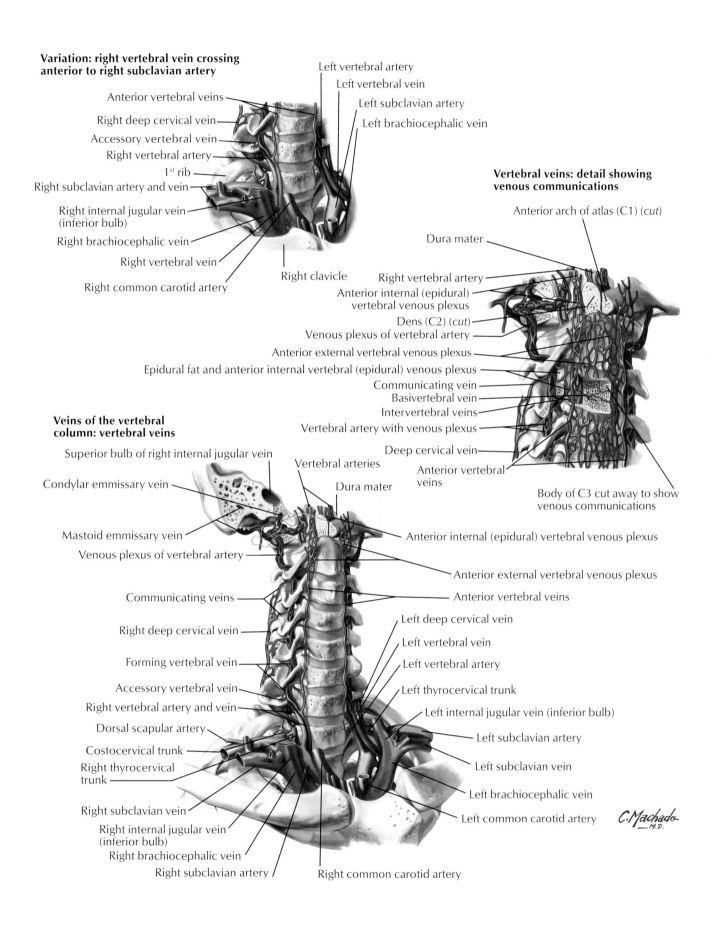

Variation: right vertebral vein crossing anterior to right subclavian artery

Anterior vertebral veins

Right deep cervical vein

Accessory vertebral vein

Right vertebral artery

1st rib

Right subclavian artery and vein

Right internal jugular vein (inferior bulb)

Right brachiocephalic vein

Right vertebral vein

Right common carotid artery

Left vertebral artery

Left vertebral vein

Left subclavian artery

Left brachiocephalic vein

Right clavicle

Vertebral veins: detail showing venous communications

Anterior arch of atlas (C1) (cut)

Dura mater

Right vertebral artery

Anterior internal (epidural) vertebral venous plexus

Dens (C2) (cut)

Venous plexus of vertebral artery

Anterior external vertebral venous plexus

Epidural fat and anterior internal vertebral (epidural) venous plexus

Communicating vein

Basivertebral vein

Intervertebral veins

Vertebral artery with venous plexus

Deep cervical vein

Anterior vertebral veins

Body of C3 cut away to show venous communications

Veins of the vertebral column: vertebral veins

Superior bulb of right internal jugular vein

Condylar emmissary vein

Mastoid emmissary vein

Venous plexus of vertebral artery

Communicating veins

Right deep cervical vein

Forming vertebral vein

Accessory vertebral vein

Right vertebral artery and vein

Dorsal scapular artery

Costocervical trunk

Right thyrocervical trunk

Right subclavian vein

Right internal jugular vein (inferior bulb)

Right brachiocephalic vein

Right subclavian artery

Vertebral arteries

Dura mater

Right common carotid artery

Anterior internal (epidural) vertebral venous plexus

Anterior external vertebral venous plexus

Anterior vertebral veins

Left deep cervical vein

Left vertebral vein

Left vertebral artery

Left thyrocervical trunk

Left internal jugular vein (inferior bulb)

Left subclavian artery

Left subclavian vein

Left brachiocephalic vein

Left common carotid artery

C. Machado —M.D.

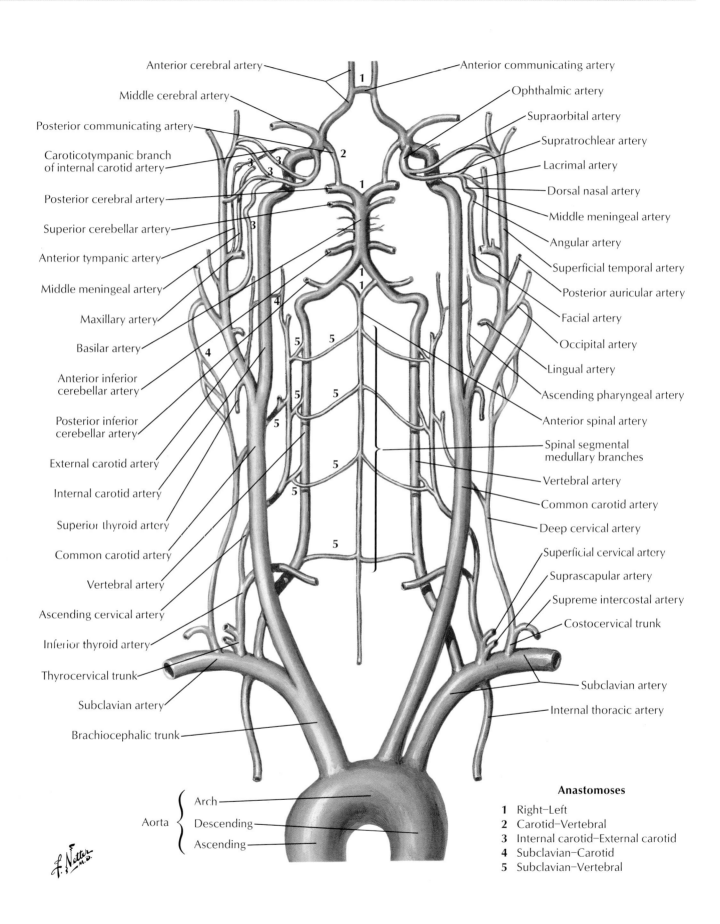

Anterior cerebral artery

Middle cerebral artery

Posterior communicating artery

Caroticotympanic branch of internal carotid artery

Posterior cerebral artery

Superior cerebellar artery

Anterior tympanic artery

Middle meningeal artery

Maxillary artery

Basilar artery

Anterior inferior cerebellar artery

Posterior inferior cerebellar artery

External carotid artery

Internal carotid artery

Superior thyroid artery

Common carotid artery

Vertebral artery

Ascending cervical artery

Inferior thyroid artery

Thyrocervical trunk

Subclavian artery

Brachiocephalic trunk

Anterior communicating artery

Ophthalmic artery

Supraorbital artery

Supratrochlear artery

Lacrimal artery

Dorsal nasal artery

Middle meningeal artery

Angular artery

Superficial temporal artery

Posterior auricular artery

Facial artery

Occipital artery

Lingual artery

Ascending pharyngeal artery

Anterior spinal artery

Spinal segmental medullary branches

Vertebral artery

Common carotid artery

Deep cervical artery

Superficial cervical artery

Suprascapular artery

Supreme intercostal artery

Costocervical trunk

Subclavian artery

Internal thoracic artery

Aorta {
Arch
Descending
Ascending
}

Anastomoses

1 Right–Left
2 Carotid–Vertebral
3 Internal carotid–External carotid
4 Subclavian–Carotid
5 Subclavian–Vertebral

Plate 138 **Cerebral Vasculature**

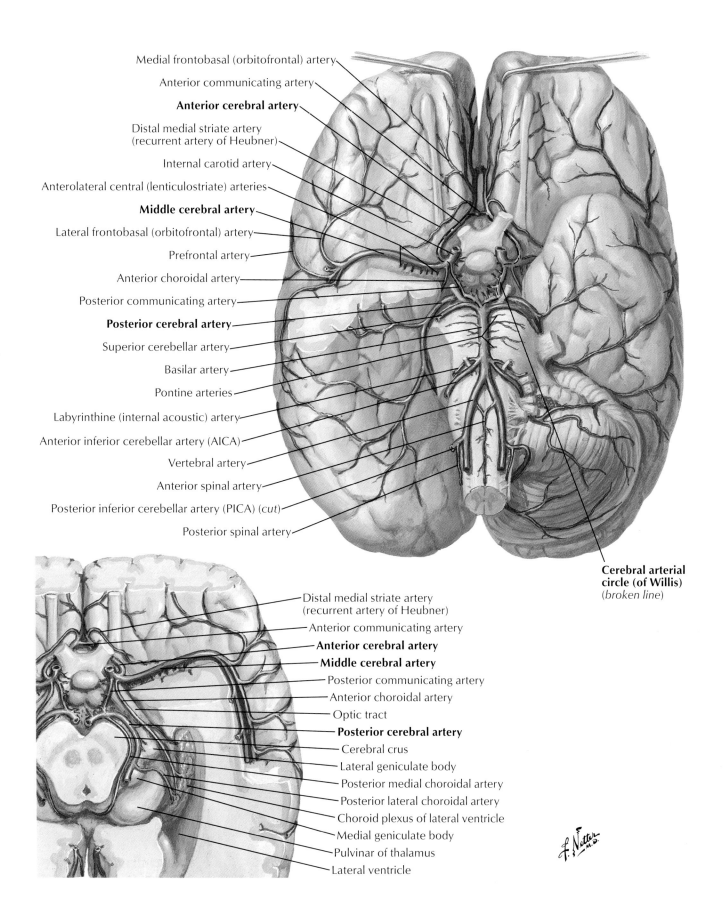

Medial frontobasal (orbitofrontal) artery

Anterior communicating artery

Anterior cerebral artery

Distal medial striate artery
(recurrent artery of Heubner)

Internal carotid artery

Anterolateral central (lenticulostriate) arteries

Middle cerebral artery

Lateral frontobasal (orbitofrontal) artery

Prefrontal artery

Anterior choroidal artery

Posterior communicating artery

Posterior cerebral artery

Superior cerebellar artery

Basilar artery

Pontine arteries

Labyrinthine (internal acoustic) artery

Anterior inferior cerebellar artery (AICA)

Vertebral artery

Anterior spinal artery

Posterior inferior cerebellar artery (PICA) (cut)

Posterior spinal artery

**Cerebral arterial
circle (of Willis)**
(broken line)

Distal medial striate artery
(recurrent artery of Heubner)

Anterior communicating artery

Anterior cerebral artery

Middle cerebral artery

Posterior communicating artery

Anterior choroidal artery

Optic tract

Posterior cerebral artery

Cerebral crus

Lateral geniculate body

Posterior medial choroidal artery

Posterior lateral choroidal artery

Choroid plexus of lateral ventricle

Medial geniculate body

Pulvinar of thalamus

Lateral ventricle

f. Netter

Vessels dissected out: inferior view

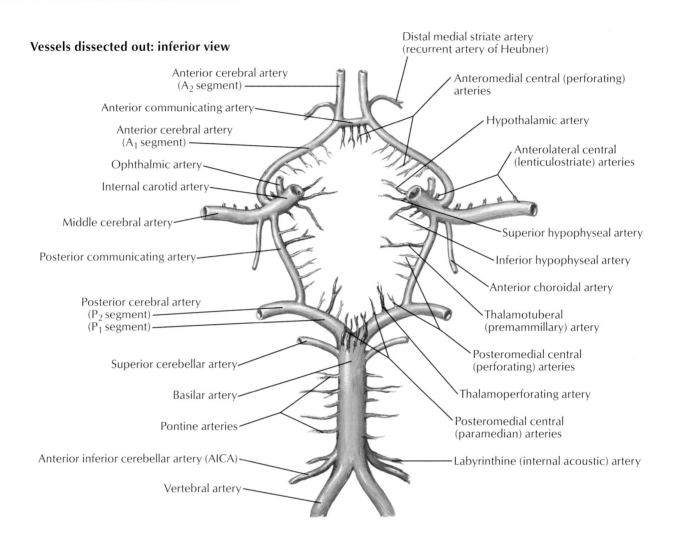

Distal medial striate artery (recurrent artery of Heubner)

Anterior cerebral artery (A_2 segment)

Anterior communicating artery

Anterior cerebral artery (A_1 segment)

Ophthalmic artery

Internal carotid artery

Middle cerebral artery

Posterior communicating artery

Posterior cerebral artery (P_2 segment) (P_1 segment)

Superior cerebellar artery

Basilar artery

Pontine arteries

Anterior inferior cerebellar artery (AICA)

Vertebral artery

Anteromedial central (perforating) arteries

Hypothalamic artery

Anterolateral central (lenticulostriate) arteries

Superior hypophyseal artery

Inferior hypophyseal artery

Anterior choroidal artery

Thalamotuberal (premammillary) artery

Posteromedial central (perforating) arteries

Thalamoperforating artery

Posteromedial central (paramedian) arteries

Labyrinthine (internal acoustic) artery

Vessels in situ: inferior view

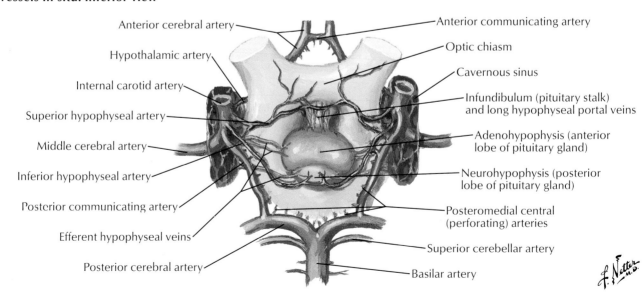

Anterior cerebral artery

Hypothalamic artery

Internal carotid artery

Superior hypophyseal artery

Middle cerebral artery

Inferior hypophyseal artery

Posterior communicating artery

Efferent hypophyseal veins

Posterior cerebral artery

Anterior communicating artery

Optic chiasm

Cavernous sinus

Infundibulum (pituitary stalk) and long hypophyseal portal veins

Adenohypophysis (anterior lobe of pituitary gland)

Neurohypophysis (posterior lobe of pituitary gland)

Posteromedial central (perforating) arteries

Superior cerebellar artery

Basilar artery

Plate 140

Cerebral Vasculature

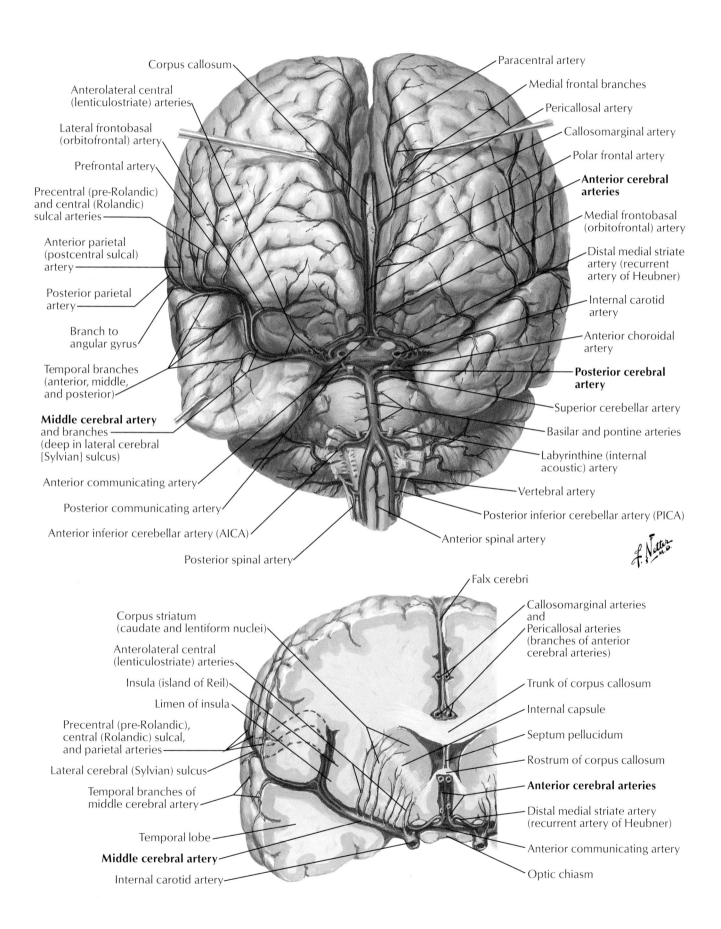

Corpus callosum

Anterolateral central (lenticulostriate) arteries

Lateral frontobasal (orbitofrontal) artery

Prefrontal artery

Precentral (pre-Rolandic) and central (Rolandic) sulcal arteries

Anterior parietal (postcentral sulcal) artery

Posterior parietal artery

Branch to angular gyrus

Temporal branches (anterior, middle, and posterior)

Middle cerebral artery and branches (deep in lateral cerebral [Sylvian] sulcus)

Anterior communicating artery

Posterior communicating artery

Anterior inferior cerebellar artery (AICA)

Posterior spinal artery

Paracentral artery

Medial frontal branches

Pericallosal artery

Callosomarginal artery

Polar frontal artery

Anterior cerebral arteries

Medial frontobasal (orbitofrontal) artery

Distal medial striate artery (recurrent artery of Heubner)

Internal carotid artery

Anterior choroidal artery

Posterior cerebral artery

Superior cerebellar artery

Basilar and pontine arteries

Labyrinthine (internal acoustic) artery

Vertebral artery

Posterior inferior cerebellar artery (PICA)

Anterior spinal artery

Corpus striatum (caudate and lentiform nuclei)

Anterolateral central (lenticulostriate) arteries

Insula (island of Reil)

Limen of insula

Precentral (pre-Rolandic), central (Rolandic) sulcal, and parietal arteries

Lateral cerebral (Sylvian) sulcus

Temporal branches of middle cerebral artery

Temporal lobe

Middle cerebral artery

Internal carotid artery

Falx cerebri

Callosomarginal arteries and Pericallosal arteries (branches of anterior cerebral arteries)

Trunk of corpus callosum

Internal capsule

Septum pellucidum

Rostrum of corpus callosum

Anterior cerebral arteries

Distal medial striate artery (recurrent artery of Heubner)

Anterior communicating artery

Optic chiasm

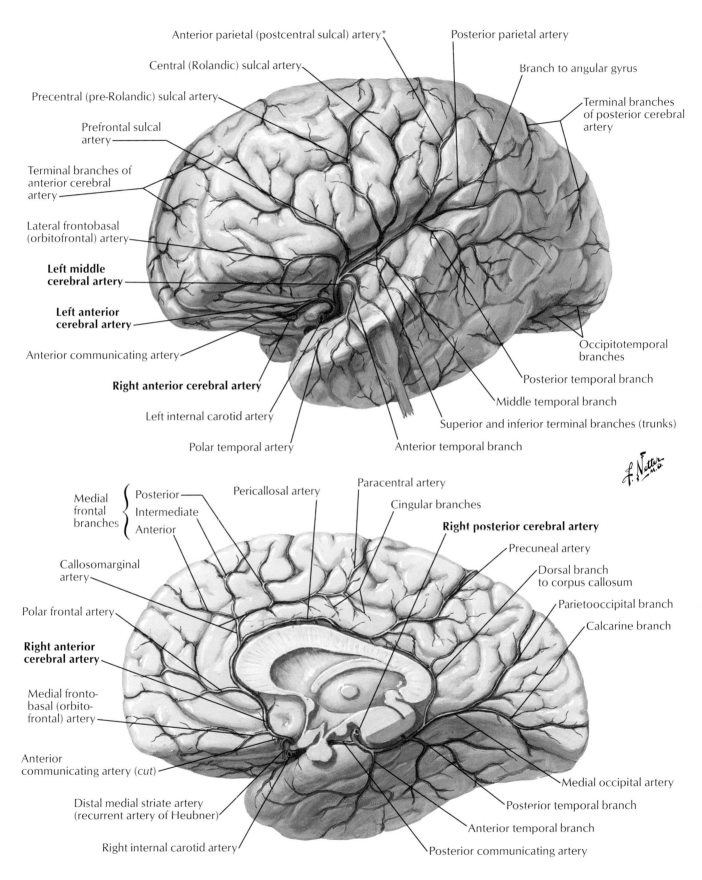

Anterior parietal (postcentral sulcal) artery*

Central (Rolandic) sulcal artery

Precentral (pre-Rolandic) sulcal artery

Prefrontal sulcal artery

Terminal branches of anterior cerebral artery

Lateral frontobasal (orbitofrontal) artery

Left middle cerebral artery

Left anterior cerebral artery

Anterior communicating artery

Right anterior cerebral artery

Left internal carotid artery

Polar temporal artery

Posterior parietal artery

Branch to angular gyrus

Terminal branches of posterior cerebral artery

Occipitotemporal branches

Posterior temporal branch

Middle temporal branch

Superior and inferior terminal branches (trunks)

Anterior temporal branch

Medial frontal branches { Posterior, Intermediate, Anterior }

Pericallosal artery

Paracentral artery

Cingular branches

Right posterior cerebral artery

Precuneal artery

Dorsal branch to corpus callosum

Parietooccipital branch

Calcarine branch

Callosomarginal artery

Polar frontal artery

Right anterior cerebral artery

Medial fronto-basal (orbito-frontal) artery

Anterior communicating artery (*cut*)

Distal medial striate artery (recurrent artery of Heubner)

Right internal carotid artery

Medial occipital artery

Posterior temporal branch

Anterior temporal branch

Posterior communicating artery

*Note: Anterior parietal (postcentral sulcal) artery also occurs as separate anterior parietal and postcentral sulcal arteries.

Plate 142   **Cerebral Vasculature**

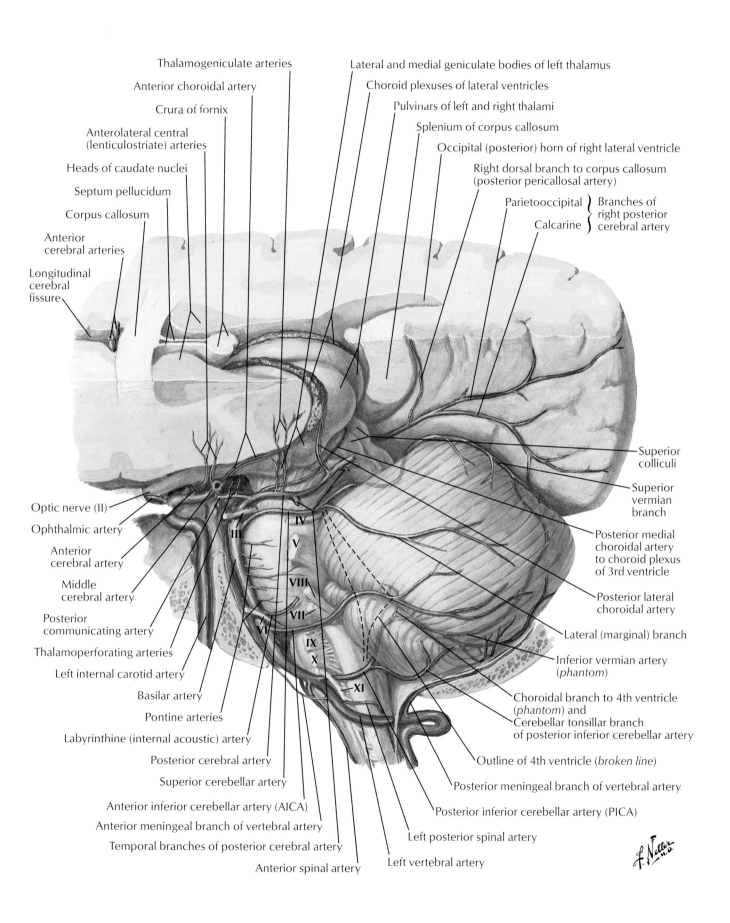

Thalamogeniculate arteries

Anterior choroidal artery

Crura of fornix

Anterolateral central
(lenticulostriate) arteries

Heads of caudate nuclei

Septum pellucidum

Corpus callosum

Anterior
cerebral arteries

Longitudinal
cerebral
fissure

Lateral and medial geniculate bodies of left thalamus

Choroid plexuses of lateral ventricles

Pulvinars of left and right thalami

Splenium of corpus callosum

Occipital (posterior) horn of right lateral ventricle

Right dorsal branch to corpus callosum
(posterior pericallosal artery)

Parietooccipital ⎫ Branches of
⎬ right posterior
Calcarine ⎭ cerebral artery

Optic nerve (II)

Ophthalmic artery

Anterior
cerebral artery

Middle
cerebral artery

Posterior
communicating artery

Thalamoperforating arteries

Left internal carotid artery

Basilar artery

Pontine arteries

Labyrinthine (internal acoustic) artery

Posterior cerebral artery

Superior cerebellar artery

Anterior inferior cerebellar artery (AICA)

Anterior meningeal branch of vertebral artery

Temporal branches of posterior cerebral artery

Anterior spinal artery

III

IV

V

VIII

VII

VI

IX

X

XI

Left vertebral artery

Left posterior spinal artery

Posterior inferior cerebellar artery (PICA)

Posterior meningeal branch of vertebral artery

Outline of 4th ventricle (broken line)

Choroidal branch to 4th ventricle
(phantom) and
Cerebellar tonsillar branch
of posterior inferior cerebellar artery

Inferior vermian artery
(phantom)

Lateral (marginal) branch

Posterior lateral
choroidal artery

Posterior medial
choroidal artery
to choroid plexus
of 3rd ventricle

Superior
vermian
branch

Superior
colliculi

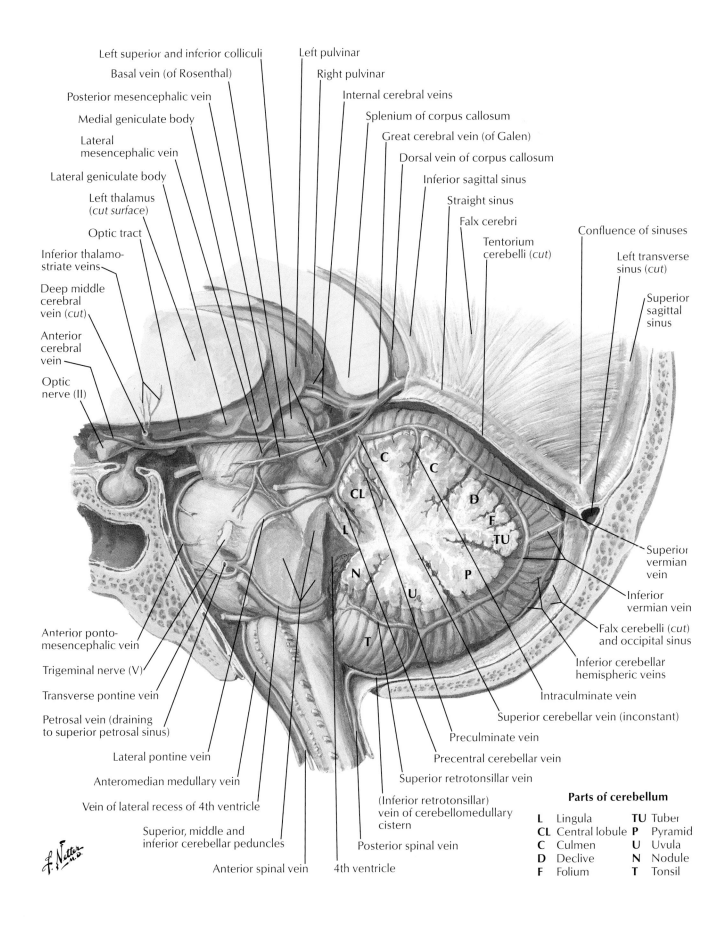

Left superior and inferior colliculi

Basal vein (of Rosenthal)

Posterior mesencephalic vein

Medial geniculate body

Lateral mesencephalic vein

Lateral geniculate body

Left thalamus (*cut surface*)

Optic tract

Inferior thalamo-striate veins

Deep middle cerebral vein (*cut*)

Anterior cerebral vein

Optic nerve (II)

Left pulvinar

Right pulvinar

Internal cerebral veins

Splenium of corpus callosum

Great cerebral vein (of Galen)

Dorsal vein of corpus callosum

Inferior sagittal sinus

Straight sinus

Falx cerebri

Tentorium cerebelli (*cut*)

Confluence of sinuses

Left transverse sinus (*cut*)

Superior sagittal sinus

Superior vermian vein

Inferior vermian vein

Falx cerebelli (*cut*) and occipital sinus

Inferior cerebellar hemispheric veins

Intraculminate vein

Superior cerebellar vein (inconstant)

Precentral cerebellar vein

Superior retrotonsillar vein

Preculminate vein

Anterior ponto-mesencephalic vein

Trigeminal nerve (V)

Transverse pontine vein

Petrosal vein (draining to superior petrosal sinus)

Lateral pontine vein

Anteromedian medullary vein

Vein of lateral recess of 4th ventricle

Superior, middle and inferior cerebellar peduncles

Anterior spinal vein

4th ventricle

Posterior spinal vein

(Inferior retrotonsillar) vein of cerebellomedullary cistern

Parts of cerebellum

L	Lingula	**TU**	Tuber
CL	Central lobule	**P**	Pyramid
C	Culmen	**U**	Uvula
D	Declive	**N**	Nodule
F	Folium	**T**	Tonsil

f. Netter m.d.

Plate 144

Cerebral Vasculature

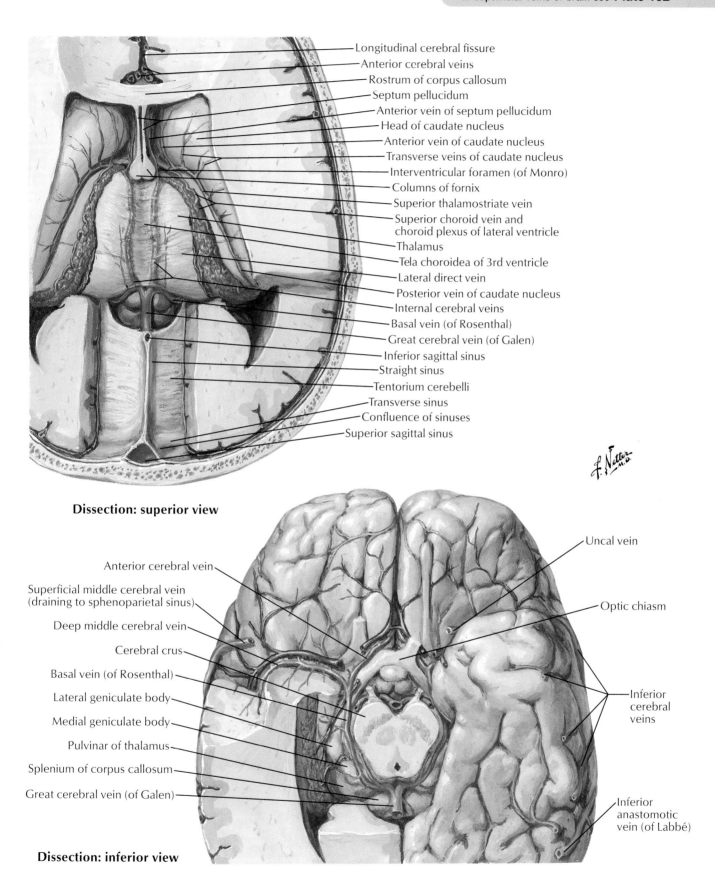

Longitudinal cerebral fissure
Anterior cerebral veins
Rostrum of corpus callosum
Septum pellucidum
Anterior vein of septum pellucidum
Head of caudate nucleus
Anterior vein of caudate nucleus
Transverse veins of caudate nucleus
Interventricular foramen (of Monro)
Columns of fornix
Superior thalamostriate vein
Superior choroid vein and choroid plexus of lateral ventricle
Thalamus
Tela choroidea of 3rd ventricle
Lateral direct vein
Posterior vein of caudate nucleus
Internal cerebral veins
Basal vein (of Rosenthal)
Great cerebral vein (of Galen)
Inferior sagittal sinus
Straight sinus
Tentorium cerebelli
Transverse sinus
Confluence of sinuses
Superior sagittal sinus

Dissection: superior view

Anterior cerebral vein
Superficial middle cerebral vein (draining to sphenoparietal sinus)
Deep middle cerebral vein
Cerebral crus
Basal vein (of Rosenthal)
Lateral geniculate body
Medial geniculate body
Pulvinar of thalamus
Splenium of corpus callosum
Great cerebral vein (of Galen)

Uncal vein
Optic chiasm
Inferior cerebral veins
Inferior anastomotic vein (of Labbé)

Dissection: inferior view

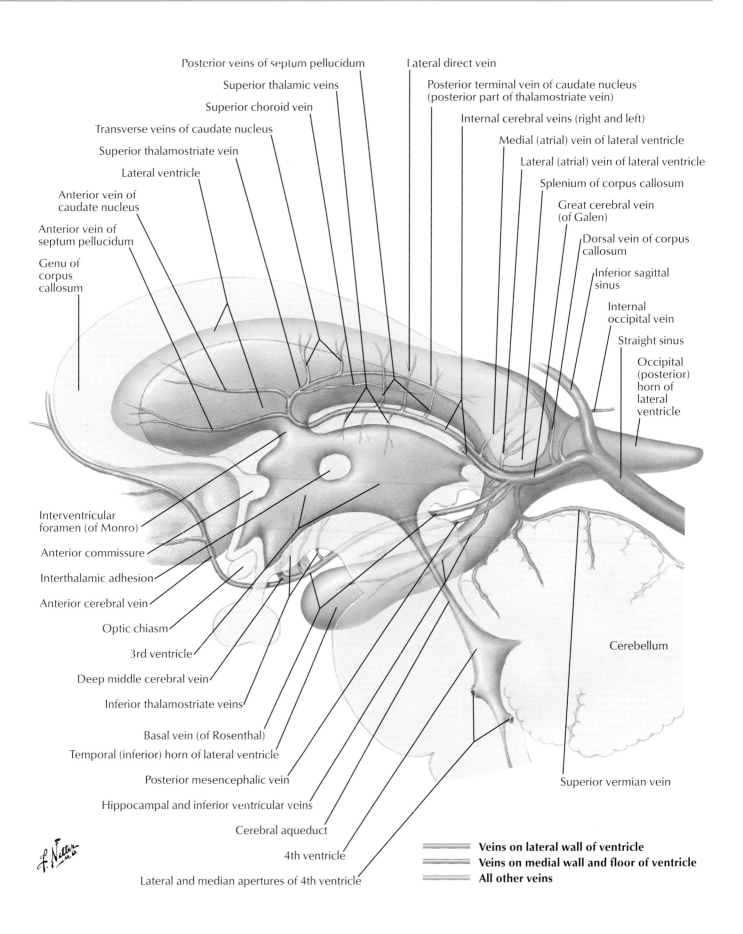

Posterior veins of septum pellucidum

Superior thalamic veins

Superior choroid vein

Transverse veins of caudate nucleus

Superior thalamostriate vein

Lateral ventricle

Anterior vein of caudate nucleus

Anterior vein of septum pellucidum

Genu of corpus callosum

Lateral direct vein

Posterior terminal vein of caudate nucleus (posterior part of thalamostriate vein)

Internal cerebral veins (right and left)

Medial (atrial) vein of lateral ventricle

Lateral (atrial) vein of lateral ventricle

Splenium of corpus callosum

Great cerebral vein (of Galen)

Dorsal vein of corpus callosum

Inferior sagittal sinus

Internal occipital vein

Straight sinus

Occipital (posterior) horn of lateral ventricle

Interventricular foramen (of Monro)

Anterior commissure

Interthalamic adhesion

Anterior cerebral vein

Optic chiasm

3rd ventricle

Deep middle cerebral vein

Inferior thalamostriate veins

Basal vein (of Rosenthal)

Temporal (inferior) horn of lateral ventricle

Posterior mesencephalic vein

Hippocampal and inferior ventricular veins

Cerebral aqueduct

4th ventricle

Lateral and median apertures of 4th ventricle

Cerebellum

Superior vermian vein

Veins on lateral wall of ventricle
Veins on medial wall and floor of ventricle
All other veins

Plate 146   *Cerebral Vasculature*

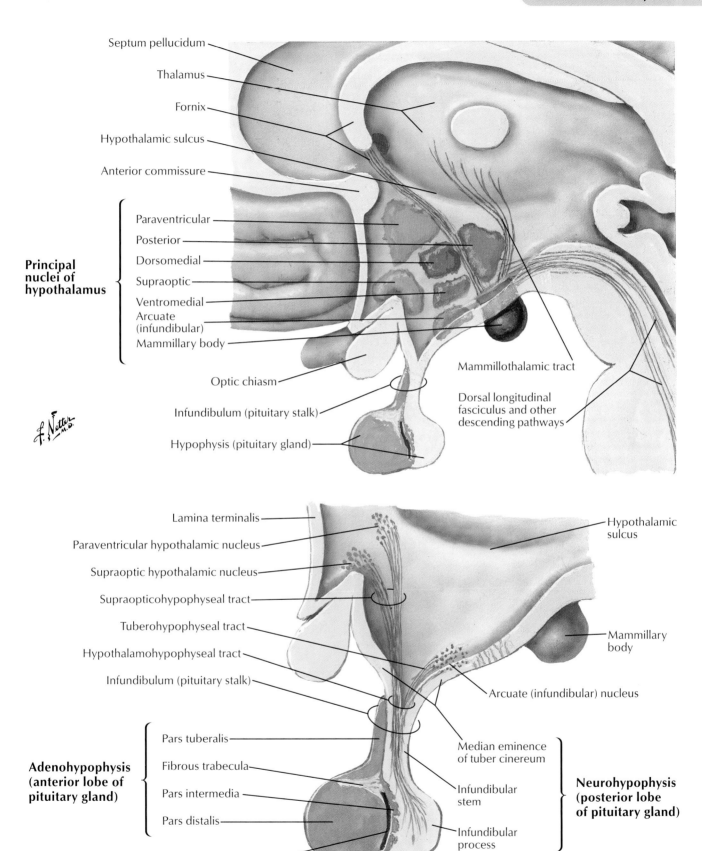

Septum pellucidum

Thalamus

Fornix

Hypothalamic sulcus

Anterior commissure

Principal nuclei of hypothalamus

Paraventricular
Posterior
Dorsomedial
Supraoptic
Ventromedial
Arcuate (infundibular)
Mammillary body

Optic chiasm

Infundibulum (pituitary stalk)

Hypophysis (pituitary gland)

Mammillothalamic tract

Dorsal longitudinal fasciculus and other descending pathways

Lamina terminalis

Paraventricular hypothalamic nucleus

Supraoptic hypothalamic nucleus

Supraopticohypophyseal tract

Tuberohypophyseal tract

Hypothalamohypophyseal tract

Infundibulum (pituitary stalk)

Adenohypophysis (anterior lobe of pituitary gland)

Pars tuberalis
Fibrous trabecula
Pars intermedia
Pars distalis

Cleft

Hypothalamic sulcus

Mammillary body

Arcuate (infundibular) nucleus

Median eminence of tuber cinereum

Infundibular stem

Infundibular process

Neurohypophysis (posterior lobe of pituitary gland)

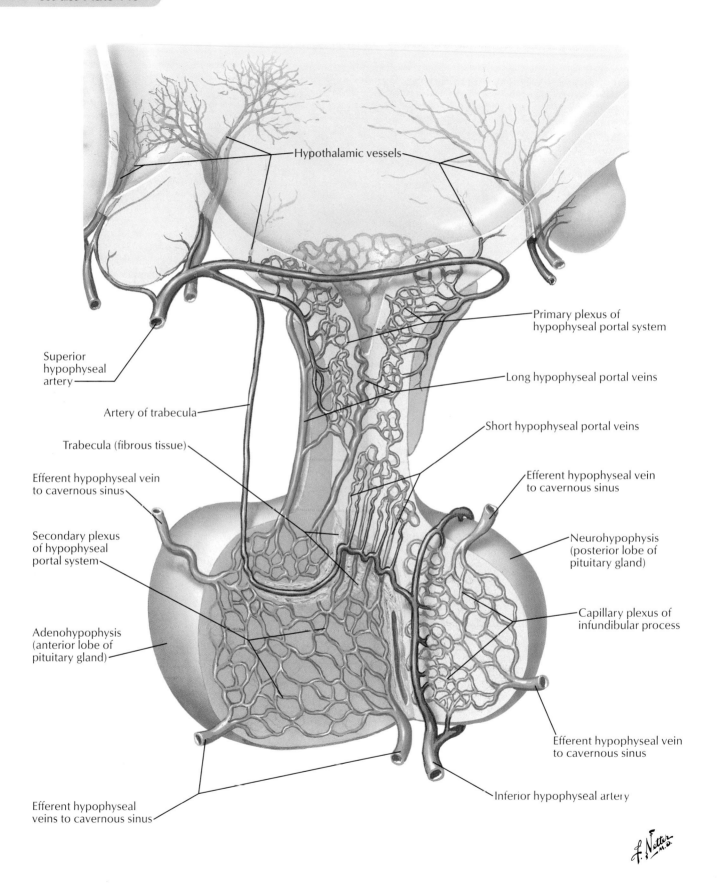

Hypothalamic vessels

Primary plexus of hypophyseal portal system

Superior hypophyseal artery

Long hypophyseal portal veins

Artery of trabecula

Short hypophyseal portal veins

Trabecula (fibrous tissue)

Efferent hypophyseal vein to cavernous sinus

Efferent hypophyseal vein to cavernous sinus

Secondary plexus of hypophyseal portal system

Neurohypophysis (posterior lobe of pituitary gland)

Capillary plexus of infundibular process

Adenohypophysis (anterior lobe of pituitary gland)

Efferent hypophyseal vein to cavernous sinus

Efferent hypophyseal veins to cavernous sinus

Inferior hypophyseal artery

Plate 148   **Cerebral Vasculature**

Median (A) and paramedian (B, C) sagittal MR images

A

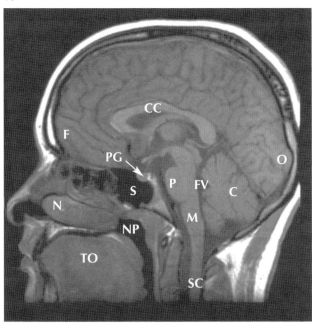

C	Cerebellum	N	Inferior nasal concha
CC	Corpus callosum	NP	Nasopharynx
E	Extraocular muscles	O	Occipital pole
F	Frontal pole	ON	Optic nerve
FV	Fourth ventricle	P	Pons
L	Lateral ventricle	PG	Pituitary gland
M	Medulla oblongata	S	Sphenoid sinus
MB	Midbrain	SC	Spinal cord
MS	Maxillary sinus	T	Thalamus
		TC	Tentorium cerebelli
		TO	Tongue

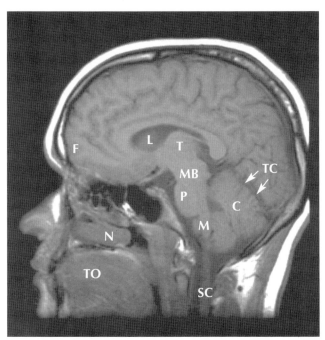

B

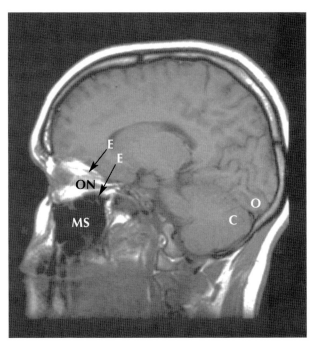

C

Axial CT images of the head from inferior (A) to superior (C)

A

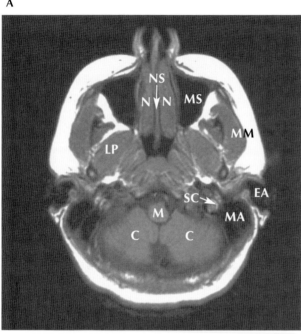

B	Basilar artery	**M**	Medulla oblongata
C	Cerebellum	**MA**	Mastoid air cells
CH	Cerebral hemisphere	**MB**	Midbrain
		MM	Masseter muscle
CS	Confluence of sinuses	**MR**	Medial rectus muscle
E	Eye	**MS**	Maxillary sinus
EA	External acoustic meatus	**N**	Nasal concha
		NS	Nasal septum
ES	Ethmoid sinus	**P**	Pons
F	Fat in orbit	**S**	Sphenoid sinus
FV	Fourth ventricle	**SC**	Semicircular canals
L	Lens		
LP	Lateral pterygoid muscle	**SS**	Superior sagittal sinus
LR	Lateral rectus muscle	**T**	Temporalis muscle
		TL	Temporal lobe

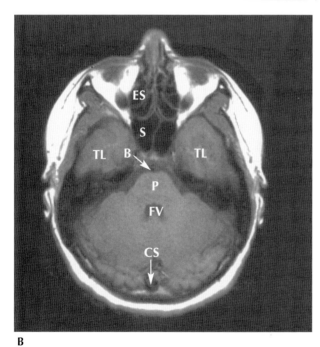

B

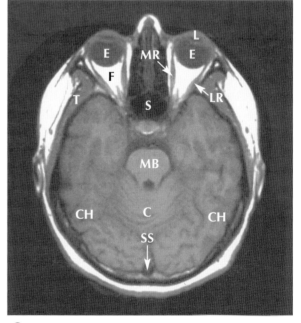

C

Plate 150

Regional Scans

Coronal CT images of the head from anterior (A) to posterior (C)

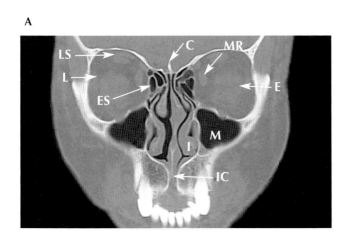

A

A	Anterior clinoid process	**L**	Lateral rectus muscle
C	Crista galli	**LS**	Levator palpebrae superioris and superior rectus muscles
E	Eye (vitreous chamber)		
ES	Ethmoid sinus	**M**	Maxillary sinus
G	Greater wing of the sphenoid	**MR**	Medial rectus muscle
I	Inferior nasal concha	**N**	Nasal septum
IC	Incisive canal	**OC**	Oral cavity
IR	Inferior rectus muscle	**S**	Sphenoid sinus
		Z	Zygomatic arch

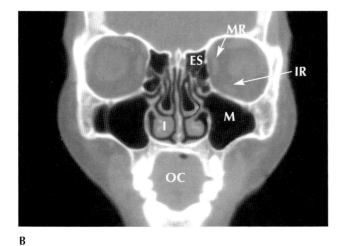

B

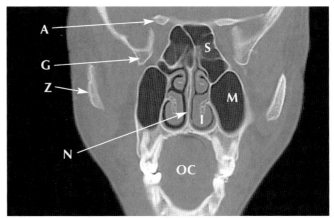

C

Section 2 **Back and Spinal Cord**

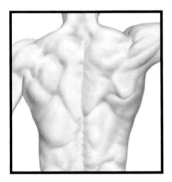
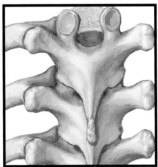
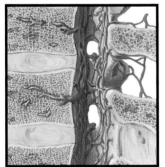
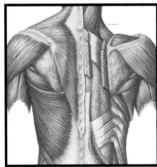

Topographic Anatomy
Plate 152

2 Back and Spinal Cord

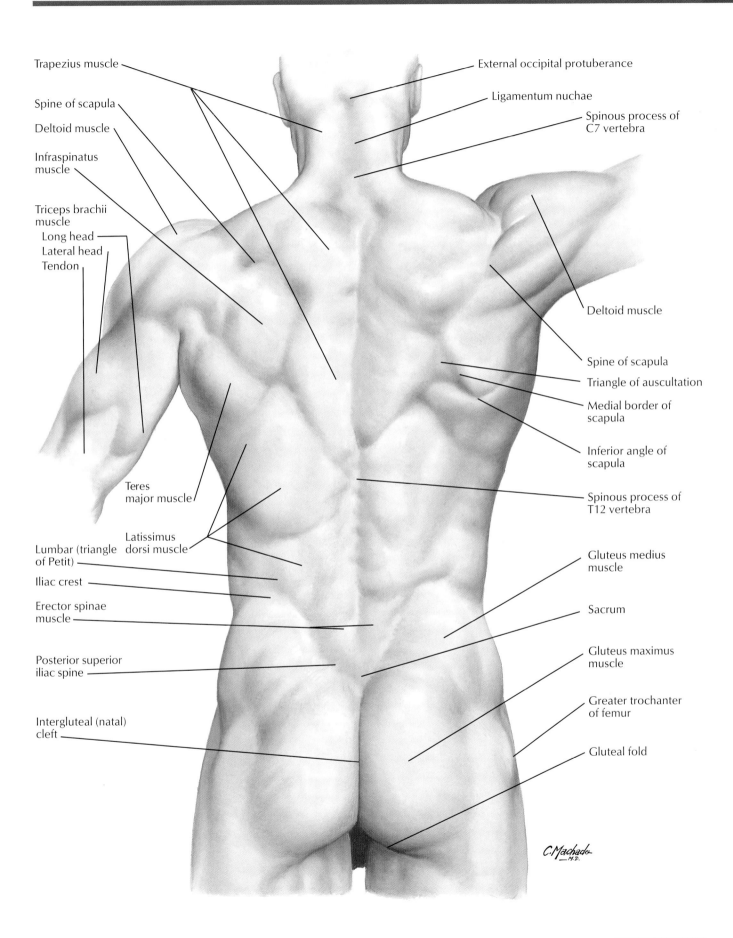

Trapezius muscle

Spine of scapula

Deltoid muscle

Infraspinatus
muscle

Triceps brachii
muscle
  Long head
  Lateral head
  Tendon

External occipital protuberance

Ligamentum nuchae

Spinous process of
C7 vertebra

Deltoid muscle

Spine of scapula

Triangle of auscultation

Medial border of
scapula

Inferior angle of
scapula

Spinous process of
T12 vertebra

Teres
major muscle

Latissimus
dorsi muscle

Lumbar (triangle
of Petit)

Iliac crest

Erector spinae
muscle

Posterior superior
iliac spine

Intergluteal (natal)
cleft

Gluteus medius
muscle

Sacrum

Gluteus maximus
muscle

Greater trochanter
of femur

Gluteal fold

C. Machado
—M.D.

See also **Plates 13, 17, 18, 154, 155, 157, 185, 248**

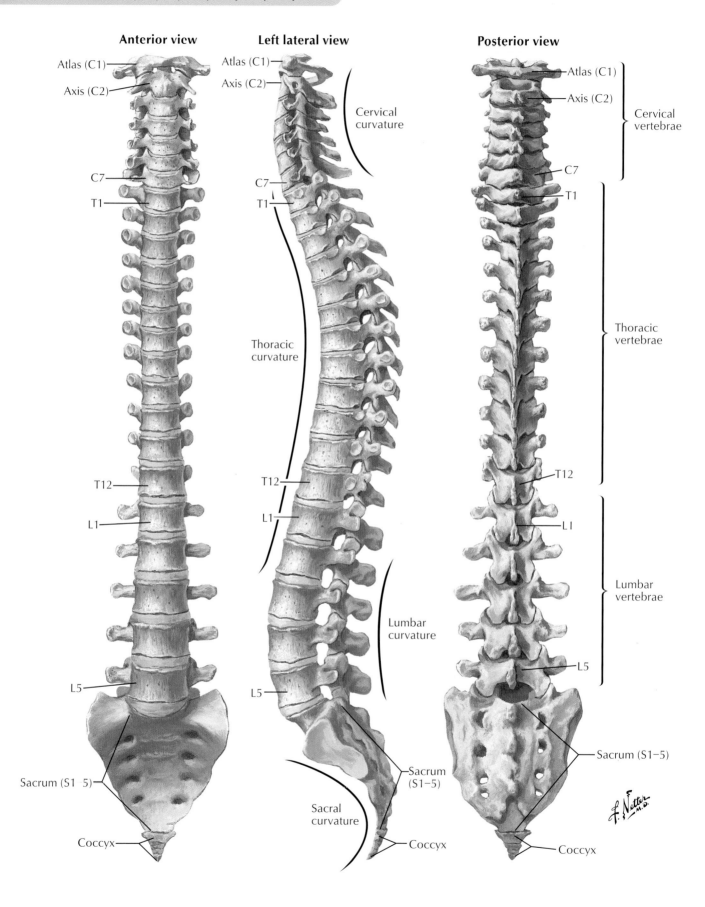

Anterior view

Atlas (C1)
Axis (C2)
C7
T1
T12
L1
L5
Sacrum (S1 5)
Coccyx

Left lateral view

Atlas (C1)
Axis (C2)
Cervical curvature
C7
T1
Thoracic curvature
T12
L1
Lumbar curvature
L5
Sacrum (S1–5)
Sacral curvature
Coccyx

Posterior view

Atlas (C1)
Axis (C2)
Cervical vertebrae
C7
T1
Thoracic vertebrae
T12
L1
Lumbar vertebrae
L5
Sacrum (S1–5)
Coccyx

Plate 153

Bones and Ligaments

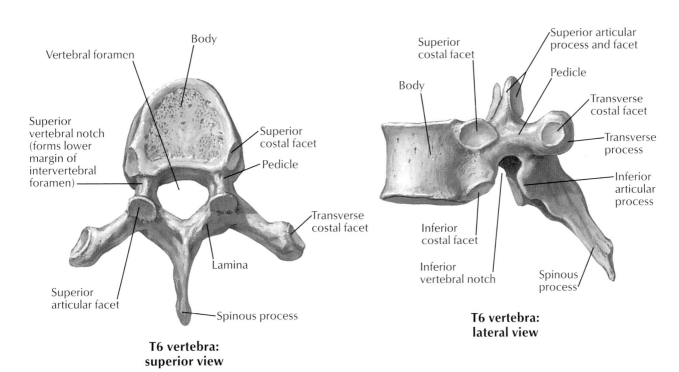

Vertebral foramen

Body

Superior
vertebral notch
(forms lower
margin of
intervertebral
foramen)

Superior
costal facet

Pedicle

Transverse
costal facet

Superior
articular facet

Lamina

Spinous process

**T6 vertebra:
superior view**

Superior
costal facet

Body

Superior articular
process and facet

Pedicle

Transverse
costal facet

Transverse
process

Inferior
articular
process

Inferior
costal facet

Inferior
vertebral notch

Spinous
process

**T6 vertebra:
lateral view**

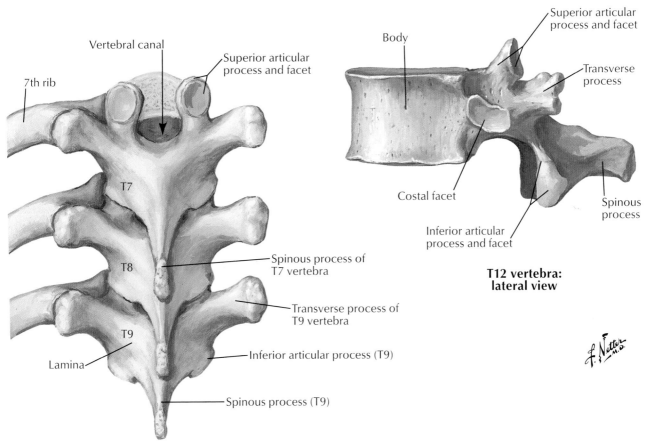

Vertebral canal

Superior articular
process and facet

7th rib

T7

T8

T9

Lamina

Spinous process of
T7 vertebra

Transverse process of
T9 vertebra

Inferior articular process (T9)

Spinous process (T9)

**T7, T8 and T9 vertebrae:
posterior view**

Body

Superior articular
process and facet

Transverse
process

Costal facet

Inferior articular
process and facet

Spinous
process

**T12 vertebra:
lateral view**

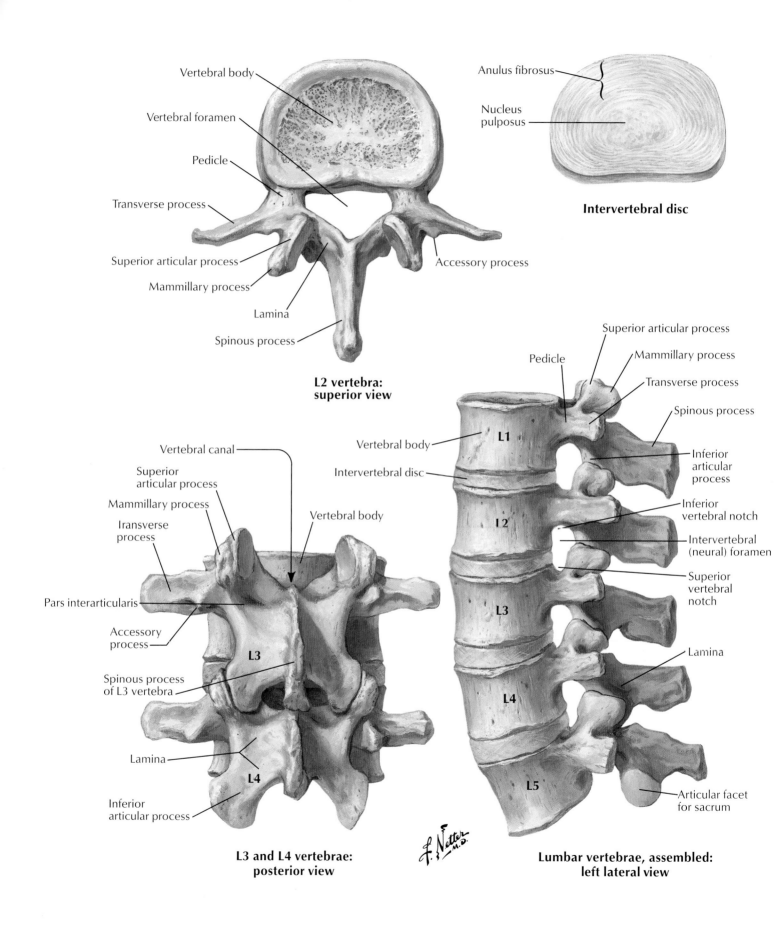

Vertebral body

Vertebral foramen

Pedicle

Transverse process

Superior articular process

Mammillary process

Lamina

Spinous process

**L2 vertebra:
superior view**

Anulus fibrosus

Nucleus
pulposus

Intervertebral disc

Vertebral canal

Superior
articular process

Mammillary process

Transverse
process

Pars interarticularis

Accessory
process

Spinous process
of L3 vertebra

Lamina

Inferior
articular process

Vertebral body

L3

L4

**L3 and L4 vertebrae:
posterior view**

Superior articular process

Mammillary process

Pedicle

Transverse process

Spinous process

Vertebral body

Intervertebral disc

L1

L2

L3

L4

L5

Inferior
articular
process

Inferior
vertebral notch

Intervertebral
(neural) foramen

Superior
vertebral
notch

Lamina

Articular facet
for sacrum

**Lumbar vertebrae, assembled:
left lateral view**

Plate 155

Bones and Ligaments

Anteroposterior radiograph

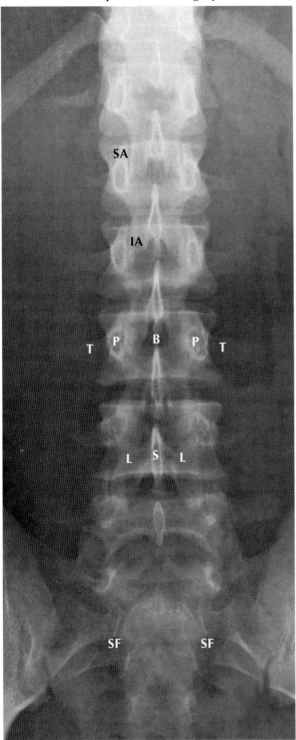

Lateral radiograph

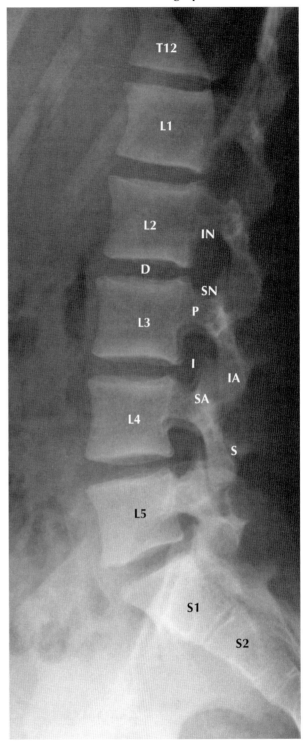

B	Body of L3 vertebra
IA	Inferior articular process of L1 vertebra
L	Lamina of L4 vertebra
P	Pedicle of L3 vertebra
S	Spinous process of L4 vertebra
SA	Superior articular process of L1 vertebra
SF	Sacral foramen
T	Transverse process of L3 vertebra

D	Intervertebral disc space
I	Intervertebral foramen
IA	Inferior articular process of L3 vertebra
IN	Inferior vertebral notch of L2 vertebra
P	Pedicle of L3 vertebra
S	Spinous process of L3 vertebra
SA	Superior articular process of L4 vertebra
SN	Superior vertebral notch of L3 vertebra
Note:	The vertebral bodies are numbered

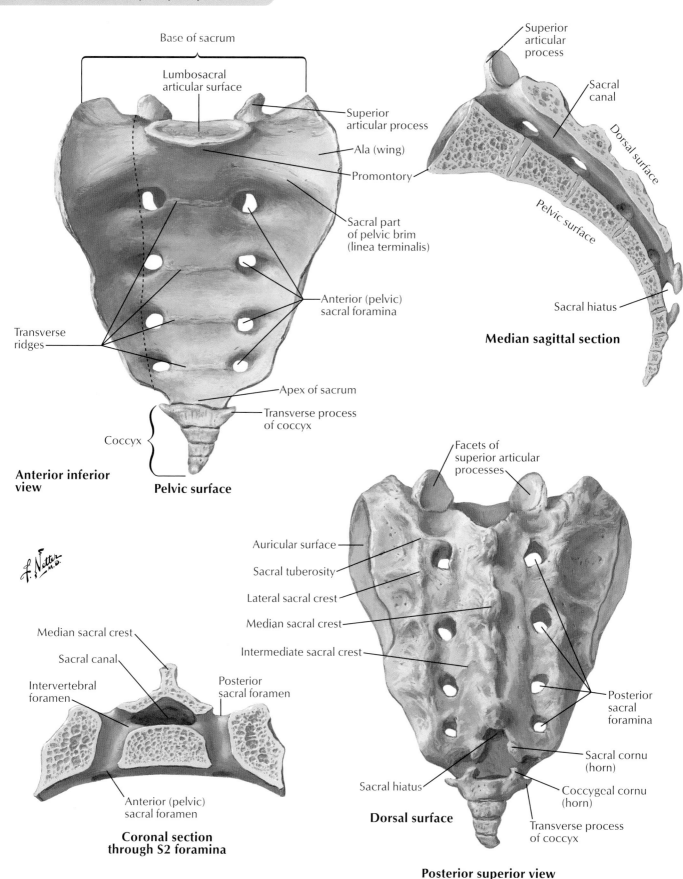

Base of sacrum

Lumbosacral
articular surface

Superior
articular process

Ala (wing)

Promontory

Sacral part
of pelvic brim
(linea terminalis)

Anterior (pelvic)
sacral foramina

Transverse
ridges

Apex of sacrum

Transverse process
of coccyx

Coccyx

**Anterior inferior
view**

Pelvic surface

Superior
articular
process

Sacral
canal

Dorsal surface

Pelvic surface

Sacral hiatus

Median sagittal section

Facets of
superior articular
processes

Auricular surface

Sacral tuberosity

Lateral sacral crest

Median sacral crest

Intermediate sacral crest

Median sacral crest

Sacral canal

Intervertebral
foramen

Posterior
sacral foramen

Anterior (pelvic)
sacral foramen

**Coronal section
through S2 foramina**

Posterior
sacral
foramina

Sacral cornu
(horn)

Coccygeal cornu
(horn)

Sacral hiatus

Transverse process
of coccyx

Dorsal surface

Posterior superior view

Plate 157

Bones and Ligaments

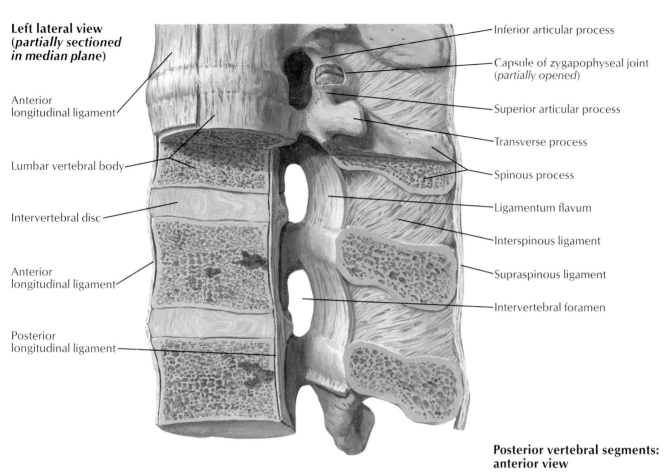

Left lateral view (*partially sectioned in median plane*)

Anterior longitudinal ligament

Lumbar vertebral body

Intervertebral disc

Anterior longitudinal ligament

Posterior longitudinal ligament

Inferior articular process

Capsule of zygapophyseal joint (*partially opened*)

Superior articular process

Transverse process

Spinous process

Ligamentum flavum

Interspinous ligament

Supraspinous ligament

Intervertebral foramen

Posterior vertebral segments: anterior view

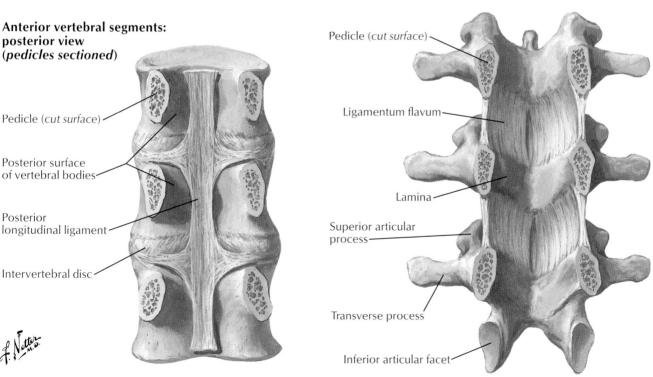

Anterior vertebral segments: posterior view (*pedicles sectioned*)

Pedicle (*cut surface*)

Posterior surface of vertebral bodies

Posterior longitudinal ligament

Intervertebral disc

Pedicle (*cut surface*)

Ligamentum flavum

Lamina

Superior articular process

Transverse process

Inferior articular facet

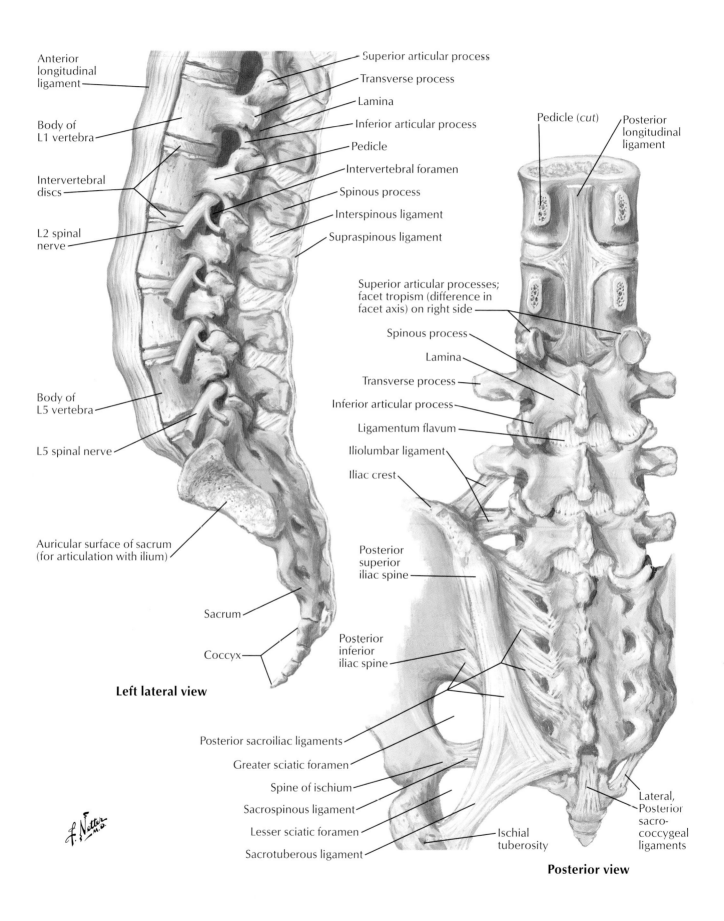

Anterior longitudinal ligament

Body of L1 vertebra

Intervertebral discs

L2 spinal nerve

Body of L5 vertebra

L5 spinal nerve

Auricular surface of sacrum (for articulation with ilium)

Sacrum

Coccyx

Left lateral view

Superior articular process

Transverse process

Lamina

Inferior articular process

Pedicle

Intervertebral foramen

Spinous process

Interspinous ligament

Supraspinous ligament

Pedicle (*cut*)

Posterior longitudinal ligament

Superior articular processes; facet tropism (difference in facet axis) on right side

Spinous process

Lamina

Transverse process

Inferior articular process

Ligamentum flavum

Iliolumbar ligament

Iliac crest

Posterior superior iliac spine

Posterior inferior iliac spine

Posterior sacroiliac ligaments

Greater sciatic foramen

Spine of ischium

Sacrospinous ligament

Lesser sciatic foramen

Sacrotuberous ligament

Ischial tuberosity

Lateral, Posterior sacro-coccygeal ligaments

Posterior view

Plate 159   **Bones and Ligaments**

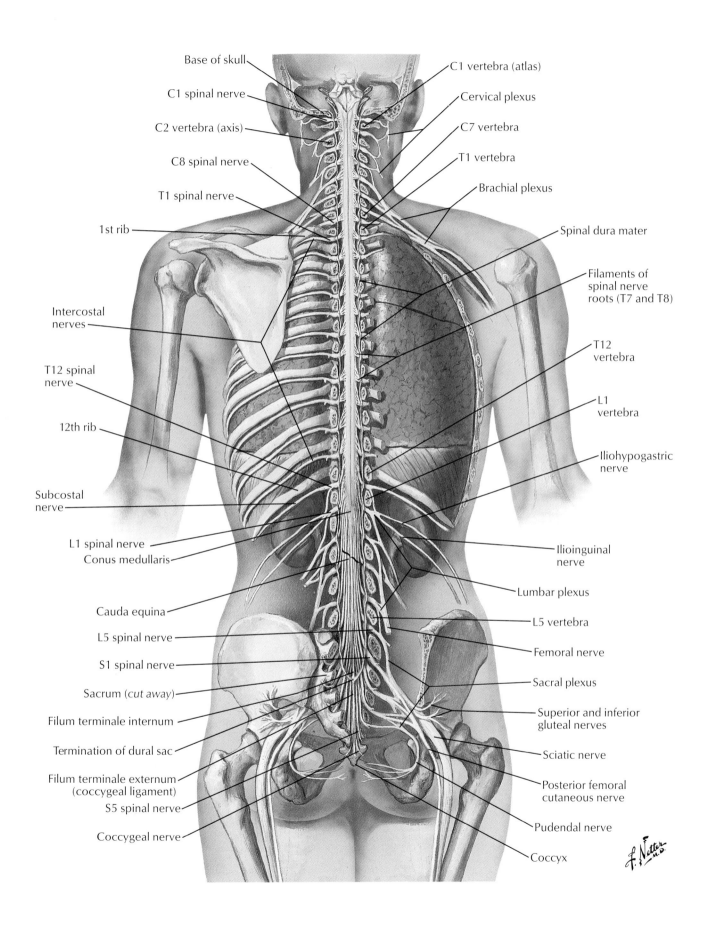

Base of skull

C1 spinal nerve

C2 vertebra (axis)

C8 spinal nerve

T1 spinal nerve

1st rib

Intercostal nerves

T12 spinal nerve

12th rib

Subcostal nerve

L1 spinal nerve

Conus medullaris

Cauda equina

L5 spinal nerve

S1 spinal nerve

Sacrum (cut away)

Filum terminale internum

Termination of dural sac

Filum terminale externum (coccygeal ligament)

S5 spinal nerve

Coccygeal nerve

C1 vertebra (atlas)

Cervical plexus

C7 vertebra

T1 vertebra

Brachial plexus

Spinal dura mater

Filaments of spinal nerve roots (T7 and T8)

T12 vertebra

L1 vertebra

Iliohypogastric nerve

Ilioinguinal nerve

Lumbar plexus

L5 vertebra

Femoral nerve

Sacral plexus

Superior and inferior gluteal nerves

Sciatic nerve

Posterior femoral cutaneous nerve

Pudendal nerve

Coccyx

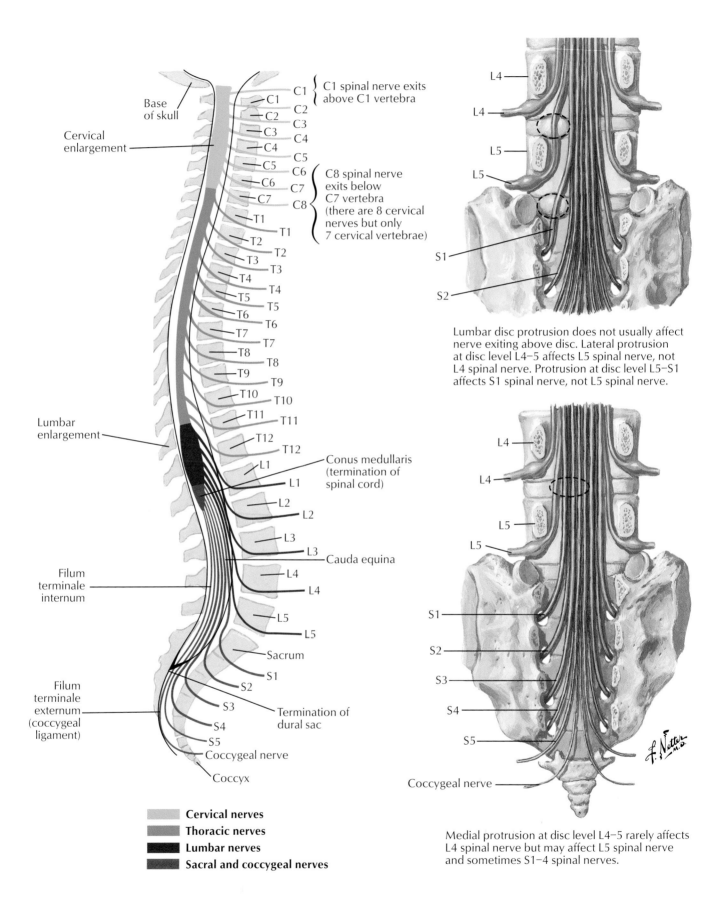

Base of skull

Cervical enlargement

C1 { C1 spinal nerve exits above C1 vertebra

C1
C2
C3
C4
C5
C6
C7
C8 { C8 spinal nerve exits below C7 vertebra (there are 8 cervical nerves but only 7 cervical vertebrae)

C1
C2
C3
C4
C5
C6
C7

T1
T2
T3
T4
T5
T6
T7
T8
T9
T10
T11
T12

T1
T2
T3
T4
T5
T6
T7
T8
T9
T10
T11
T12

Lumbar enlargement

Conus medullaris (termination of spinal cord)

L1
L2
L3
L4
L5

L1
L2
L3
L4
L5

Cauda equina

Filum terminale internum

Sacrum

S1
S2
S3
S4
S5

Termination of dural sac

Filum terminale externum (coccygeal ligament)

Coccygeal nerve

Coccyx

Cervical nerves
Thoracic nerves
Lumbar nerves
Sacral and coccygeal nerves

L4
L4
L5
L5
S1
S2

Lumbar disc protrusion does not usually affect nerve exiting above disc. Lateral protrusion at disc level L4–5 affects L5 spinal nerve, not L4 spinal nerve. Protrusion at disc level L5–S1 affects S1 spinal nerve, not L5 spinal nerve.

L4
L4
L5
L5
S1
S2
S3
S4
S5

Coccygeal nerve

Medial protrusion at disc level L4–5 rarely affects L4 spinal nerve but may affect L5 spinal nerve and sometimes S1–4 spinal nerves.

Plate 161   **Spinal Cord**

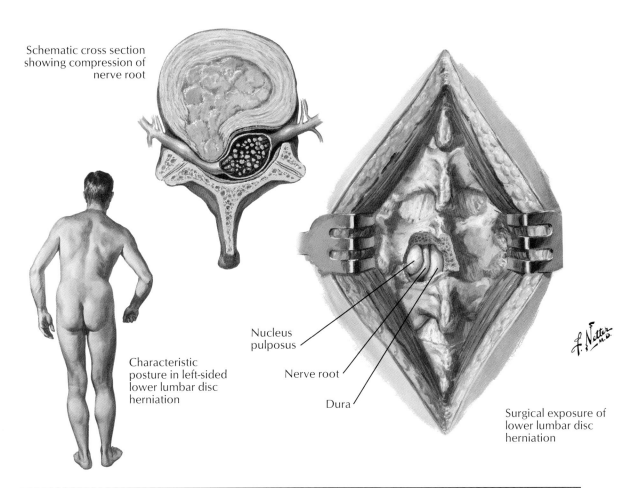

Schematic cross section showing compression of nerve root

Characteristic posture in left-sided lower lumbar disc herniation

Nucleus pulposus

Nerve root

Dura

Surgical exposure of lower lumbar disc herniation

Clinical features of herniated lumbar nucleus pulposus					
Level of herniation	Pain	Numbness	Weakness	Atrophy	Reflexes
L3 L4 L5 L5 S **L4—5 disc; 5th lumbar nerve root**	Over sacro-iliac joint, hip, lateral thigh and leg	Lateral leg, first 3 toes	Dorsiflexion of great toe and foot; difficulty walking on heels; foot drop may occur	Minor	Changes uncommon in knee and ankle jerks, but internal hamstring reflex diminished or absent
L4 L5 S **L5—S1 disc; 1st sacral nerve root**	Over sacro-iliac joint, hip, postero-lateral thigh and leg to heel	Back of calf, lateral heel, foot to toe	Plantar flexion of foot and great toe may be affected; difficulty walking on toes	Gastrocnemi-us and soleus	Ankle jerk diminished or absent

Lumbar puncture

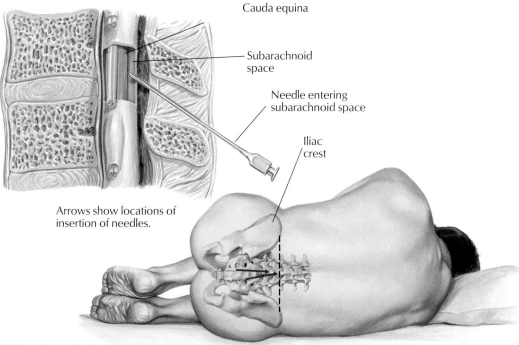

Cauda equina

Subarachnoid space

Needle entering subarachnoid space

Iliac crest

Arrows show locations of insertion of needles.

Epidural anesthesia

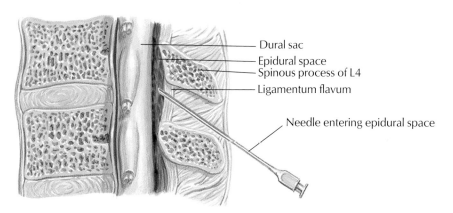

Dural sac
Epidural space
Spinous process of L4
Ligamentum flavum

Needle entering epidural space

Epidural anesthesia and lumbar puncture are performed by inserting a needle above or below the L4 vertebral spine, which lies at the level of the iliac crest. For epidural anesthesia, the needle passes into the epidural space, and anesthetic agent bathes the nerve roots in proximity. Lumbar puncture, on the other hand, is performed in order to collect a sample of cerebrospinal fluid (CSF) or to introduce an anesthetic agent into the CSF (spinal anesthesia), so therefore the needle penetrates the dural sac to enter the subarachnoid space.

C. Machado
—M.D.

Plate 163

Spinal Cord

See also **Plates 483, 543**; for maps of cutaneous nerves see **Plates 24, 472, 474–476, 478, 481, 538–542**

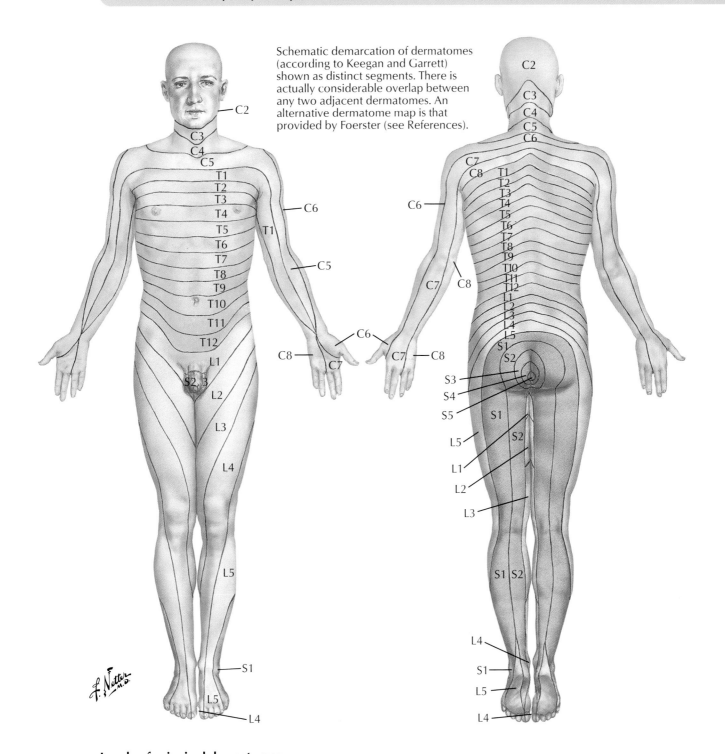

Schematic demarcation of dermatomes (according to Keegan and Garrett) shown as distinct segments. There is actually considerable overlap between any two adjacent dermatomes. An alternative dermatome map is that provided by Foerster (see References).

Levels of principal dermatomes

C5	Clavicles
C5, 6, 7	Lateral parts of upper limbs
C8, T1	Medial sides of upper limbs
C6	Thumb
C6, 7, 8	Hand
C8	Ring and little fingers
T4	Level of nipples
T10	Level of umbilicus
L1	Inguinal or groin regions
L1, 2, 3, 4	Anterior and inner surfaces of lower limbs
L4, 5, S1	Foot
L4	Medial side of great toe
S1, 2, L5	Posterior and outer surfaces of lower limbs
S1	Lateral margin of foot and little toe
S2, 3, 4	Perineum

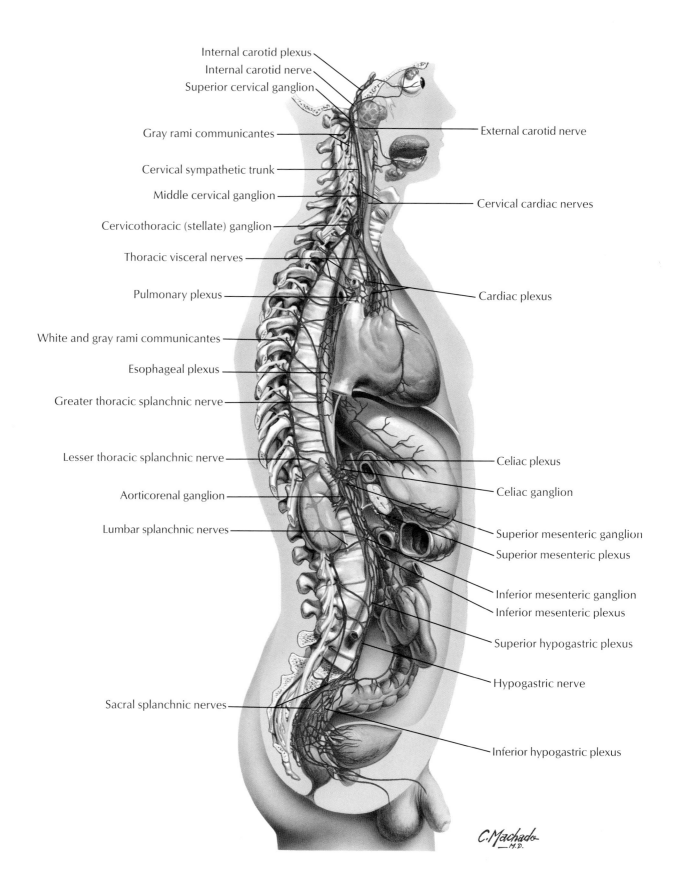

Internal carotid plexus

Internal carotid nerve

Superior cervical ganglion

Gray rami communicantes

Cervical sympathetic trunk

Middle cervical ganglion

Cervicothoracic (stellate) ganglion

Thoracic visceral nerves

Pulmonary plexus

White and gray rami communicantes

Esophageal plexus

Greater thoracic splanchnic nerve

Lesser thoracic splanchnic nerve

Aorticorenal ganglion

Lumbar splanchnic nerves

Sacral splanchnic nerves

External carotid nerve

Cervical cardiac nerves

Cardiac plexus

Celiac plexus

Celiac ganglion

Superior mesenteric ganglion

Superior mesenteric plexus

Inferior mesenteric ganglion

Inferior mesenteric plexus

Superior hypogastric plexus

Hypogastric nerve

Inferior hypogastric plexus

C. Machado
M.D.

Plate 165

Spinal Cord

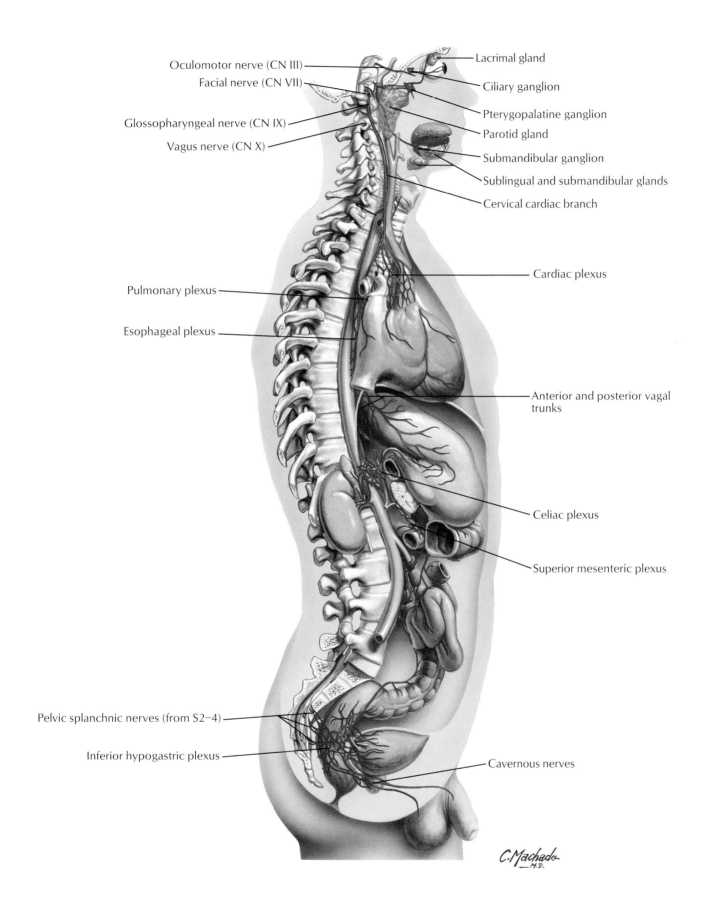

Oculomotor nerve (CN III)

Facial nerve (CN VII)

Glossopharyngeal nerve (CN IX)

Vagus nerve (CN X)

Lacrimal gland

Ciliary ganglion

Pterygopalatine ganglion

Parotid gland

Submandibular ganglion

Sublingual and submandibular glands

Cervical cardiac branch

Cardiac plexus

Pulmonary plexus

Esophageal plexus

Anterior and posterior vagal trunks

Celiac plexus

Superior mesenteric plexus

Pelvic splanchnic nerves (from S2–4)

Inferior hypogastric plexus

Cavernous nerves

C. Machado
_M.D._

Sympathetic Nervous System: Schema

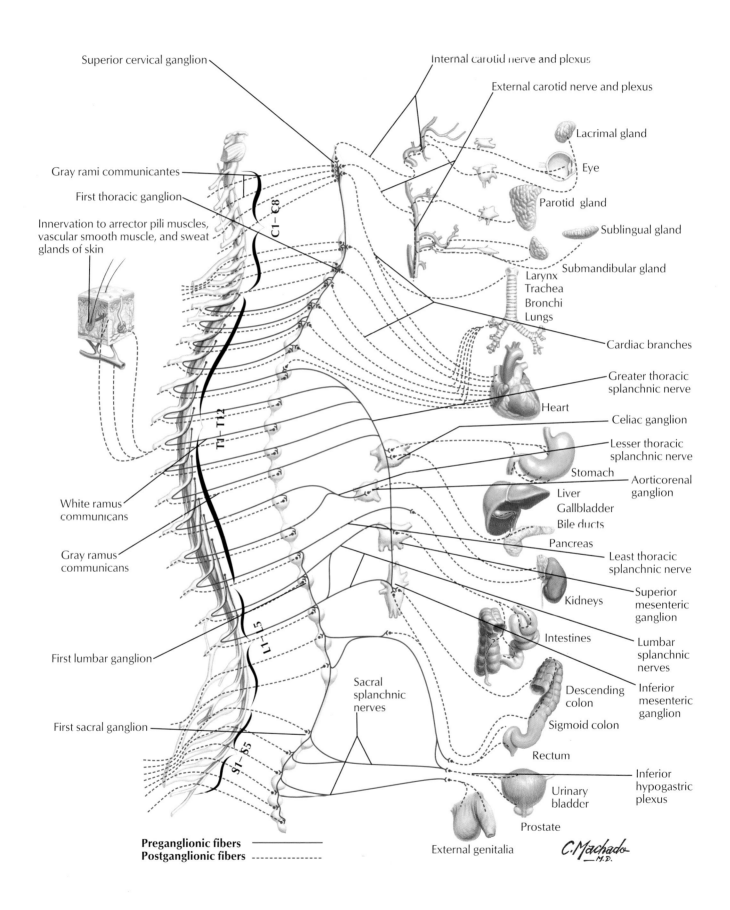

Superior cervical ganglion

Internal carotid nerve and plexus

External carotid nerve and plexus

Lacrimal gland

Eye

Gray rami communicantes

Parotid gland

First thoracic ganglion

Sublingual gland

Innervation to arrector pili muscles, vascular smooth muscle, and sweat glands of skin

Submandibular gland

Larynx
Trachea
Bronchi
Lungs

C1–C8

Cardiac branches

Greater thoracic splanchnic nerve

Heart

Celiac ganglion

T1–T12

Lesser thoracic splanchnic nerve

Stomach

Aorticorenal ganglion

Liver
Gallbladder
Bile ducts

White ramus communicans

Pancreas

Least thoracic splanchnic nerve

Gray ramus communicans

Kidneys

Superior mesenteric ganglion

Intestines

Lumbar splanchnic nerves

L1–L5

First lumbar ganglion

Inferior mesenteric ganglion

Sacral splanchnic nerves

Descending colon

Sigmoid colon

First sacral ganglion

Rectum

Inferior hypogastric plexus

S1–S5

Urinary bladder

Prostate

External genitalia

C. Machado
—M.D.

Preganglionic fibers ——————
Postganglionic fibers - - - - - - -

Plate 167

Spinal Cord

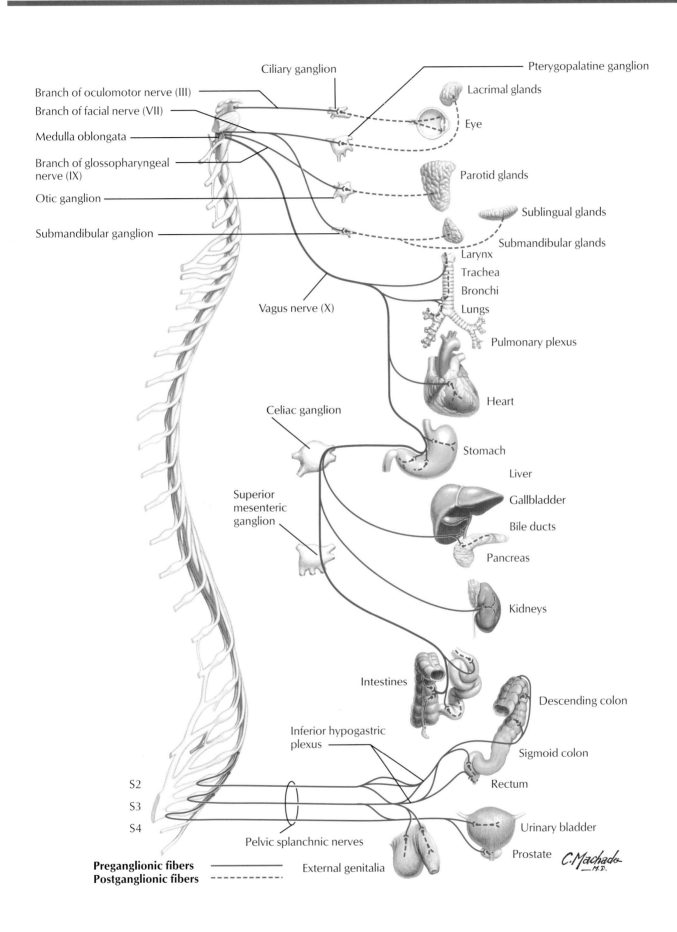

Ciliary ganglion

Pterygopalatine ganglion

Branch of oculomotor nerve (III)

Lacrimal glands

Branch of facial nerve (VII)

Eye

Medulla oblongata

Branch of glossopharyngeal nerve (IX)

Parotid glands

Otic ganglion

Sublingual glands

Submandibular ganglion

Submandibular glands

Larynx

Trachea

Bronchi

Lungs

Vagus nerve (X)

Pulmonary plexus

Heart

Celiac ganglion

Stomach

Liver

Gallbladder

Superior mesenteric ganglion

Bile ducts

Pancreas

Kidneys

Intestines

Descending colon

Inferior hypogastric plexus

Sigmoid colon

Rectum

S2

S3

S4

Urinary bladder

Pelvic splanchnic nerves

Prostate

Preganglionic fibers
Postganglionic fibers

External genitalia

C. Machado
M.D.

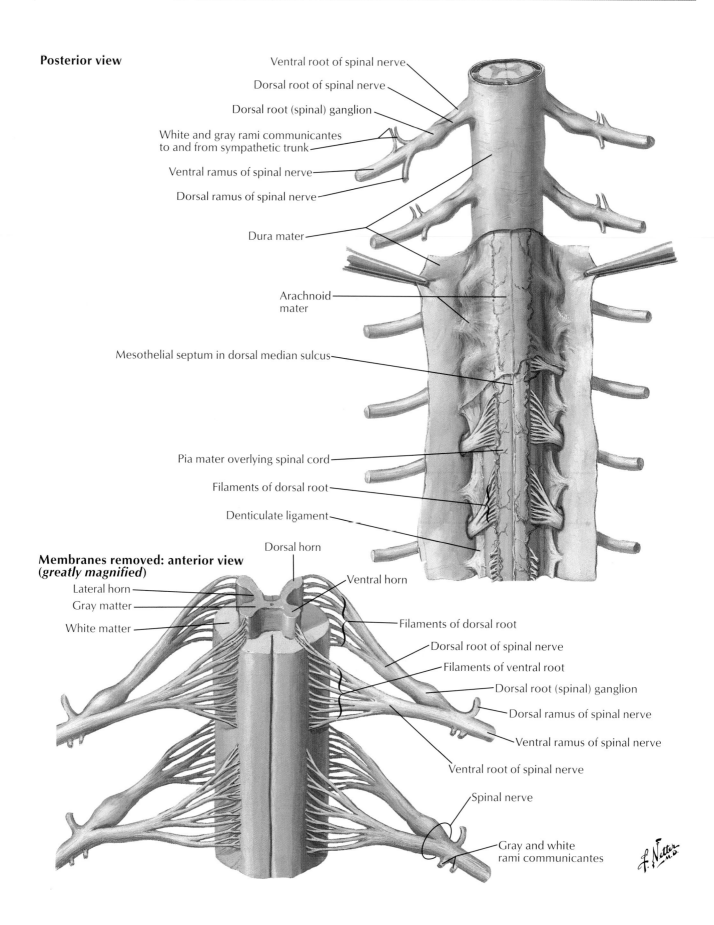

Posterior view

Ventral root of spinal nerve

Dorsal root of spinal nerve

Dorsal root (spinal) ganglion

White and gray rami communicantes
to and from sympathetic trunk

Ventral ramus of spinal nerve

Dorsal ramus of spinal nerve

Dura mater

Arachnoid mater

Mesothelial septum in dorsal median sulcus

Pia mater overlying spinal cord

Filaments of dorsal root

Denticulate ligament

Dorsal horn

Membranes removed: anterior view
(*greatly magnified*)

Lateral horn

Gray matter

White matter

Ventral horn

Filaments of dorsal root

Dorsal root of spinal nerve

Filaments of ventral root

Dorsal root (spinal) ganglion

Dorsal ramus of spinal nerve

Ventral ramus of spinal nerve

Ventral root of spinal nerve

Spinal nerve

Gray and white
rami communicantes

Plate 169   **Spinal Cord**

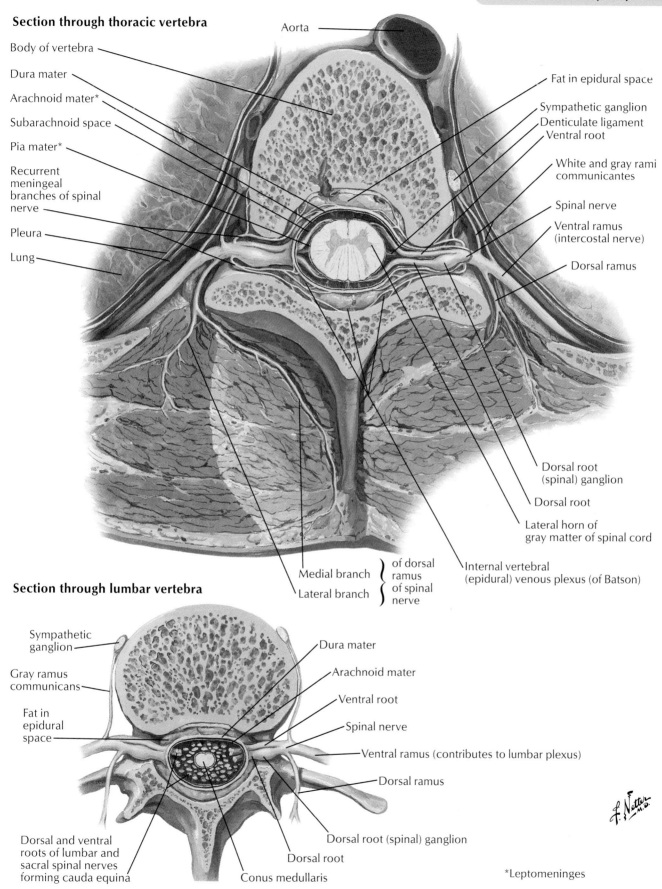

Section through thoracic vertebra

Aorta

Body of vertebra

Dura mater

Arachnoid mater*

Subarachnoid space

Pia mater*

Recurrent meningeal branches of spinal nerve

Pleura

Lung

Fat in epidural space

Sympathetic ganglion

Denticulate ligament

Ventral root

White and gray rami communicantes

Spinal nerve

Ventral ramus (intercostal nerve)

Dorsal ramus

Dorsal root (spinal) ganglion

Dorsal root

Lateral horn of gray matter of spinal cord

Internal vertebral (epidural) venous plexus (of Batson)

Medial branch } of dorsal ramus
Lateral branch } of spinal nerve

Section through lumbar vertebra

Sympathetic ganglion

Gray ramus communicans

Fat in epidural space

Dura mater

Arachnoid mater

Ventral root

Spinal nerve

Ventral ramus (contributes to lumbar plexus)

Dorsal ramus

Dorsal root (spinal) ganglion

Dorsal root

Conus medullaris

Dorsal and ventral roots of lumbar and sacral spinal nerves forming cauda equina

*Leptomeninges

Arteries of Spinal Cord: Schema

See also **Plate 138**

Anterior view

Posterior view

Posterior cerebral artery

Superior cerebellar artery

Basilar artery

Anterior inferior cerebellar artery (AICA)

Posterior inferior cerebellar artery (PICA)

Anterior spinal artery

Vertebral artery

Anterior segmental medullary arteries

Ascending cervical artery

Deep cervical artery

Subclavian artery

Anterior segmental medullary artery

Posterior intercostal artery

Pial plexus

Major anterior segmental medullary artery (great radicular artery of Adamkiewicz)

Posterior intercostal artery

Anterior segmental medullary artery

Lumbar artery

Anastomotic loops to posterior spinal arteries

Cauda equina arteries

Lateral (or medial) sacral arteries

Cervical vertebrae

Thoracic vertebrae

Lumbar vertebrae

Sacrum

Posterior inferior cerebellar artery

Posterior spinal arteries

Vertebral artery

Posterior segmental medullary arteries

Deep cervical artery

Ascending cervical artery

Subclavian artery

Posterior segmental medullary arteries

Posterior intercostal arteries

Posterior segmental medullary arteries

Anastomotic loops to anterior spinal artery

Lumbar arteries

Lateral (or medial) sacral arteries

Note: All spinal nerve roots have associated **radicular** or **segmental medullary arteries**. Most roots have radicular arteries (see Plate 172). Both types of arteries run along roots, but radicular arteries end before reaching anterior or posterior spinal arteries; larger segmental medullary arteries continue on to supply a segment of these arteries.

f. Netter
M.D.

Plate 171

Spinal Cord

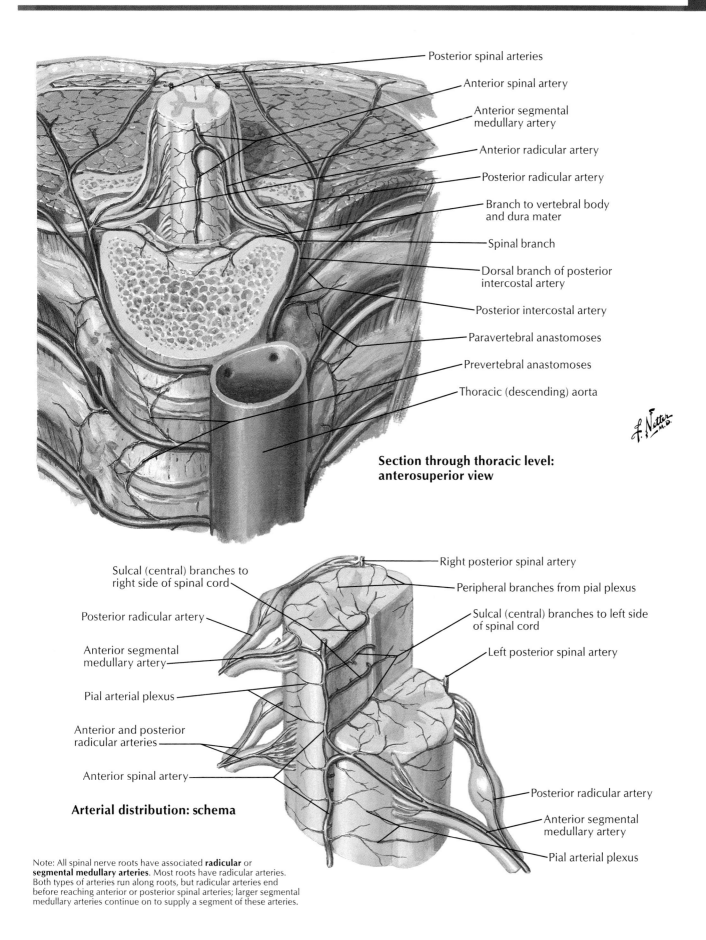

Posterior spinal arteries

Anterior spinal artery

Anterior segmental medullary artery

Anterior radicular artery

Posterior radicular artery

Branch to vertebral body and dura mater

Spinal branch

Dorsal branch of posterior intercostal artery

Posterior intercostal artery

Paravertebral anastomoses

Prevertebral anastomoses

Thoracic (descending) aorta

Section through thoracic level: anterosuperior view

Sulcal (central) branches to right side of spinal cord

Posterior radicular artery

Anterior segmental medullary artery

Pial arterial plexus

Anterior and posterior radicular arteries

Anterior spinal artery

Arterial distribution: schema

Right posterior spinal artery

Peripheral branches from pial plexus

Sulcal (central) branches to left side of spinal cord

Left posterior spinal artery

Posterior radicular artery

Anterior segmental medullary artery

Pial arterial plexus

Note: All spinal nerve roots have associated **radicular** or **segmental medullary arteries**. Most roots have radicular arteries. Both types of arteries run along roots, but radicular arteries end before reaching anterior or posterior spinal arteries; larger segmental medullary arteries continue on to supply a segment of these arteries.

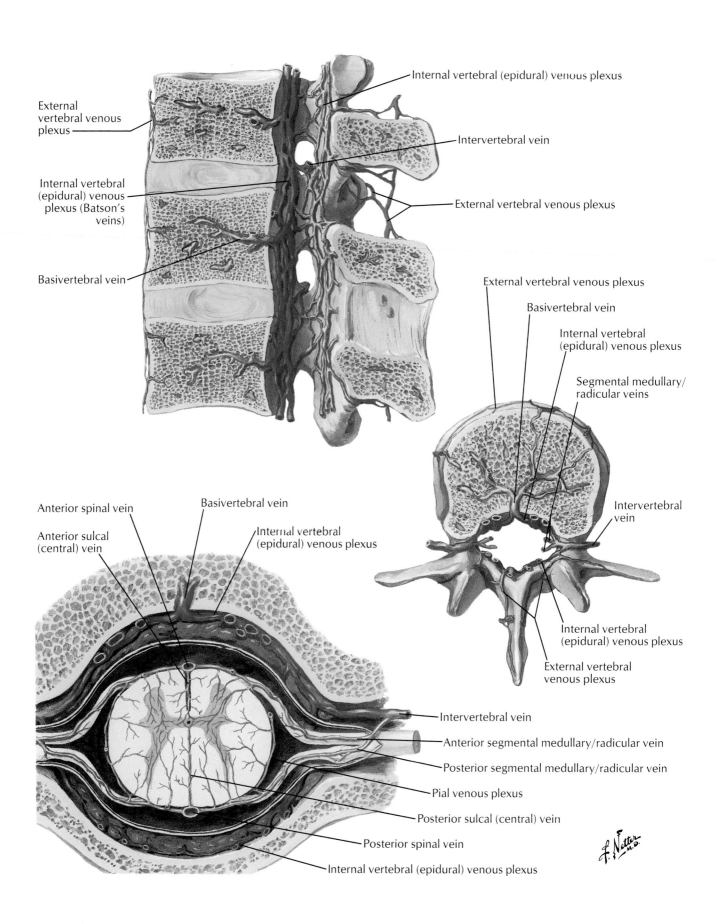

External vertebral venous plexus

Internal vertebral (epidural) venous plexus

Internal vertebral (epidural) venous plexus (Batson's veins)

Intervertebral vein

External vertebral venous plexus

Basivertebral vein

External vertebral venous plexus

Basivertebral vein

Internal vertebral (epidural) venous plexus

Segmental medullary/radicular veins

Intervertebral vein

Internal vertebral (epidural) venous plexus

External vertebral venous plexus

Anterior spinal vein

Basivertebral vein

Anterior sulcal (central) vein

Internal vertebral (epidural) venous plexus

Intervertebral vein

Anterior segmental medullary/radicular vein

Posterior segmental medullary/radicular vein

Pial venous plexus

Posterior sulcal (central) vein

Posterior spinal vein

Internal vertebral (epidural) venous plexus

Plate 173   **Spinal Cord**

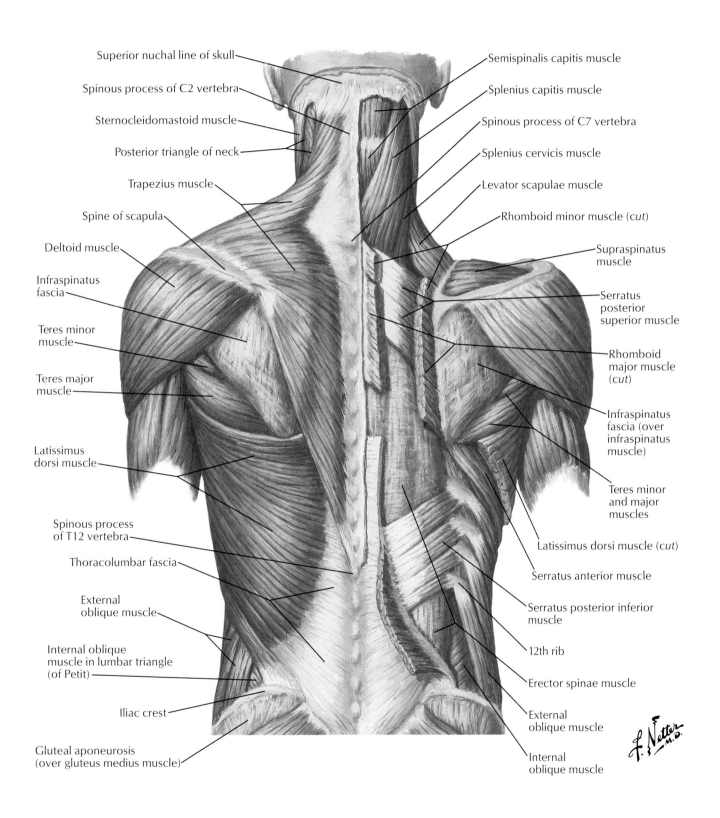

Superior nuchal line of skull

Spinous process of C2 vertebra

Sternocleidomastoid muscle

Posterior triangle of neck

Trapezius muscle

Spine of scapula

Deltoid muscle

Infraspinatus fascia

Teres minor muscle

Teres major muscle

Latissimus dorsi muscle

Spinous process of T12 vertebra

Thoracolumbar fascia

External oblique muscle

Internal oblique muscle in lumbar triangle (of Petit)

Iliac crest

Gluteal aponeurosis (over gluteus medius muscle)

Semispinalis capitis muscle

Splenius capitis muscle

Spinous process of C7 vertebra

Splenius cervicis muscle

Levator scapulae muscle

Rhomboid minor muscle (cut)

Supraspinatus muscle

Serratus posterior superior muscle

Rhomboid major muscle (cut)

Infraspinatus fascia (over infraspinatus muscle)

Teres minor and major muscles

Latissimus dorsi muscle (cut)

Serratus anterior muscle

Serratus posterior inferior muscle

12th rib

Erector spinae muscle

External oblique muscle

Internal oblique muscle

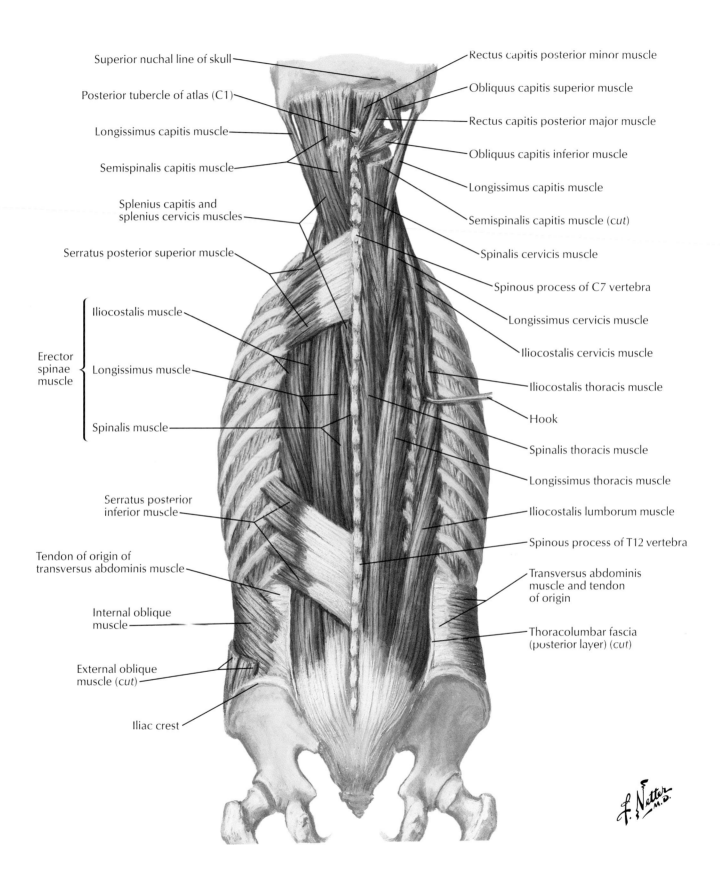

Superior nuchal line of skull

Posterior tubercle of atlas (C1)

Longissimus capitis muscle

Semispinalis capitis muscle

Splenius capitis and splenius cervicis muscles

Serratus posterior superior muscle

Erector spinae muscle
- Iliocostalis muscle
- Longissimus muscle
- Spinalis muscle

Serratus posterior inferior muscle

Tendon of origin of transversus abdominis muscle

Internal oblique muscle

External oblique muscle (cut)

Iliac crest

Rectus capitis posterior minor muscle

Obliquus capitis superior muscle

Rectus capitis posterior major muscle

Obliquus capitis inferior muscle

Longissimus capitis muscle

Semispinalis capitis muscle (cut)

Spinalis cervicis muscle

Spinous process of C7 vertebra

Longissimus cervicis muscle

Iliocostalis cervicis muscle

Iliocostalis thoracis muscle

Hook

Spinalis thoracis muscle

Longissimus thoracis muscle

Iliocostalis lumborum muscle

Spinous process of T12 vertebra

Transversus abdominis muscle and tendon of origin

Thoracolumbar fascia (posterior layer) (cut)

Plate 175   **Muscles and Nerves**

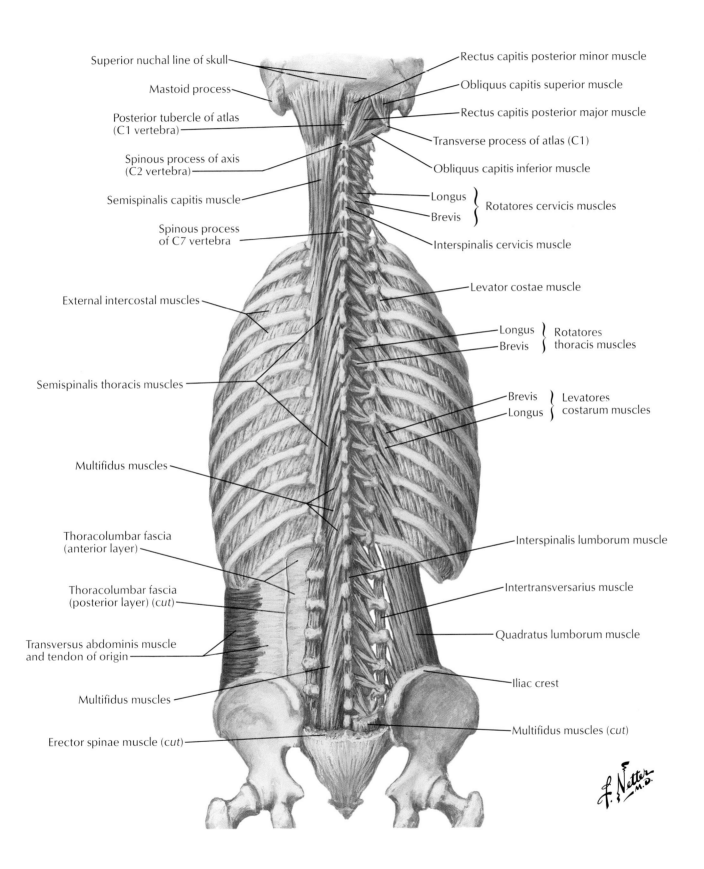

Superior nuchal line of skull

Mastoid process

Posterior tubercle of atlas (C1 vertebra)

Spinous process of axis (C2 vertebra)

Semispinalis capitis muscle

Spinous process of C7 vertebra

External intercostal muscles

Semispinalis thoracis muscles

Multifidus muscles

Thoracolumbar fascia (anterior layer)

Thoracolumbar fascia (posterior layer) (cut)

Transversus abdominis muscle and tendon of origin

Multifidus muscles

Erector spinae muscle (cut)

Rectus capitis posterior minor muscle

Obliquus capitis superior muscle

Rectus capitis posterior major muscle

Transverse process of atlas (C1)

Obliquus capitis inferior muscle

Longus
Brevis } Rotatores cervicis muscles

Interspinalis cervicis muscle

Levator costae muscle

Longus
Brevis } Rotatores thoracis muscles

Brevis
Longus } Levatores costarum muscles

Interspinalis lumborum muscle

Intertransversarius muscle

Quadratus lumborum muscle

Iliac crest

Multifidus muscles (cut)

f. Netter
m.d.

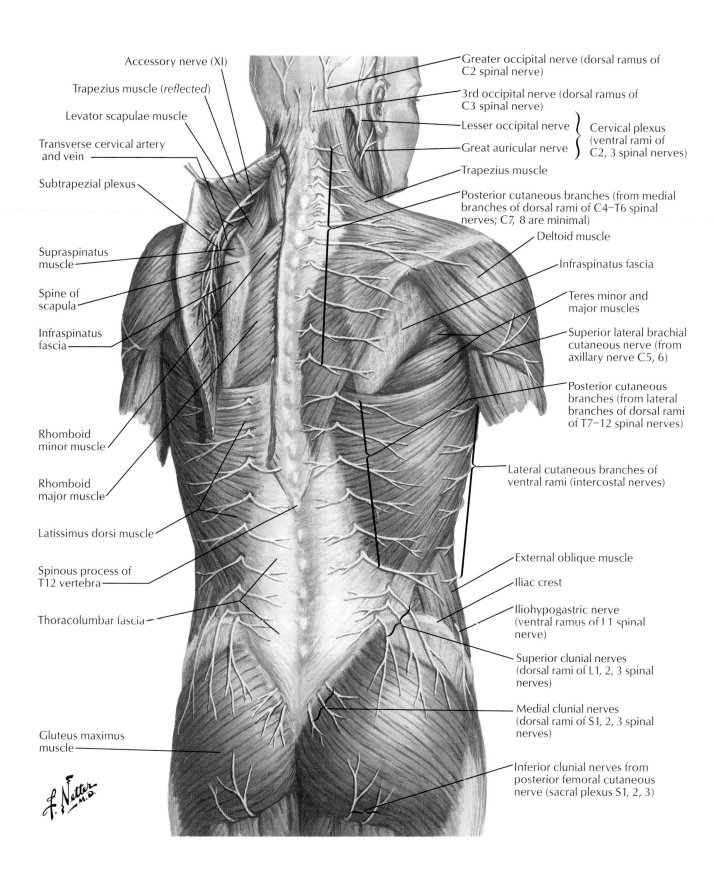

Accessory nerve (XI)

Trapezius muscle (*reflected*)

Levator scapulae muscle

Transverse cervical artery and vein

Subtrapezial plexus

Supraspinatus muscle

Spine of scapula

Infraspinatus fascia

Rhomboid minor muscle

Rhomboid major muscle

Latissimus dorsi muscle

Spinous process of T12 vertebra

Thoracolumbar fascia

Gluteus maximus muscle

Greater occipital nerve (dorsal ramus of C2 spinal nerve)

3rd occipital nerve (dorsal ramus of C3 spinal nerve)

Lesser occipital nerve

Great auricular nerve

Cervical plexus (ventral rami of C2, 3 spinal nerves)

Trapezius muscle

Posterior cutaneous branches (from medial branches of dorsal rami of C4–T6 spinal nerves; C7, 8 are minimal)

Deltoid muscle

Infraspinatus fascia

Teres minor and major muscles

Superior lateral brachial cutaneous nerve (from axillary nerve C5, 6)

Posterior cutaneous branches (from lateral branches of dorsal rami of T7–12 spinal nerves)

Lateral cutaneous branches of ventral rami (intercostal nerves)

External oblique muscle

Iliac crest

Iliohypogastric nerve (ventral ramus of L1 spinal nerve)

Superior clunial nerves (dorsal rami of L1, 2, 3 spinal nerves)

Medial clunial nerves (dorsal rami of S1, 2, 3 spinal nerves)

Inferior clunial nerves from posterior femoral cutaneous nerve (sacral plexus S1, 2, 3)

Plate 177

Muscles and Nerves

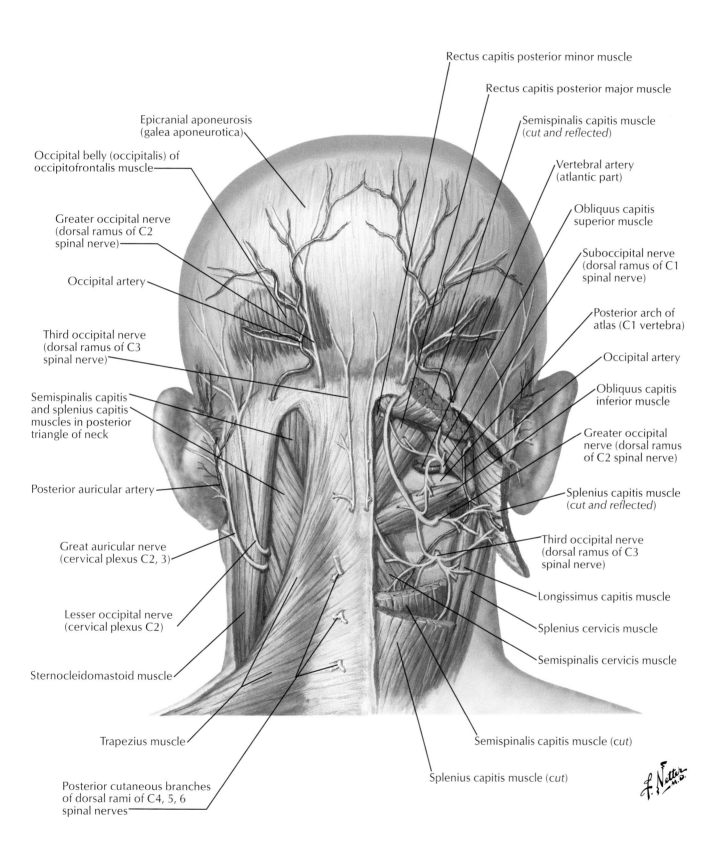

Rectus capitis posterior minor muscle

Rectus capitis posterior major muscle

Semispinalis capitis muscle
(*cut and reflected*)

Vertebral artery
(atlantic part)

Obliquus capitis
superior muscle

Suboccipital nerve
(dorsal ramus of C1
spinal nerve)

Posterior arch of
atlas (C1 vertebra)

Occipital artery

Obliquus capitis
inferior muscle

Greater occipital
nerve (dorsal ramus
of C2 spinal nerve)

Splenius capitis muscle
(*cut and reflected*)

Third occipital nerve
(dorsal ramus of C3
spinal nerve)

Longissimus capitis muscle

Splenius cervicis muscle

Semispinalis cervicis muscle

Semispinalis capitis muscle (*cut*)

Splenius capitis muscle (*cut*)

Epicranial aponeurosis
(galea aponeurotica)

Occipital belly (occipitalis) of
occipitofrontalis muscle

Greater occipital nerve
(dorsal ramus of C2
spinal nerve)

Occipital artery

Third occipital nerve
(dorsal ramus of C3
spinal nerve)

Semispinalis capitis
and splenius capitis
muscles in posterior
triangle of neck

Posterior auricular artery

Great auricular nerve
(cervical plexus C2, 3)

Lesser occipital nerve
(cervical plexus C2)

Sternocleidomastoid muscle

Trapezius muscle

Posterior cutaneous branches
of dorsal rami of C4, 5, 6
spinal nerves

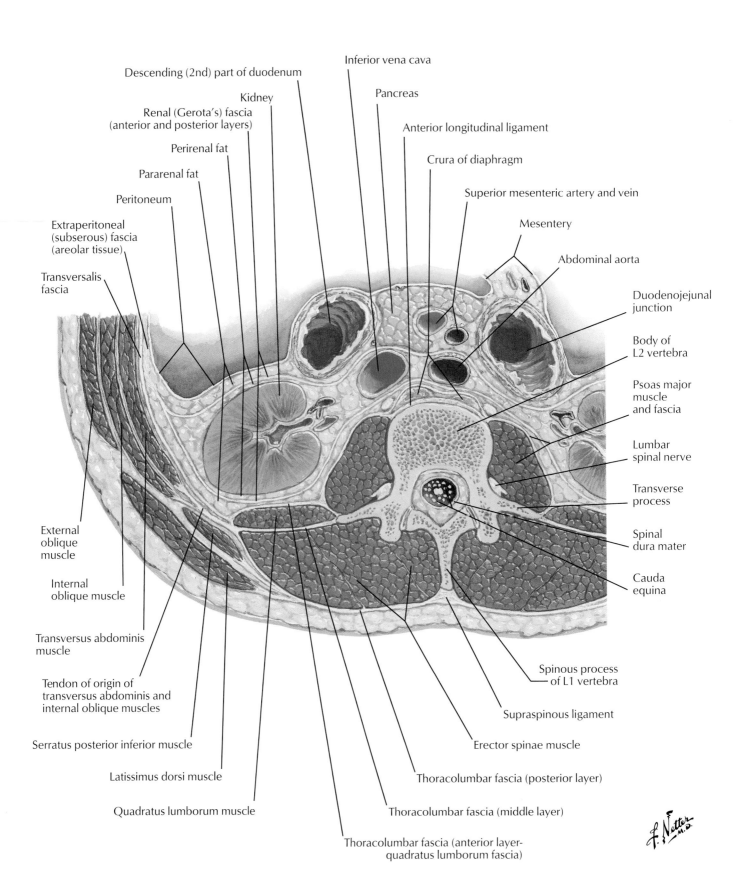

Descending (2nd) part of duodenum

Kidney

Renal (Gerota's) fascia
(anterior and posterior layers)

Perirenal fat

Pararenal fat

Peritoneum

Extraperitoneal
(subserous) fascia
(areolar tissue)

Transversalis
fascia

Inferior vena cava

Pancreas

Anterior longitudinal ligament

Crura of diaphragm

Superior mesenteric artery and vein

Mesentery

Abdominal aorta

Duodenojejunal
junction

Body of
L2 vertebra

Psoas major
muscle
and fascia

Lumbar
spinal nerve

Transverse
process

Spinal
dura mater

Cauda
equina

External
oblique
muscle

Internal
oblique muscle

Transversus abdominis
muscle

Tendon of origin of
transversus abdominis and
internal oblique muscles

Serratus posterior inferior muscle

Latissimus dorsi muscle

Quadratus lumborum muscle

Spinous process
of L1 vertebra

Supraspinous ligament

Erector spinae muscle

Thoracolumbar fascia (posterior layer)

Thoracolumbar fascia (middle layer)

Thoracolumbar fascia (anterior layer-
quadratus lumborum fascia)

F. Netter
M.D.

Plate 179   **Muscles and Nerves**

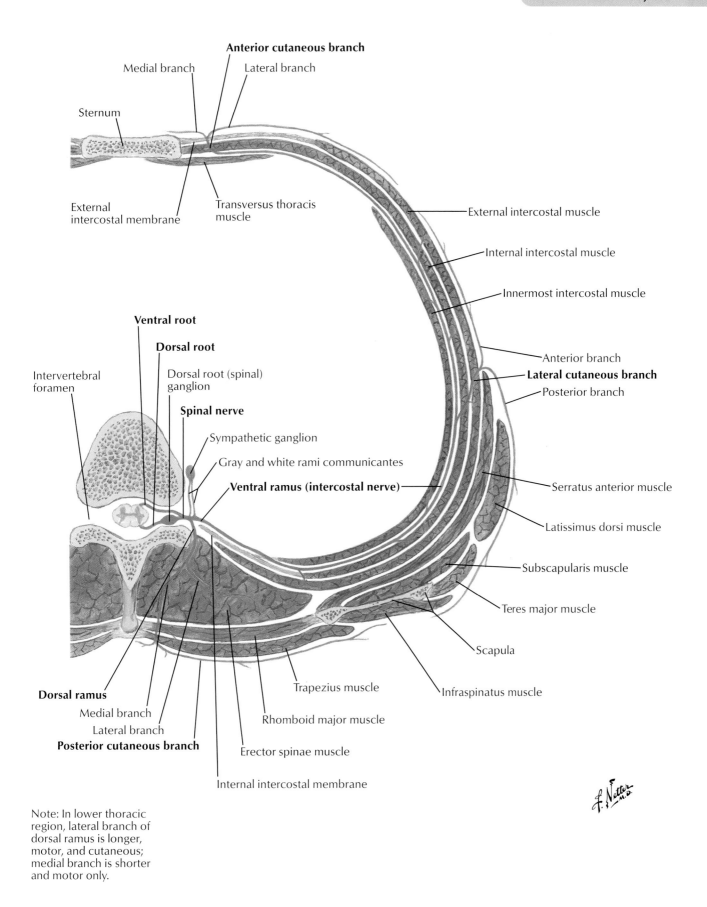

Anterior cutaneous branch

Medial branch

Lateral branch

Sternum

External intercostal muscle

External intercostal membrane

Transversus thoracis muscle

Internal intercostal muscle

Innermost intercostal muscle

Ventral root

Dorsal root

Anterior branch

Lateral cutaneous branch

Posterior branch

Intervertebral foramen

Dorsal root (spinal) ganglion

Spinal nerve

Sympathetic ganglion

Gray and white rami communicantes

Ventral ramus (intercostal nerve)

Serratus anterior muscle

Latissimus dorsi muscle

Subscapularis muscle

Teres major muscle

Scapula

Infraspinatus muscle

Dorsal ramus

Medial branch

Lateral branch

Posterior cutaneous branch

Internal intercostal membrane

Erector spinae muscle

Rhomboid major muscle

Trapezius muscle

Note: In lower thoracic region, lateral branch of dorsal ramus is longer, motor, and cutaneous; medial branch is shorter and motor only.

Section 3 **Thorax**

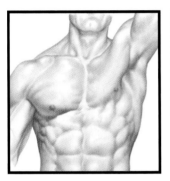
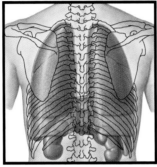
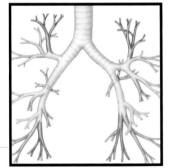
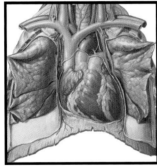

Topographic Anatomy
Plates 181

Mammary Gland
Plates 182–184

Body Wall
Plates 185–195

Lungs
Plates 196–210

3 Thorax

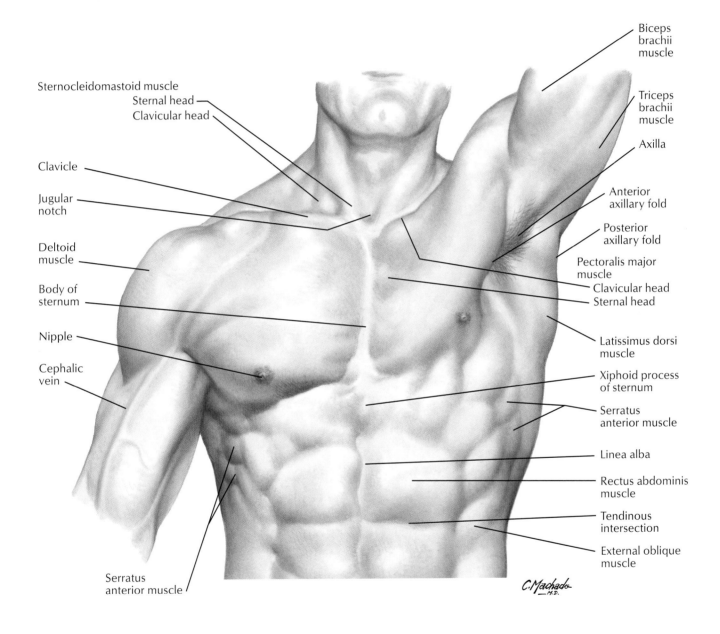

Biceps
brachii
muscle

Triceps
brachii
muscle

Axilla

Anterior
axillary fold

Posterior
axillary fold

Pectoralis major
muscle

Clavicular head

Sternal head

Latissimus dorsi
muscle

Xiphoid process
of sternum

Serratus
anterior muscle

Linea alba

Rectus abdominis
muscle

Tendinous
intersection

External oblique
muscle

Sternocleidomastoid muscle

Sternal head

Clavicular head

Clavicle

Jugular
notch

Deltoid
muscle

Body of
sternum

Nipple

Cephalic
vein

Serratus
anterior muscle

C.Machado
—M.D.

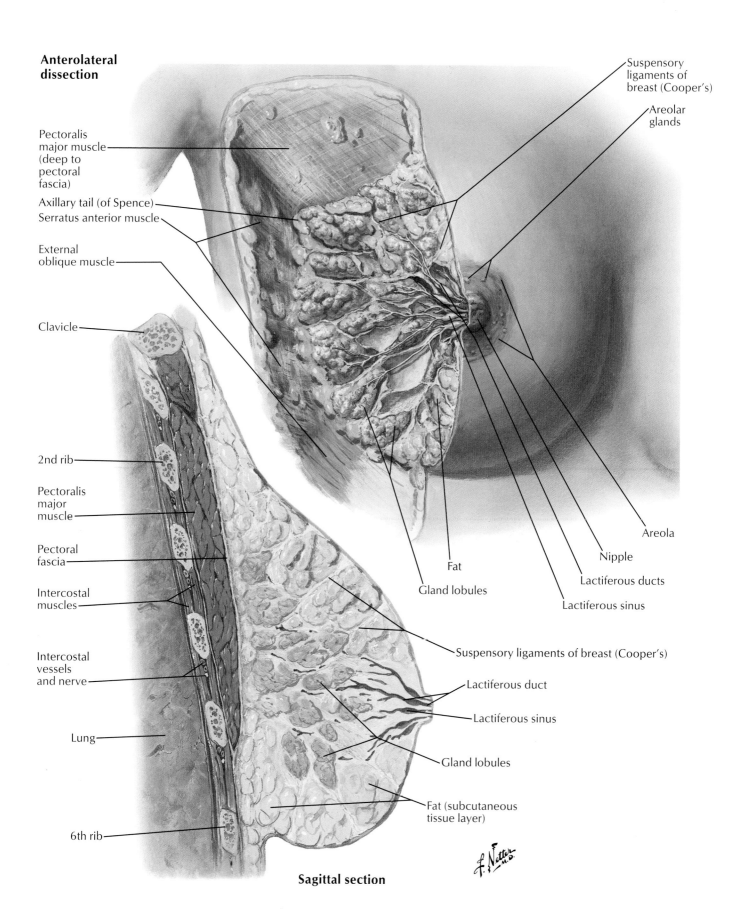

Anterolateral dissection

Pectoralis major muscle (deep to pectoral fascia)

Axillary tail (of Spence)

Serratus anterior muscle

External oblique muscle

Clavicle

2nd rib

Pectoralis major muscle

Pectoral fascia

Intercostal muscles

Intercostal vessels and nerve

Lung

6th rib

Suspensory ligaments of breast (Cooper's)

Areolar glands

Areola

Nipple

Lactiferous ducts

Lactiferous sinus

Fat

Gland lobules

Suspensory ligaments of breast (Cooper's)

Lactiferous duct

Lactiferous sinus

Gland lobules

Fat (subcutaneous tissue layer)

Sagittal section

Plate 182   **Mammary Gland**

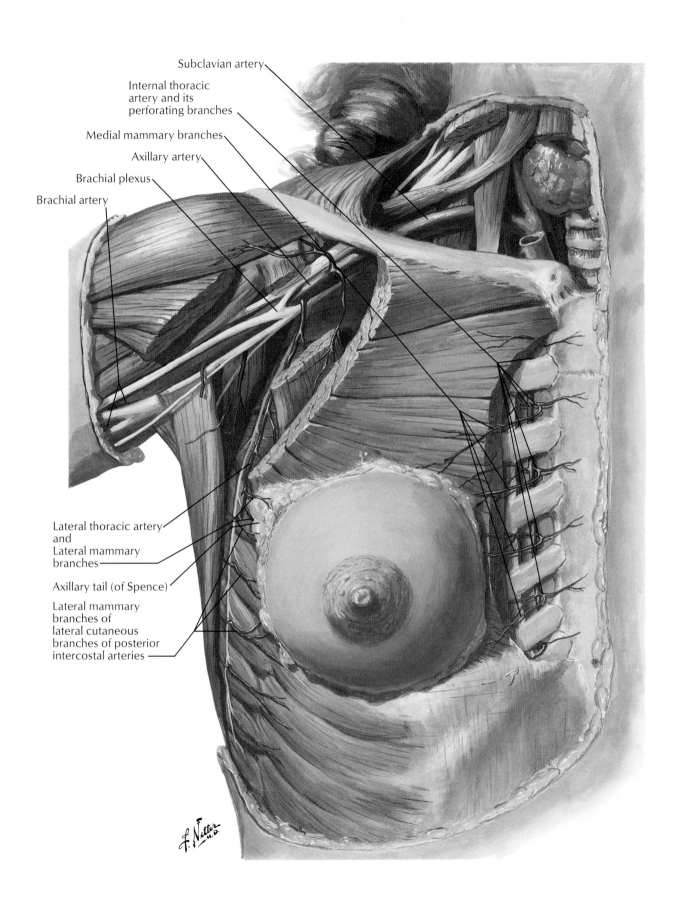

Subclavian artery

Internal thoracic artery and its perforating branches

Medial mammary branches

Axillary artery

Brachial plexus

Brachial artery

Lateral thoracic artery and
Lateral mammary branches

Axillary tail (of Spence)

Lateral mammary branches of lateral cutaneous branches of posterior intercostal arteries

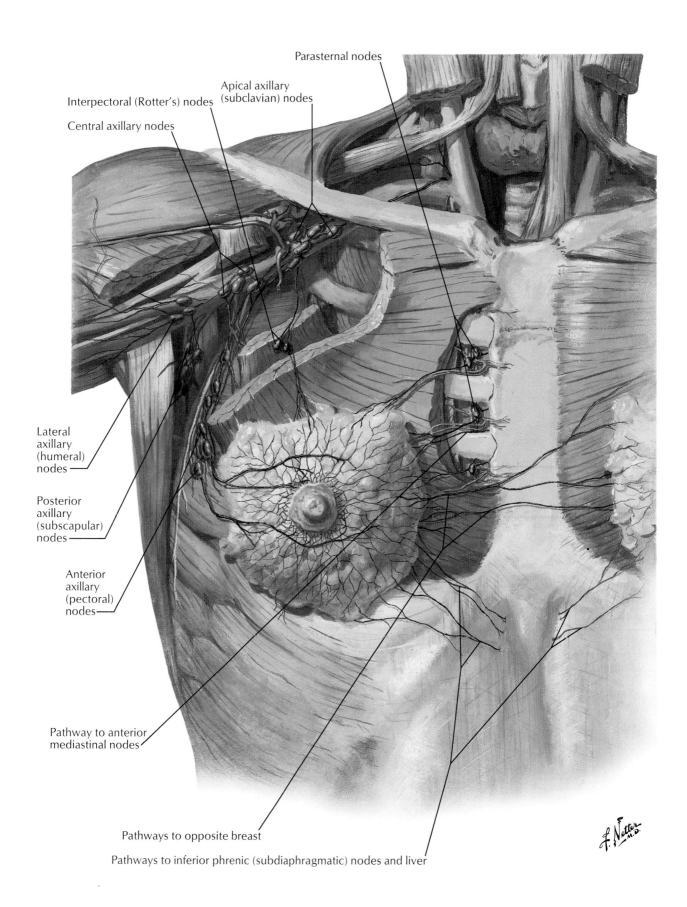

Parasternal nodes

Apical axillary
(subclavian) nodes

Interpectoral (Rotter's) nodes

Central axillary nodes

Lateral
axillary
(humeral)
nodes

Posterior
axillary
(subscapular)
nodes

Anterior
axillary
(pectoral)
nodes

Pathway to anterior
mediastinal nodes

Pathways to opposite breast

Pathways to inferior phrenic (subdiaphragmatic) nodes and liver

Plate 184 **Mammary Gland**

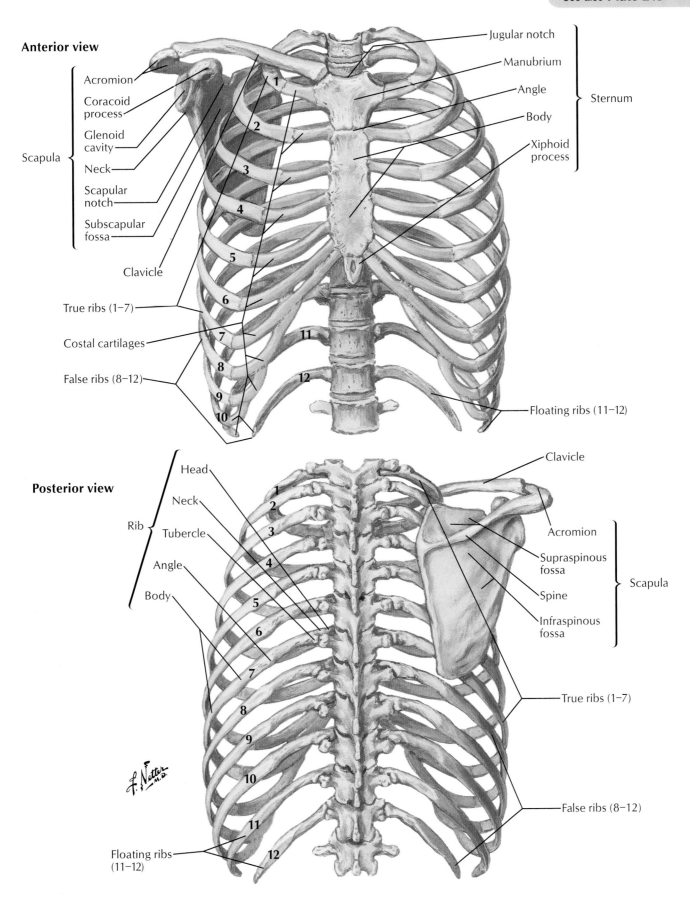

Anterior view

Scapula
- Acromion
- Coracoid process
- Glenoid cavity
- Neck
- Scapular notch
- Subscapular fossa

Clavicle

True ribs (1–7)

Costal cartilages

False ribs (8–12)

Jugular notch

Manubrium

Angle

Body — Sternum

Xiphoid process

1
2
3
4
5
6
7
8
9
10
11
12

Floating ribs (11–12)

Posterior view

Rib
- Head
- Neck
- Tubercle
- Angle
- Body

1
2
3
4
5
6
7
8
9
10
11
12

Clavicle

Acromion

Supraspinous fossa

Spine — Scapula

Infraspinous fossa

True ribs (1–7)

False ribs (8–12)

Floating ribs (11–12)

F. Netter M.D.

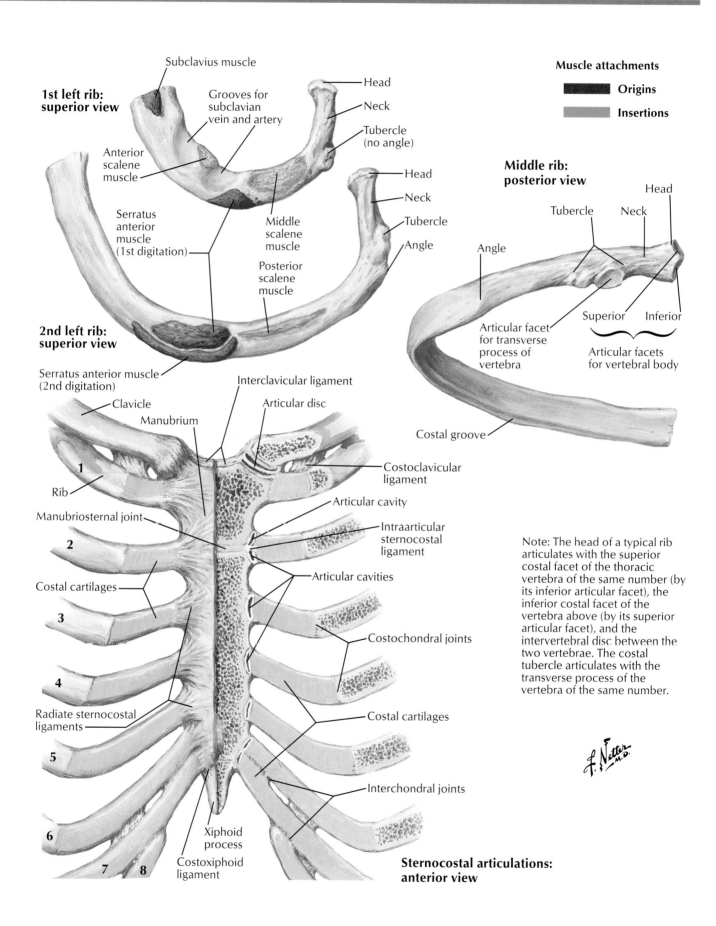

1st left rib: superior view

Subclavius muscle

Grooves for subclavian vein and artery

Anterior scalene muscle

Serratus anterior muscle (1st digitation)

Head

Neck

Tubercle (no angle)

2nd left rib: superior view

Head

Neck

Tubercle

Angle

Middle scalene muscle

Posterior scalene muscle

Serratus anterior muscle (2nd digitation)

Muscle attachments

■ Origins

▨ Insertions

Middle rib: posterior view

Tubercle

Neck

Head

Angle

Superior   Inferior

Articular facet for transverse process of vertebra

Articular facets for vertebral body

Costal groove

Interclavicular ligament

Articular disc

Clavicle

Manubrium

1

Rib

Manubriosternal joint

2

Costal cartilages

3

4

Radiate sternocostal ligaments

5

6

7   8

Xiphoid process

Costoxiphoid ligament

Costoclavicular ligament

Articular cavity

Intraarticular sternocostal ligament

Articular cavities

Costochondral joints

Costal cartilages

Interchondral joints

Note: The head of a typical rib articulates with the superior costal facet of the thoracic vertebra of the same number (by its inferior articular facet), the inferior costal facet of the vertebra above (by its superior articular facet), and the intervertebral disc between the two vertebrae. The costal tubercle articulates with the transverse process of the vertebra of the same number.

Sternocostal articulations: anterior view

Plate 186   **Body Wall**

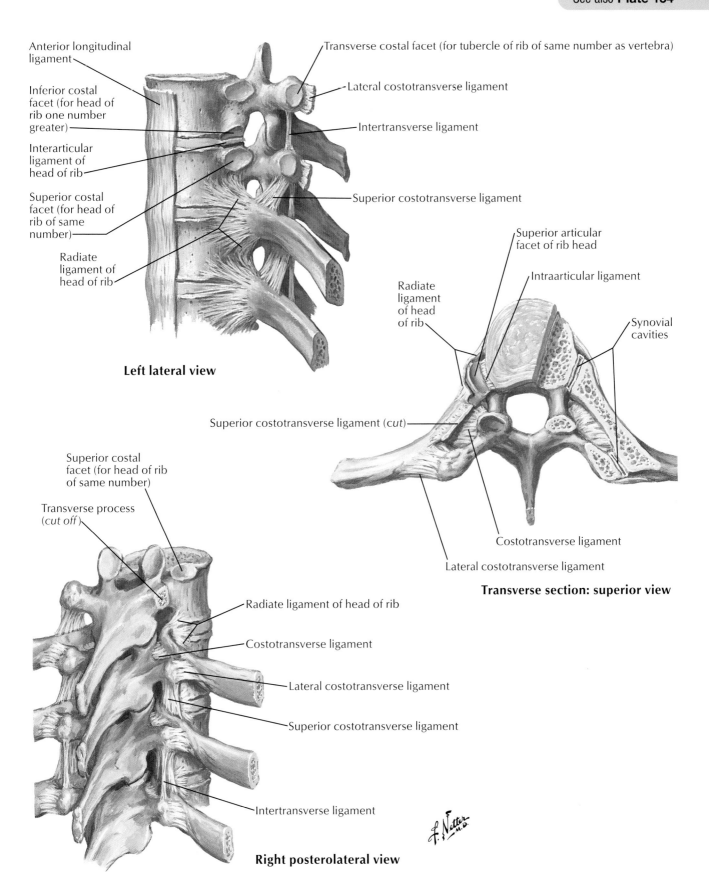

Anterior longitudinal ligament

Inferior costal facet (for head of rib one number greater)

Interarticular ligament of head of rib

Superior costal facet (for head of rib of same number)

Radiate ligament of head of rib

Transverse costal facet (for tubercle of rib of same number as vertebra)

Lateral costotransverse ligament

Intertransverse ligament

Superior costotransverse ligament

Left lateral view

Radiate ligament of head of rib

Superior articular facet of rib head

Intraarticular ligament

Synovial cavities

Superior costotransverse ligament (*cut*)

Costotransverse ligament

Lateral costotransverse ligament

Transverse section: superior view

Superior costal facet (for head of rib of same number)

Transverse process (*cut off*)

Radiate ligament of head of rib

Costotransverse ligament

Lateral costotransverse ligament

Superior costotransverse ligament

Intertransverse ligament

Right posterolateral view

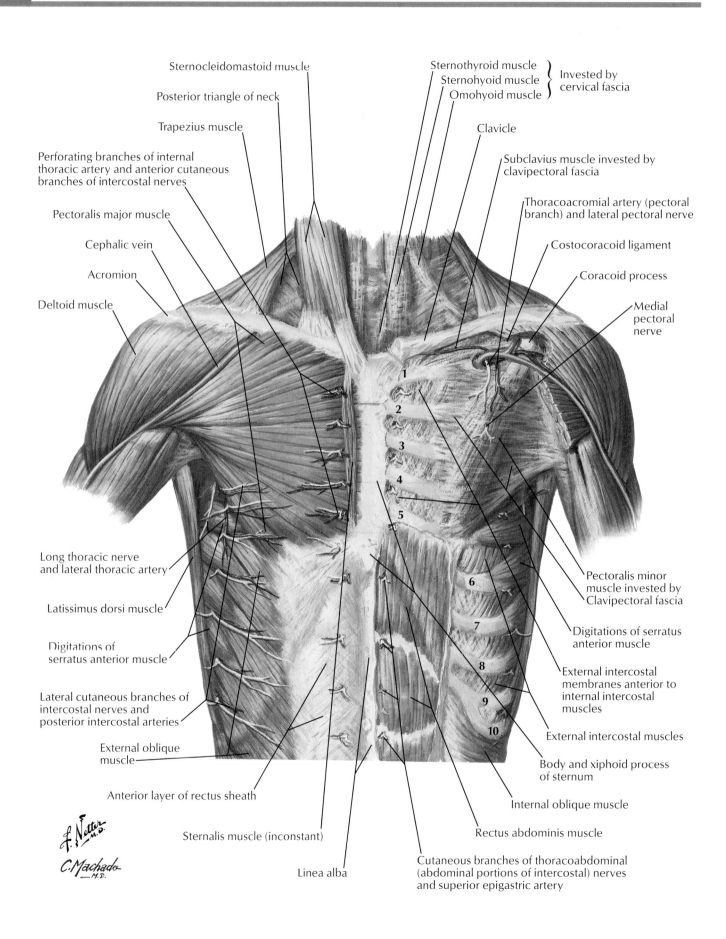

Sternocleidomastoid muscle

Posterior triangle of neck

Trapezius muscle

Perforating branches of internal thoracic artery and anterior cutaneous branches of intercostal nerves

Pectoralis major muscle

Cephalic vein

Acromion

Deltoid muscle

Sternothyroid muscle
Sternohyoid muscle
Omohyoid muscle
} Invested by cervical fascia

Clavicle

Subclavius muscle invested by clavipectoral fascia

Thoracoacromial artery (pectoral branch) and lateral pectoral nerve

Costocoracoid ligament

Coracoid process

Medial pectoral nerve

Long thoracic nerve and lateral thoracic artery

Latissimus dorsi muscle

Digitations of serratus anterior muscle

Lateral cutaneous branches of intercostal nerves and posterior intercostal arteries

External oblique muscle

Anterior layer of rectus sheath

Sternalis muscle (inconstant)

Linea alba

Pectoralis minor muscle invested by Clavipectoral fascia

Digitations of serratus anterior muscle

External intercostal membranes anterior to internal intercostal muscles

External intercostal muscles

Body and xiphoid process of sternum

Internal oblique muscle

Rectus abdominis muscle

Cutaneous branches of thoracoabdominal (abdominal portions of intercostal) nerves and superior epigastric artery

Plate 188   **Body Wall**

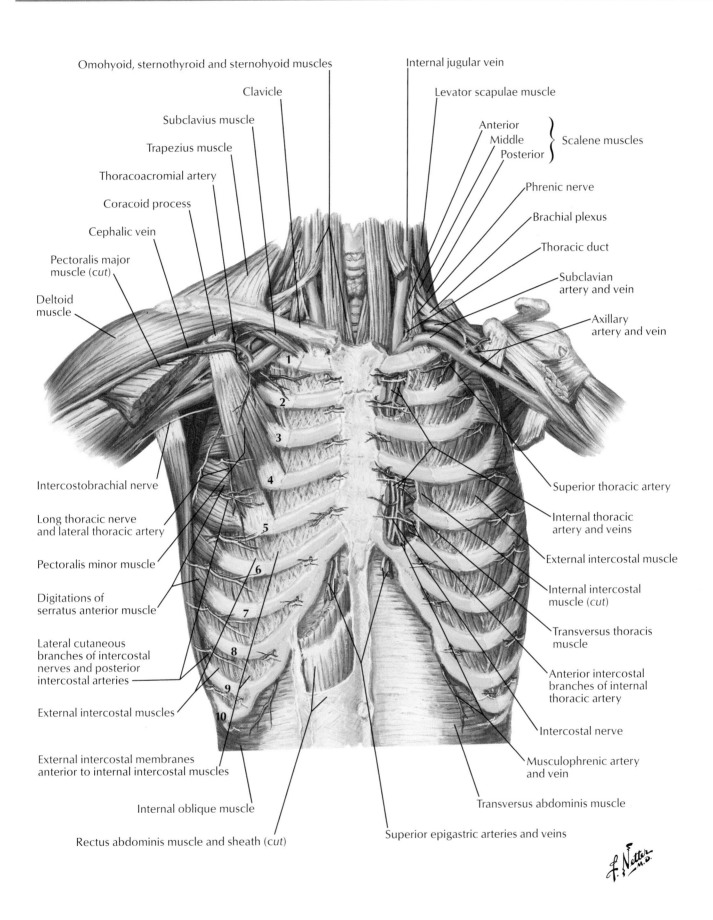

Omohyoid, sternothyroid and sternohyoid muscles

Clavicle

Subclavius muscle

Trapezius muscle

Thoracoacromial artery

Coracoid process

Cephalic vein

Pectoralis major muscle (cut)

Deltoid muscle

Intercostobrachial nerve

Long thoracic nerve and lateral thoracic artery

Pectoralis minor muscle

Digitations of serratus anterior muscle

Lateral cutaneous branches of intercostal nerves and posterior intercostal arteries

External intercostal muscles

External intercostal membranes anterior to internal intercostal muscles

Internal oblique muscle

Rectus abdominis muscle and sheath (cut)

Internal jugular vein

Levator scapulae muscle

Anterior
Middle
Posterior } Scalene muscles

Phrenic nerve

Brachial plexus

Thoracic duct

Subclavian artery and vein

Axillary artery and vein

Superior thoracic artery

Internal thoracic artery and veins

External intercostal muscle

Internal intercostal muscle (cut)

Transversus thoracis muscle

Anterior intercostal branches of internal thoracic artery

Intercostal nerve

Musculophrenic artery and vein

Transversus abdominis muscle

Superior epigastric arteries and veins

1 2 3 4 5 6 7 8 9 10

Preferred sites
1. For pneumothorax (2nd or 3rd interspace at midclavicular line)
2. For hemothorax (5th interspace at midaxillary line)

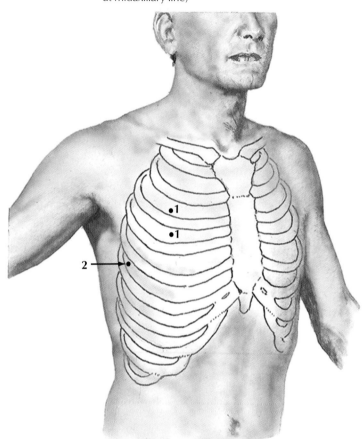

A. Trocar and cannula pushed through intercostal space

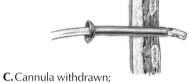

B. Trocar withdrawn; tube passed into chest through cannula

C. Cannula withdrawn; tube connected to underwater seal (with suction if indicated)

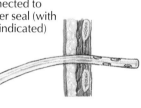

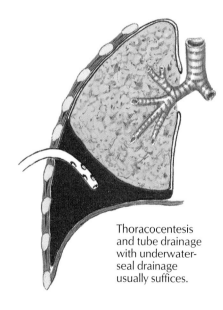

Thoracocentesis and tube drainage with underwater-seal drainage usually suffices.

D. Intercostal space is pierced above rib to avoid damage to neurovascular bundle lying in costal groove

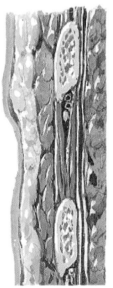

Plate 190

Body Wall

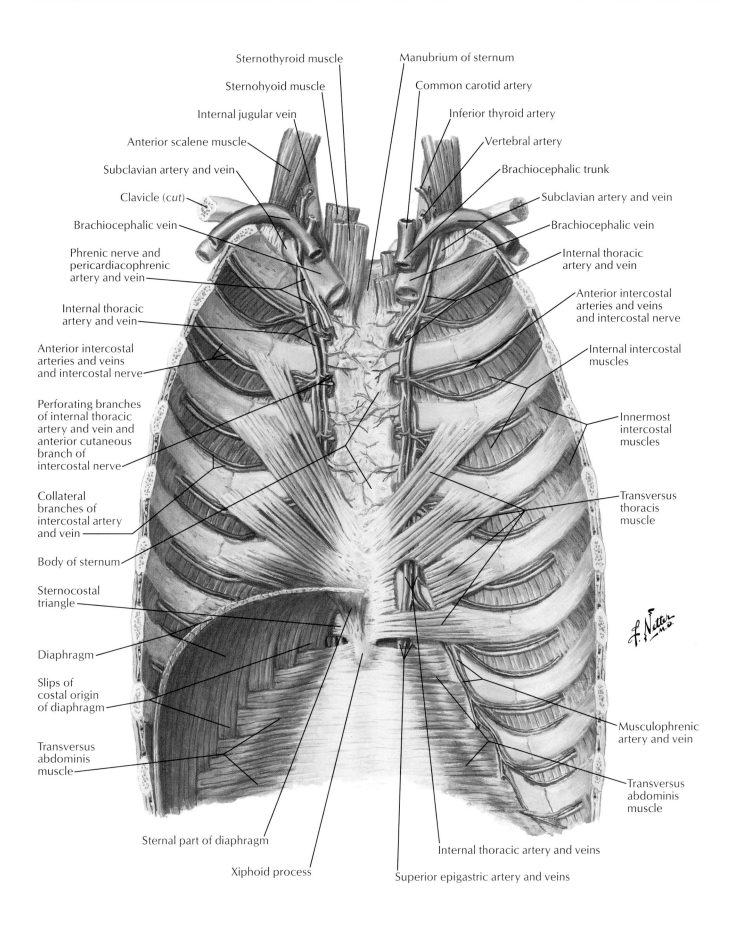

Sternothyroid muscle

Sternohyoid muscle

Internal jugular vein

Anterior scalene muscle

Subclavian artery and vein

Clavicle (*cut*)

Brachiocephalic vein

Phrenic nerve and pericardiacophrenic artery and vein

Internal thoracic artery and vein

Anterior intercostal arteries and veins and intercostal nerve

Perforating branches of internal thoracic artery and vein and anterior cutaneous branch of intercostal nerve

Collateral branches of intercostal artery and vein

Body of sternum

Sternocostal triangle

Diaphragm

Slips of costal origin of diaphragm

Transversus abdominis muscle

Manubrium of sternum

Common carotid artery

Inferior thyroid artery

Vertebral artery

Brachiocephalic trunk

Subclavian artery and vein

Brachiocephalic vein

Internal thoracic artery and vein

Anterior intercostal arteries and veins and intercostal nerve

Internal intercostal muscles

Innermost intercostal muscles

Transversus thoracis muscle

Musculophrenic artery and vein

Transversus abdominis muscle

Sternal part of diaphragm

Xiphoid process

Internal thoracic artery and veins

Superior epigastric artery and veins

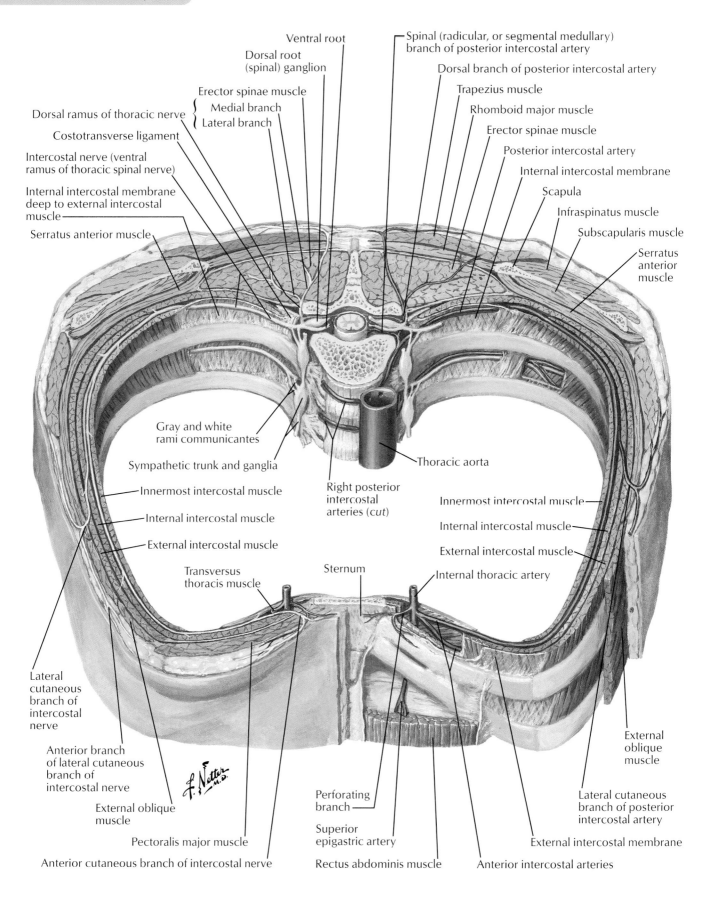

Ventral root

Dorsal root (spinal) ganglion

Spinal (radicular, or segmental medullary) branch of posterior intercostal artery

Dorsal branch of posterior intercostal artery

Erector spinae muscle

Trapezius muscle

Dorsal ramus of thoracic nerve { Medial branch { Lateral branch

Rhomboid major muscle

Erector spinae muscle

Costotransverse ligament

Posterior intercostal artery

Intercostal nerve (ventral ramus of thoracic spinal nerve)

Internal intercostal membrane

Scapula

Internal intercostal membrane deep to external intercostal muscle

Infraspinatus muscle

Subscapularis muscle

Serratus anterior muscle

Serratus anterior muscle

Gray and white rami communicantes

Sympathetic trunk and ganglia

Thoracic aorta

Innermost intercostal muscle

Right posterior intercostal arteries (cut)

Innermost intercostal muscle

Internal intercostal muscle

Internal intercostal muscle

External intercostal muscle

External intercostal muscle

Transversus thoracis muscle

Sternum

Internal thoracic artery

Lateral cutaneous branch of intercostal nerve

Anterior branch of lateral cutaneous branch of intercostal nerve

External oblique muscle

External oblique muscle

Lateral cutaneous branch of posterior intercostal artery

Pectoralis major muscle

Perforating branch

Superior epigastric artery

Rectus abdominis muscle

External intercostal membrane

Anterior cutaneous branch of intercostal nerve

Anterior intercostal arteries

Plate 192

Body Wall

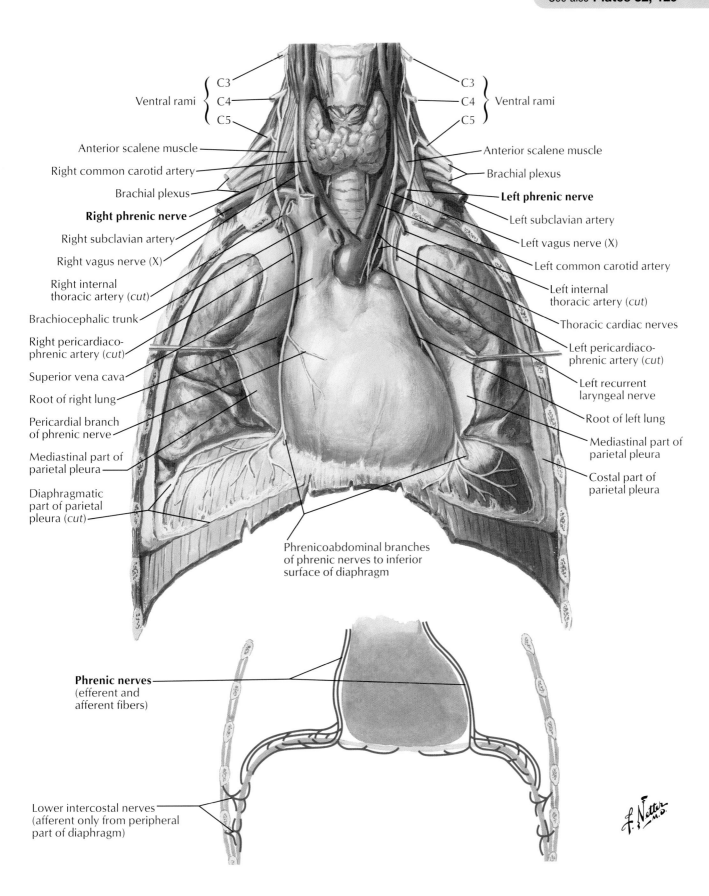

Ventral rami { C3
C4
C5

C3 } Ventral rami
C4
C5

Anterior scalene muscle

Right common carotid artery

Brachial plexus

Right phrenic nerve

Right subclavian artery

Right vagus nerve (X)

Right internal thoracic artery (*cut*)

Brachiocephalic trunk

Right pericardiaco-phrenic artery (*cut*)

Superior vena cava

Root of right lung

Pericardial branch of phrenic nerve

Mediastinal part of parietal pleura

Diaphragmatic part of parietal pleura (*cut*)

Anterior scalene muscle

Brachial plexus

Left phrenic nerve

Left subclavian artery

Left vagus nerve (X)

Left common carotid artery

Left internal thoracic artery (*cut*)

Thoracic cardiac nerves

Left pericardiaco-phrenic artery (*cut*)

Left recurrent laryngeal nerve

Root of left lung

Mediastinal part of parietal pleura

Costal part of parietal pleura

Phrenicoabdominal branches of phrenic nerves to inferior surface of diaphragm

Phrenic nerves (efferent and afferent fibers)

Lower intercostal nerves (afferent only from peripheral part of diaphragm)

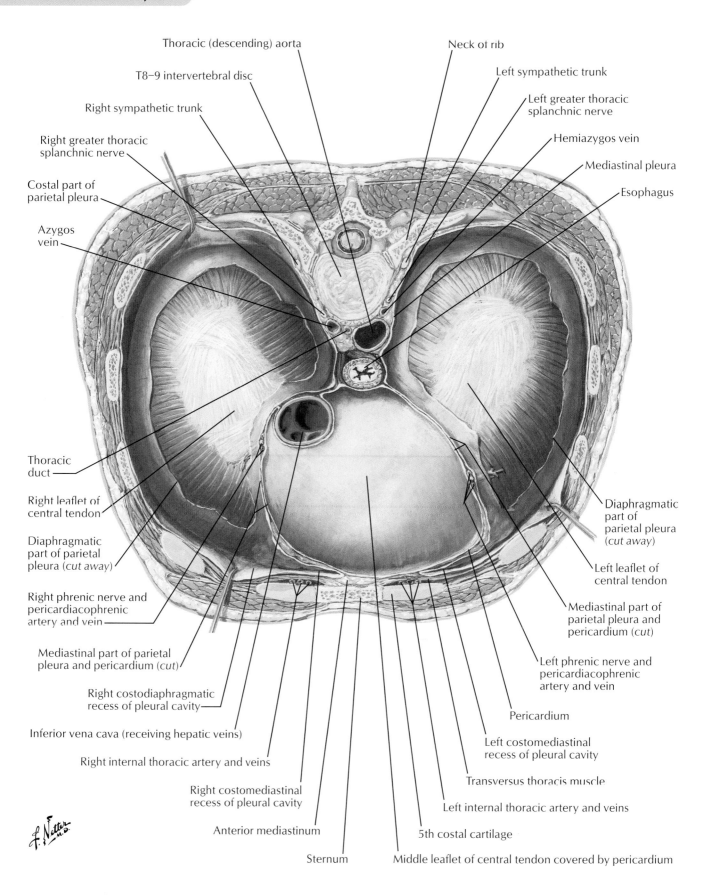

Thoracic (descending) aorta

Neck of rib

T8–9 intervertebral disc

Left sympathetic trunk

Right sympathetic trunk

Left greater thoracic splanchnic nerve

Right greater thoracic splanchnic nerve

Hemiazygos vein

Mediastinal pleura

Costal part of parietal pleura

Esophagus

Azygos vein

Thoracic duct

Right leaflet of central tendon

Diaphragmatic part of parietal pleura (cut away)

Left leaflet of central tendon

Right phrenic nerve and pericardiacophrenic artery and vein

Mediastinal part of parietal pleura and pericardium (cut)

Mediastinal part of parietal pleura and pericardium (cut)

Left phrenic nerve and pericardiacophrenic artery and vein

Right costodiaphragmatic recess of pleural cavity

Pericardium

Inferior vena cava (receiving hepatic veins)

Left costomediastinal recess of pleural cavity

Right internal thoracic artery and veins

Transversus thoracis muscle

Right costomediastinal recess of pleural cavity

Left internal thoracic artery and veins

Anterior mediastinum

5th costal cartilage

Sternum

Middle leaflet of central tendon covered by pericardium

Plate 194

Body Wall

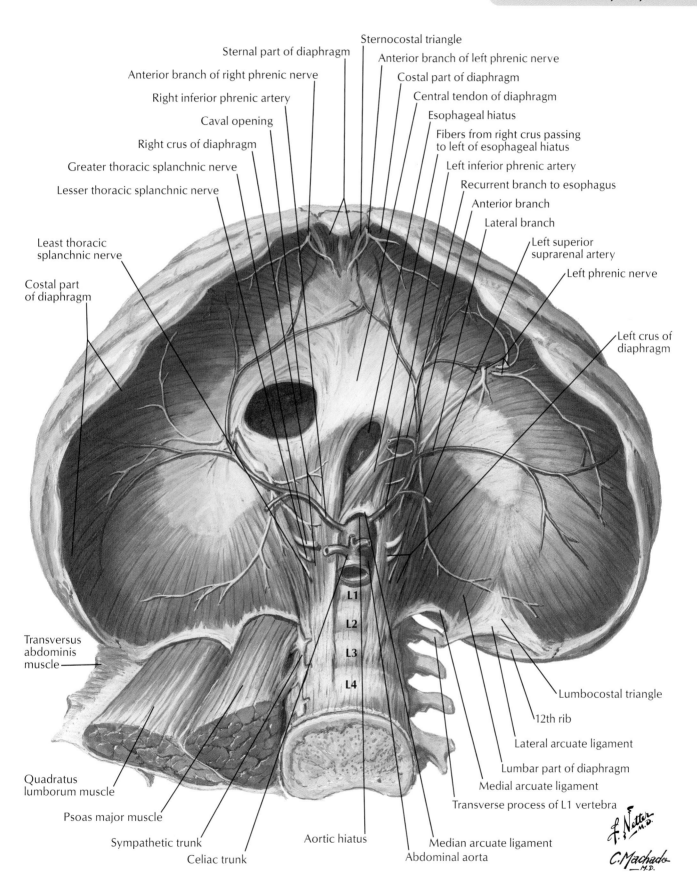

Sternocostal triangle

Sternal part of diaphragm

Anterior branch of left phrenic nerve

Anterior branch of right phrenic nerve

Costal part of diaphragm

Right inferior phrenic artery

Central tendon of diaphragm

Caval opening

Esophageal hiatus

Right crus of diaphragm

Fibers from right crus passing to left of esophageal hiatus

Greater thoracic splanchnic nerve

Left inferior phrenic artery

Lesser thoracic splanchnic nerve

Recurrent branch to esophagus

Anterior branch

Lateral branch

Least thoracic splanchnic nerve

Left superior suprarenal artery

Left phrenic nerve

Costal part of diaphragm

Left crus of diaphragm

Transversus abdominis muscle

L1

L2

L3

L4

Lumbocostal triangle

12th rib

Lateral arcuate ligament

Lumbar part of diaphragm

Quadratus lumborum muscle

Medial arcuate ligament

Psoas major muscle

Transverse process of L1 vertebra

Sympathetic trunk

Median arcuate ligament

Celiac trunk

Aortic hiatus

Abdominal aorta

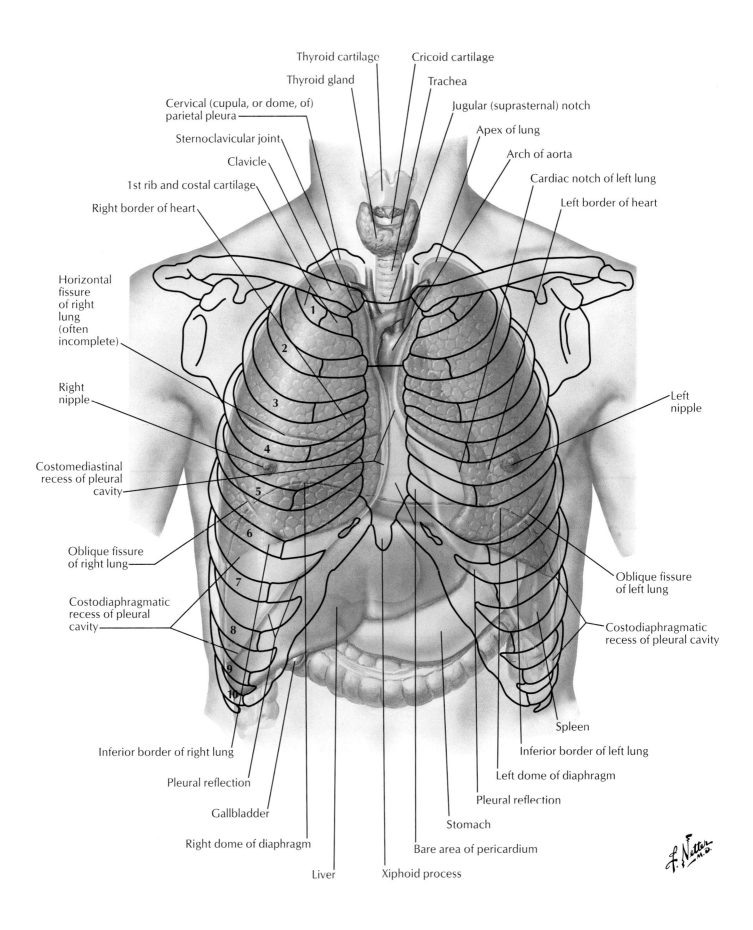

Thyroid cartilage

Cricoid cartilage

Thyroid gland

Trachea

Cervical (cupula, or dome, of) parietal pleura

Jugular (suprasternal) notch

Sternoclavicular joint

Apex of lung

Clavicle

Arch of aorta

1st rib and costal cartilage

Cardiac notch of left lung

Right border of heart

Left border of heart

Horizontal fissure of right lung (often incomplete)

Right nipple

Left nipple

Costomediastinal recess of pleural cavity

Oblique fissure of right lung

Oblique fissure of left lung

Costodiaphragmatic recess of pleural cavity

Costodiaphragmatic recess of pleural cavity

Spleen

Inferior border of right lung

Inferior border of left lung

Pleural reflection

Left dome of diaphragm

Gallbladder

Pleural reflection

Right dome of diaphragm

Stomach

Liver

Xiphoid process

Bare area of pericardium

Plate 196

Lungs

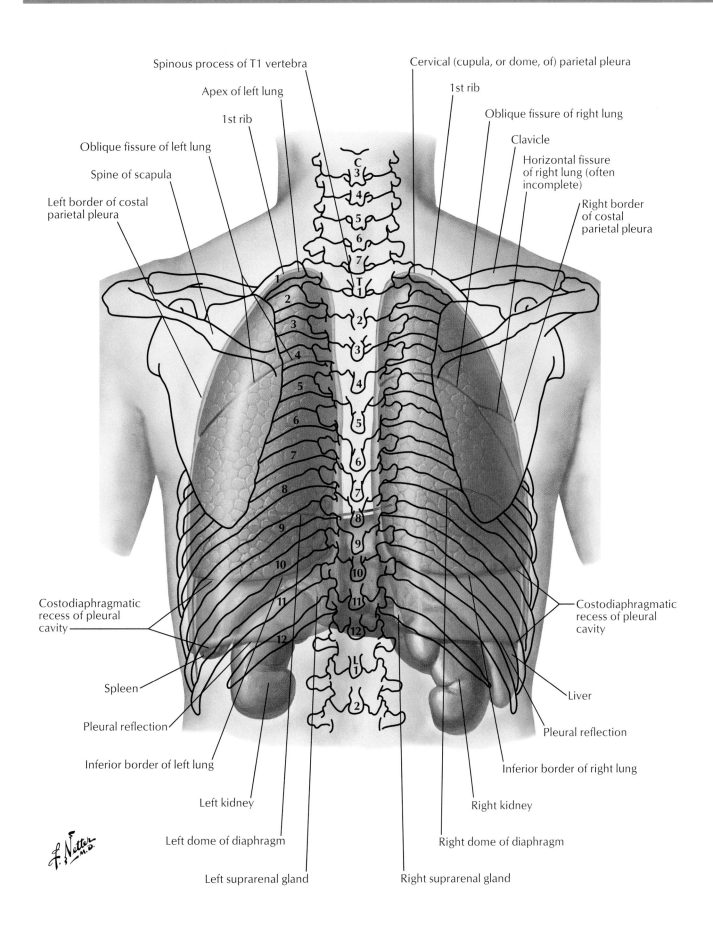

Spinous process of T1 vertebra

Apex of left lung

1st rib

Oblique fissure of left lung

Spine of scapula

Left border of costal parietal pleura

Cervical (cupula, or dome, of) parietal pleura

1st rib

Oblique fissure of right lung

Clavicle

Horizontal fissure of right lung (often incomplete)

Right border of costal parietal pleura

Costodiaphragmatic recess of pleural cavity

Costodiaphragmatic recess of pleural cavity

Spleen

Liver

Pleural reflection

Pleural reflection

Inferior border of left lung

Inferior border of right lung

Left kidney

Right kidney

Left dome of diaphragm

Right dome of diaphragm

Left suprarenal gland

Right suprarenal gland

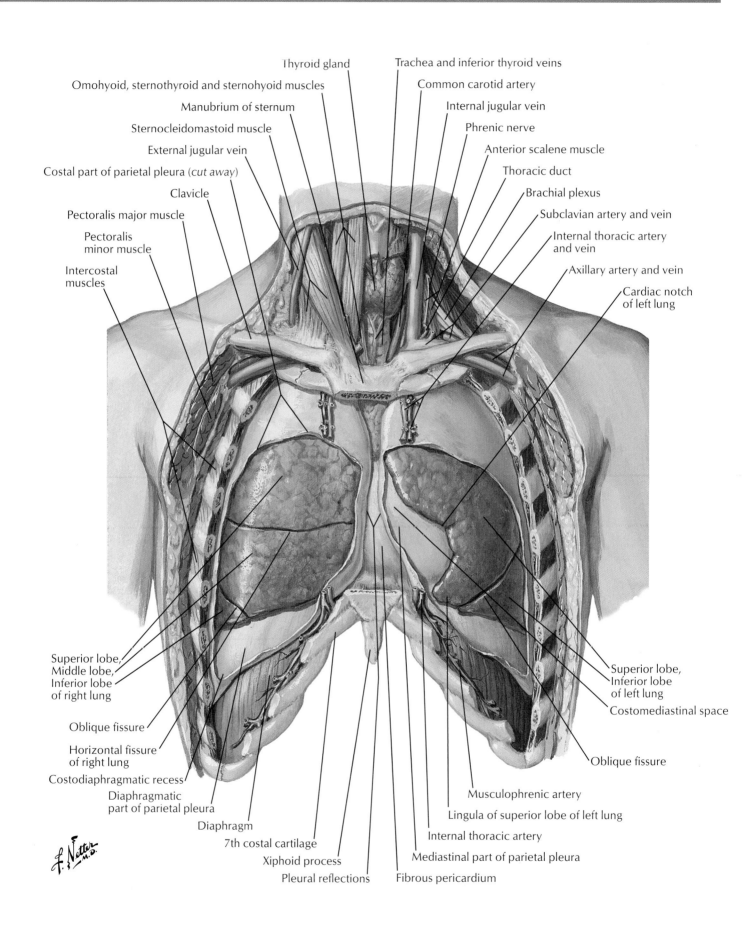

Thyroid gland

Trachea and inferior thyroid veins

Omohyoid, sternothyroid and sternohyoid muscles

Common carotid artery

Manubrium of sternum

Internal jugular vein

Sternocleidomastoid muscle

Phrenic nerve

External jugular vein

Anterior scalene muscle

Costal part of parietal pleura (*cut away*)

Thoracic duct

Clavicle

Brachial plexus

Pectoralis major muscle

Subclavian artery and vein

Pectoralis minor muscle

Internal thoracic artery and vein

Intercostal muscles

Axillary artery and vein

Cardiac notch of left lung

Superior lobe, Middle lobe, Inferior lobe of right lung

Superior lobe, Inferior lobe of left lung

Oblique fissure

Costomediastinal space

Horizontal fissure of right lung

Costodiaphragmatic recess

Oblique fissure

Diaphragmatic part of parietal pleura

Musculophrenic artery

Diaphragm

Lingula of superior lobe of left lung

7th costal cartilage

Internal thoracic artery

Xiphoid process

Mediastinal part of parietal pleura

Pleural reflections

Fibrous pericardium

Plate 198

Lungs

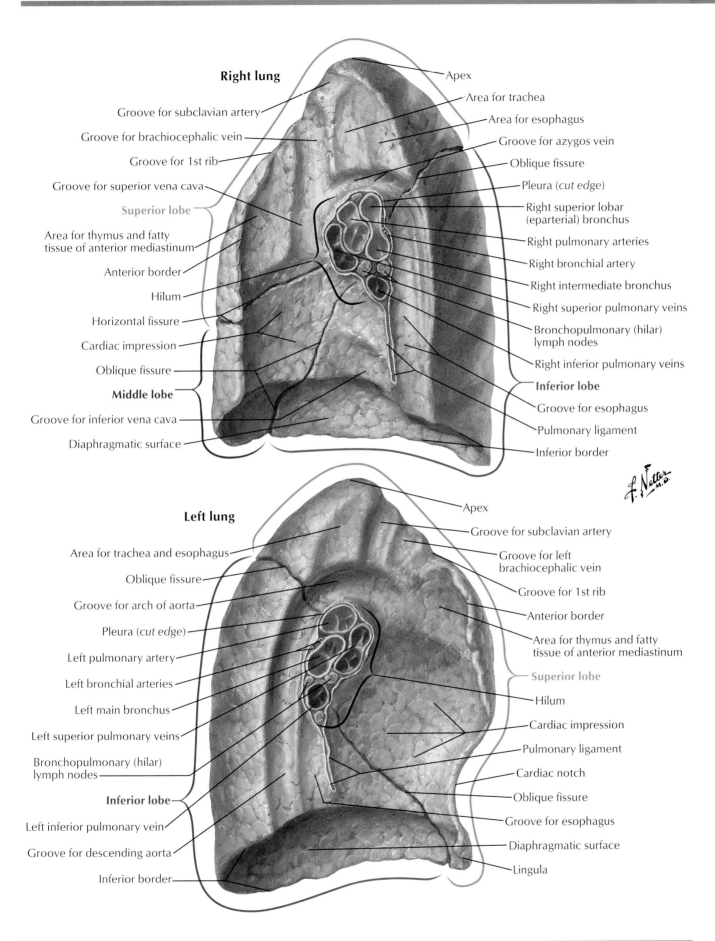

Right lung

Groove for subclavian artery

Groove for brachiocephalic vein

Groove for 1st rib

Groove for superior vena cava

Superior lobe

Area for thymus and fatty tissue of anterior mediastinum

Anterior border

Hilum

Horizontal fissure

Cardiac impression

Oblique fissure

Middle lobe

Groove for inferior vena cava

Diaphragmatic surface

Apex

Area for trachea

Area for esophagus

Groove for azygos vein

Oblique fissure

Pleura (cut edge)

Right superior lobar (eparterial) bronchus

Right pulmonary arteries

Right bronchial artery

Right intermediate bronchus

Right superior pulmonary veins

Bronchopulmonary (hilar) lymph nodes

Right inferior pulmonary veins

Inferior lobe

Groove for esophagus

Pulmonary ligament

Inferior border

Left lung

Area for trachea and esophagus

Oblique fissure

Groove for arch of aorta

Pleura (cut edge)

Left pulmonary artery

Left bronchial arteries

Left main bronchus

Left superior pulmonary veins

Bronchopulmonary (hilar) lymph nodes

Inferior lobe

Left inferior pulmonary vein

Groove for descending aorta

Inferior border

Apex

Groove for subclavian artery

Groove for left brachiocephalic vein

Groove for 1st rib

Anterior border

Area for thymus and fatty tissue of anterior mediastinum

Superior lobe

Hilum

Cardiac impression

Pulmonary ligament

Cardiac notch

Oblique fissure

Groove for esophagus

Diaphragmatic surface

Lingula

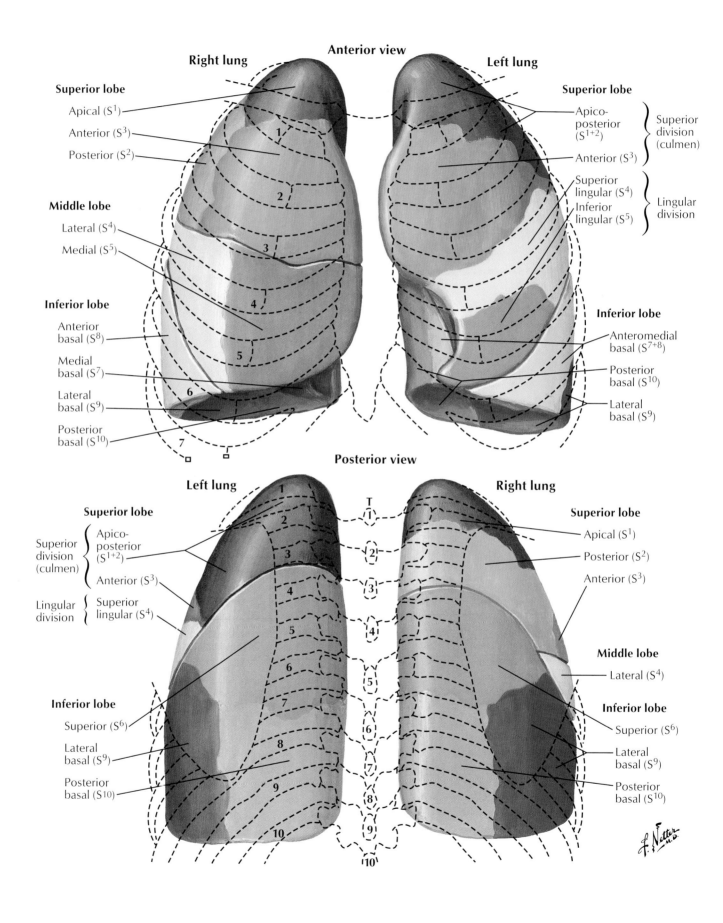

Anterior view

Right lung

Left lung

Superior lobe
- Apical (S^1)
- Anterior (S^3)
- Posterior (S^2)

Middle lobe
- Lateral (S^4)
- Medial (S^5)

Inferior lobe
- Anterior basal (S^8)
- Medial basal (S^7)
- Lateral basal (S^9)
- Posterior basal (S^{10})

Superior lobe
- Apico-posterior (S^{1+2}) } Superior division (culmen)
- Anterior (S^3) }
- Superior lingular (S^4) } Lingular division
- Inferior lingular (S^5) }

Inferior lobe
- Anteromedial basal (S^{7+8})
- Posterior basal (S^{10})
- Lateral basal (S^9)

Posterior view

Left lung

Right lung

Superior lobe
- Superior division (culmen) { Apico-posterior (S^{1+2})
- Anterior (S^3)
- Lingular division { Superior lingular (S^4)

Inferior lobe
- Superior (S^6)
- Lateral basal (S^9)
- Posterior basal (S^{10})

Superior lobe
- Apical (S^1)
- Posterior (S^2)
- Anterior (S^3)

Middle lobe
- Lateral (S^4)

Inferior lobe
- Superior (S^6)
- Lateral basal (S^9)
- Posterior basal (S^{10})

Plate 200

Lungs

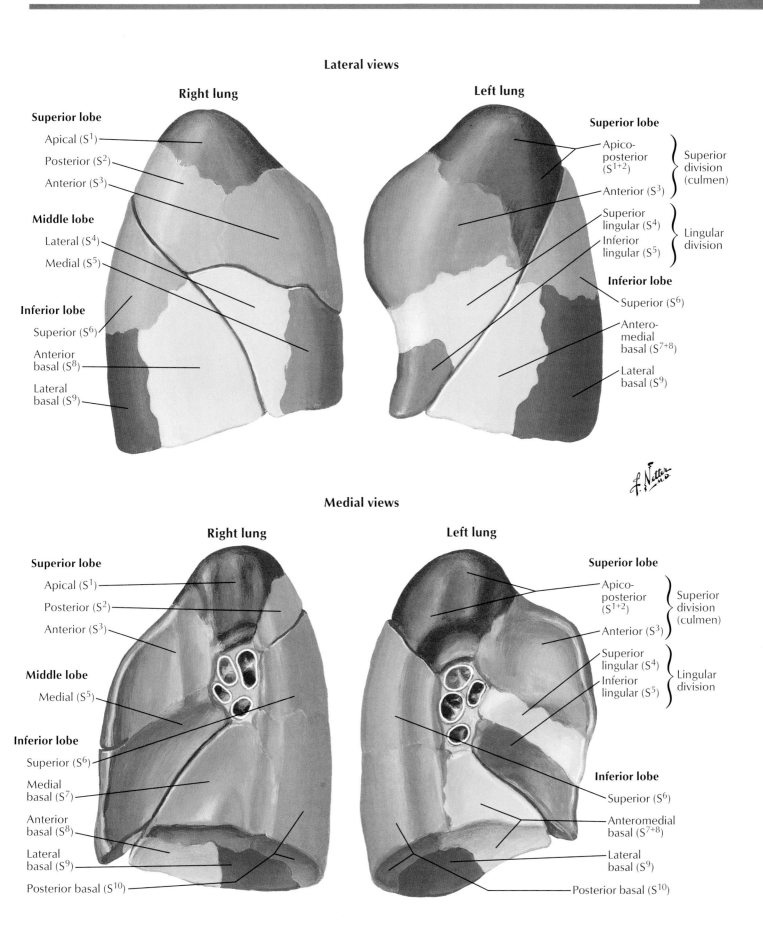

Lateral views

Right lung

Left lung

Superior lobe
Apical (S^1)
Posterior (S^2)
Anterior (S^3)

Middle lobe
Lateral (S^4)
Medial (S^5)

Inferior lobe
Superior (S^6)
Anterior basal (S^8)
Lateral basal (S^9)

Superior lobe
Apico-posterior (S^{1+2}) } Superior division (culmen)
Anterior (S^3) }
Superior lingular (S^4) } Lingular division
Inferior lingular (S^5) }

Inferior lobe
Superior (S^6)
Antero-medial basal (S^{7+8})
Lateral basal (S^9)

Medial views

Right lung

Left lung

Superior lobe
Apical (S^1)
Posterior (S^2)
Anterior (S^3)

Middle lobe
Medial (S^5)

Inferior lobe
Superior (S^6)
Medial basal (S^7)
Anterior basal (S^8)
Lateral basal (S^9)
Posterior basal (S^{10})

Superior lobe
Apico-posterior (S^{1+2}) } Superior division (culmen)
Anterior (S^3) }
Superior lingular (S^4) } Lingular division
Inferior lingular (S^5) }

Inferior lobe
Superior (S^6)
Anteromedial basal (S^{7+8})
Lateral basal (S^9)
Posterior basal (S^{10})

Lungs

Plate 201

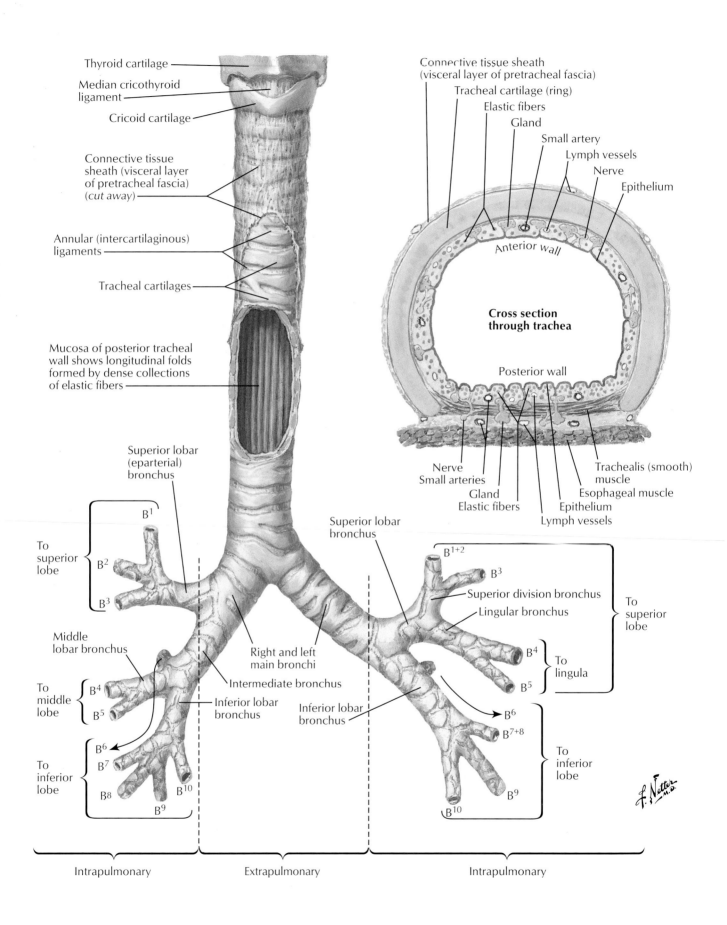

Thyroid cartilage

Median cricothyroid ligament

Cricoid cartilage

Connective tissue sheath (visceral layer of pretracheal fascia) (cut away)

Annular (intercartilaginous) ligaments

Tracheal cartilages

Mucosa of posterior tracheal wall shows longitudinal folds formed by dense collections of elastic fibers

Connective tissue sheath (visceral layer of pretracheal fascia)

Tracheal cartilage (ring)

Elastic fibers

Gland

Small artery

Lymph vessels

Nerve

Epithelium

Anterior wall

Cross section through trachea

Posterior wall

Nerve
Small arteries
Gland
Elastic fibers

Trachealis (smooth) muscle

Esophageal muscle

Epithelium

Lymph vessels

Superior lobar (eparterial) bronchus

Superior lobar bronchus

B^1

To superior lobe

B^2

B^3

B^{1+2}

B^3

Superior division bronchus

Lingular bronchus

To superior lobe

Middle lobar bronchus

Right and left main bronchi

B^4

To lingula

To middle lobe

B^4

Intermediate bronchus

B^5

B^5

Inferior lobar bronchus

Inferior lobar bronchus

B^6

B^6

B^{7+8}

To inferior lobe

B^7

To inferior lobe

B^8

B^{10}

B^9

B^9

B^{10}

Intrapulmonary

Extrapulmonary

Intrapulmonary

Plate 202

Lungs

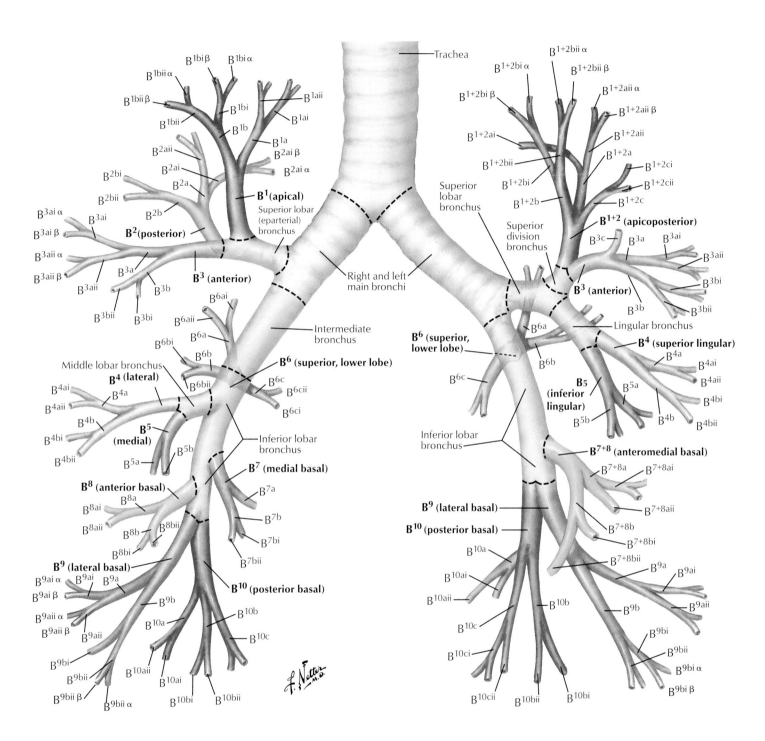

Nomenclature in common usage for bronchopulmonary segments (Plates 200 and 201) is that of Jackson and Huber, and segmental bronchi are named accordingly. Ikeda proposed nomenclature (as demonstrated here) for bronchial subdivisions as far as 6th generation. For simplification on this illustration, only some bronchial subdivisions are labeled as far as 5th or 6th generation. Segmental bronchi (B) are numbered from 1 to 10 in each lung, corresponding to pulmonary segments. In left lung,

B^1 and B^2 are combined as are B^7 and B^8. Subsegmental, or 4th order, bronchi are indicated by addition of lower-case letters a, b, or c when an additional branch is present. Fifth order bronchi are designated by Roman numerals i (anterior) or ii (posterior) and 6th order bronchi by Greek letters α or β. Several texts use alternate numbers (as proposed by Boyden) for segmental bronchi.

Variations of standard bronchial pattern shown here are common, especially in peripheral airways.

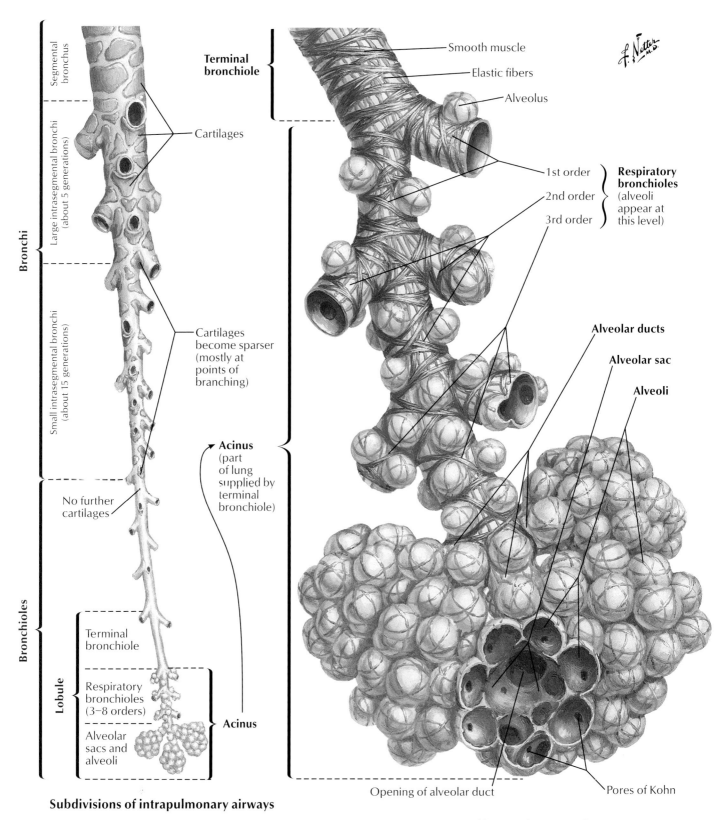

Terminal bronchiole

Cartilages

Smooth muscle

Elastic fibers

Alveolus

1st order

2nd order

3rd order

Respiratory bronchioles (alveoli appear at this level)

Cartilages become sparser (mostly at points of branching)

Segmental bronchus

Large intrasegmental bronchi (about 5 generations)

Bronchi

Small intrasegmental bronchi (about 15 generations)

No further cartilages

Acinus (part of lung supplied by terminal bronchiole)

Alveolar ducts

Alveolar sac

Alveoli

Bronchioles

Lobule

Terminal bronchiole

Respiratory bronchioles (3–8 orders)

Alveolar sacs and alveoli

Acinus

Opening of alveolar duct

Pores of Kohn

Subdivisions of intrapulmonary airways

Structure of intrapulmonary airways

Plate 204

Lungs

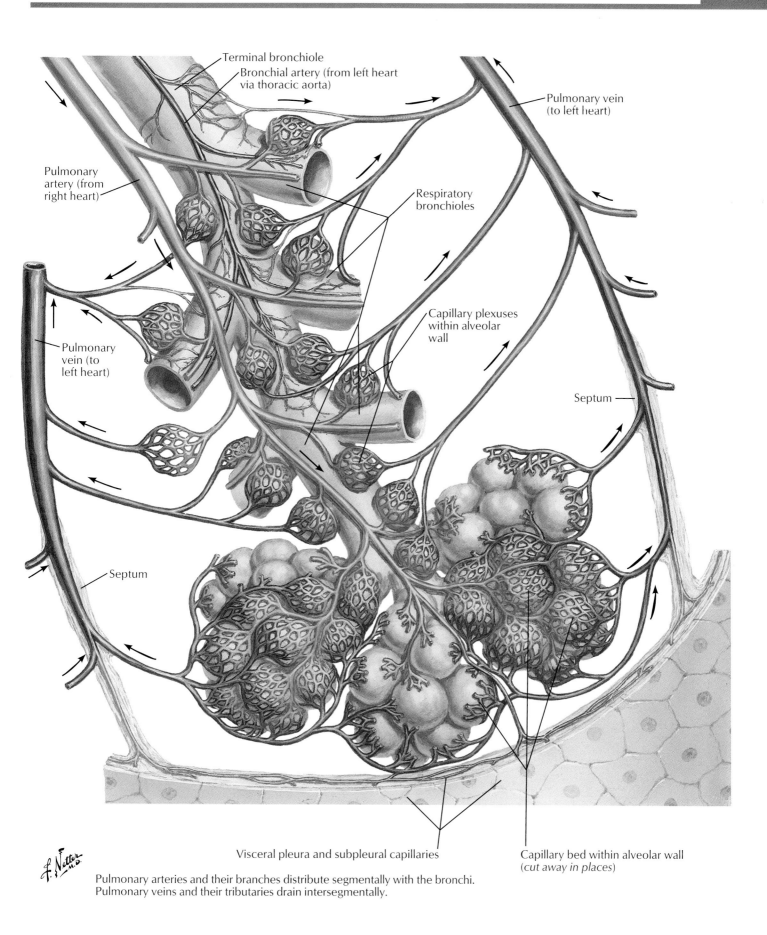

Terminal bronchiole

Bronchial artery (from left heart via thoracic aorta)

Pulmonary vein (to left heart)

Pulmonary artery (from right heart)

Respiratory bronchioles

Capillary plexuses within alveolar wall

Pulmonary vein (to left heart)

Septum

Septum

Visceral pleura and subpleural capillaries

Capillary bed within alveolar wall (*cut away in places*)

Pulmonary arteries and their branches distribute segmentally with the bronchi. Pulmonary veins and their tributaries drain intersegmentally.

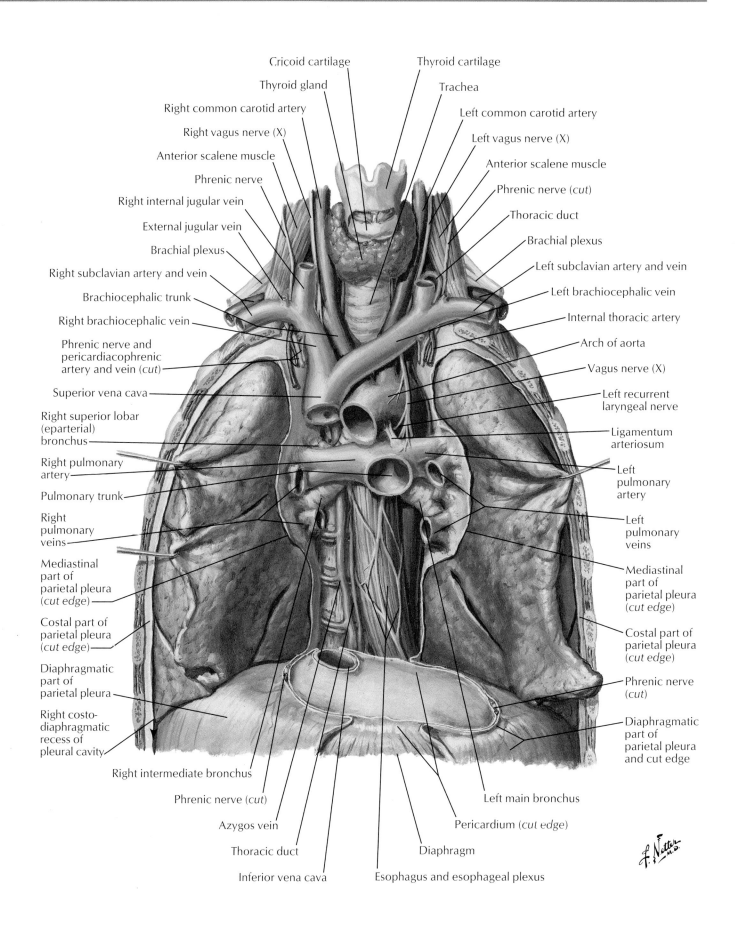

Cricoid cartilage

Thyroid cartilage

Thyroid gland

Trachea

Right common carotid artery

Left common carotid artery

Right vagus nerve (X)

Left vagus nerve (X)

Anterior scalene muscle

Anterior scalene muscle

Phrenic nerve

Phrenic nerve (cut)

Right internal jugular vein

Thoracic duct

External jugular vein

Brachial plexus

Brachial plexus

Left subclavian artery and vein

Right subclavian artery and vein

Left brachiocephalic vein

Brachiocephalic trunk

Internal thoracic artery

Right brachiocephalic vein

Arch of aorta

Phrenic nerve and pericardiacophrenic artery and vein (cut)

Vagus nerve (X)

Superior vena cava

Left recurrent laryngeal nerve

Right superior lobar (eparterial) bronchus

Ligamentum arteriosum

Right pulmonary artery

Left pulmonary artery

Pulmonary trunk

Right pulmonary veins

Left pulmonary veins

Mediastinal part of parietal pleura (cut edge)

Mediastinal part of parietal pleura (cut edge)

Costal part of parietal pleura (cut edge)

Costal part of parietal pleura (cut edge)

Diaphragmatic part of parietal pleura

Phrenic nerve (cut)

Right costo-diaphragmatic recess of pleural cavity

Diaphragmatic part of parietal pleura and cut edge

Right intermediate bronchus

Left main bronchus

Phrenic nerve (cut)

Pericardium (cut edge)

Azygos vein

Diaphragm

Thoracic duct

Inferior vena cava

Esophagus and esophageal plexus

Plate 206

Lungs

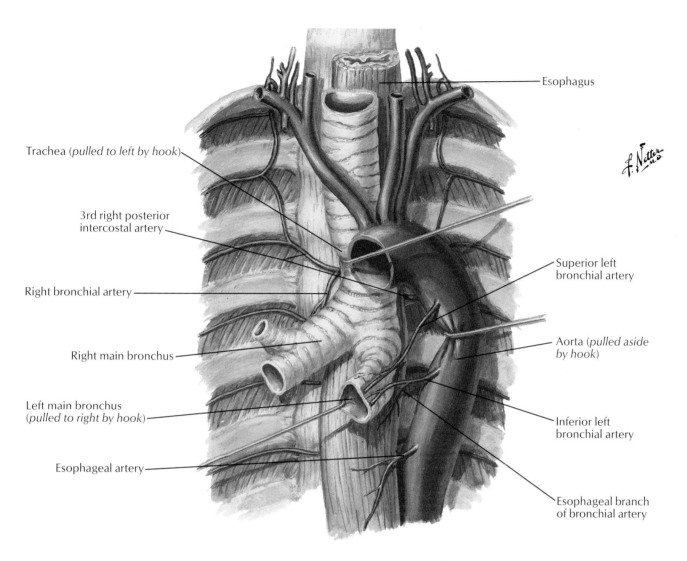

Esophagus

Trachea (*pulled to left by hook*)

3rd right posterior intercostal artery

Right bronchial artery

Right main bronchus

Left main bronchus (*pulled to right by hook*)

Esophageal artery

Superior left bronchial artery

Aorta (*pulled aside by hook*)

Inferior left bronchial artery

Esophageal branch of bronchial artery

Variations in bronchial arteries

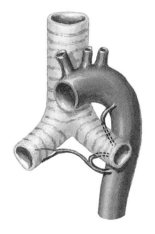

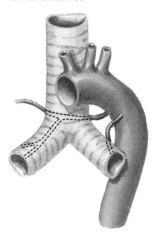

Right and left bronchial arteries originating from aorta by single stem

Only single bronchial artery to each bronchus (normally, two to left bronchus)

Bronchial veins

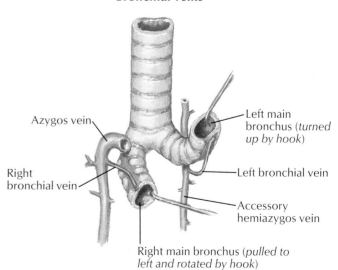

Azygos vein

Right bronchial vein

Left main bronchus (*turned up by hook*)

Left bronchial vein

Accessory hemiazygos vein

Right main bronchus (*pulled to left and rotated by hook*)

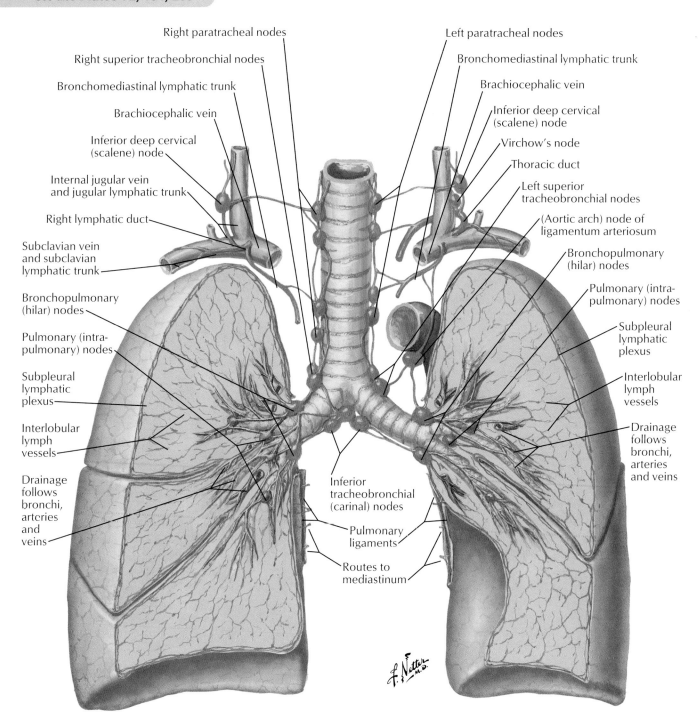

Right paratracheal nodes

Right superior tracheobronchial nodes

Bronchomediastinal lymphatic trunk

Brachiocephalic vein

Inferior deep cervical (scalene) node

Internal jugular vein and jugular lymphatic trunk

Right lymphatic duct

Subclavian vein and subclavian lymphatic trunk

Bronchopulmonary (hilar) nodes

Pulmonary (intra-pulmonary) nodes

Subpleural lymphatic plexus

Interlobular lymph vessels

Drainage follows bronchi, arteries and veins

Left paratracheal nodes

Bronchomediastinal lymphatic trunk

Brachiocephalic vein

Inferior deep cervical (scalene) node

Virchow's node

Thoracic duct

Left superior tracheobronchial nodes

(Aortic arch) node of ligamentum arteriosum

Bronchopulmonary (hilar) nodes

Pulmonary (intra-pulmonary) nodes

Subpleural lymphatic plexus

Interlobular lymph vessels

Drainage follows bronchi, arteries and veins

Inferior tracheobronchial (carinal) nodes

Pulmonary ligaments

Routes to mediastinum

Drainage routes

Right lung: All lobes drain to pulmonary and broncho-pulmonary (hilar) nodes, then to inferior tracheobronchial (carinal) nodes, right superior tracheobronchial nodes, and right paratracheal nodes on way to brachiocephalic vein via bronchomediastinal lymphatic trunk and/or inferior deep cervical (scalene) node.

Left lung: Superior lobe drains to pulmonary and broncho-pulmonary (hilar) nodes, inferior tracheobronchial (carinal) nodes, left superior tracheobronchial nodes, left paratracheal nodes and/or (aortic arch) node of ligamentum arteriosum, then to brachiocephalic vein via left bronchomediastinal trunk and thoracic duct. Left inferior lobe drains also to pulmonary and bronchopulmonary (hilar) nodes and to inferior tracheo-bronchial (carinal) nodes, but then mostly to right superior tracheobronchial nodes, where it follows same route as lymph from right lung.

Plate 208

Lungs

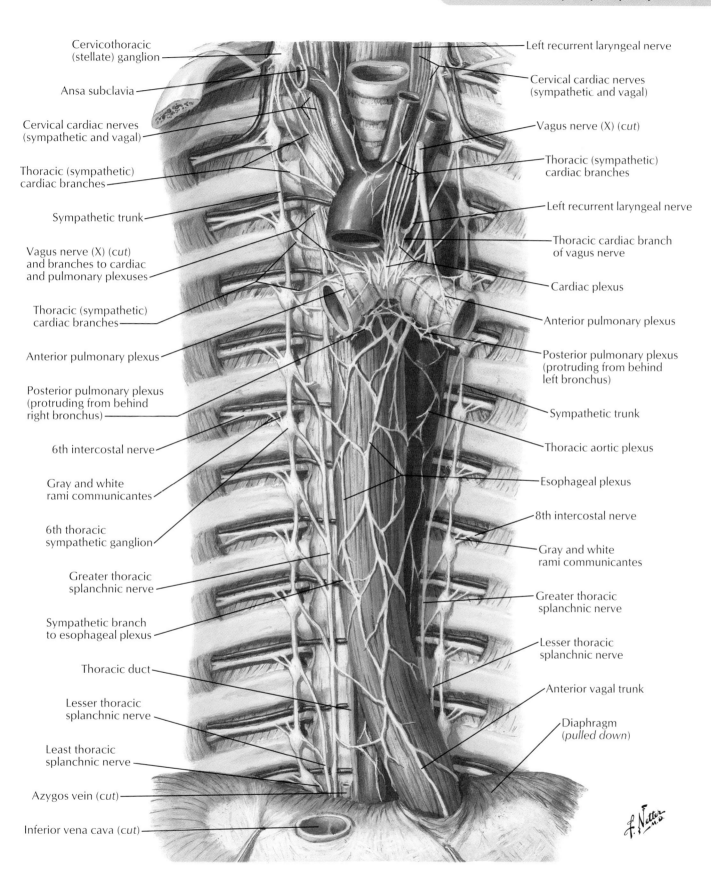

Cervicothoracic (stellate) ganglion

Ansa subclavia

Cervical cardiac nerves (sympathetic and vagal)

Thoracic (sympathetic) cardiac branches

Sympathetic trunk

Vagus nerve (X) (cut) and branches to cardiac and pulmonary plexuses

Thoracic (sympathetic) cardiac branches

Anterior pulmonary plexus

Posterior pulmonary plexus (protruding from behind right bronchus)

6th intercostal nerve

Gray and white rami communicantes

6th thoracic sympathetic ganglion

Greater thoracic splanchnic nerve

Sympathetic branch to esophageal plexus

Thoracic duct

Lesser thoracic splanchnic nerve

Least thoracic splanchnic nerve

Azygos vein (cut)

Inferior vena cava (cut)

Left recurrent laryngeal nerve

Cervical cardiac nerves (sympathetic and vagal)

Vagus nerve (X) (cut)

Thoracic (sympathetic) cardiac branches

Left recurrent laryngeal nerve

Thoracic cardiac branch of vagus nerve

Cardiac plexus

Anterior pulmonary plexus

Posterior pulmonary plexus (protruding from behind left bronchus)

Sympathetic trunk

Thoracic aortic plexus

Esophageal plexus

8th intercostal nerve

Gray and white rami communicantes

Greater thoracic splanchnic nerve

Lesser thoracic splanchnic nerve

Anterior vagal trunk

Diaphragm (pulled down)

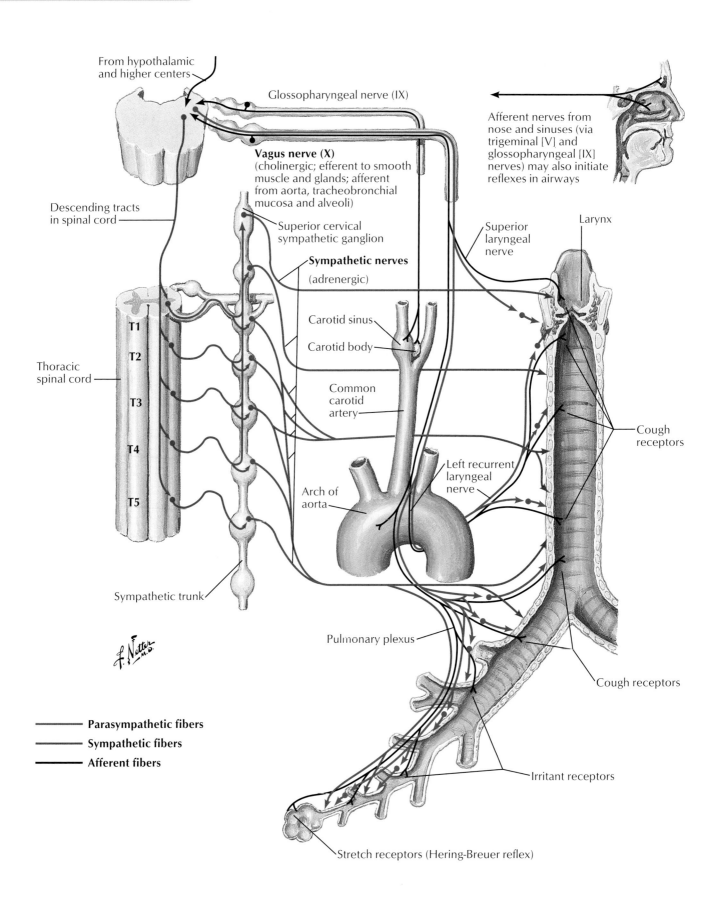

From hypothalamic and higher centers

Glossopharyngeal nerve (IX)

Afferent nerves from nose and sinuses (via trigeminal [V] and glossopharyngeal [IX] nerves) may also initiate reflexes in airways

Vagus nerve (X) (cholinergic; efferent to smooth muscle and glands; afferent from aorta, tracheobronchial mucosa and alveoli)

Descending tracts in spinal cord

Superior cervical sympathetic ganglion

Superior laryngeal nerve

Larynx

Sympathetic nerves (adrenergic)

T1

T2

Thoracic spinal cord

T3

Carotid sinus

Carotid body

Common carotid artery

Cough receptors

T4

T5

Left recurrent laryngeal nerve

Arch of aorta

Sympathetic trunk

Pulmonary plexus

Cough receptors

Irritant receptors

Parasympathetic fibers

Sympathetic fibers

Afferent fibers

Stretch receptors (Hering-Breuer reflex)

Plate 210

Lungs

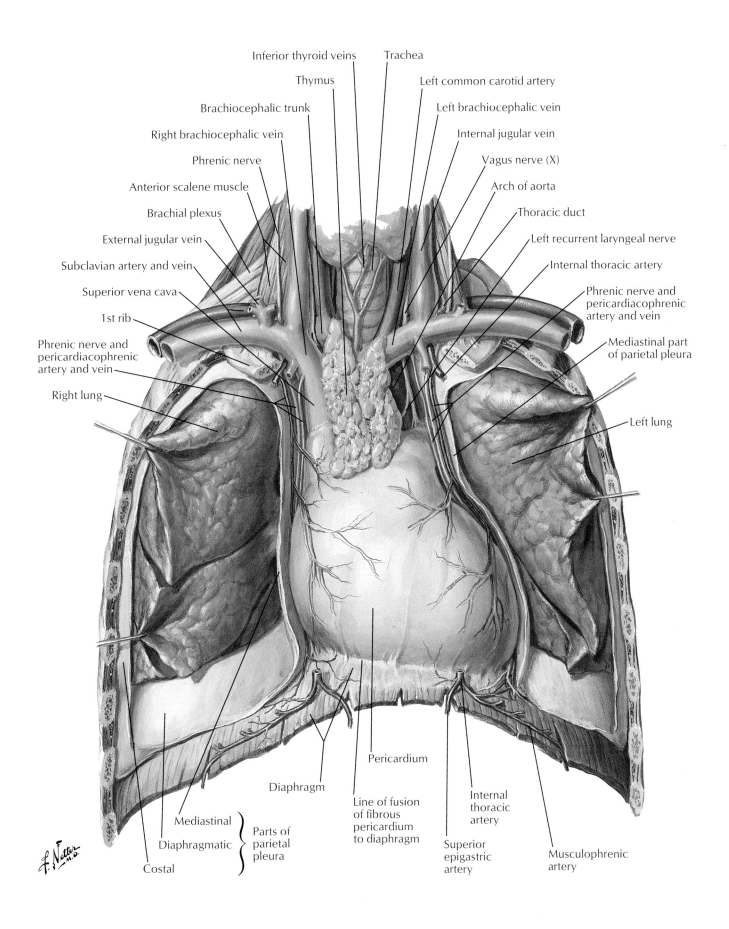

Inferior thyroid veins

Trachea

Thymus

Left common carotid artery

Brachiocephalic trunk

Left brachiocephalic vein

Right brachiocephalic vein

Internal jugular vein

Phrenic nerve

Vagus nerve (X)

Anterior scalene muscle

Arch of aorta

Brachial plexus

Thoracic duct

External jugular vein

Left recurrent laryngeal nerve

Subclavian artery and vein

Internal thoracic artery

Superior vena cava

Phrenic nerve and pericardiacophrenic artery and vein

1st rib

Mediastinal part of parietal pleura

Phrenic nerve and pericardiacophrenic artery and vein

Right lung

Left lung

Pericardium

Diaphragm

Line of fusion of fibrous pericardium to diaphragm

Internal thoracic artery

Mediastinal

Diaphragmatic

} Parts of parietal pleura

Costal

Superior epigastric artery

Musculophrenic artery

f. Netter m.o.

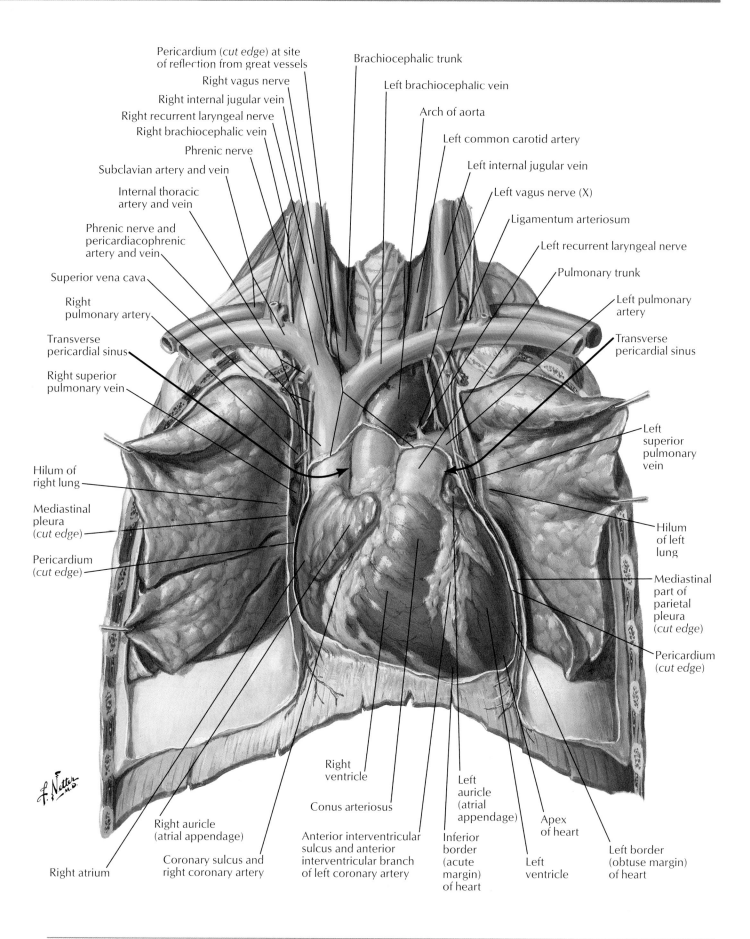

Pericardium (*cut edge*) at site of reflection from great vessels

Right vagus nerve

Right internal jugular vein

Right recurrent laryngeal nerve

Right brachiocephalic vein

Phrenic nerve

Subclavian artery and vein

Internal thoracic artery and vein

Phrenic nerve and pericardiacophrenic artery and vein

Superior vena cava

Right pulmonary artery

Transverse pericardial sinus

Right superior pulmonary vein

Hilum of right lung

Mediastinal pleura (*cut edge*)

Pericardium (*cut edge*)

Brachiocephalic trunk

Left brachiocephalic vein

Arch of aorta

Left common carotid artery

Left internal jugular vein

Left vagus nerve (X)

Ligamentum arteriosum

Left recurrent laryngeal nerve

Pulmonary trunk

Left pulmonary artery

Transverse pericardial sinus

Left superior pulmonary vein

Hilum of left lung

Mediastinal part of parietal pleura (*cut edge*)

Pericardium (*cut edge*)

Right atrium

Right auricle (atrial appendage)

Coronary sulcus and right coronary artery

Right ventricle

Conus arteriosus

Anterior interventricular sulcus and anterior interventricular branch of left coronary artery

Inferior border (acute margin) of heart

Left auricle (atrial appendage)

Left ventricle

Apex of heart

Left border (obtuse margin) of heart

Plate 212   **Heart**

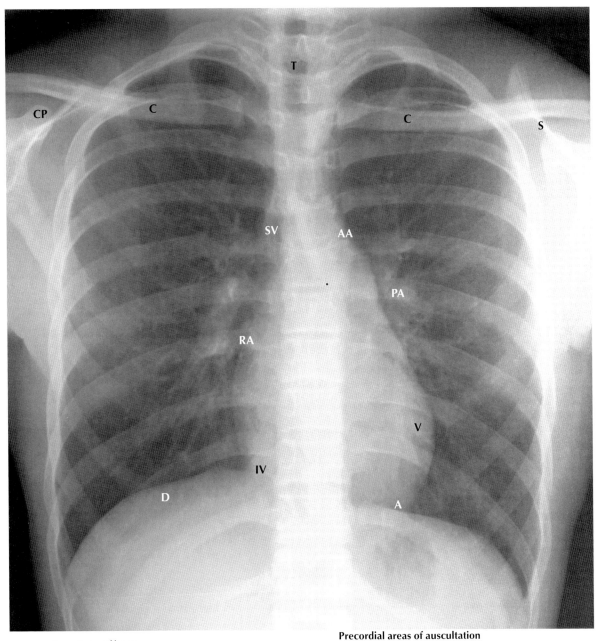

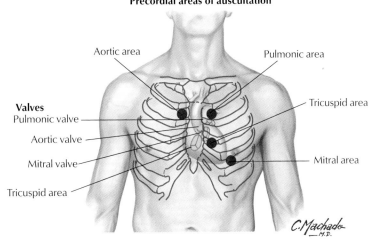

Precordial areas of auscultation

A	Apex of heart
AA	Aortic arch
C	Clavicle
CP	Coracoid process of scapula
D	Dome of diaphragm (right)
IV	Inferior vena cava
PA	Pulmonary artery (left)
RA	Right atrium
S	Spine of scapula
SV	Superior vena cava
T	Trachea (air)
V	Left ventricle

Heart

Plate 213

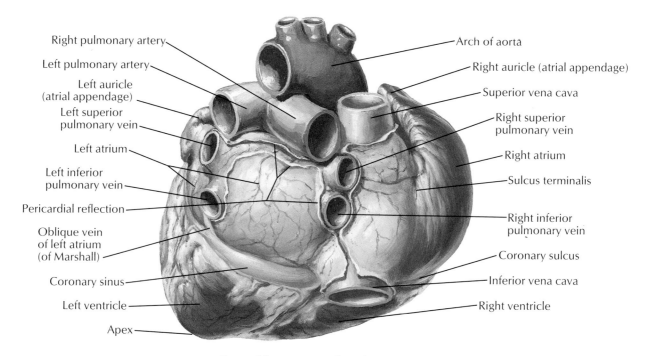

Right pulmonary artery

Left pulmonary artery

Left auricle (atrial appendage)

Left superior pulmonary vein

Left atrium

Left inferior pulmonary vein

Pericardial reflection

Oblique vein of left atrium (of Marshall)

Coronary sinus

Left ventricle

Apex

Arch of aorta

Right auricle (atrial appendage)

Superior vena cava

Right superior pulmonary vein

Right atrium

Sulcus terminalis

Right inferior pulmonary vein

Coronary sulcus

Inferior vena cava

Right ventricle

Base of heart: posterior view

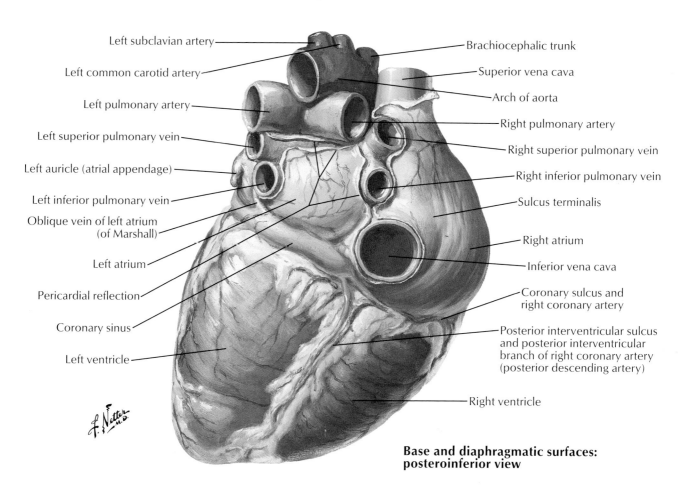

Left subclavian artery

Left common carotid artery

Left pulmonary artery

Left superior pulmonary vein

Left auricle (atrial appendage)

Left inferior pulmonary vein

Oblique vein of left atrium (of Marshall)

Left atrium

Pericardial reflection

Coronary sinus

Left ventricle

Brachiocephalic trunk

Superior vena cava

Arch of aorta

Right pulmonary artery

Right superior pulmonary vein

Right inferior pulmonary vein

Sulcus terminalis

Right atrium

Inferior vena cava

Coronary sulcus and right coronary artery

Posterior interventricular sulcus and posterior interventricular branch of right coronary artery (posterior descending artery)

Right ventricle

Base and diaphragmatic surfaces: posteroinferior view

Plate 214

Heart

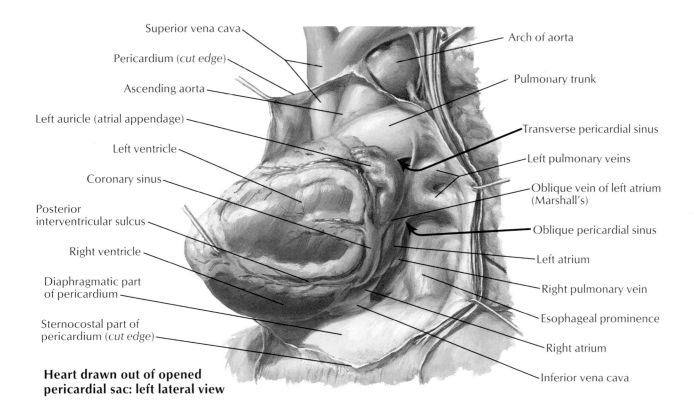

Superior vena cava

Pericardium (*cut edge*)

Ascending aorta

Left auricle (atrial appendage)

Left ventricle

Coronary sinus

Posterior interventricular sulcus

Right ventricle

Diaphragmatic part of pericardium

Sternocostal part of pericardium (*cut edge*)

Arch of aorta

Pulmonary trunk

Transverse pericardial sinus

Left pulmonary veins

Oblique vein of left atrium (Marshall's)

Oblique pericardial sinus

Left atrium

Right pulmonary vein

Esophageal prominence

Right atrium

Inferior vena cava

Heart drawn out of opened pericardial sac: left lateral view

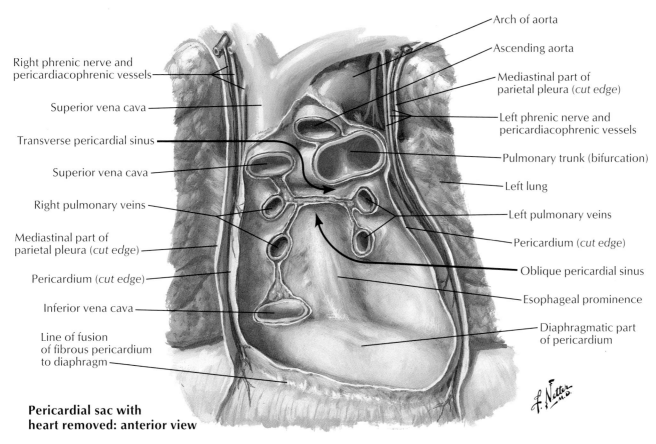

Right phrenic nerve and pericardiacophrenic vessels

Superior vena cava

Transverse pericardial sinus

Superior vena cava

Right pulmonary veins

Mediastinal part of parietal pleura (*cut edge*)

Pericardium (*cut edge*)

Inferior vena cava

Line of fusion of fibrous pericardium to diaphragm

Arch of aorta

Ascending aorta

Mediastinal part of parietal pleura (*cut edge*)

Left phrenic nerve and pericardiacophrenic vessels

Pulmonary trunk (bifurcation)

Left lung

Left pulmonary veins

Pericardium (*cut edge*)

Oblique pericardial sinus

Esophageal prominence

Diaphragmatic part of pericardium

Pericardial sac with heart removed: anterior view

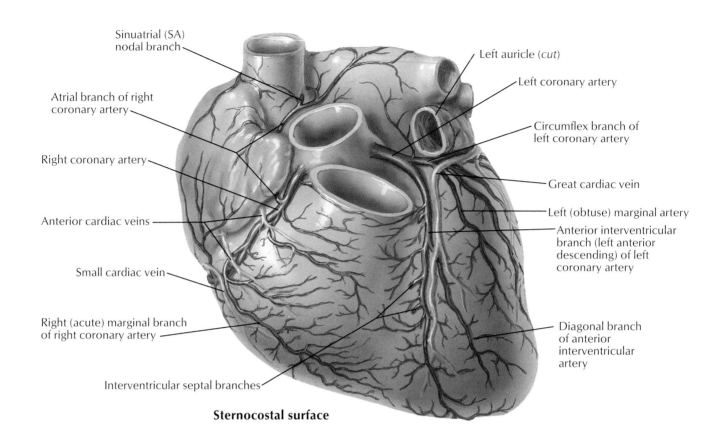

Sinuatrial (SA) nodal branch

Atrial branch of right coronary artery

Right coronary artery

Anterior cardiac veins

Small cardiac vein

Right (acute) marginal branch of right coronary artery

Interventricular septal branches

Left auricle (*cut*)

Left coronary artery

Circumflex branch of left coronary artery

Great cardiac vein

Left (obtuse) marginal artery

Anterior interventricular branch (left anterior descending) of left coronary artery

Diagonal branch of anterior interventricular artery

Sternocostal surface

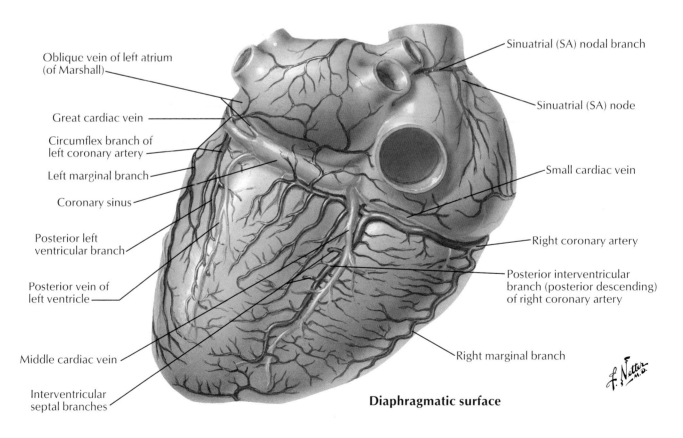

Oblique vein of left atrium (of Marshall)

Great cardiac vein

Circumflex branch of left coronary artery

Left marginal branch

Coronary sinus

Posterior left ventricular branch

Posterior vein of left ventricle

Middle cardiac vein

Interventricular septal branches

Sinuatrial (SA) nodal branch

Sinuatrial (SA) node

Small cardiac vein

Right coronary artery

Posterior interventricular branch (posterior descending) of right coronary artery

Right marginal branch

Diaphragmatic surface

Plate 216   **Heart**

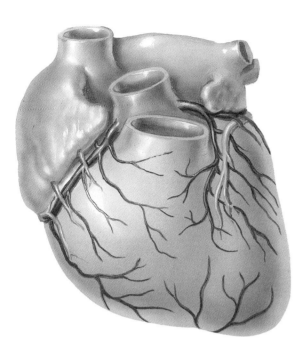

Anterior interventricular (left anterior descending) branch of left coronary artery is very short. Apical part of anterior (sternocostal) surface supplied by branches from posterior interventricular (posterior descending) branch of right coronary artery curving around apex.

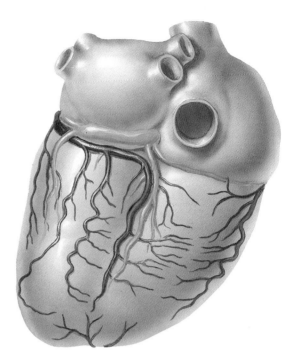

Posterior interventricular (posterior descending) branch is derived from circumflex branch of left coronary artery instead of from right coronary artery.

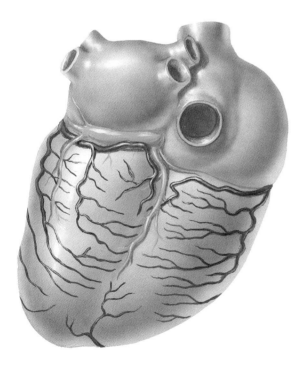

Posterior interventricular (posterior descending) branch is absent. Area supplied chiefly by small branches from circumflex branch of left coronary artery and from right coronary artery.

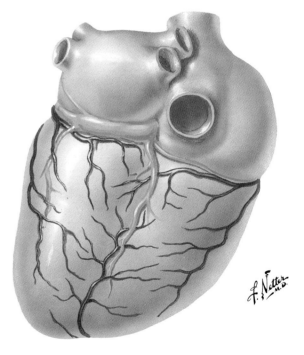

Posterior interventricular (posterior descending) branch is absent. Area supplied chiefly by elongated anterior interventricular (left anterior descending) branch curving around apex.

Right coronary artery: left anterior oblique view

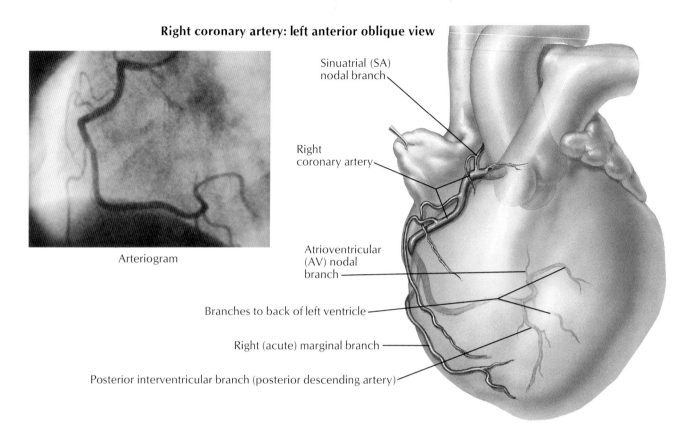

Arteriogram

Sinuatrial (SA) nodal branch

Right coronary artery

Atrioventricular (AV) nodal branch

Branches to back of left ventricle

Right (acute) marginal branch

Posterior interventricular branch (posterior descending artery)

Right coronary artery: right anterior oblique view

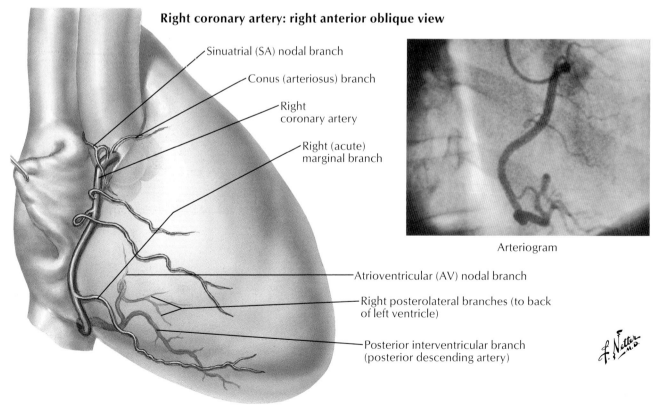

Sinuatrial (SA) nodal branch

Conus (arteriosus) branch

Right coronary artery

Right (acute) marginal branch

Arteriogram

Atrioventricular (AV) nodal branch

Right posterolateral branches (to back of left ventricle)

Posterior interventricular branch (posterior descending artery)

Plate 218   **Heart**

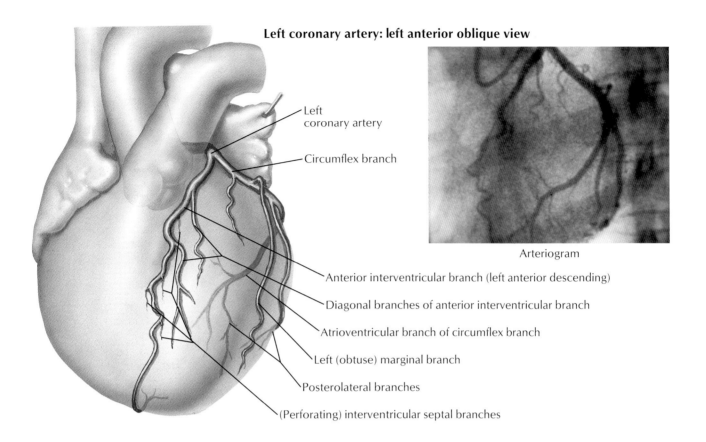

Left coronary artery: left anterior oblique view

Left coronary artery

Circumflex branch

Arteriogram

Anterior interventricular branch (left anterior descending)

Diagonal branches of anterior interventricular branch

Atrioventricular branch of circumflex branch

Left (obtuse) marginal branch

Posterolateral branches

(Perforating) interventricular septal branches

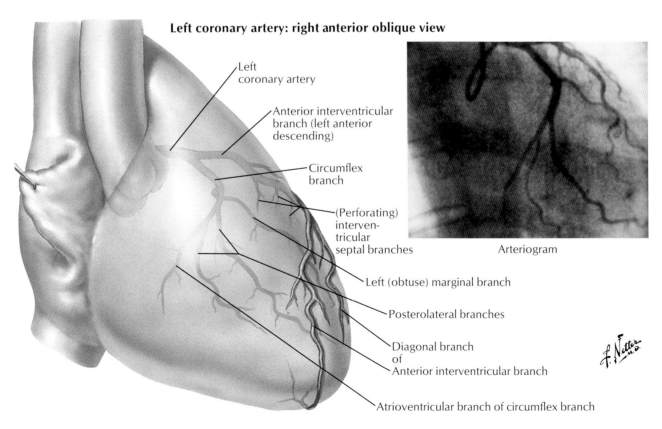

Left coronary artery: right anterior oblique view

Left coronary artery

Anterior interventricular branch (left anterior descending)

Circumflex branch

(Perforating) interventricular septal branches

Arteriogram

Left (obtuse) marginal branch

Posterolateral branches

Diagonal branch of Anterior interventricular branch

Atrioventricular branch of circumflex branch

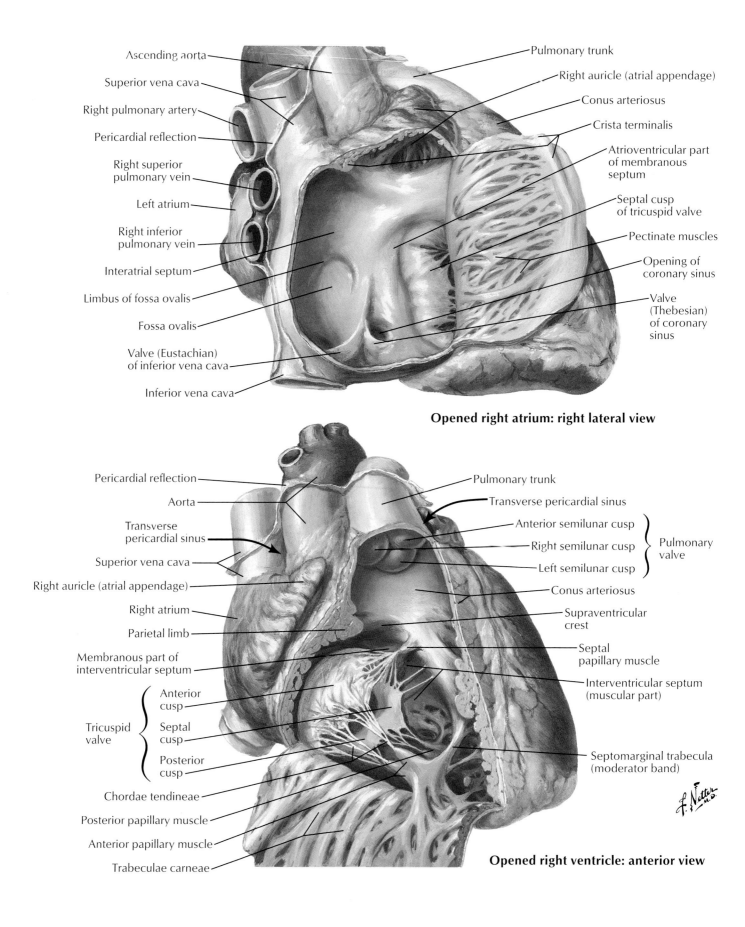

Ascending aorta
Superior vena cava
Right pulmonary artery
Pericardial reflection
Right superior pulmonary vein
Left atrium
Right inferior pulmonary vein
Interatrial septum
Limbus of fossa ovalis
Fossa ovalis
Valve (Eustachian) of inferior vena cava
Inferior vena cava

Pulmonary trunk
Right auricle (atrial appendage)
Conus arteriosus
Crista terminalis
Atrioventricular part of membranous septum
Septal cusp of tricuspid valve
Pectinate muscles
Opening of coronary sinus
Valve (Thebesian) of coronary sinus

Opened right atrium: right lateral view

Pericardial reflection
Aorta
Transverse pericardial sinus
Superior vena cava
Right auricle (atrial appendage)
Right atrium
Parietal limb
Membranous part of interventricular septum
Tricuspid valve { Anterior cusp
Septal cusp
Posterior cusp }
Chordae tendineae
Posterior papillary muscle
Anterior papillary muscle
Trabeculae carneae

Pulmonary trunk
Transverse pericardial sinus
Anterior semilunar cusp
Right semilunar cusp   Pulmonary valve
Left semilunar cusp
Conus arteriosus
Supraventricular crest
Septal papillary muscle
Interventricular septum (muscular part)
Septomarginal trabecula (moderator band)

Opened right ventricle: anterior view

Plate 220   **Heart**

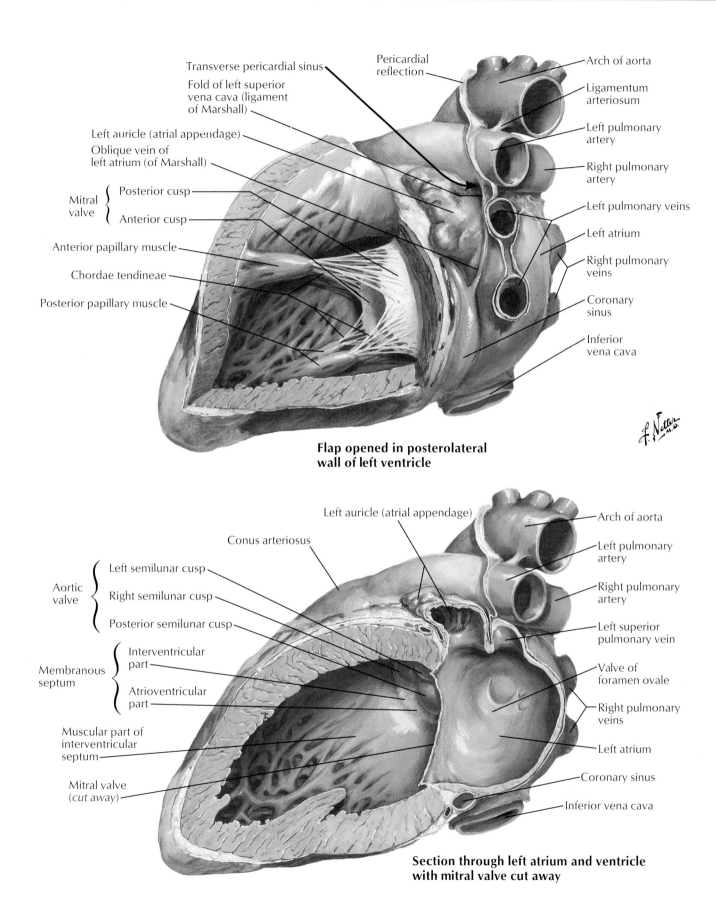

Transverse pericardial sinus

Pericardial reflection

Arch of aorta

Fold of left superior vena cava (ligament of Marshall)

Ligamentum arteriosum

Left auricle (atrial appendage)

Left pulmonary artery

Oblique vein of left atrium (of Marshall)

Right pulmonary artery

Mitral valve { Posterior cusp

Left pulmonary veins

Anterior cusp

Left atrium

Anterior papillary muscle

Right pulmonary veins

Chordae tendineae

Coronary sinus

Posterior papillary muscle

Inferior vena cava

F. Netter M.D.

Flap opened in posterolateral wall of left ventricle

Left auricle (atrial appendage)

Conus arteriosus

Arch of aorta

Left pulmonary artery

Aortic valve { Left semilunar cusp

Right semilunar cusp

Right pulmonary artery

Posterior semilunar cusp

Left superior pulmonary vein

Membranous septum { Interventricular part

Valve of foramen ovale

Atrioventricular part

Right pulmonary veins

Muscular part of interventricular septum

Left atrium

Mitral valve (*cut away*)

Coronary sinus

Inferior vena cava

Section through left atrium and ventricle with mitral valve cut away

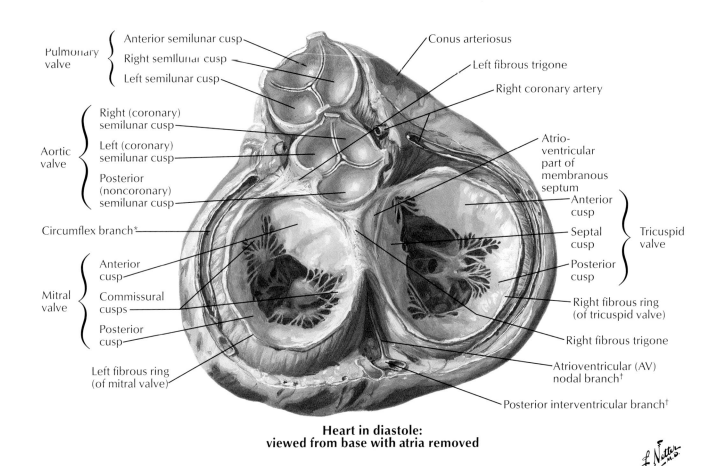

Pulmonary valve
- Anterior semilunar cusp
- Right semilunar cusp
- Left semilunar cusp

Aortic valve
- Right (coronary) semilunar cusp
- Left (coronary) semilunar cusp
- Posterior (noncoronary) semilunar cusp

Circumflex branch*

Mitral valve
- Anterior cusp
- Commissural cusps
- Posterior cusp

Left fibrous ring (of mitral valve)

Conus arteriosus

Left fibrous trigone

Right coronary artery

Atrio-ventricular part of membranous septum

Tricuspid valve
- Anterior cusp
- Septal cusp
- Posterior cusp

Right fibrous ring (of tricuspid valve)

Right fibrous trigone

Atrioventricular (AV) nodal branch[†]

Posterior interventricular branch[†]

Heart in diastole: viewed from base with atria removed

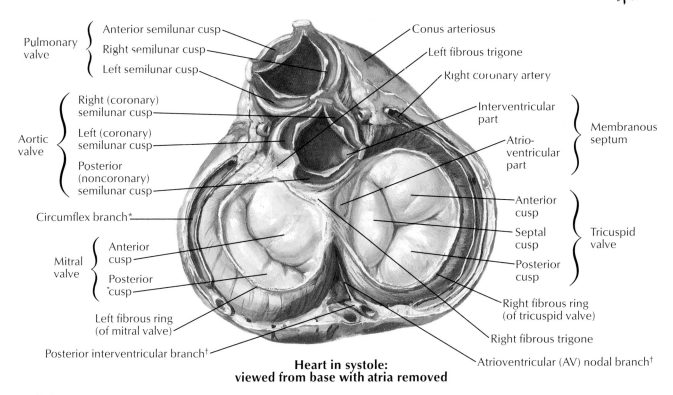

Pulmonary valve
- Anterior semilunar cusp
- Right semilunar cusp
- Left semilunar cusp

Aortic valve
- Right (coronary) semilunar cusp
- Left (coronary) semilunar cusp
- Posterior (noncoronary) semilunar cusp

Circumflex branch*

Mitral valve
- Anterior cusp
- Posterior cusp

Left fibrous ring (of mitral valve)

Posterior interventricular branch[†]

Conus arteriosus

Left fibrous trigone

Right coronary artery

Membranous septum
- Interventricular part
- Atrio-ventricular part

Tricuspid valve
- Anterior cusp
- Septal cusp
- Posterior cusp

Right fibrous ring (of tricuspid valve)

Right fibrous trigone

Atrioventricular (AV) nodal branch[†]

Heart in systole: viewed from base with atria removed

*Of left coronary artery
[†]Of right coronary artery

Plate 222

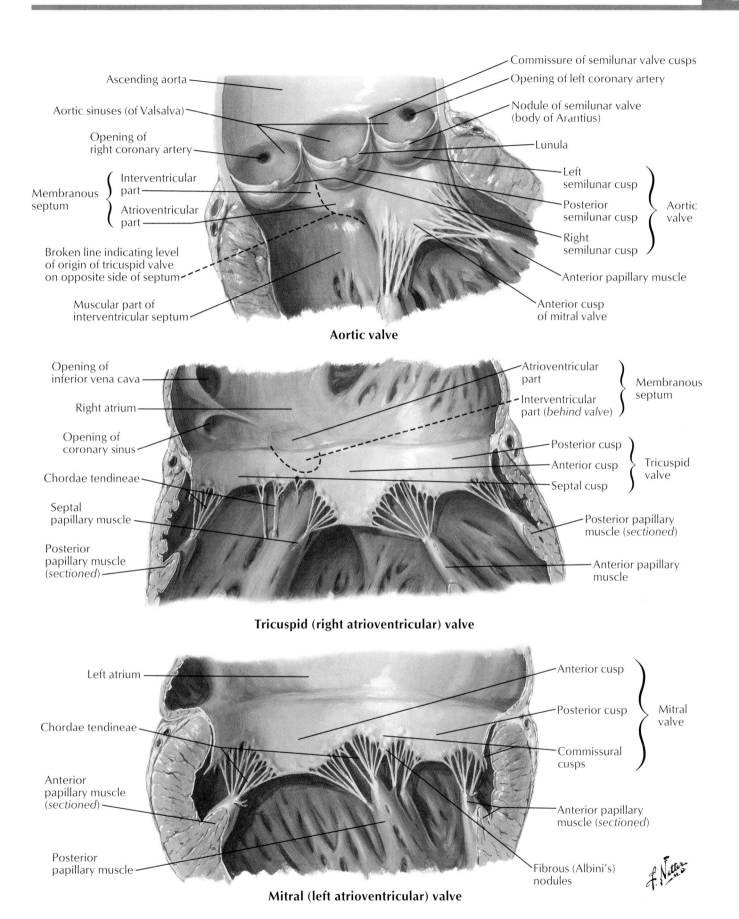

Aortic valve

Ascending aorta

Aortic sinuses (of Valsalva)

Opening of right coronary artery

Membranous septum
- Interventricular part
- Atrioventricular part

Broken line indicating level of origin of tricuspid valve on opposite side of septum

Muscular part of interventricular septum

Commissure of semilunar valve cusps

Opening of left coronary artery

Nodule of semilunar valve (body of Arantius)

Lunula

Aortic valve
- Left semilunar cusp
- Posterior semilunar cusp
- Right semilunar cusp

Anterior papillary muscle

Anterior cusp of mitral valve

Tricuspid (right atrioventricular) valve

Opening of inferior vena cava

Right atrium

Opening of coronary sinus

Chordae tendineae

Septal papillary muscle

Posterior papillary muscle (sectioned)

Membranous septum
- Atrioventricular part
- Interventricular part (behind valve)

Tricuspid valve
- Posterior cusp
- Anterior cusp
- Septal cusp

Posterior papillary muscle (sectioned)

Anterior papillary muscle

Mitral (left atrioventricular) valve

Left atrium

Chordae tendineae

Anterior papillary muscle (sectioned)

Posterior papillary muscle

Mitral valve
- Anterior cusp
- Posterior cusp
- Commissural cusps

Anterior papillary muscle (sectioned)

Fibrous (Albini's) nodules

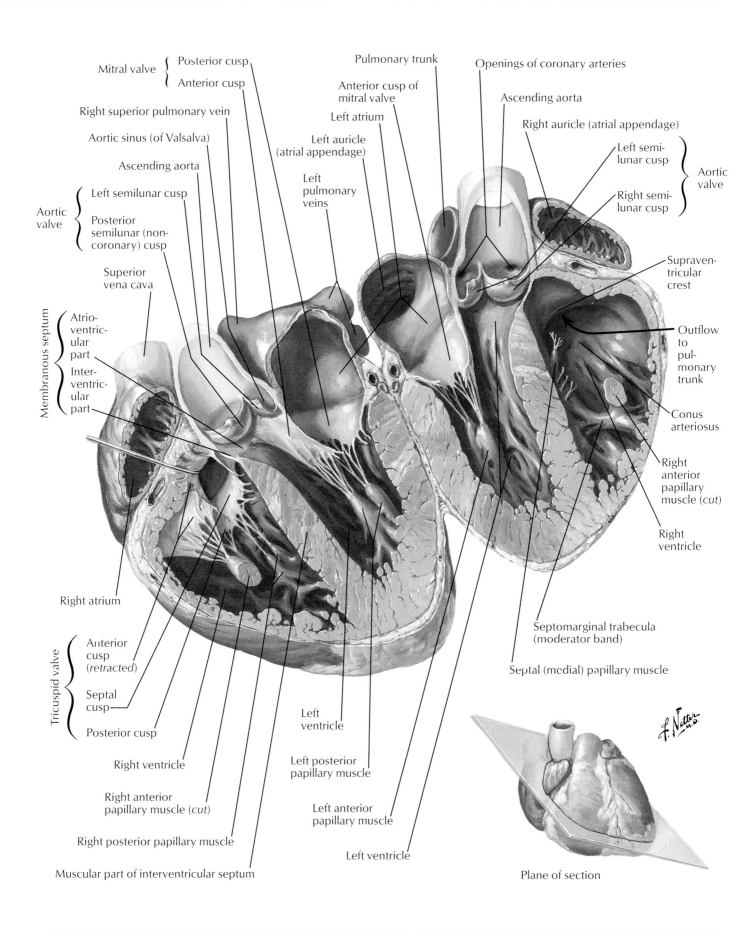

Mitral valve { Posterior cusp
Anterior cusp

Right superior pulmonary vein

Aortic sinus (of Valsalva)

Ascending aorta

Aortic valve { Left semilunar cusp
Posterior semilunar (non-coronary) cusp

Superior vena cava

Membranous septum { Atrio-ventricular part
Inter-ventricular part

Right atrium

Tricuspid valve { Anterior cusp (retracted)
Septal cusp
Posterior cusp

Right ventricle

Right anterior papillary muscle (cut)

Right posterior papillary muscle

Muscular part of interventricular septum

Pulmonary trunk

Anterior cusp of mitral valve

Left atrium

Left auricle (atrial appendage)

Left pulmonary veins

Openings of coronary arteries

Ascending aorta

Right auricle (atrial appendage)

Left semilunar cusp
Right semilunar cusp
} Aortic valve

Supraventricular crest

Outflow to pulmonary trunk

Conus arteriosus

Right anterior papillary muscle (cut)

Right ventricle

Septomarginal trabecula (moderator band)

Septal (medial) papillary muscle

Left ventricle

Left posterior papillary muscle

Left anterior papillary muscle

Left ventricle

Plane of section

Plate 224   **Heart**

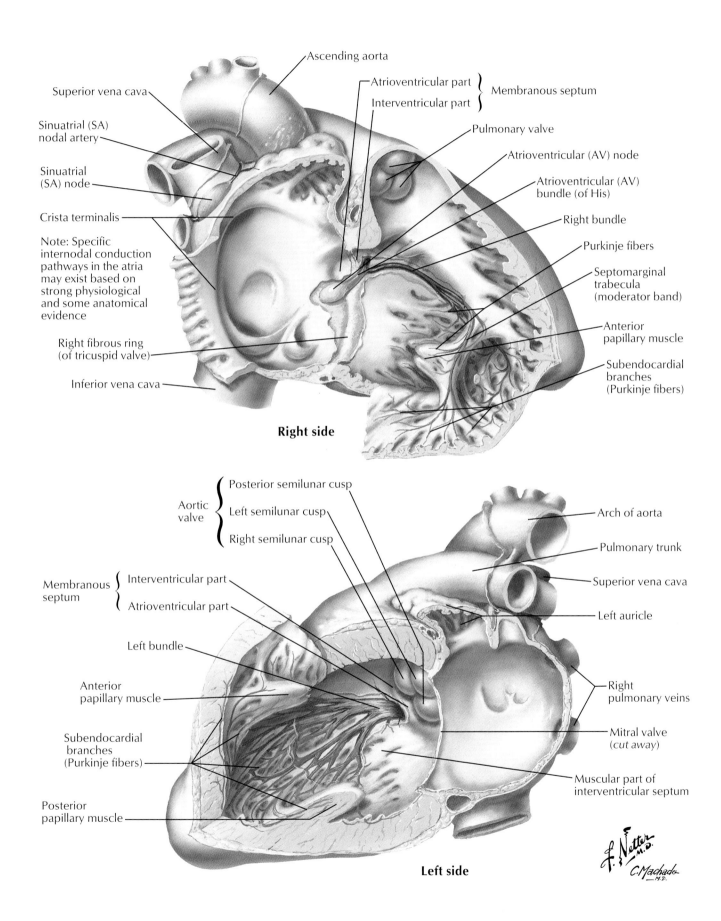

Ascending aorta

Superior vena cava

Sinuatrial (SA) nodal artery

Sinuatrial (SA) node

Crista terminalis

Note: Specific internodal conduction pathways in the atria may exist based on strong physiological and some anatomical evidence

Right fibrous ring (of tricuspid valve)

Inferior vena cava

Atrioventricular part
Interventricular part
} Membranous septum

Pulmonary valve

Atrioventricular (AV) node

Atrioventricular (AV) bundle (of His)

Right bundle

Purkinje fibers

Septomarginal trabecula (moderator band)

Anterior papillary muscle

Subendocardial branches (Purkinje fibers)

Right side

Aortic valve {
Posterior semilunar cusp
Left semilunar cusp
Right semilunar cusp

Membranous septum {
Interventricular part
Atrioventricular part

Left bundle

Anterior papillary muscle

Subendocardial branches (Purkinje fibers)

Posterior papillary muscle

Arch of aorta

Pulmonary trunk

Superior vena cava

Left auricle

Right pulmonary veins

Mitral valve (cut away)

Muscular part of interventricular septum

Left side

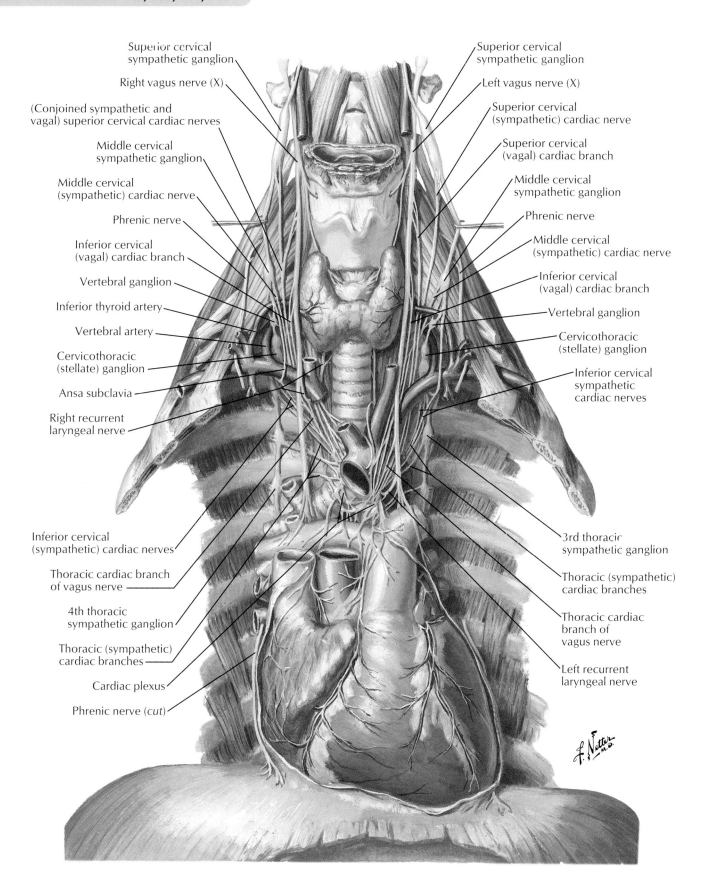

Superior cervical sympathetic ganglion

Right vagus nerve (X)

(Conjoined sympathetic and vagal) superior cervical cardiac nerves

Middle cervical sympathetic ganglion

Middle cervical (sympathetic) cardiac nerve

Phrenic nerve

Inferior cervical (vagal) cardiac branch

Vertebral ganglion

Inferior thyroid artery

Vertebral artery

Cervicothoracic (stellate) ganglion

Ansa subclavia

Right recurrent laryngeal nerve

Inferior cervical (sympathetic) cardiac nerves

Thoracic cardiac branch of vagus nerve

4th thoracic sympathetic ganglion

Thoracic (sympathetic) cardiac branches

Cardiac plexus

Phrenic nerve (*cut*)

Superior cervical sympathetic ganglion

Left vagus nerve (X)

Superior cervical (sympathetic) cardiac nerve

Superior cervical (vagal) cardiac branch

Middle cervical sympathetic ganglion

Phrenic nerve

Middle cervical (sympathetic) cardiac nerve

Inferior cervical (vagal) cardiac branch

Vertebral ganglion

Cervicothoracic (stellate) ganglion

Inferior cervical sympathetic cardiac nerves

3rd thoracic sympathetic ganglion

Thoracic (sympathetic) cardiac branches

Thoracic cardiac branch of vagus nerve

Left recurrent laryngeal nerve

Plate 226   **Heart**

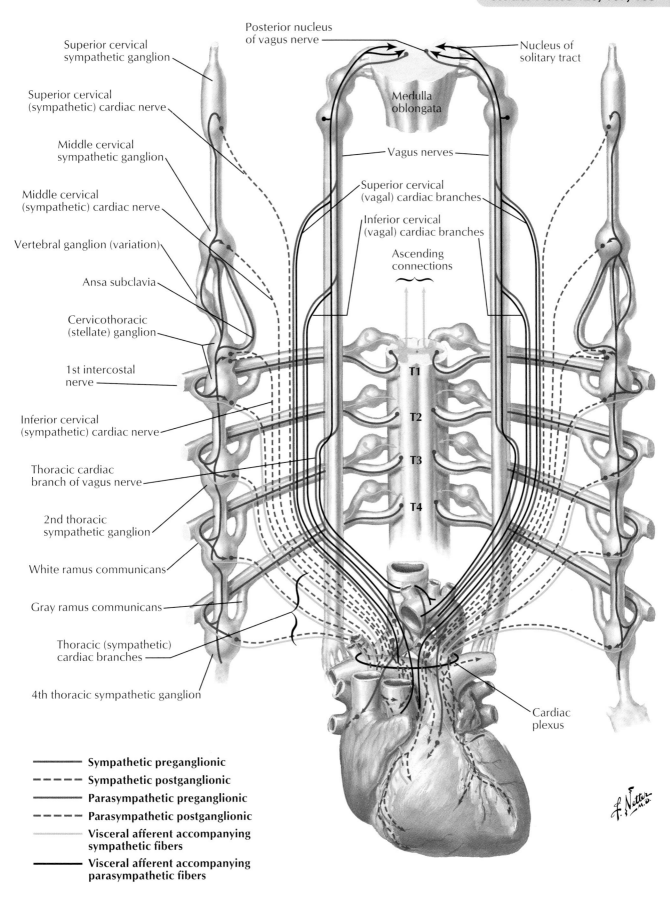

Posterior nucleus of vagus nerve

Nucleus of solitary tract

Superior cervical sympathetic ganglion

Superior cervical (sympathetic) cardiac nerve

Middle cervical sympathetic ganglion

Middle cervical (sympathetic) cardiac nerve

Vertebral ganglion (variation)

Ansa subclavia

Cervicothoracic (stellate) ganglion

1st intercostal nerve

Inferior cervical (sympathetic) cardiac nerve

Thoracic cardiac branch of vagus nerve

2nd thoracic sympathetic ganglion

White ramus communicans

Gray ramus communicans

Thoracic (sympathetic) cardiac branches

4th thoracic sympathetic ganglion

Medulla oblongata

Vagus nerves

Superior cervical (vagal) cardiac branches

Inferior cervical (vagal) cardiac branches

Ascending connections

T1

T2

T3

T4

Cardiac plexus

——————— Sympathetic preganglionic
— — — — — Sympathetic postganglionic
——————— Parasympathetic preganglionic
— — — — — Parasympathetic postganglionic
——————— Visceral afferent accompanying sympathetic fibers
——————— Visceral afferent accompanying parasympathetic fibers

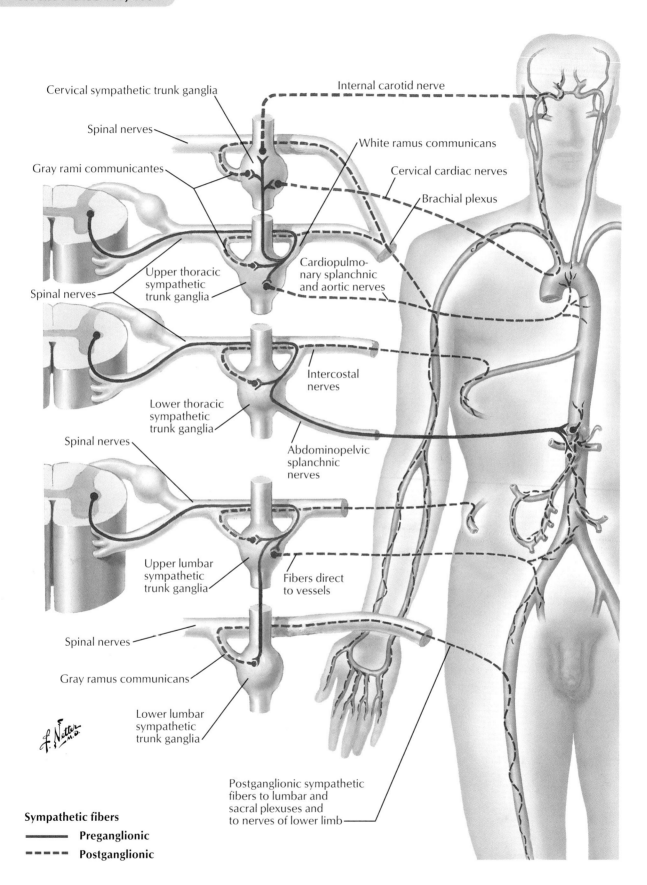

Cervical sympathetic trunk ganglia

Internal carotid nerve

Spinal nerves

White ramus communicans

Gray rami communicantes

Cervical cardiac nerves

Brachial plexus

Upper thoracic sympathetic trunk ganglia

Cardiopulmo-nary splanchnic and aortic nerves

Spinal nerves

Intercostal nerves

Lower thoracic sympathetic trunk ganglia

Abdominopelvic splanchnic nerves

Spinal nerves

Upper lumbar sympathetic trunk ganglia

Fibers direct to vessels

Spinal nerves

Gray ramus communicans

Lower lumbar sympathetic trunk ganglia

Postganglionic sympathetic fibers to lumbar and sacral plexuses and to nerves of lower limb

Sympathetic fibers

——————— **Preganglionic**

- - - - - - **Postganglionic**

Plate 228

Heart

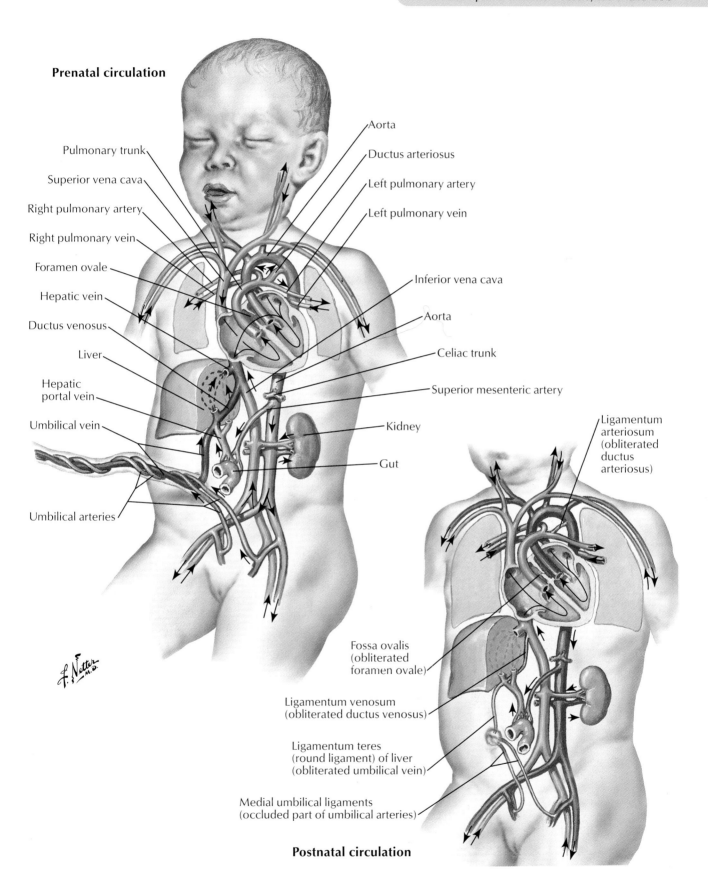

Prenatal circulation

Pulmonary trunk

Superior vena cava

Right pulmonary artery

Right pulmonary vein

Foramen ovale

Hepatic vein

Ductus venosus

Liver

Hepatic portal vein

Umbilical vein

Umbilical arteries

Aorta

Ductus arteriosus

Left pulmonary artery

Left pulmonary vein

Inferior vena cava

Aorta

Celiac trunk

Superior mesenteric artery

Kidney

Gut

Ligamentum arteriosum (obliterated ductus arteriosus)

Fossa ovalis (obliterated foramen ovale)

Ligamentum venosum (obliterated ductus venosus)

Ligamentum teres (round ligament) of liver (obliterated umbilical vein)

Medial umbilical ligaments (occluded part of umbilical arteries)

Postnatal circulation

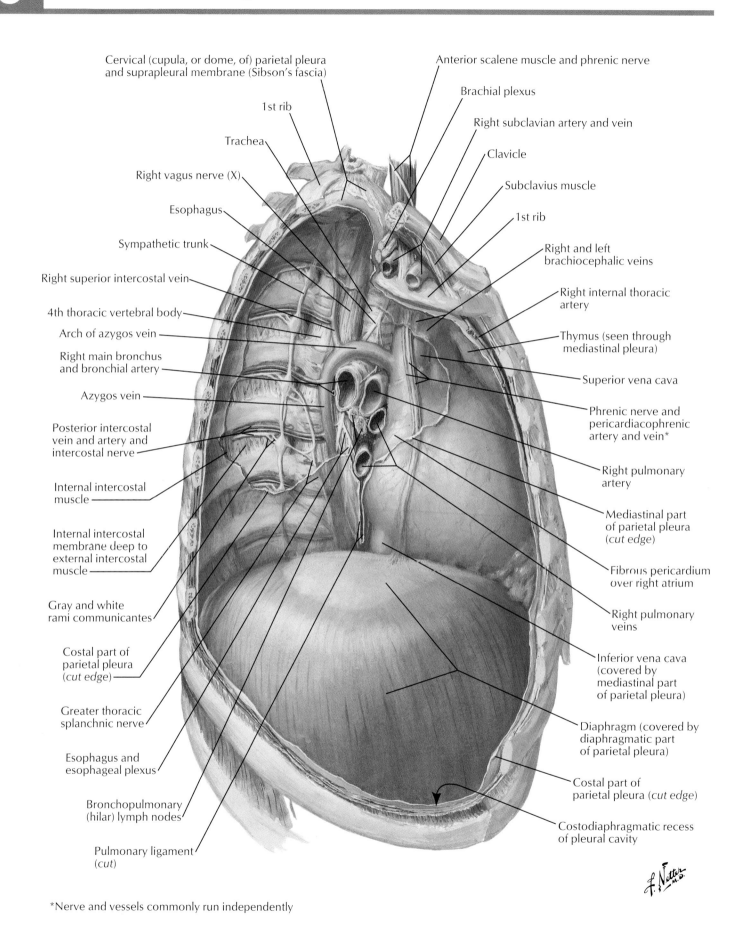

Cervical (cupula, or dome, of) parietal pleura and suprapleural membrane (Sibson's fascia)

1st rib

Trachea

Right vagus nerve (X)

Esophagus

Sympathetic trunk

Right superior intercostal vein

4th thoracic vertebral body

Arch of azygos vein

Right main bronchus and bronchial artery

Azygos vein

Posterior intercostal vein and artery and intercostal nerve

Internal intercostal muscle

Internal intercostal membrane deep to external intercostal muscle

Gray and white rami communicantes

Costal part of parietal pleura (cut edge)

Greater thoracic splanchnic nerve

Esophagus and esophageal plexus

Bronchopulmonary (hilar) lymph nodes

Pulmonary ligament (cut)

Anterior scalene muscle and phrenic nerve

Brachial plexus

Right subclavian artery and vein

Clavicle

Subclavius muscle

1st rib

Right and left brachiocephalic veins

Right internal thoracic artery

Thymus (seen through mediastinal pleura)

Superior vena cava

Phrenic nerve and pericardiacophrenic artery and vein*

Right pulmonary artery

Mediastinal part of parietal pleura (cut edge)

Fibrous pericardium over right atrium

Right pulmonary veins

Inferior vena cava (covered by mediastinal part of parietal pleura)

Diaphragm (covered by diaphragmatic part of parietal pleura)

Costal part of parietal pleura (cut edge)

Costodiaphragmatic recess of pleural cavity

*Nerve and vessels commonly run independently

Plate 230

Mediastinum

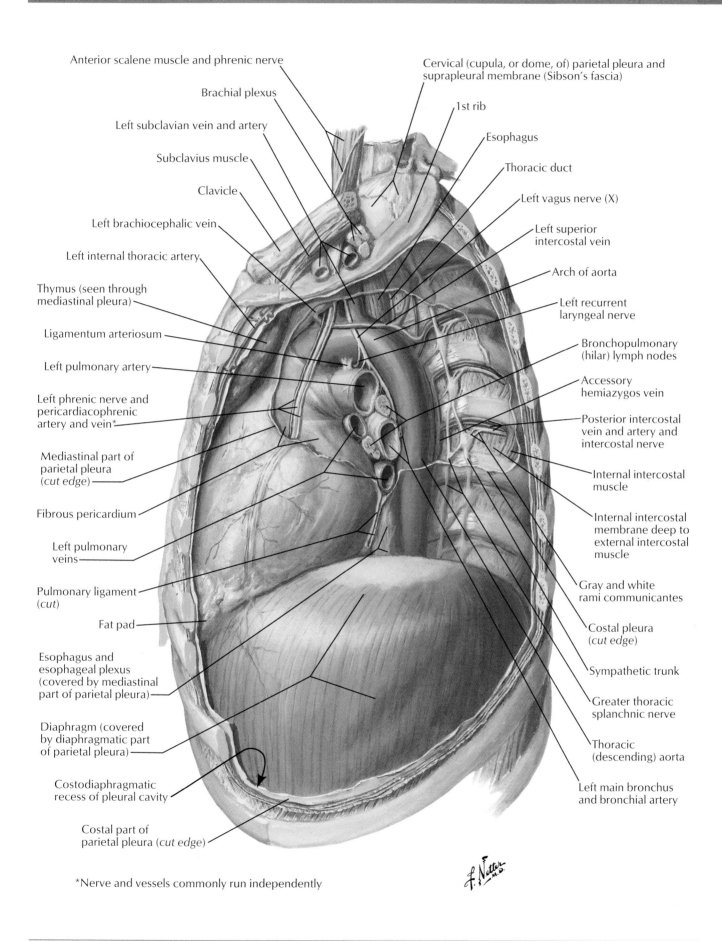

Anterior scalene muscle and phrenic nerve

Brachial plexus

Left subclavian vein and artery

Subclavius muscle

Clavicle

Left brachiocephalic vein

Left internal thoracic artery

Thymus (seen through mediastinal pleura)

Ligamentum arteriosum

Left pulmonary artery

Left phrenic nerve and pericardiacophrenic artery and vein*

Mediastinal part of parietal pleura (*cut edge*)

Fibrous pericardium

Left pulmonary veins

Pulmonary ligament (*cut*)

Fat pad

Esophagus and esophageal plexus (covered by mediastinal part of parietal pleura)

Diaphragm (covered by diaphragmatic part of parietal pleura)

Costodiaphragmatic recess of pleural cavity

Costal part of parietal pleura (*cut edge*)

Cervical (cupula, or dome, of) parietal pleura and suprapleural membrane (Sibson's fascia)

1st rib

Esophagus

Thoracic duct

Left vagus nerve (X)

Left superior intercostal vein

Arch of aorta

Left recurrent laryngeal nerve

Bronchopulmonary (hilar) lymph nodes

Accessory hemiazygos vein

Posterior intercostal vein and artery and intercostal nerve

Internal intercostal muscle

Internal intercostal membrane deep to external intercostal muscle

Gray and white rami communicantes

Costal pleura (*cut edge*)

Sympathetic trunk

Greater thoracic splanchnic nerve

Thoracic (descending) aorta

Left main bronchus and bronchial artery

*Nerve and vessels commonly run independently

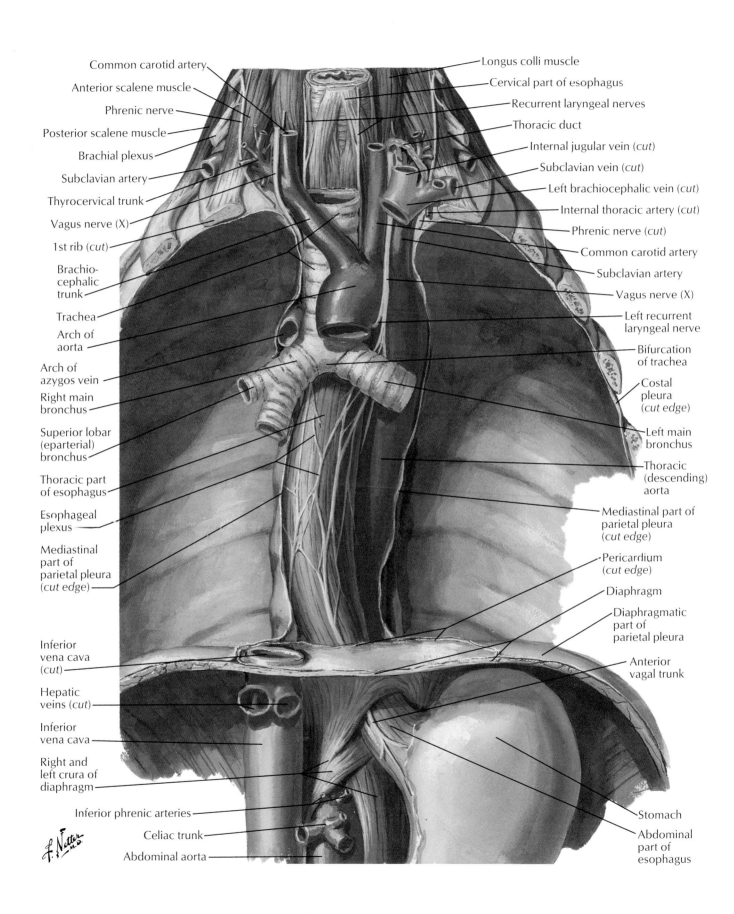

Common carotid artery

Anterior scalene muscle

Phrenic nerve

Posterior scalene muscle

Brachial plexus

Subclavian artery

Thyrocervical trunk

Vagus nerve (X)

1st rib (cut)

Brachio-cephalic trunk

Trachea

Arch of aorta

Arch of azygos vein

Right main bronchus

Superior lobar (eparterial) bronchus

Thoracic part of esophagus

Esophageal plexus

Mediastinal part of parietal pleura (cut edge)

Inferior vena cava (cut)

Hepatic veins (cut)

Inferior vena cava

Right and left crura of diaphragm

Inferior phrenic arteries

Celiac trunk

Abdominal aorta

Longus colli muscle

Cervical part of esophagus

Recurrent laryngeal nerves

Thoracic duct

Internal jugular vein (cut)

Subclavian vein (cut)

Left brachiocephalic vein (cut)

Internal thoracic artery (cut)

Phrenic nerve (cut)

Common carotid artery

Subclavian artery

Vagus nerve (X)

Left recurrent laryngeal nerve

Bifurcation of trachea

Costal pleura (cut edge)

Left main bronchus

Thoracic (descending) aorta

Mediastinal part of parietal pleura (cut edge)

Pericardium (cut edge)

Diaphragm

Diaphragmatic part of parietal pleura

Anterior vagal trunk

Stomach

Abdominal part of esophagus

Plate 232 **Mediastinum**

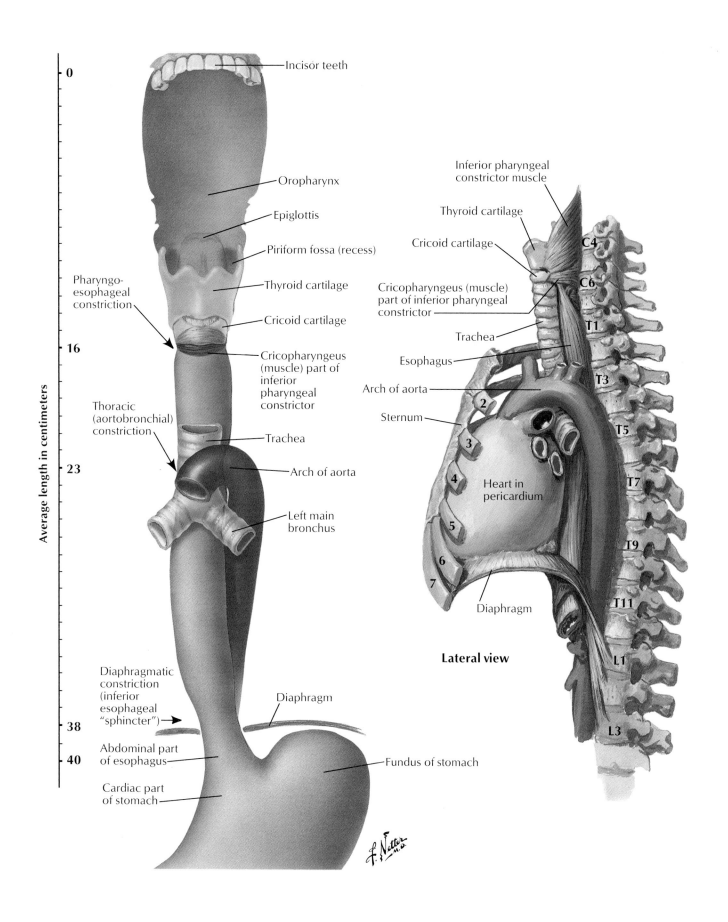

Incisor teeth

Oropharynx

Epiglottis

Piriform fossa (recess)

Thyroid cartilage

Cricoid cartilage

Pharyngo-
esophageal
constriction

Cricopharyngeus
(muscle) part of
inferior
pharyngeal
constrictor

Thoracic
(aortobronchial)
constriction

Trachea

Arch of aorta

Left main
bronchus

Diaphragmatic
constriction
(inferior
esophageal
"sphincter")

Diaphragm

Abdominal part
of esophagus

Fundus of stomach

Cardiac part
of stomach

Average length in centimeters

0

16

23

38

40

Inferior pharyngeal
constrictor muscle

Thyroid cartilage

Cricoid cartilage

Cricopharyngeus (muscle)
part of inferior pharyngeal
constrictor

Trachea

Esophagus

Arch of aorta

Sternum

Heart in
pericardium

Diaphragm

Lateral view

C4

C6

T1

T3

T5

T7

T9

T11

L1

L3

2

3

4

5

6

7

f. Netter
M.D.

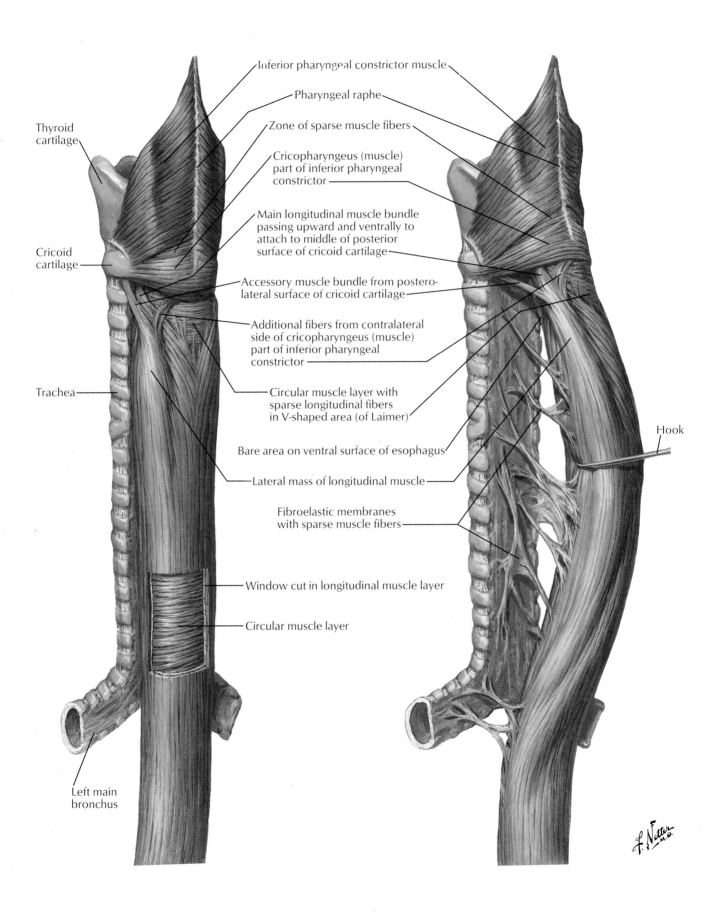

Inferior pharyngeal constrictor muscle

Pharyngeal raphe

Zone of sparse muscle fibers

Cricopharyngeus (muscle) part of inferior pharyngeal constrictor

Main longitudinal muscle bundle passing upward and ventrally to attach to middle of posterior surface of cricoid cartilage

Accessory muscle bundle from postero-lateral surface of cricoid cartilage

Additional fibers from contralateral side of cricopharyngeus (muscle) part of inferior pharyngeal constrictor

Circular muscle layer with sparse longitudinal fibers in V-shaped area (of Laimer)

Bare area on ventral surface of esophagus

Lateral mass of longitudinal muscle

Fibroelastic membranes with sparse muscle fibers

Window cut in longitudinal muscle layer

Circular muscle layer

Thyroid cartilage

Cricoid cartilage

Trachea

Left main bronchus

Hook

Plate 234 **Mediastinum**

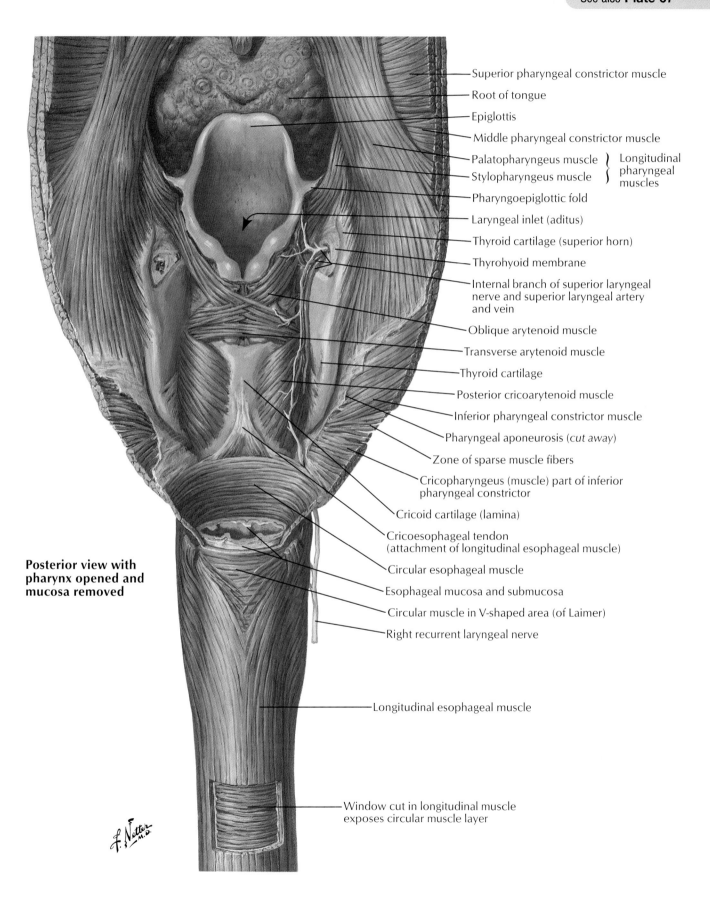

Superior pharyngeal constrictor muscle

Root of tongue

Epiglottis

Middle pharyngeal constrictor muscle

Palatopharyngeus muscle ⎫ Longitudinal
pharyngeal
Stylopharyngeus muscle ⎭ muscles

Pharyngoepiglottic fold

Laryngeal inlet (aditus)

Thyroid cartilage (superior horn)

Thyrohyoid membrane

Internal branch of superior laryngeal
nerve and superior laryngeal artery
and vein

Oblique arytenoid muscle

Transverse arytenoid muscle

Thyroid cartilage

Posterior cricoarytenoid muscle

Inferior pharyngeal constrictor muscle

Pharyngeal aponeurosis (*cut away*)

Zone of sparse muscle fibers

Cricopharyngeus (muscle) part of inferior
pharyngeal constrictor

Cricoid cartilage (lamina)

Cricoesophageal tendon
(attachment of longitudinal esophageal muscle)

Circular esophageal muscle

Esophageal mucosa and submucosa

Circular muscle in V-shaped area (of Laimer)

Right recurrent laryngeal nerve

Longitudinal esophageal muscle

Window cut in longitudinal muscle
exposes circular muscle layer

**Posterior view with
pharynx opened and
mucosa removed**

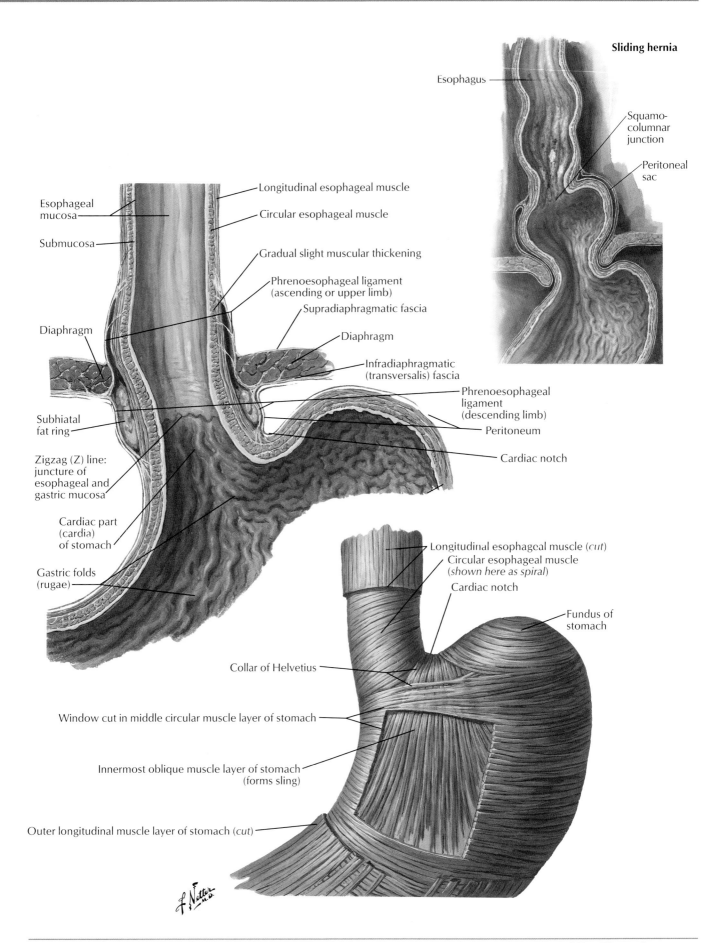

Sliding hernia

Esophagus

Squamo-columnar junction

Peritoneal sac

Esophageal mucosa

Submucosa

Longitudinal esophageal muscle

Circular esophageal muscle

Gradual slight muscular thickening

Phrenoesophageal ligament (ascending or upper limb)

Supradiaphragmatic fascia

Diaphragm

Diaphragm

Infradiaphragmatic (transversalis) fascia

Phrenoesophageal ligament (descending limb)

Peritoneum

Subhiatal fat ring

Cardiac notch

Zigzag (Z) line: juncture of esophageal and gastric mucosa

Cardiac part (cardia) of stomach

Gastric folds (rugae)

Longitudinal esophageal muscle (*cut*)

Circular esophageal muscle (*shown here as spiral*)

Cardiac notch

Fundus of stomach

Collar of Helvetius

Window cut in middle circular muscle layer of stomach

Innermost oblique muscle layer of stomach (forms sling)

Outer longitudinal muscle layer of stomach (*cut*)

Plate 236   **Mediastinum**

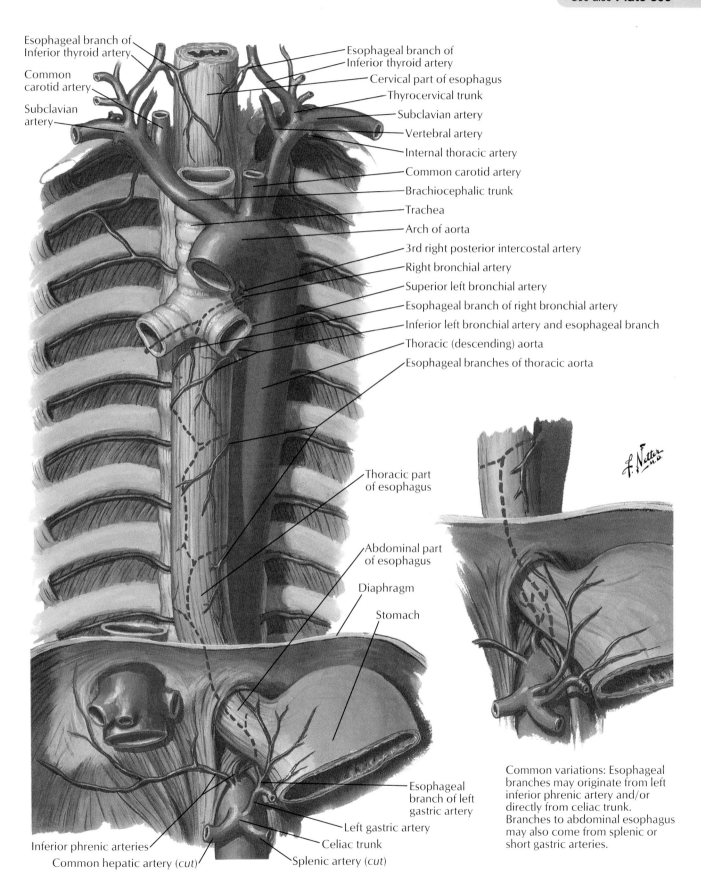

Esophageal branch of Inferior thyroid artery

Common carotid artery

Subclavian artery

Esophageal branch of Inferior thyroid artery

Cervical part of esophagus

Thyrocervical trunk

Subclavian artery

Vertebral artery

Internal thoracic artery

Common carotid artery

Brachiocephalic trunk

Trachea

Arch of aorta

3rd right posterior intercostal artery

Right bronchial artery

Superior left bronchial artery

Esophageal branch of right bronchial artery

Inferior left bronchial artery and esophageal branch

Thoracic (descending) aorta

Esophageal branches of thoracic aorta

Thoracic part of esophagus

Abdominal part of esophagus

Diaphragm

Stomach

Esophageal branch of left gastric artery

Left gastric artery

Celiac trunk

Splenic artery (*cut*)

Inferior phrenic arteries

Common hepatic artery (*cut*)

Common variations: Esophageal branches may originate from left inferior phrenic artery and/or directly from celiac trunk. Branches to abdominal esophagus may also come from splenic or short gastric arteries.

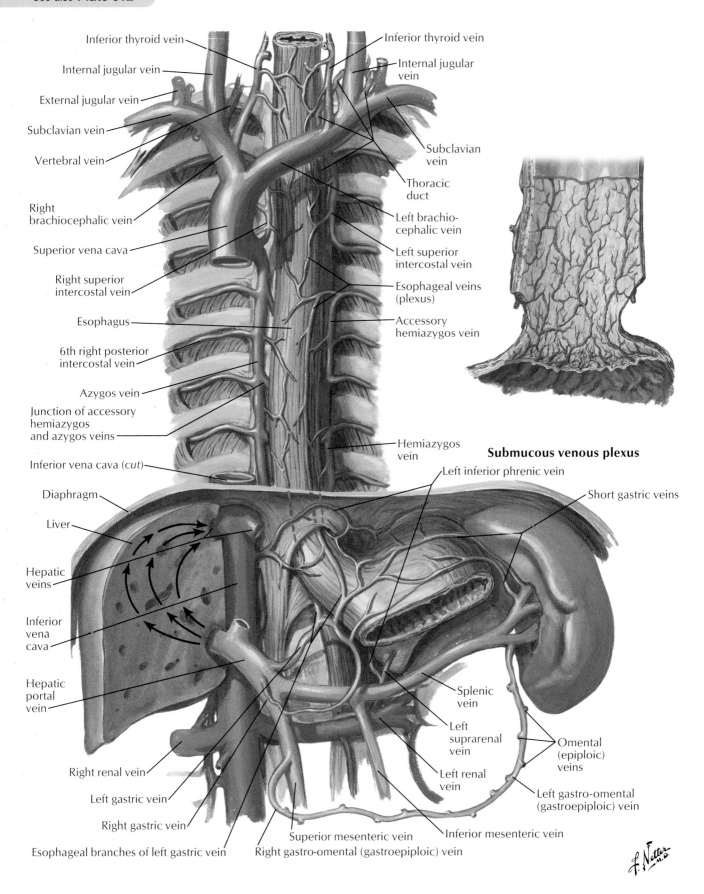

Inferior thyroid vein

Internal jugular vein

External jugular vein

Subclavian vein

Vertebral vein

Right brachiocephalic vein

Superior vena cava

Right superior intercostal vein

Esophagus

6th right posterior intercostal vein

Azygos vein

Junction of accessory hemiazygos and azygos veins

Inferior vena cava (*cut*)

Diaphragm

Liver

Hepatic veins

Inferior vena cava

Hepatic portal vein

Right renal vein

Left gastric vein

Right gastric vein

Esophageal branches of left gastric vein

Inferior thyroid vein

Internal jugular vein

Subclavian vein

Thoracic duct

Left brachio-cephalic vein

Left superior intercostal vein

Esophageal veins (plexus)

Accessory hemiazygos vein

Hemiazygos vein

Submucous venous plexus

Left inferior phrenic vein

Short gastric veins

Splenic vein

Left suprarenal vein

Left renal vein

Omental (epiploic) veins

Left gastro-omental (gastroepiploic) vein

Inferior mesenteric vein

Superior mesenteric vein

Right gastro-omental (gastroepiploic) vein

Plate 238

Mediastinum

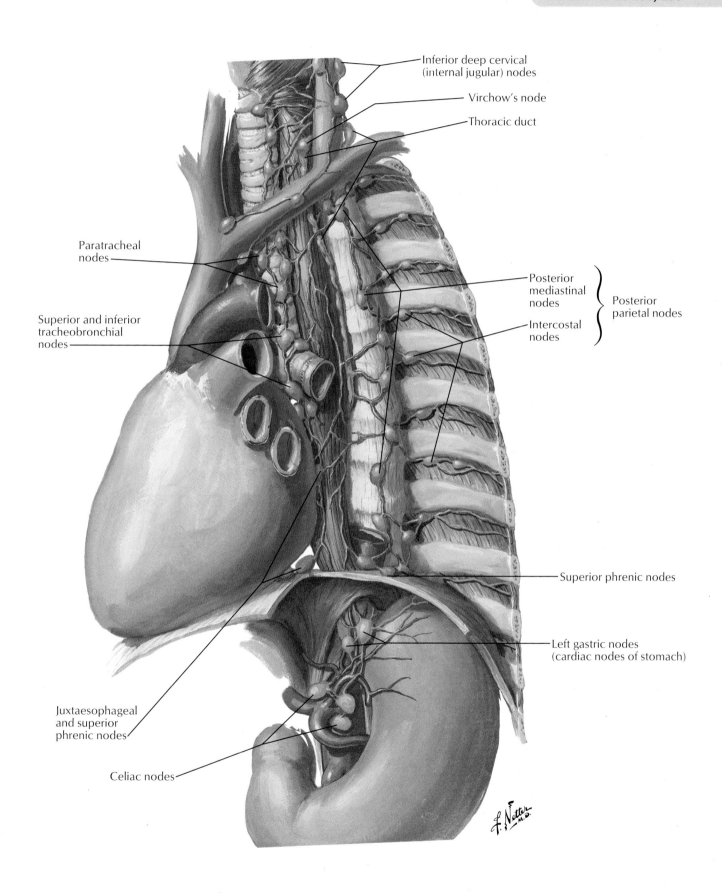

Inferior deep cervical (internal jugular) nodes

Virchow's node

Thoracic duct

Paratracheal nodes

Posterior mediastinal nodes

Posterior parietal nodes

Intercostal nodes

Superior and inferior tracheobronchial nodes

Superior phrenic nodes

Left gastric nodes (cardiac nodes of stomach)

Juxtaesophageal and superior phrenic nodes

Celiac nodes

Nerves of Esophagus

See also **Plates 165, 166, 209**

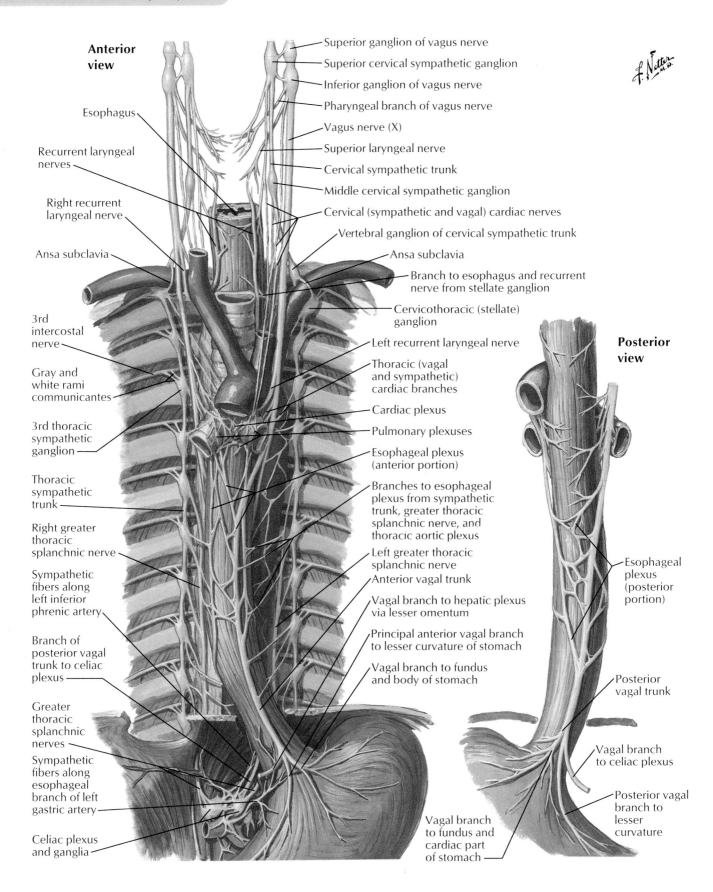

Anterior view

Esophagus

Recurrent laryngeal nerves

Right recurrent laryngeal nerve

Ansa subclavia

3rd intercostal nerve

Gray and white rami communicantes

3rd thoracic sympathetic ganglion

Thoracic sympathetic trunk

Right greater thoracic splanchnic nerve

Sympathetic fibers along left inferior phrenic artery

Branch of posterior vagal trunk to celiac plexus

Greater thoracic splanchnic nerves

Sympathetic fibers along esophageal branch of left gastric artery

Celiac plexus and ganglia

Superior ganglion of vagus nerve

Superior cervical sympathetic ganglion

Inferior ganglion of vagus nerve

Pharyngeal branch of vagus nerve

Vagus nerve (X)

Superior laryngeal nerve

Cervical sympathetic trunk

Middle cervical sympathetic ganglion

Cervical (sympathetic and vagal) cardiac nerves

Vertebral ganglion of cervical sympathetic trunk

Ansa subclavia

Branch to esophagus and recurrent nerve from stellate ganglion

Cervicothoracic (stellate) ganglion

Left recurrent laryngeal nerve

Thoracic (vagal and sympathetic) cardiac branches

Cardiac plexus

Pulmonary plexuses

Esophageal plexus (anterior portion)

Branches to esophageal plexus from sympathetic trunk, greater thoracic splanchnic nerve, and thoracic aortic plexus

Left greater thoracic splanchnic nerve

Anterior vagal trunk

Vagal branch to hepatic plexus via lesser omentum

Principal anterior vagal branch to lesser curvature of stomach

Vagal branch to fundus and body of stomach

Posterior view

Esophageal plexus (posterior portion)

Posterior vagal trunk

Vagal branch to celiac plexus

Posterior vagal branch to lesser curvature

Vagal branch to fundus and cardiac part of stomach

Plate 240

Mediastinum

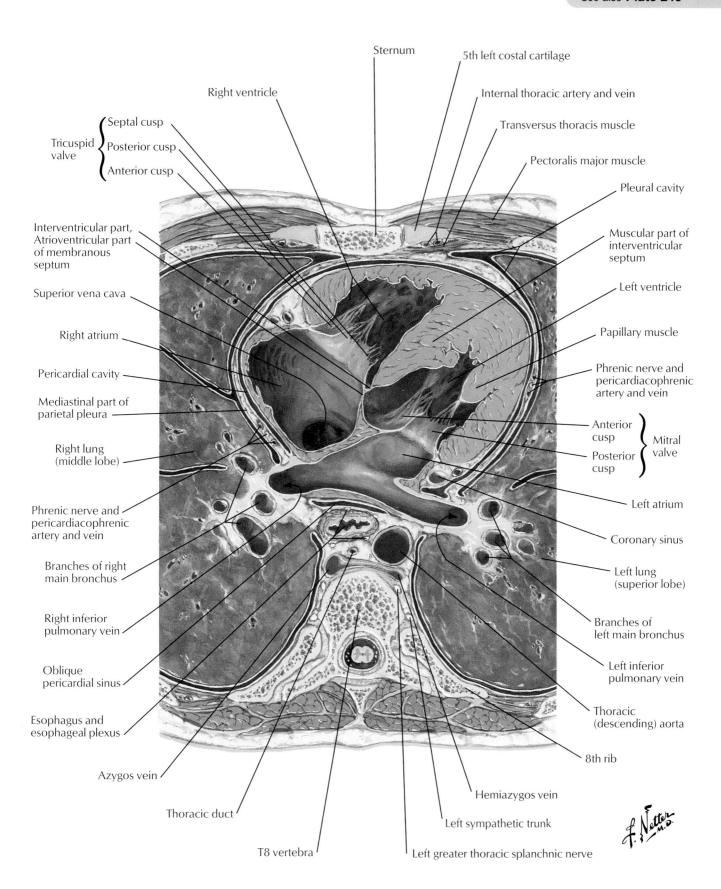

Sternum

5th left costal cartilage

Right ventricle

Internal thoracic artery and vein

Transversus thoracis muscle

Tricuspid valve
{ Septal cusp
Posterior cusp
Anterior cusp }

Pectoralis major muscle

Pleural cavity

Interventricular part,
Atrioventricular part
of membranous
septum

Muscular part of
interventricular
septum

Superior vena cava

Left ventricle

Right atrium

Papillary muscle

Pericardial cavity

Phrenic nerve and
pericardiacophrenic
artery and vein

Mediastinal part of
parietal pleura

Anterior
cusp
} Mitral
valve
Posterior
cusp

Right lung
(middle lobe)

Left atrium

Phrenic nerve and
pericardiacophrenic
artery and vein

Coronary sinus

Branches of right
main bronchus

Left lung
(superior lobe)

Right inferior
pulmonary vein

Branches of
left main bronchus

Oblique
pericardial sinus

Left inferior
pulmonary vein

Esophagus and
esophageal plexus

Thoracic
(descending) aorta

8th rib

Azygos vein

Hemiazygos vein

Thoracic duct

Left sympathetic trunk

T8 vertebra

Left greater thoracic splanchnic nerve

Chest Scans: Axial CT Images

Series of chest axial CT images from superior (A) to inferior (C)

A

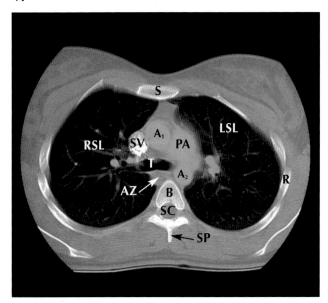

B

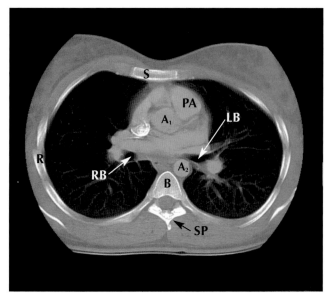

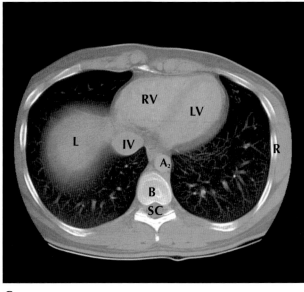

C

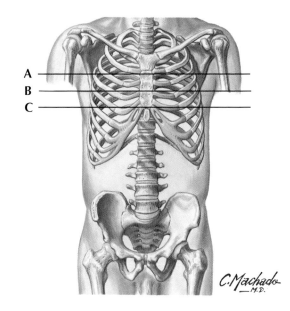

A₁	Ascending aorta	**R**	Rib
A₂	Descending aorta	**RB**	Right (main stem) bronchus
AZ	Azygos vein	**RSL**	Right superior lobe of lung
B	Body of vertebra	**RV**	Right ventricle
IV	Inferior vena cava	**S**	Sternum
L	Liver	**SC**	Spinal cord
LB	Left (main stem) bronchus	**SP**	Spinous process of vertebra
LSL	Left superior lobe of lung	**SV**	Superior vena cava
LV	Left ventricle	**T**	Trachea (bifurcation)
PA	Pulmonary artery		

Plate 242   **Regional Scans**

Transverse Section: Lower Level of T3, Sternoclavicular Joint

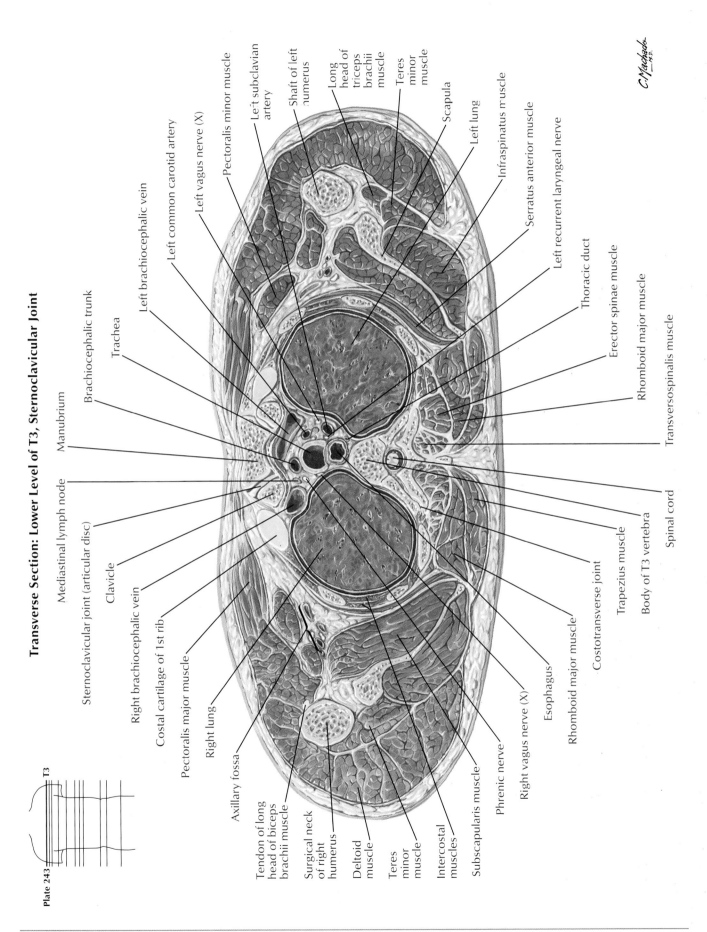

Mediastinal lymph node

Manubrium

Brachiocephalic trunk

Trachea

Left brachiocephalic vein

Left common carotid artery

Left vagus nerve (X)

Pectoralis minor muscle

Left subclavian artery

Shaft of left humerus

Long head of triceps brachii muscle

Teres minor muscle

Scapula

Left lung

Infraspinatus muscle

Serratus anterior muscle

Left recurrent laryngeal nerve

Thoracic duct

Erector spinae muscle

Rhomboid major muscle

Transversospinalis muscle

Sternoclavicular joint (articular disc)

Clavicle

Right brachiocephalic vein

Costal cartilage of 1st rib

Pectoralis major muscle

Right lung

Axillary fossa

Tendon of long head of biceps brachii muscle

Surgical neck of right humerus

Deltoid muscle

Teres minor muscle

Intercostal muscles

Subscapularis muscle

Phrenic nerve

Right vagus nerve (X)

Esophagus

Rhomboid major muscle

Costotransverse joint

Trapezius muscle

Body of T3 vertebra

Spinal cord

T3

Plate 243

Transverse Section: T3–4 Intervertebral Disc, Manubrium

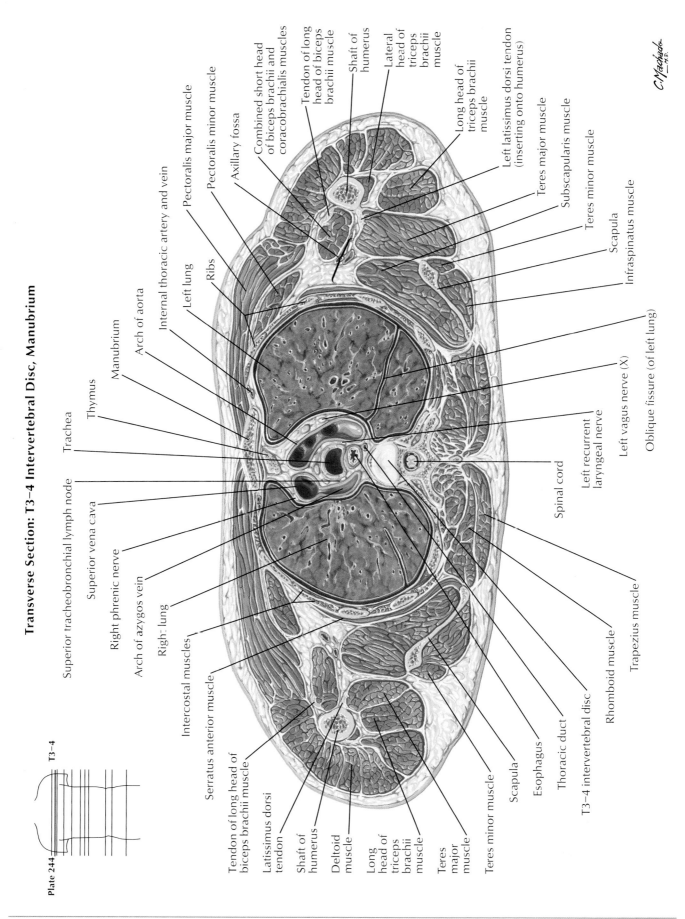

Superior tracheobronchial lymph node

Trachea

Thymus

Manubrium

Arch of aorta

Internal thoracic artery and vein

Left lung

Ribs

Pectoralis major muscle

Pectoralis minor muscle

Axillary fossa

Combined short head of biceps brachii and coracobrachialis muscles

Tendon of long head of biceps brachii muscle

Shaft of humerus

Lateral head of triceps brachii muscle

Long head of triceps brachii muscle

Left latissimus dorsi tendon (inserting onto humerus)

Teres major muscle

Subscapularis muscle

Teres minor muscle

Scapula

Infraspinatus muscle

Oblique fissure (of left lung)

Left vagus nerve (X)

Left recurrent laryngeal nerve

Spinal cord

Trapezius muscle

Rhomboid muscle

T3–4 intervertebral disc

Thoracic duct

Esophagus

Scapula

Teres minor muscle

Teres major muscle

Long head of triceps brachii muscle

Deltoid muscle

Shaft of humerus

Latissimus dorsi tendon

Tendon of long head of biceps brachii muscle

Serratus anterior muscle

Intercostal muscles

Right lung

Arch of azygos vein

Right phrenic nerve

Superior vena cava

T3–4

Plate 244

Plate 244

Cross-Sectional Anatomy

Transverse Section: T4–5 Intervertebral Disc, Sternal Angle

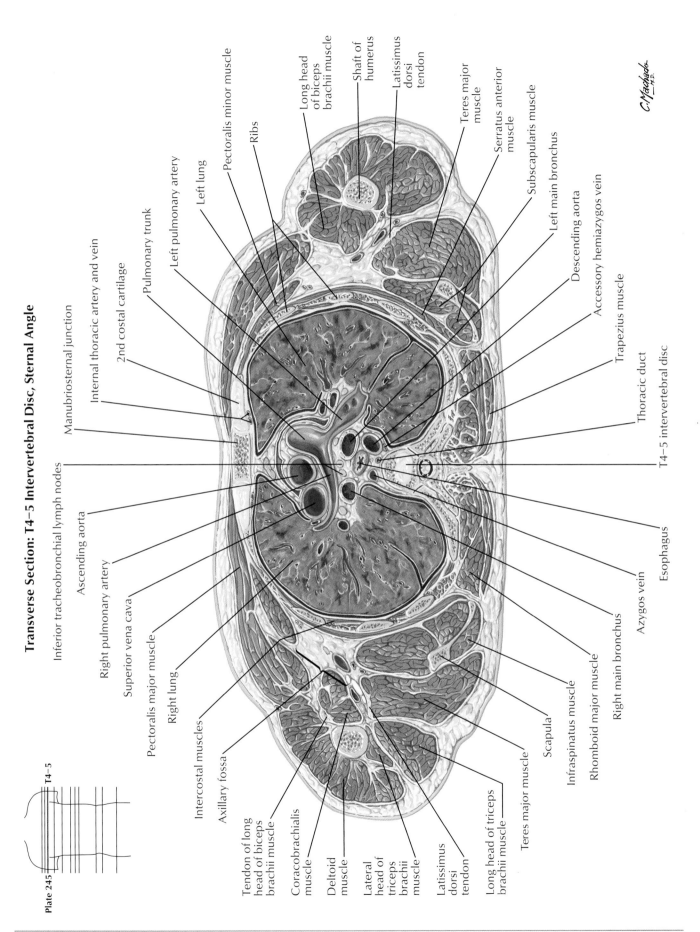

Inferior tracheobronchial lymph nodes

Manubriosternal junction

Internal thoracic artery and vein

2nd costal cartilage

Pulmonary trunk

Left pulmonary artery

Left lung

Pectoralis minor muscle

Ribs

Long head of biceps brachii muscle

Shaft of humerus

Latissimus dorsi tendon

Teres major muscle

Serratus anterior muscle

Subscapularis muscle

Left main bronchus

Descending aorta

Accessory hemiazygos vein

Trapezius muscle

Thoracic duct

T4–5 intervertebral disc

Ascending aorta

Right pulmonary artery

Superior vena cava

Pectoralis major muscle

Right lung

Intercostal muscles

Axillary fossa

Tendon of long head of biceps brachii muscle

Coracobrachialis muscle

Deltoid muscle

Lateral head of triceps brachii muscle

Latissimus dorsi tendon

Long head of triceps brachii muscle

Teres major muscle

Scapula

Infraspinatus muscle

Rhomboid major muscle

Right main bronchus

Azygos vein

Esophagus

T4–5

Plate 245

Transverse Section: Level of T7, 3rd Interchondral Space

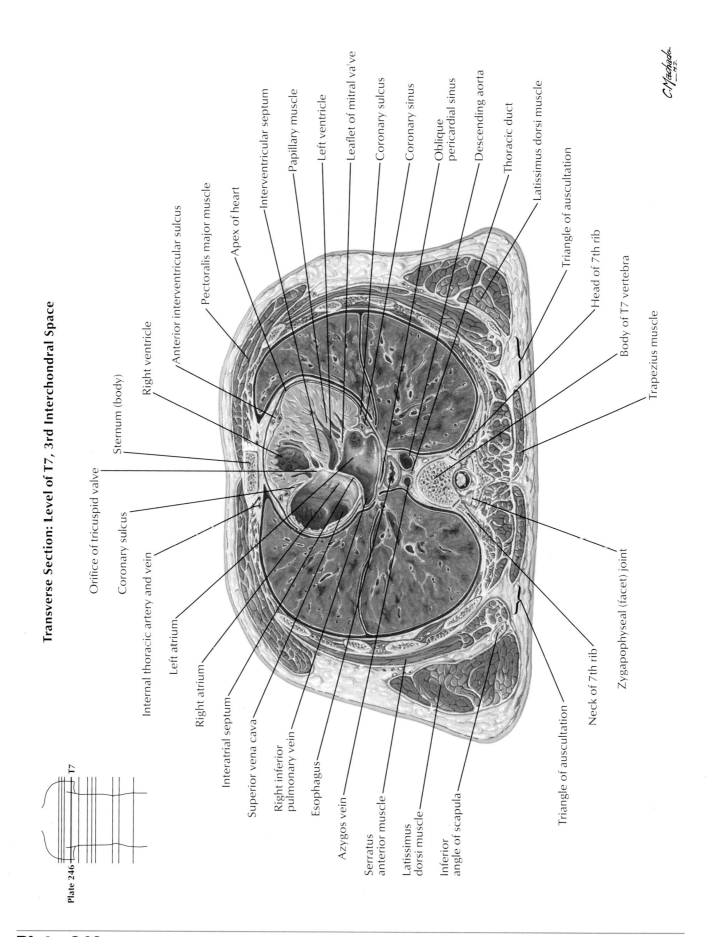

Orifice of tricuspid valve
Coronary sulcus
Internal thoracic artery and vein
Sternum (body)
Right ventricle
Anterior interventricular sulcus
Pectoralis major muscle
Apex of heart
Interventricular septum
Papillary muscle
Left ventricle
Leaflet of mitral valve
Coronary sulcus
Coronary sinus
Oblique pericardial sinus
Descending aorta
Thoracic duct
Latissimus dorsi muscle
Triangle of auscultation
Head of 7th rib
Body of T7 vertebra
Trapezius muscle

Left atrium
Right atrium
Interatrial septum
Superior vena cava
Right inferior pulmonary vein
Esophagus
Azygos vein
Serratus anterior muscle
Latissimus dorsi muscle
Inferior angle of scapula
Triangle of auscultation
Neck of 7th rib
Zygapophyseal (facet) joint

T7

Plate 246

Plate 246   **Cross-Sectional Anatomy**

Section 4 **Abdomen**

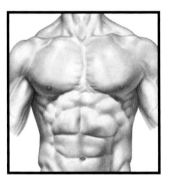
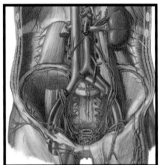
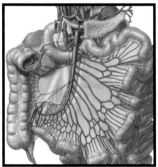
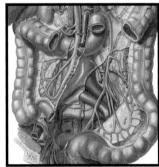

Topographic Anatomy
Plate 217

Body Wall
Plates 248–267

4 Abdomen

Abdominal Sections
Plates 348–349

Regional Scans
Plate 350

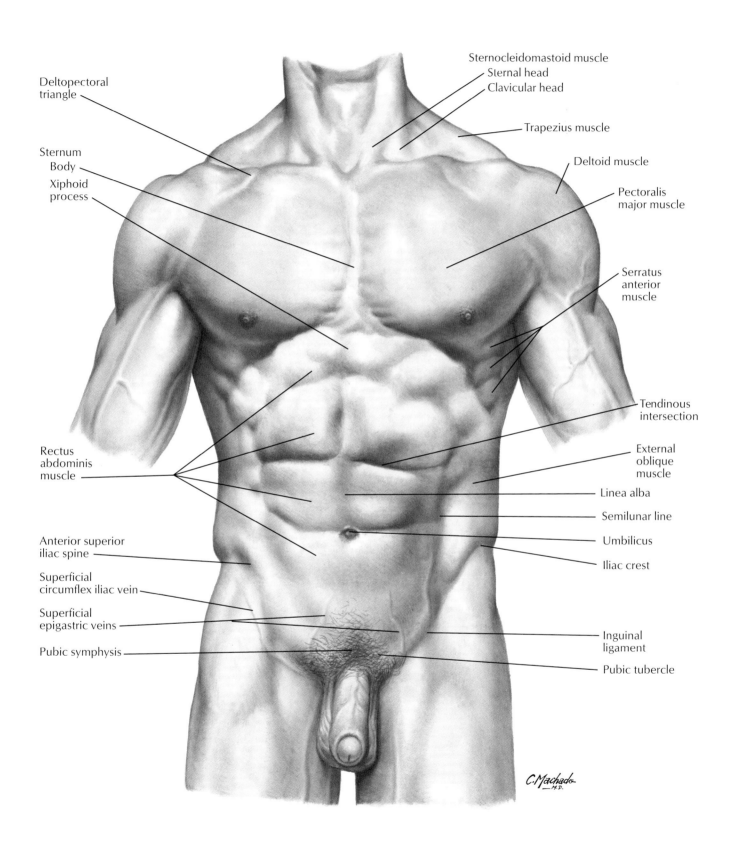

Deltopectoral triangle

Sternum
Body
Xiphoid process

Rectus abdominis muscle

Anterior superior iliac spine

Superficial circumflex iliac vein

Superficial epigastric veins

Pubic symphysis

Sternocleidomastoid muscle
Sternal head
Clavicular head

Trapezius muscle

Deltoid muscle

Pectoralis major muscle

Serratus anterior muscle

Tendinous intersection

External oblique muscle

Linea alba

Semilunar line

Umbilicus

Iliac crest

Inguinal ligament

Pubic tubercle

C. Machado
M.D.

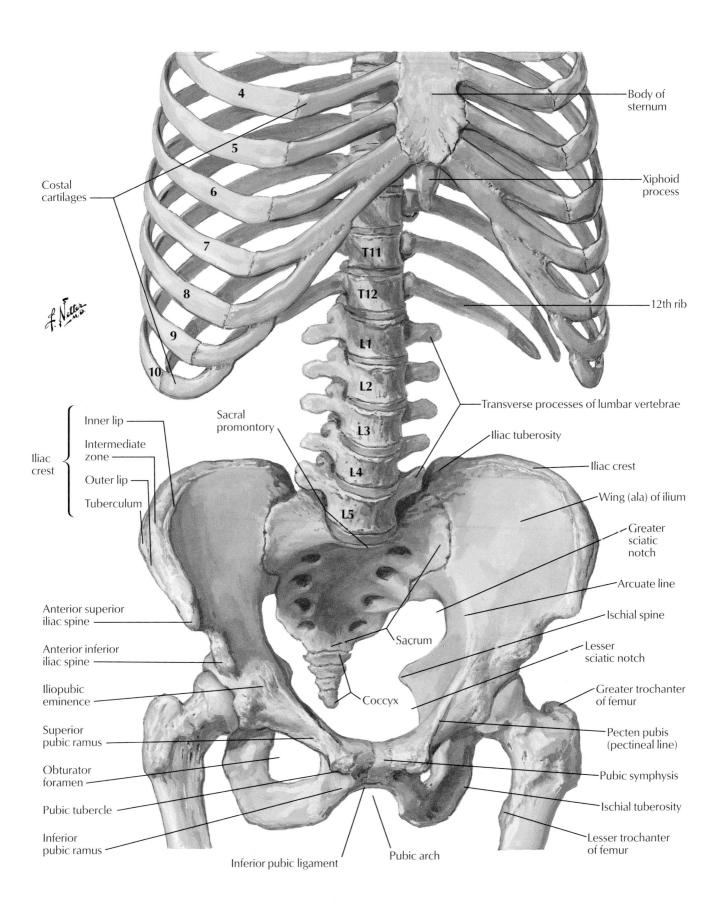

Body of sternum

Xiphoid process

12th rib

Transverse processes of lumbar vertebrae

Iliac tuberosity

Iliac crest

Wing (ala) of ilium

Greater sciatic notch

Arcuate line

Ischial spine

Lesser sciatic notch

Greater trochanter of femur

Pecten pubis (pectineal line)

Pubic symphysis

Ischial tuberosity

Lesser trochanter of femur

Costal cartilages

4
5
6
7
8
9
10

T11
T12
L1
L2
L3
L4
L5

Sacral promontory

Sacrum

Coccyx

Iliac crest
Inner lip
Intermediate zone
Outer lip
Tuberculum

Anterior superior iliac spine

Anterior inferior iliac spine

Iliopubic eminence

Superior pubic ramus

Obturator foramen

Pubic tubercle

Inferior pubic ramus

Inferior pubic ligament

Pubic arch

Plate 248

Body Wall

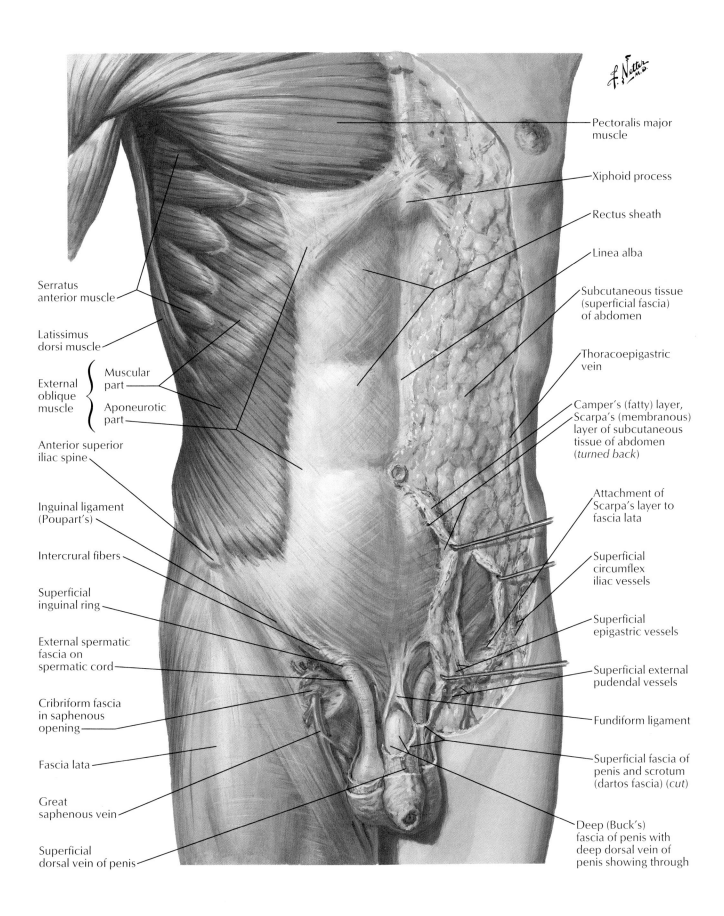

Serratus
anterior muscle

Latissimus
dorsi muscle

External
oblique
muscle { Muscular
part
Aponeurotic
part

Anterior superior
iliac spine

Inguinal ligament
(Poupart's)

Intercrural fibers

Superficial
inguinal ring

External spermatic
fascia on
spermatic cord

Cribriform fascia
in saphenous
opening

Fascia lata

Great
saphenous vein

Superficial
dorsal vein of penis

Pectoralis major
muscle

Xiphoid process

Rectus sheath

Linea alba

Subcutaneous tissue
(superficial fascia)
of abdomen

Thoracoepigastric
vein

Camper's (fatty) layer,
Scarpa's (membranous)
layer of subcutaneous
tissue of abdomen
(turned back)

Attachment of
Scarpa's layer to
fascia lata

Superficial
circumflex
iliac vessels

Superficial
epigastric vessels

Superficial external
pudendal vessels

Fundiform ligament

Superficial fascia of
penis and scrotum
(dartos fascia) (cut)

Deep (Buck's)
fascia of penis with
deep dorsal vein of
penis showing through

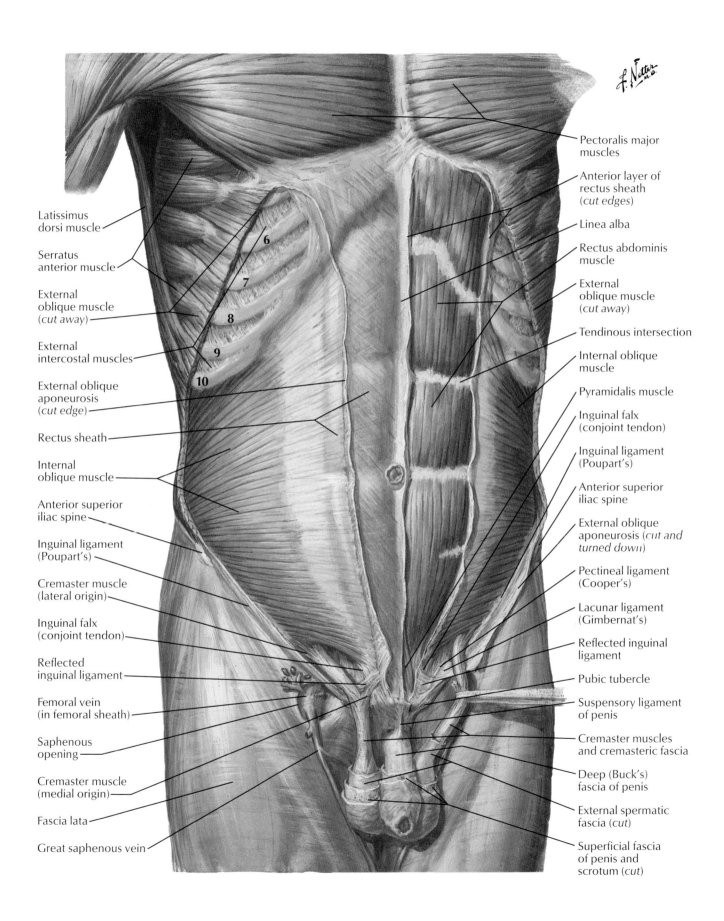

Pectoralis major muscles

Anterior layer of rectus sheath (*cut edges*)

Linea alba

Rectus abdominis muscle

External oblique muscle (*cut away*)

Tendinous intersection

Internal oblique muscle

Pyramidalis muscle

Inguinal falx (conjoint tendon)

Inguinal ligament (Poupart's)

Anterior superior iliac spine

External oblique aponeurosis (*cut and turned down*)

Pectineal ligament (Cooper's)

Lacunar ligament (Gimbernat's)

Reflected inguinal ligament

Pubic tubercle

Suspensory ligament of penis

Cremaster muscles and cremasteric fascia

Deep (Buck's) fascia of penis

External spermatic fascia (*cut*)

Superficial fascia of penis and scrotum (*cut*)

Latissimus dorsi muscle

Serratus anterior muscle

External oblique muscle (*cut away*)

External intercostal muscles

External oblique aponeurosis (*cut edge*)

Rectus sheath

Internal oblique muscle

Anterior superior iliac spine

Inguinal ligament (Poupart's)

Cremaster muscle (lateral origin)

Inguinal falx (conjoint tendon)

Reflected inguinal ligament

Femoral vein (in femoral sheath)

Saphenous opening

Cremaster muscle (medial origin)

Fascia lata

Great saphenous vein

Plate 250   **Body Wall**

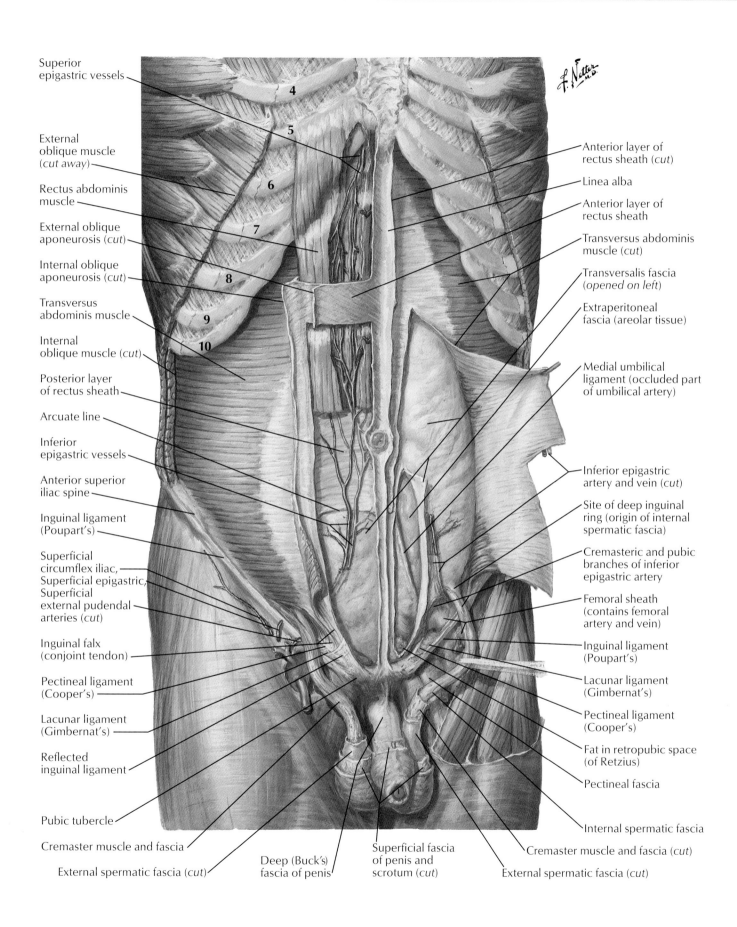

Superior epigastric vessels

External oblique muscle (*cut away*)

Rectus abdominis muscle

External oblique aponeurosis (*cut*)

Internal oblique aponeurosis (*cut*)

Transversus abdominis muscle

Internal oblique muscle (*cut*)

Posterior layer of rectus sheath

Arcuate line

Inferior epigastric vessels

Anterior superior iliac spine

Inguinal ligament (Poupart's)

Superficial circumflex iliac, Superficial epigastric, Superficial external pudendal arteries (*cut*)

Inguinal falx (conjoint tendon)

Pectineal ligament (Cooper's)

Lacunar ligament (Gimbernat's)

Reflected inguinal ligament

Pubic tubercle

Cremaster muscle and fascia

External spermatic fascia (*cut*)

Deep (Buck's) fascia of penis

Superficial fascia of penis and scrotum (*cut*)

Anterior layer of rectus sheath (*cut*)

Linea alba

Anterior layer of rectus sheath

Transversus abdominis muscle (*cut*)

Transversalis fascia (*opened on left*)

Extraperitoneal fascia (areolar tissue)

Medial umbilical ligament (occluded part of umbilical artery)

Inferior epigastric artery and vein (*cut*)

Site of deep inguinal ring (origin of internal spermatic fascia)

Cremasteric and pubic branches of inferior epigastric artery

Femoral sheath (contains femoral artery and vein)

Inguinal ligament (Poupart's)

Lacunar ligament (Gimbernat's)

Pectineal ligament (Cooper's)

Fat in retropubic space (of Retzius)

Pectineal fascia

Internal spermatic fascia

Cremaster muscle and fascia (*cut*)

External spermatic fascia (*cut*)

Rectus Sheath: Cross Sections

Section above arcuate line

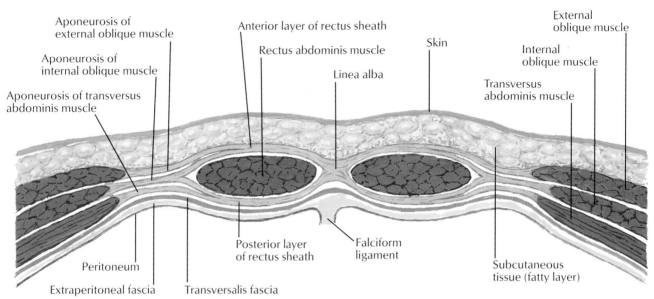

Aponeurosis of external oblique muscle

Aponeurosis of internal oblique muscle

Aponeurosis of transversus abdominis muscle

Anterior layer of rectus sheath

Rectus abdominis muscle

Linea alba

Skin

External oblique muscle

Internal oblique muscle

Transversus abdominis muscle

Posterior layer of rectus sheath

Falciform ligament

Peritoneum

Extraperitoneal fascia

Transversalis fascia

Subcutaneous tissue (fatty layer)

Aponeurosis of internal oblique muscle splits to form anterior and posterior layers of rectus sheath. Aponeurosis of external oblique muscle joins anterior layer of sheath; aponeurosis of transversus abdominis muscle joins posterior layer. Anterior and posterior layers of rectus sheath unite medially to form linea alba.

Section below arcuate line

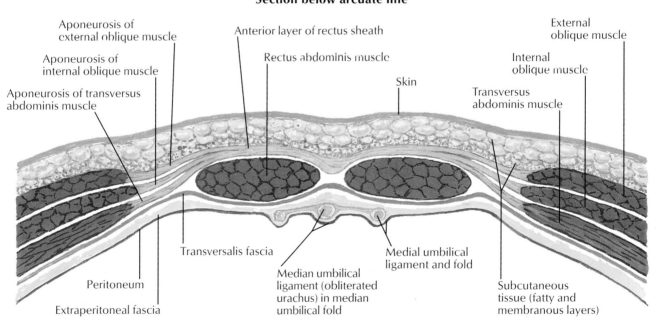

Aponeurosis of external oblique muscle

Aponeurosis of internal oblique muscle

Aponeurosis of transversus abdominis muscle

Anterior layer of rectus sheath

Rectus abdominis muscle

Skin

External oblique muscle

Internal oblique muscle

Transversus abdominis muscle

Transversalis fascia

Median umbilical ligament (obliterated urachus) in median umbilical fold

Medial umbilical ligament and fold

Peritoneum

Extraperitoneal fascia

Subcutaneous tissue (fatty and membranous layers)

Aponeurosis of internal oblique muscle does not split at this level but passes completely anterior to rectus abdominis muscle and is fused there with both aponeurosis of external oblique muscle and that of transversus abdominis muscle. Thus, posterior wall of rectus sheath is absent below arcuate line, and rectus abdominis muscle lies on transversalis fascia.

Plate 252

Body Wall

For umbilical vessels see **Plate 229**

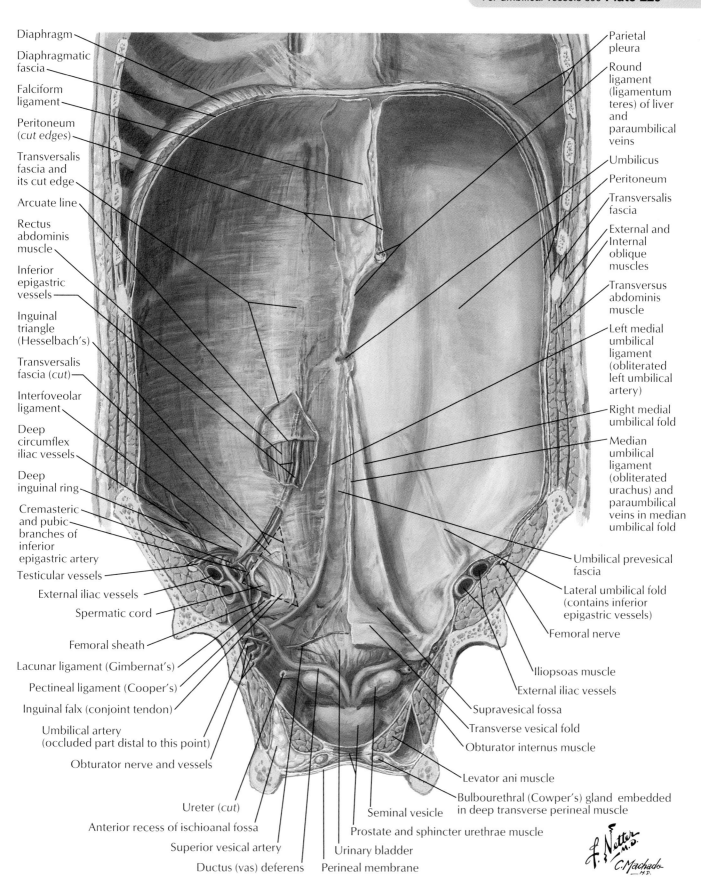

Diaphragm

Diaphragmatic fascia

Falciform ligament

Peritoneum (*cut edges*)

Transversalis fascia and its cut edge

Arcuate line

Rectus abdominis muscle

Inferior epigastric vessels

Inguinal triangle (Hesselbach's)

Transversalis fascia (*cut*)

Interfoveolar ligament

Deep circumflex iliac vessels

Deep inguinal ring

Cremasteric and pubic branches of inferior epigastric artery

Testicular vessels

External iliac vessels

Spermatic cord

Femoral sheath

Lacunar ligament (Gimbernat's)

Pectineal ligament (Cooper's)

Inguinal falx (conjoint tendon)

Umbilical artery (occluded part distal to this point)

Obturator nerve and vessels

Ureter (*cut*)

Anterior recess of ischioanal fossa

Superior vesical artery

Ductus (vas) deferens

Parietal pleura

Round ligament (ligamentum teres) of liver and paraumbilical veins

Umbilicus

Peritoneum

Transversalis fascia

External and Internal oblique muscles

Transversus abdominis muscle

Left medial umbilical ligament (obliterated left umbilical artery)

Right medial umbilical fold

Median umbilical ligament (obliterated urachus) and paraumbilical veins in median umbilical fold

Umbilical prevesical fascia

Lateral umbilical fold (contains inferior epigastric vessels)

Femoral nerve

Iliopsoas muscle

External iliac vessels

Supravesical fossa

Transverse vesical fold

Obturator internus muscle

Levator ani muscle

Bulbourethral (Cowper's) gland embedded in deep transverse perineal muscle

Prostate and sphincter urethrae muscle

Urinary bladder

Perineal membrane

Seminal vesicle

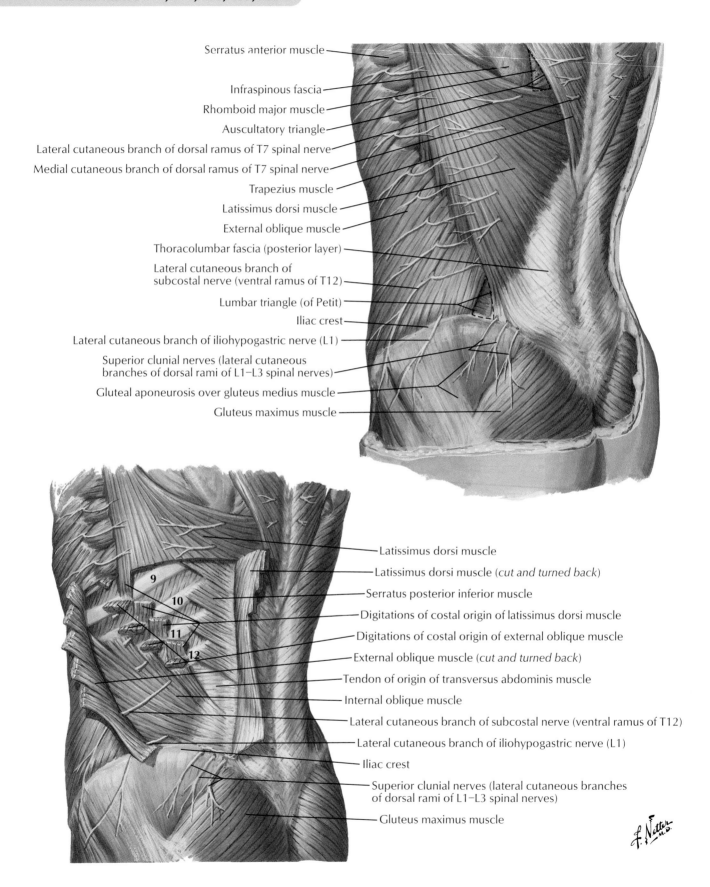

Serratus anterior muscle

Infraspinous fascia

Rhomboid major muscle

Auscultatory triangle

Lateral cutaneous branch of dorsal ramus of T7 spinal nerve

Medial cutaneous branch of dorsal ramus of T7 spinal nerve

Trapezius muscle

Latissimus dorsi muscle

External oblique muscle

Thoracolumbar fascia (posterior layer)

Lateral cutaneous branch of subcostal nerve (ventral ramus of T12)

Lumbar triangle (of Petit)

Iliac crest

Lateral cutaneous branch of iliohypogastric nerve (L1)

Superior clunial nerves (lateral cutaneous branches of dorsal rami of L1–L3 spinal nerves)

Gluteal aponeurosis over gluteus medius muscle

Gluteus maximus muscle

Latissimus dorsi muscle

Latissimus dorsi muscle (*cut and turned back*)

Serratus posterior inferior muscle

Digitations of costal origin of latissimus dorsi muscle

Digitations of costal origin of external oblique muscle

External oblique muscle (*cut and turned back*)

Tendon of origin of transversus abdominis muscle

Internal oblique muscle

Lateral cutaneous branch of subcostal nerve (ventral ramus of T12)

Lateral cutaneous branch of iliohypogastric nerve (L1)

Iliac crest

Superior clunial nerves (lateral cutaneous branches of dorsal rami of L1–L3 spinal nerves)

Gluteus maximus muscle

Plate 254

Body Wall

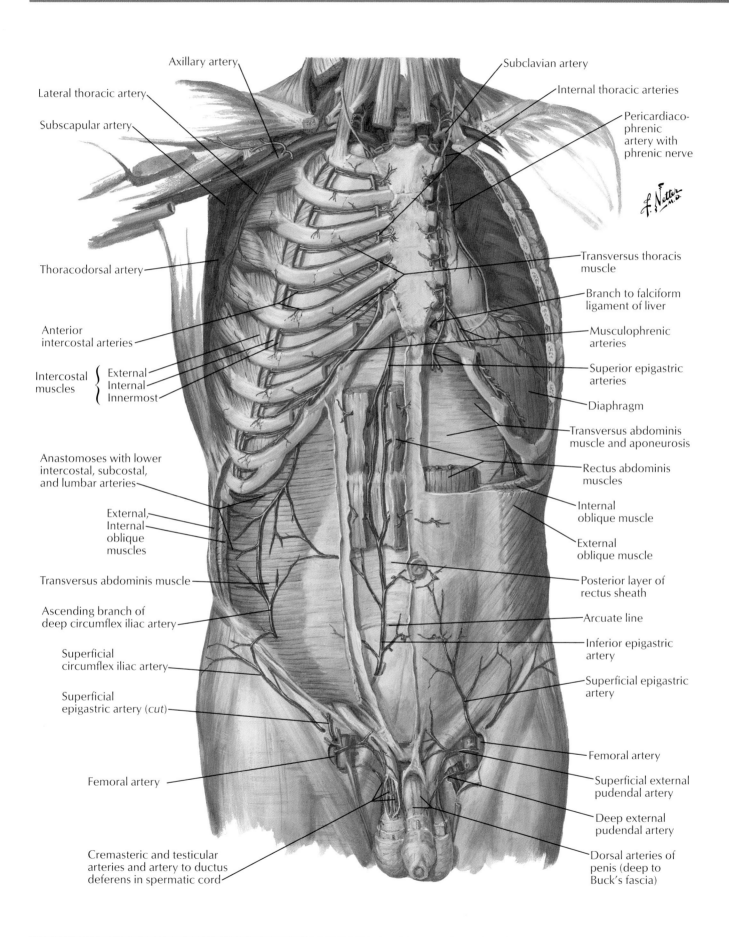

Axillary artery

Subclavian artery

Lateral thoracic artery

Internal thoracic arteries

Subscapular artery

Pericardiaco-phrenic artery with phrenic nerve

Thoracodorsal artery

Transversus thoracis muscle

Branch to falciform ligament of liver

Anterior intercostal arteries

Musculophrenic arteries

Intercostal muscles { External Internal Innermost }

Superior epigastric arteries

Diaphragm

Transversus abdominis muscle and aponeurosis

Anastomoses with lower intercostal, subcostal, and lumbar arteries

Rectus abdominis muscles

External, Internal oblique muscles

Internal oblique muscle

Transversus abdominis muscle

External oblique muscle

Ascending branch of deep circumflex iliac artery

Posterior layer of rectus sheath

Arcuate line

Superficial circumflex iliac artery

Inferior epigastric artery

Superficial epigastric artery (cut)

Superficial epigastric artery

Femoral artery

Femoral artery

Superficial external pudendal artery

Deep external pudendal artery

Cremasteric and testicular arteries and artery to ductus deferens in spermatic cord

Dorsal arteries of penis (deep to Buck's fascia)

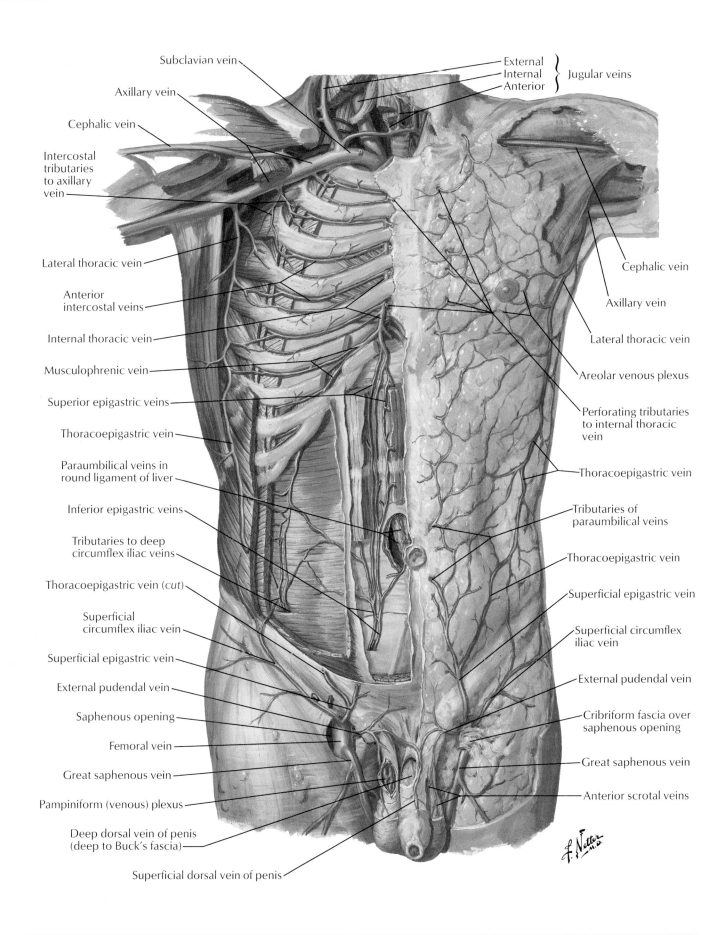

Subclavian vein

Axillary vein

Cephalic vein

Intercostal tributaries to axillary vein

Lateral thoracic vein

Anterior intercostal veins

Internal thoracic vein

Musculophrenic vein

Superior epigastric veins

Thoracoepigastric vein

Paraumbilical veins in round ligament of liver

Inferior epigastric veins

Tributaries to deep circumflex iliac veins

Thoracoepigastric vein (cut)

Superficial circumflex iliac vein

Superficial epigastric vein

External pudendal vein

Saphenous opening

Femoral vein

Great saphenous vein

Pampiniform (venous) plexus

Deep dorsal vein of penis (deep to Buck's fascia)

Superficial dorsal vein of penis

External
Internal   } Jugular veins
Anterior

Cephalic vein

Axillary vein

Lateral thoracic vein

Areolar venous plexus

Perforating tributaries to internal thoracic vein

Thoracoepigastric vein

Tributaries of paraumbilical veins

Thoracoepigastric vein

Superficial epigastric vein

Superficial circumflex iliac vein

External pudendal vein

Cribriform fascia over saphenous opening

Great saphenous vein

Anterior scrotal veins

Plate 256　　　　　　　　　　　　　　　　　　　　　**Body Wall**

See also **Plates 177, 254, 267, 498**

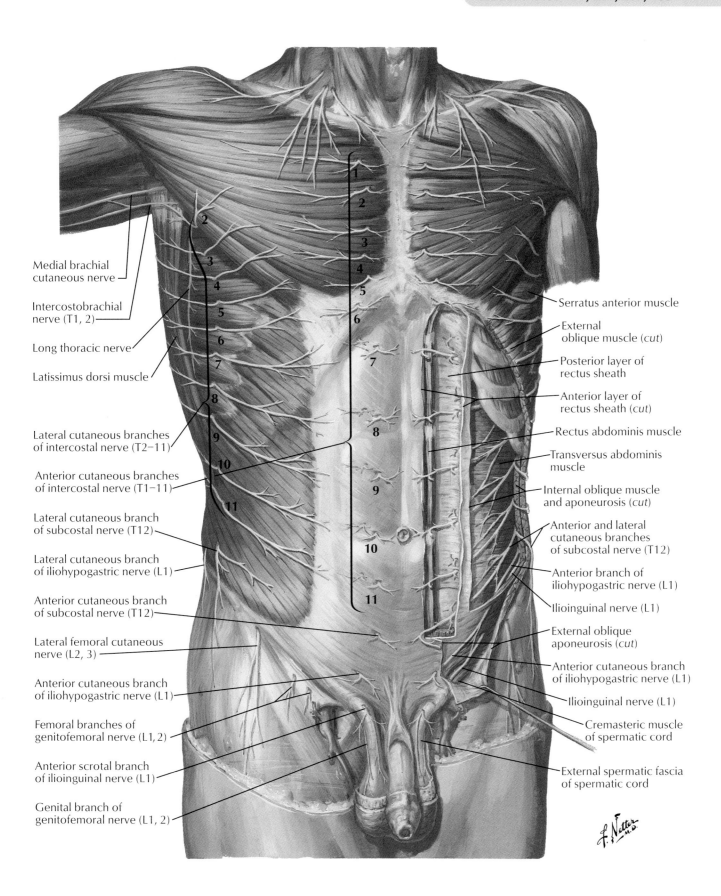

Medial brachial
cutaneous nerve

Intercostobrachial
nerve (T1, 2)

Long thoracic nerve

Latissimus dorsi muscle

Lateral cutaneous branches
of intercostal nerve (T2–11)

Anterior cutaneous branches
of intercostal nerve (T1–11)

Lateral cutaneous branch
of subcostal nerve (T12)

Lateral cutaneous branch
of iliohypogastric nerve (L1)

Anterior cutaneous branch
of subcostal nerve (T12)

Lateral femoral cutaneous
nerve (L2, 3)

Anterior cutaneous branch
of iliohypogastric nerve (L1)

Femoral branches of
genitofemoral nerve (L1, 2)

Anterior scrotal branch
of ilioinguinal nerve (L1)

Genital branch of
genitofemoral nerve (L1, 2)

Serratus anterior muscle

External
oblique muscle (*cut*)

Posterior layer of
rectus sheath

Anterior layer of
rectus sheath (*cut*)

Rectus abdominis muscle

Transversus abdominis
muscle

Internal oblique muscle
and aponeurosis (*cut*)

Anterior and lateral
cutaneous branches
of subcostal nerve (T12)

Anterior branch of
iliohypogastric nerve (L1)

Ilioinguinal nerve (L1)

External oblique
aponeurosis (*cut*)

Anterior cutaneous branch
of iliohypogastric nerve (L1)

Ilioinguinal nerve (L1)

Cremasteric muscle
of spermatic cord

External spermatic fascia
of spermatic cord

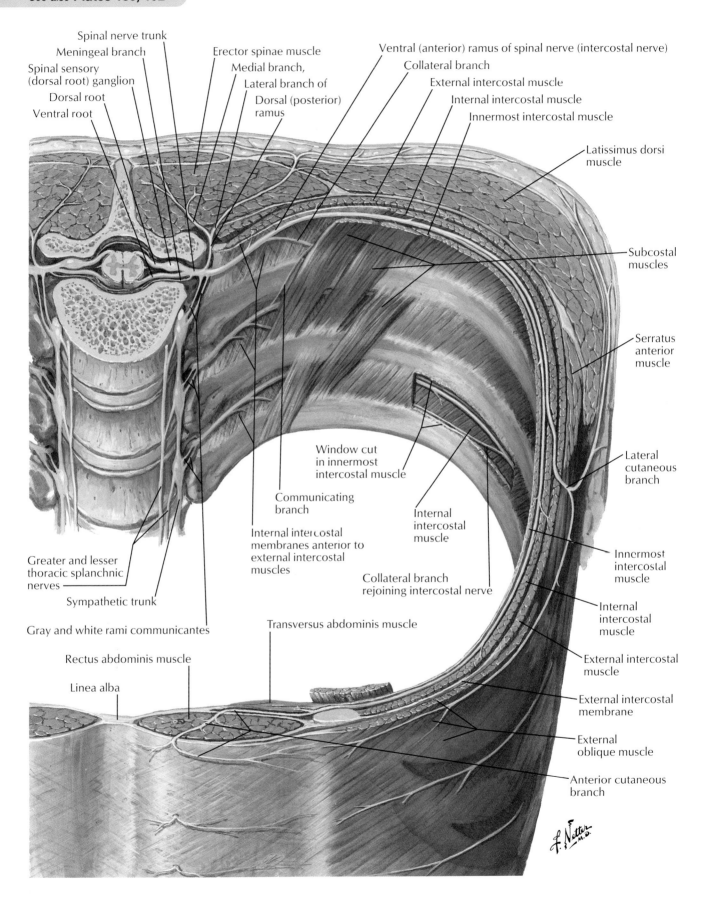

Spinal nerve trunk
Meningeal branch
Spinal sensory (dorsal root) ganglion
Dorsal root
Ventral root
Erector spinae muscle
Medial branch,
Lateral branch of
Dorsal (posterior) ramus
Ventral (anterior) ramus of spinal nerve (intercostal nerve)
Collateral branch
External intercostal muscle
Internal intercostal muscle
Innermost intercostal muscle
Latissimus dorsi muscle
Subcostal muscles
Serratus anterior muscle
Window cut in innermost intercostal muscle
Communicating branch
Internal intercostal membranes anterior to external intercostal muscles
Internal intercostal muscle
Collateral branch rejoining intercostal nerve
Lateral cutaneous branch
Innermost intercostal muscle
Internal intercostal muscle
Greater and lesser thoracic splanchnic nerves
Sympathetic trunk
Gray and white rami communicantes
Transversus abdominis muscle
External intercostal muscle
External intercostal membrane
Rectus abdominis muscle
Linea alba
External oblique muscle
Anterior cutaneous branch

Plate 258 **Body Wall**

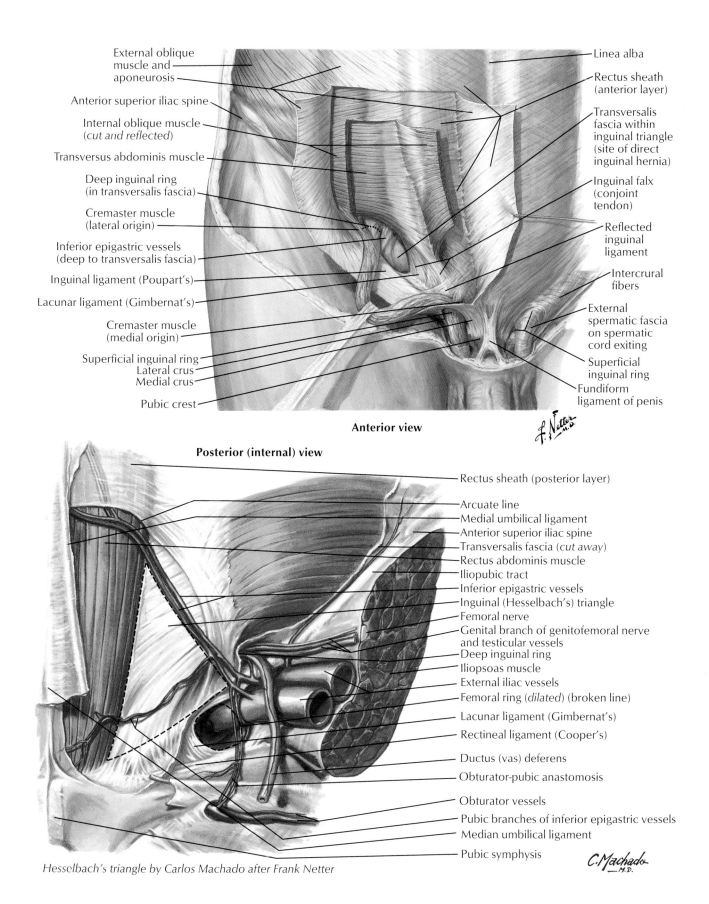

External oblique muscle and aponeurosis

Anterior superior iliac spine

Internal oblique muscle (*cut and reflected*)

Transversus abdominis muscle

Deep inguinal ring (in transversalis fascia)

Cremaster muscle (lateral origin)

Inferior epigastric vessels (deep to transversalis fascia)

Inguinal ligament (Poupart's)

Lacunar ligament (Gimbernat's)

Cremaster muscle (medial origin)

Superficial inguinal ring
Lateral crus
Medial crus

Pubic crest

Linea alba

Rectus sheath (anterior layer)

Transversalis fascia within inguinal triangle (site of direct inguinal hernia)

Inguinal falx (conjoint tendon)

Reflected inguinal ligament

Intercrural fibers

External spermatic fascia on spermatic cord exiting

Superficial inguinal ring

Fundiform ligament of penis

Anterior view

Posterior (internal) view

Rectus sheath (posterior layer)
Arcuate line
Medial umbilical ligament
Anterior superior iliac spine
Transversalis fascia (*cut away*)
Rectus abdominis muscle
Iliopubic tract
Inferior epigastric vessels
Inguinal (Hesselbach's) triangle
Femoral nerve
Genital branch of genitofemoral nerve and testicular vessels
Deep inguinal ring
Iliopsoas muscle
External iliac vessels
Femoral ring (*dilated*) (broken line)
Lacunar ligament (Gimbernat's)
Rectineal ligament (Cooper's)
Ductus (vas) deferens
Obturator-pubic anastomosis
Obturator vessels
Pubic branches of inferior epigastric vessels
Median umbilical ligament
Pubic symphysis

Hesselbach's triangle by Carlos Machado after Frank Netter

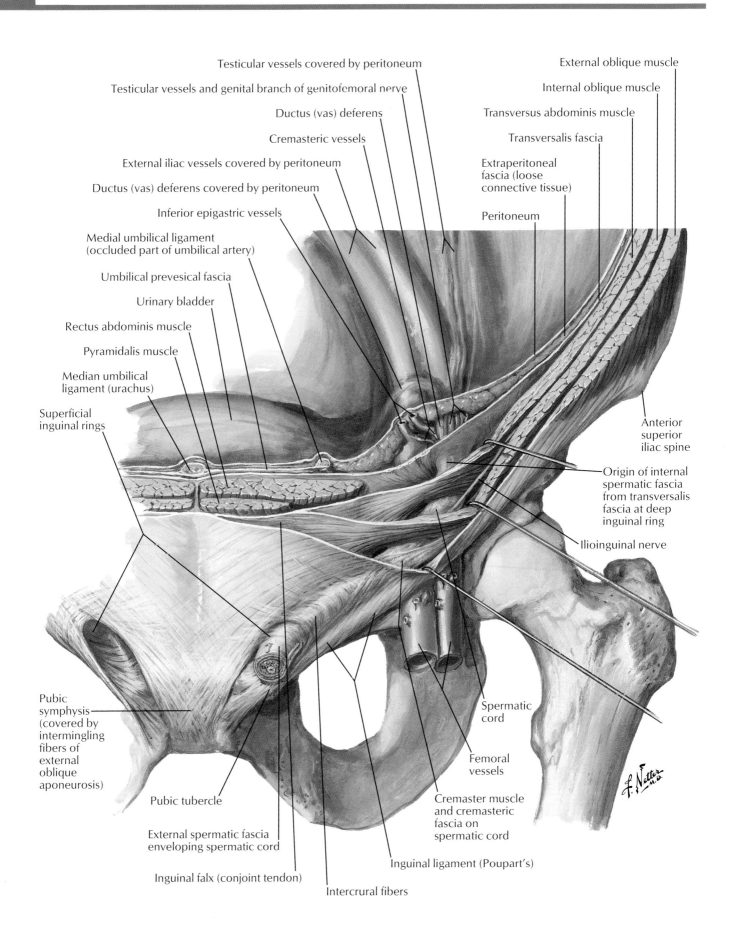

Testicular vessels covered by peritoneum

Testicular vessels and genital branch of genitofemoral nerve

Ductus (vas) deferens

Cremasteric vessels

External iliac vessels covered by peritoneum

Ductus (vas) deferens covered by peritoneum

Inferior epigastric vessels

Medial umbilical ligament (occluded part of umbilical artery)

Umbilical prevesical fascia

Urinary bladder

Rectus abdominis muscle

Pyramidalis muscle

Median umbilical ligament (urachus)

Superficial inguinal rings

External oblique muscle

Internal oblique muscle

Transversus abdominis muscle

Transversalis fascia

Extraperitoneal fascia (loose connective tissue)

Peritoneum

Anterior superior iliac spine

Origin of internal spermatic fascia from transversalis fascia at deep inguinal ring

Ilioinguinal nerve

Spermatic cord

Femoral vessels

Pubic symphysis (covered by intermingling fibers of external oblique aponeurosis)

Pubic tubercle

External spermatic fascia enveloping spermatic cord

Inguinal falx (conjoint tendon)

Intercrural fibers

Inguinal ligament (Poupart's)

Cremaster muscle and cremasteric fascia on spermatic cord

Plate 260 **Body Wall**

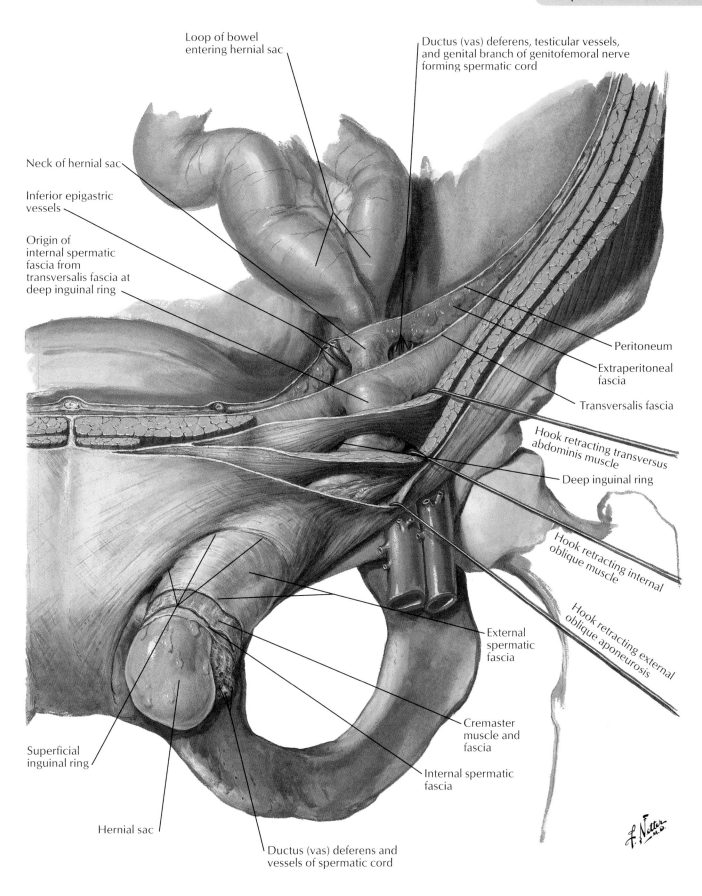

Loop of bowel entering hernial sac

Ductus (vas) deferens, testicular vessels, and genital branch of genitofemoral nerve forming spermatic cord

Neck of hernial sac

Inferior epigastric vessels

Origin of internal spermatic fascia from transversalis fascia at deep inguinal ring

Peritoneum

Extraperitoneal fascia

Transversalis fascia

Hook retracting transversus abdominis muscle

Deep inguinal ring

Hook retracting internal oblique muscle

Hook retracting external oblique aponeurosis

External spermatic fascia

Cremaster muscle and fascia

Internal spermatic fascia

Superficial inguinal ring

Hernial sac

Ductus (vas) deferens and vessels of spermatic cord

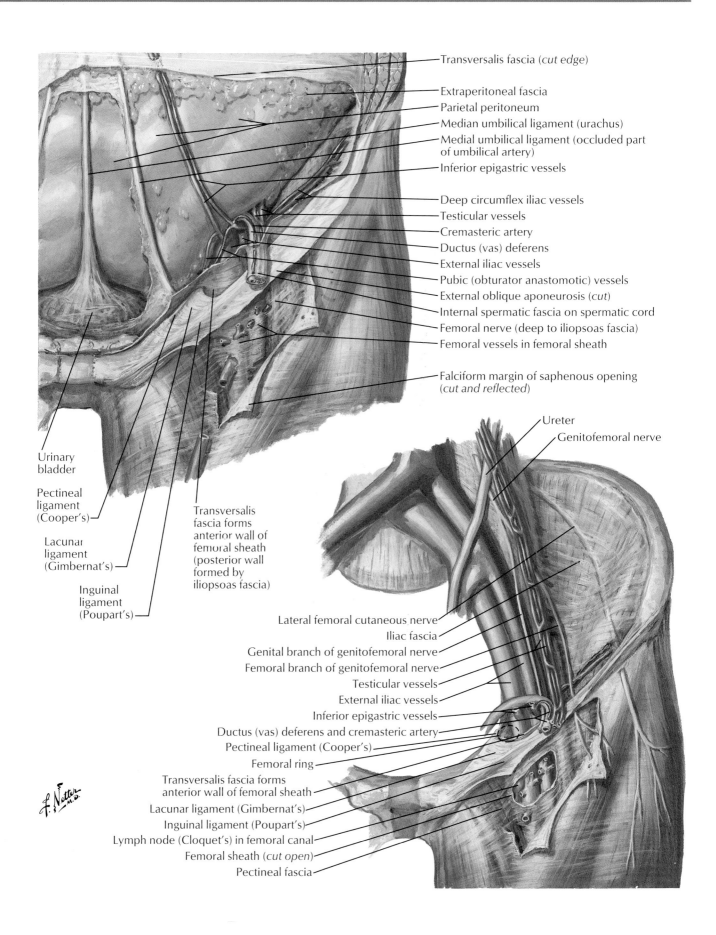

Transversalis fascia (*cut edge*)

Extraperitoneal fascia

Parietal peritoneum

Median umbilical ligament (urachus)

Medial umbilical ligament (occluded part of umbilical artery)

Inferior epigastric vessels

Deep circumflex iliac vessels

Testicular vessels

Cremasteric artery

Ductus (vas) deferens

External iliac vessels

Pubic (obturator anastomotic) vessels

External oblique aponeurosis (*cut*)

Internal spermatic fascia on spermatic cord

Femoral nerve (deep to iliopsoas fascia)

Femoral vessels in femoral sheath

Falciform margin of saphenous opening (*cut and reflected*)

Ureter

Genitofemoral nerve

Urinary bladder

Pectineal ligament (Cooper's)

Lacunar ligament (Gimbernat's)

Inguinal ligament (Poupart's)

Transversalis fascia forms anterior wall of femoral sheath (posterior wall formed by iliopsoas fascia)

Lateral femoral cutaneous nerve

Iliac fascia

Genital branch of genitofemoral nerve

Femoral branch of genitofemoral nerve

Testicular vessels

External iliac vessels

Inferior epigastric vessels

Ductus (vas) deferens and cremasteric artery

Pectineal ligament (Cooper's)

Femoral ring

Transversalis fascia forms anterior wall of femoral sheath

Lacunar ligament (Gimbernat's)

Inguinal ligament (Poupart's)

Lymph node (Cloquet's) in femoral canal

Femoral sheath (*cut open*)

Pectineal fascia

Plate 262 **Body Wall**

For diaphragm see also **Plate 195**

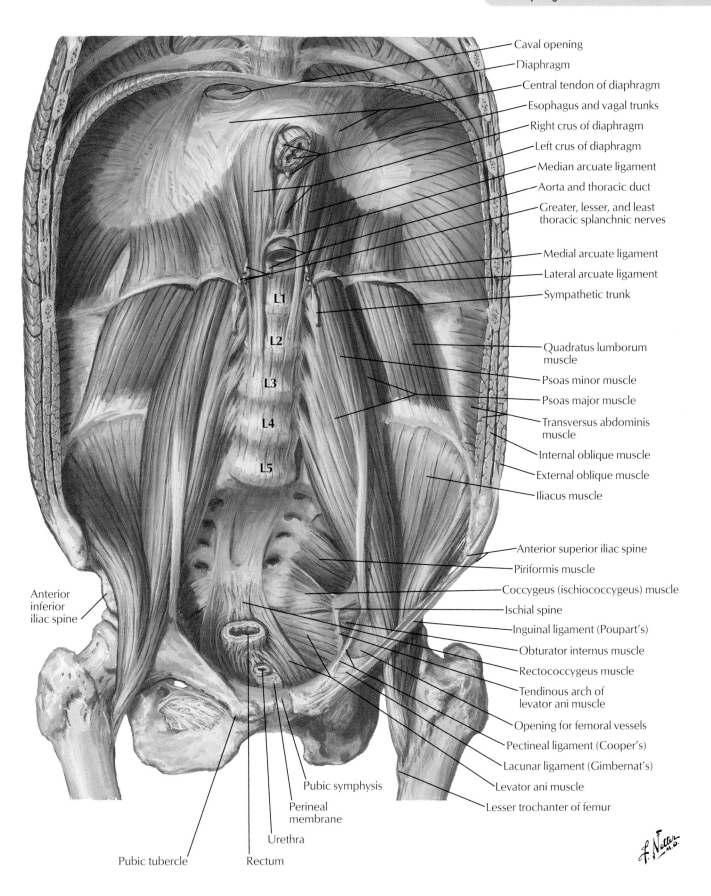

Caval opening

Diaphragm

Central tendon of diaphragm

Esophagus and vagal trunks

Right crus of diaphragm

Left crus of diaphragm

Median arcuate ligament

Aorta and thoracic duct

Greater, lesser, and least thoracic splanchnic nerves

Medial arcuate ligament

Lateral arcuate ligament

Sympathetic trunk

Quadratus lumborum muscle

Psoas minor muscle

Psoas major muscle

Transversus abdominis muscle

Internal oblique muscle

External oblique muscle

Iliacus muscle

Anterior superior iliac spine

Piriformis muscle

Coccygeus (ischiococcygeus) muscle

Ischial spine

Inguinal ligament (Poupart's)

Obturator internus muscle

Rectococcygeus muscle

Tendinous arch of levator ani muscle

Opening for femoral vessels

Pectineal ligament (Cooper's)

Lacunar ligament (Gimbernat's)

Levator ani muscle

Lesser trochanter of femur

L1

L2

L3

L4

L5

Anterior inferior iliac spine

Pubic symphysis

Perineal membrane

Urethra

Rectum

Pubic tubercle

Body Wall

Plate 263

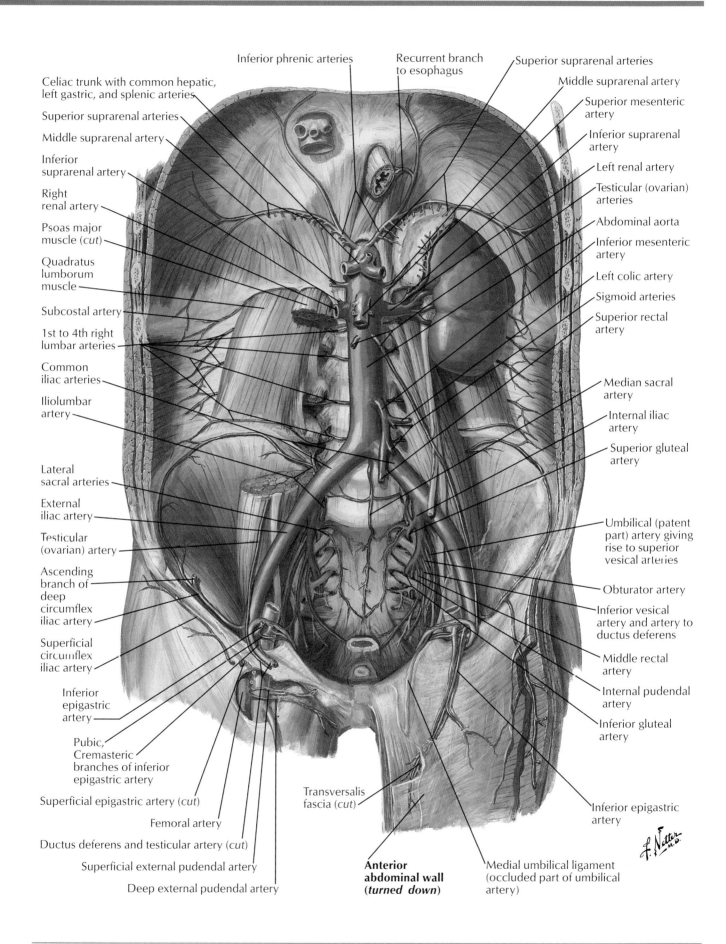

Inferior phrenic arteries

Recurrent branch to esophagus

Superior suprarenal arteries

Middle suprarenal artery

Celiac trunk with common hepatic, left gastric, and splenic arteries

Superior suprarenal arteries

Middle suprarenal artery

Inferior suprarenal artery

Right renal artery

Psoas major muscle (*cut*)

Quadratus lumborum muscle

Subcostal artery

1st to 4th right lumbar arteries

Common iliac arteries

Iliolumbar artery

Lateral sacral arteries

External iliac artery

Testicular (ovarian) artery

Ascending branch of deep circumflex iliac artery

Superficial circumflex iliac artery

Inferior epigastric artery

Pubic, Cremasteric branches of inferior epigastric artery

Superficial epigastric artery (*cut*)

Femoral artery

Ductus deferens and testicular artery (*cut*)

Superficial external pudendal artery

Deep external pudendal artery

Superior mesenteric artery

Inferior suprarenal artery

Left renal artery

Testicular (ovarian) arteries

Abdominal aorta

Inferior mesenteric artery

Left colic artery

Sigmoid arteries

Superior rectal artery

Median sacral artery

Internal iliac artery

Superior gluteal artery

Umbilical (patent part) artery giving rise to superior vesical arteries

Obturator artery

Inferior vesical artery and artery to ductus deferens

Middle rectal artery

Internal pudendal artery

Inferior gluteal artery

Inferior epigastric artery

Anterior abdominal wall (*turned down*)

Transversalis fascia (*cut*)

Medial umbilical ligament (occluded part of umbilical artery)

f. Netter M.D.

Plate 264　　　　　　　　　　　　　　　　　　　　**Body Wall**

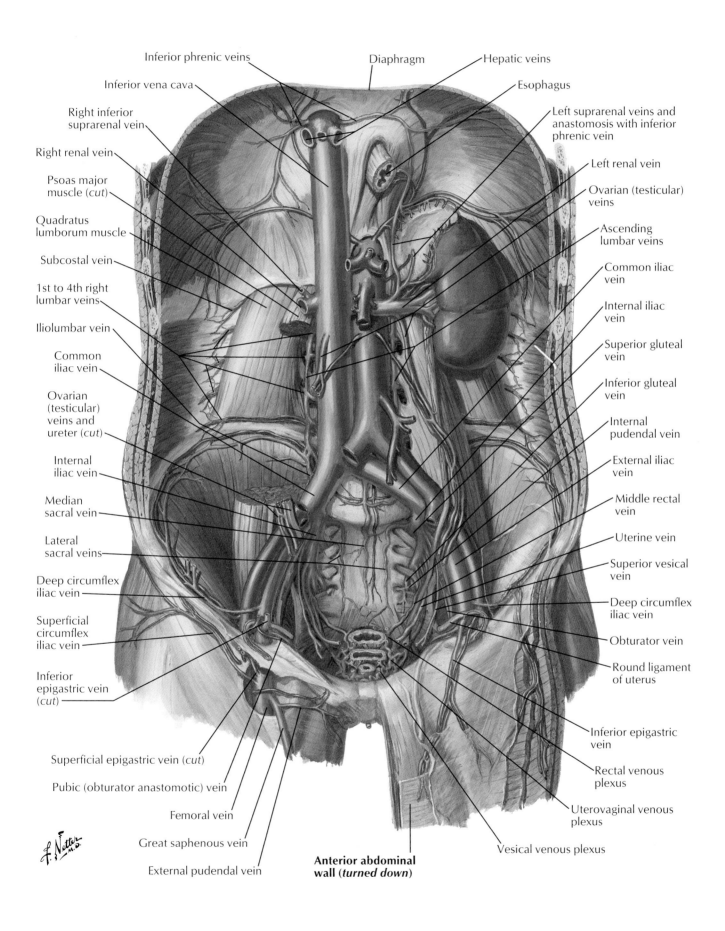

Inferior phrenic veins

Diaphragm

Hepatic veins

Inferior vena cava

Esophagus

Right inferior suprarenal vein

Left suprarenal veins and anastomosis with inferior phrenic vein

Right renal vein

Left renal vein

Psoas major muscle (cut)

Ovarian (testicular) veins

Quadratus lumborum muscle

Ascending lumbar veins

Subcostal vein

Common iliac vein

1st to 4th right lumbar veins

Internal iliac vein

Iliolumbar vein

Superior gluteal vein

Common iliac vein

Inferior gluteal vein

Ovarian (testicular) veins and ureter (cut)

Internal pudendal vein

Internal iliac vein

External iliac vein

Median sacral vein

Middle rectal vein

Lateral sacral veins

Uterine vein

Deep circumflex iliac vein

Superior vesical vein

Superficial circumflex iliac vein

Deep circumflex iliac vein

Obturator vein

Inferior epigastric vein (cut)

Round ligament of uterus

Inferior epigastric vein

Superficial epigastric vein (cut)

Rectal venous plexus

Pubic (obturator anastomotic) vein

Uterovaginal venous plexus

Femoral vein

Great saphenous vein

Vesical venous plexus

External pudendal vein

Anterior abdominal wall (turned down)

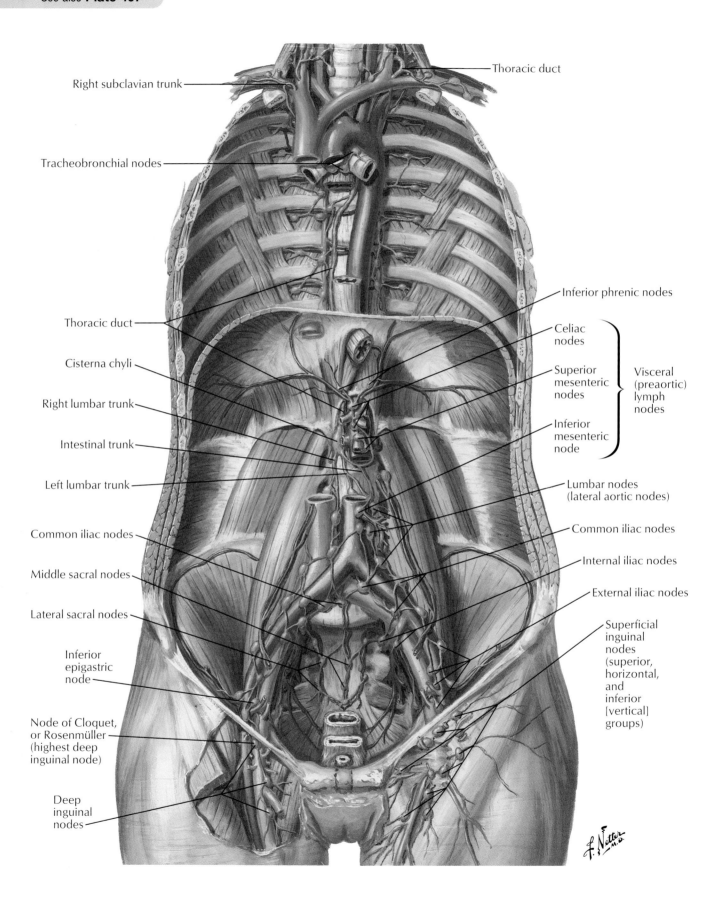

Thoracic duct

Right subclavian trunk

Tracheobronchial nodes

Inferior phrenic nodes

Thoracic duct

Celiac nodes

Cisterna chyli

Superior mesenteric nodes

Visceral (preaortic) lymph nodes

Right lumbar trunk

Intestinal trunk

Inferior mesenteric node

Left lumbar trunk

Lumbar nodes (lateral aortic nodes)

Common iliac nodes

Common iliac nodes

Middle sacral nodes

Internal iliac nodes

Lateral sacral nodes

External iliac nodes

Inferior epigastric node

Superficial inguinal nodes (superior, horizontal, and inferior [vertical] groups)

Node of Cloquet, or Rosenmüller (highest deep inguinal node)

Deep inguinal nodes

Plate 266

Body Wall

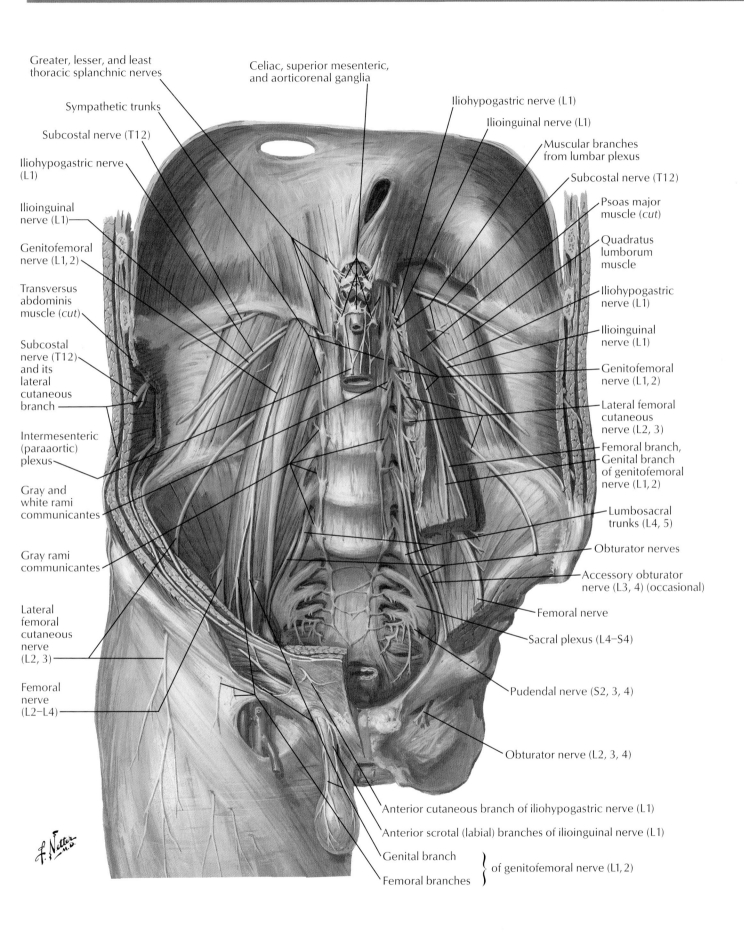

Greater, lesser, and least thoracic splanchnic nerves

Celiac, superior mesenteric, and aorticorenal ganglia

Iliohypogastric nerve (L1)

Sympathetic trunks

Ilioinguinal nerve (L1)

Subcostal nerve (T12)

Muscular branches from lumbar plexus

Iliohypogastric nerve (L1)

Subcostal nerve (T12)

Psoas major muscle (*cut*)

Ilioinguinal nerve (L1)

Quadratus lumborum muscle

Genitofemoral nerve (L1, 2)

Iliohypogastric nerve (L1)

Transversus abdominis muscle (*cut*)

Ilioinguinal nerve (L1)

Subcostal nerve (T12) and its lateral cutaneous branch

Genitofemoral nerve (L1, 2)

Lateral femoral cutaneous nerve (L2, 3)

Intermesenteric (paraaortic) plexus

Femoral branch, Genital branch of genitofemoral nerve (L1, 2)

Gray and white rami communicantes

Lumbosacral trunks (L4, 5)

Gray rami communicantes

Obturator nerves

Accessory obturator nerve (L3, 4) (occasional)

Femoral nerve

Lateral femoral cutaneous nerve (L2, 3)

Sacral plexus (L4–S4)

Femoral nerve (L2–L4)

Pudendal nerve (S2, 3, 4)

Obturator nerve (L2, 3, 4)

Anterior cutaneous branch of iliohypogastric nerve (L1)

Anterior scrotal (labial) branches of ilioinguinal nerve (L1)

Genital branch

Femoral branches

of genitofemoral nerve (L1, 2)

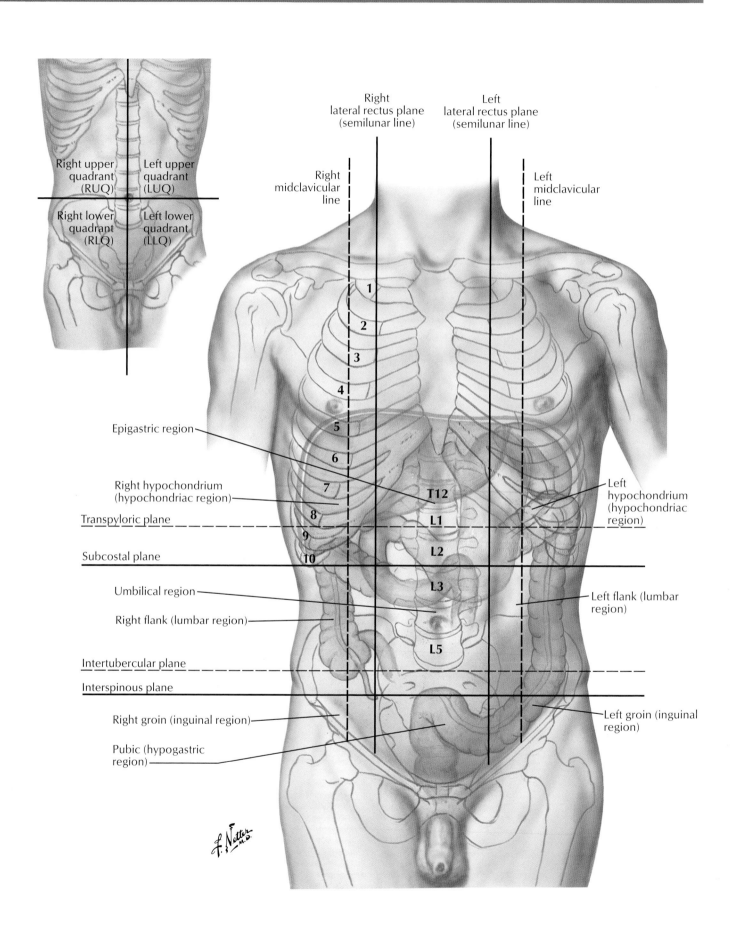

Right upper quadrant (RUQ)

Left upper quadrant (LUQ)

Right lower quadrant (RLQ)

Left lower quadrant (LLQ)

Right lateral rectus plane (semilunar line)

Left lateral rectus plane (semilunar line)

Right midclavicular line

Left midclavicular line

1
2
3
4
5
6
7
8
9
10

T12
L1
L2
L3
L5

Epigastric region

Right hypochondrium (hypochondriac region)

Transpyloric plane

Subcostal plane

Umbilical region

Right flank (lumbar region)

Intertubercular plane

Interspinous plane

Right groin (inguinal region)

Pubic (hypogastric region)

Left hypochondrium (hypochondriac region)

Left flank (lumbar region)

Left groin (inguinal region)

Plate 268   **Peritoneal Cavity**

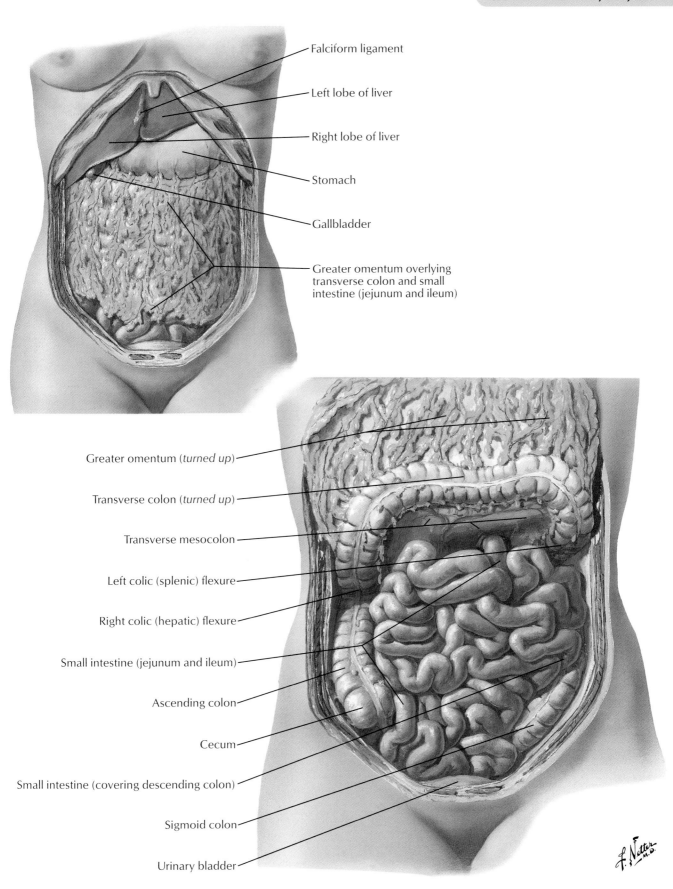

Falciform ligament

Left lobe of liver

Right lobe of liver

Stomach

Gallbladder

Greater omentum overlying transverse colon and small intestine (jejunum and ileum)

Greater omentum (*turned up*)

Transverse colon (*turned up*)

Transverse mesocolon

Left colic (splenic) flexure

Right colic (hepatic) flexure

Small intestine (jejunum and ileum)

Ascending colon

Cecum

Small intestine (covering descending colon)

Sigmoid colon

Urinary bladder

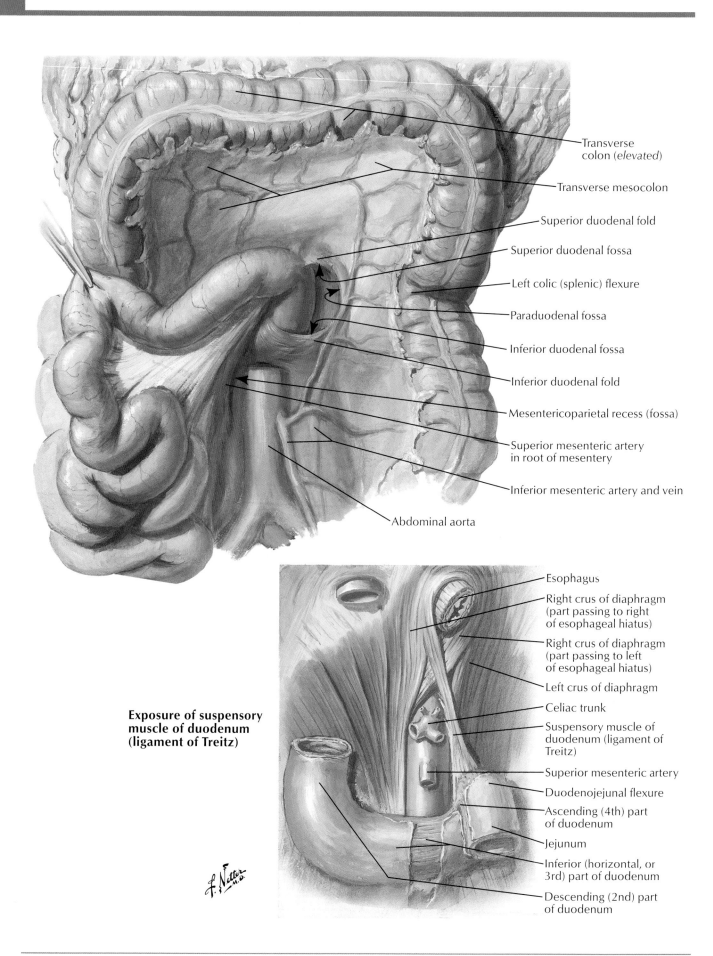

Transverse colon (*elevated*)

Transverse mesocolon

Superior duodenal fold

Superior duodenal fossa

Left colic (splenic) flexure

Paraduodenal fossa

Inferior duodenal fossa

Inferior duodenal fold

Mesentericoparietal recess (fossa)

Superior mesenteric artery in root of mesentery

Inferior mesenteric artery and vein

Abdominal aorta

Esophagus

Right crus of diaphragm (part passing to right of esophageal hiatus)

Right crus of diaphragm (part passing to left of esophageal hiatus)

Left crus of diaphragm

Celiac trunk

Suspensory muscle of duodenum (ligament of Treitz)

Superior mesenteric artery

Duodenojejunal flexure

Ascending (4th) part of duodenum

Jejunum

Inferior (horizontal, or 3rd) part of duodenum

Descending (2nd) part of duodenum

Exposure of suspensory muscle of duodenum (ligament of Treitz)

Plate 270   **Peritoneal Cavity**

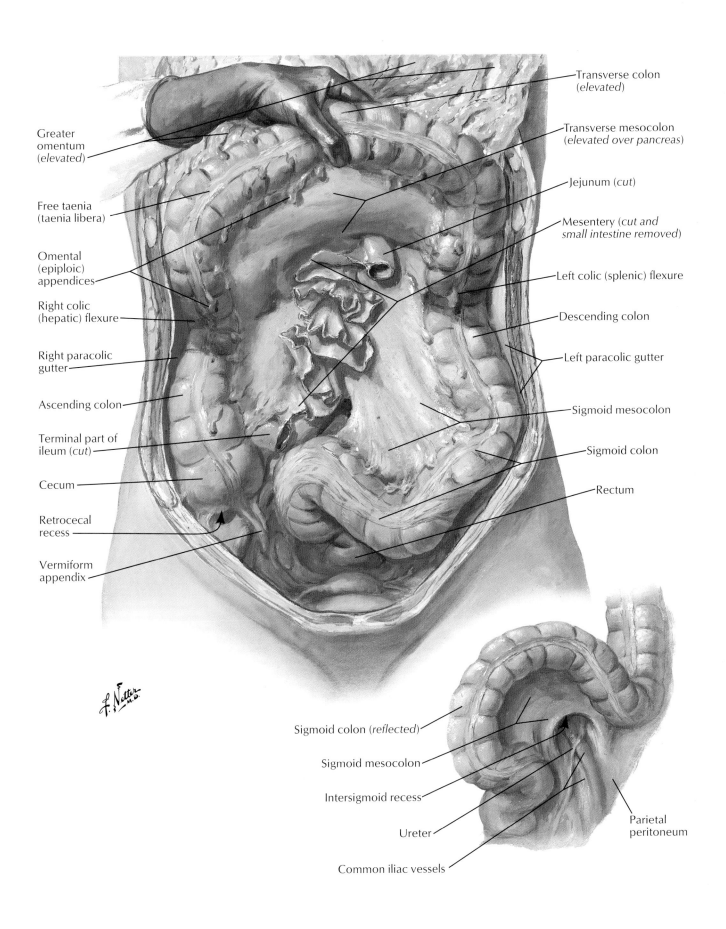

Greater omentum (*elevated*)

Free taenia (taenia libera)

Omental (epiploic) appendices

Right colic (hepatic) flexure

Right paracolic gutter

Ascending colon

Terminal part of ileum (*cut*)

Cecum

Retrocecal recess

Vermiform appendix

Transverse colon (*elevated*)

Transverse mesocolon (*elevated over pancreas*)

Jejunum (*cut*)

Mesentery (*cut and small intestine removed*)

Left colic (splenic) flexure

Descending colon

Left paracolic gutter

Sigmoid mesocolon

Sigmoid colon

Rectum

Sigmoid colon (*reflected*)

Sigmoid mesocolon

Intersigmoid recess

Ureter

Common iliac vessels

Parietal peritoneum

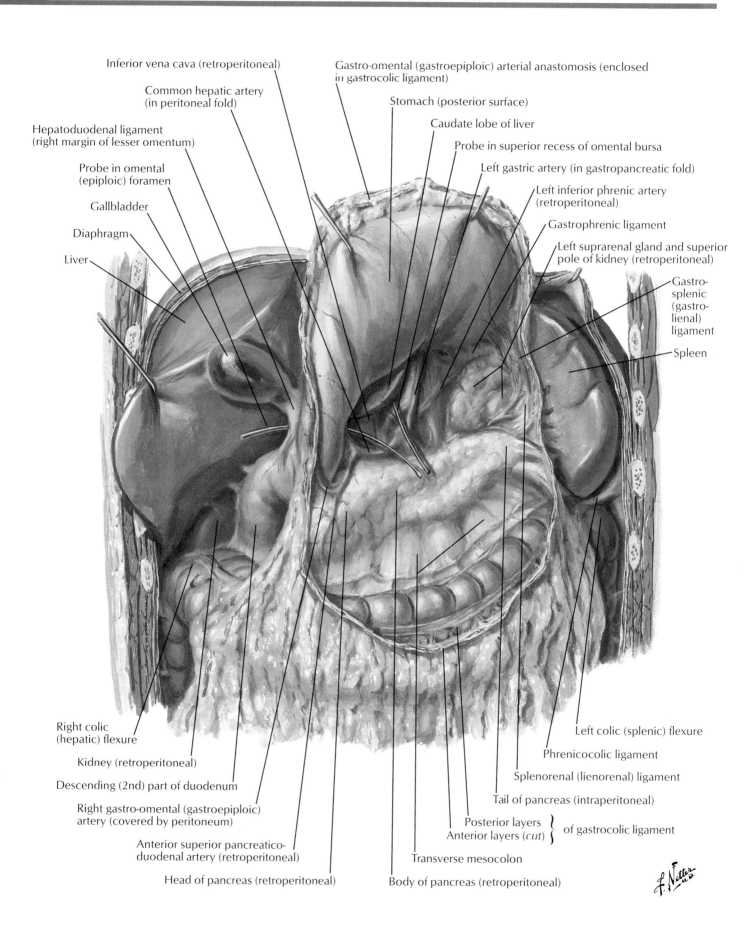

Inferior vena cava (retroperitoneal)

Common hepatic artery
(in peritoneal fold)

Hepatoduodenal ligament
(right margin of lesser omentum)

Probe in omental
(epiploic) foramen

Gallbladder

Diaphragm

Liver

Gastro-omental (gastroepiploic) arterial anastomosis (enclosed
in gastrocolic ligament)

Stomach (posterior surface)

Caudate lobe of liver

Probe in superior recess of omental bursa

Left gastric artery (in gastropancreatic fold)

Left inferior phrenic artery
(retroperitoneal)

Gastrophrenic ligament

Left suprarenal gland and superior
pole of kidney (retroperitoneal)

Gastro-
splenic
(gastro-
lienal)
ligament

Spleen

Right colic
(hepatic) flexure

Kidney (retroperitoneal)

Descending (2nd) part of duodenum

Right gastro-omental (gastroepiploic)
artery (covered by peritoneum)

Anterior superior pancreaticoduodenal artery (retroperitoneal)

Head of pancreas (retroperitoneal)

Body of pancreas (retroperitoneal)

Transverse mesocolon

Posterior layers ⎫
Anterior layers (cut) ⎬ of gastrocolic ligament

Tail of pancreas (intraperitoneal)

Splenorenal (lienorenal) ligament

Phrenicocolic ligament

Left colic (splenic) flexure

Plate 272

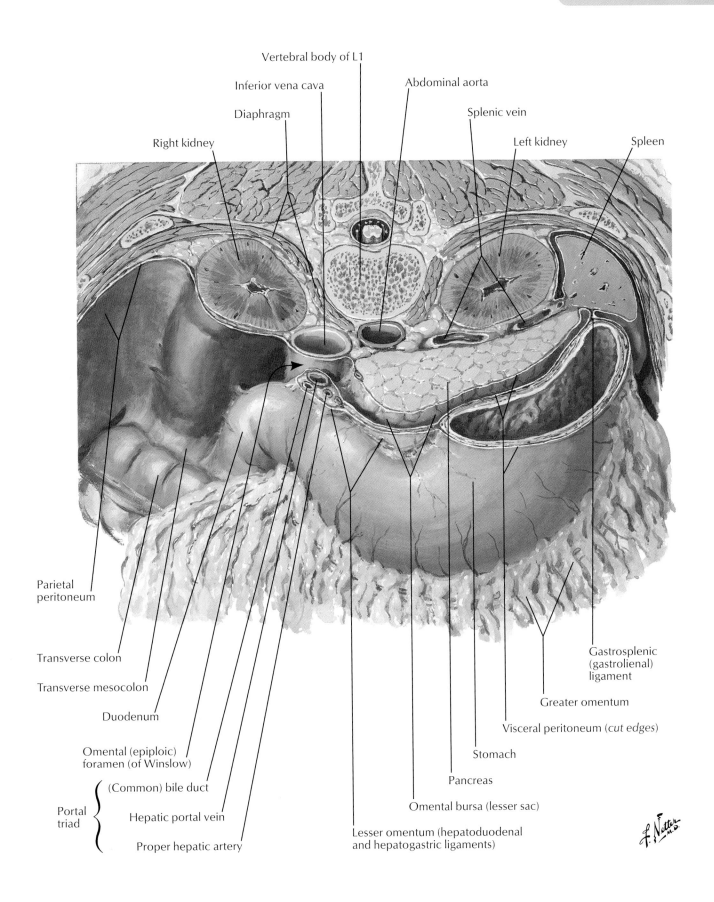

Vertebral body of L1

Inferior vena cava

Abdominal aorta

Diaphragm

Splenic vein

Right kidney

Left kidney

Spleen

Parietal
peritoneum

Transverse colon

Transverse mesocolon

Duodenum

Omental (epiploic)
foramen (of Winslow)

Portal
triad {

(Common) bile duct

Hepatic portal vein

Proper hepatic artery

Lesser omentum (hepatoduodenal
and hepatogastric ligaments)

Omental bursa (lesser sac)

Pancreas

Stomach

Visceral peritoneum (*cut edges*)

Greater omentum

Gastrosplenic
(gastrolienal)
ligament

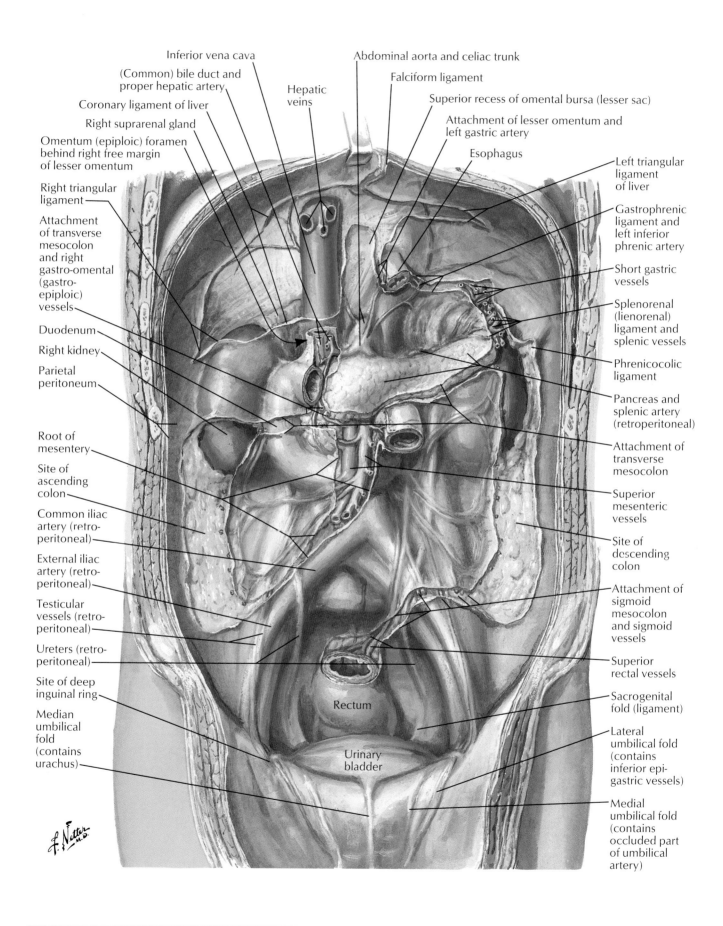

Inferior vena cava

(Common) bile duct and proper hepatic artery

Coronary ligament of liver

Right suprarenal gland

Omentum (epiploic) foramen behind right free margin of lesser omentum

Right triangular ligament

Attachment of transverse mesocolon and right gastro-omental (gastro-epiploic) vessels

Duodenum

Right kidney

Parietal peritoneum

Root of mesentery

Site of ascending colon

Common iliac artery (retro-peritoneal)

External iliac artery (retro-peritoneal)

Testicular vessels (retro-peritoneal)

Ureters (retro-peritoneal)

Site of deep inguinal ring

Median umbilical fold (contains urachus)

Hepatic veins

Abdominal aorta and celiac trunk

Falciform ligament

Superior recess of omental bursa (lesser sac)

Attachment of lesser omentum and left gastric artery

Esophagus

Left triangular ligament of liver

Gastrophrenic ligament and left inferior phrenic artery

Short gastric vessels

Splenorenal (lienorenal) ligament and splenic vessels

Phrenicocolic ligament

Pancreas and splenic artery (retroperitoneal)

Attachment of transverse mesocolon

Superior mesenteric vessels

Site of descending colon

Attachment of sigmoid mesocolon and sigmoid vessels

Superior rectal vessels

Sacrogenital fold (ligament)

Lateral umbilical fold (contains inferior epigastric vessels)

Medial umbilical fold (contains occluded part of umbilical artery)

Rectum

Urinary bladder

Plate 274

Peritoneal Cavity

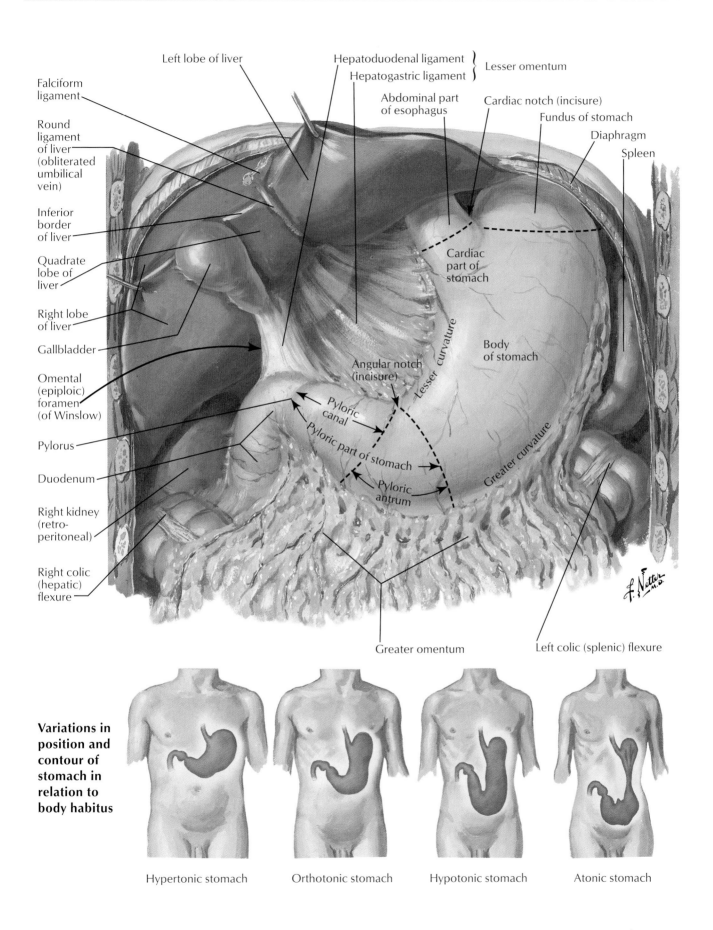

Left lobe of liver

Hepatoduodenal ligament ⎫
Hepatogastric ligament ⎬ Lesser omentum

Falciform ligament

Abdominal part of esophagus

Cardiac notch (incisure)

Fundus of stomach

Round ligament of liver (obliterated umbilical vein)

Diaphragm

Spleen

Inferior border of liver

Cardiac part of stomach

Quadrate lobe of liver

Body of stomach

Right lobe of liver

Lesser curvature

Gallblader

Angular notch (incisure)

Omental (epiploic) foramen (of Winslow)

Pyloric canal

Pylorus

Pyloric part of stomach

Duodenum

Pyloric antrum

Greater curvature

Right kidney (retroperitoneal)

Right colic (hepatic) flexure

Greater omentum

Left colic (splenic) flexure

Variations in position and contour of stomach in relation to body habitus

Hypertonic stomach

Orthotonic stomach

Hypotonic stomach

Atonic stomach

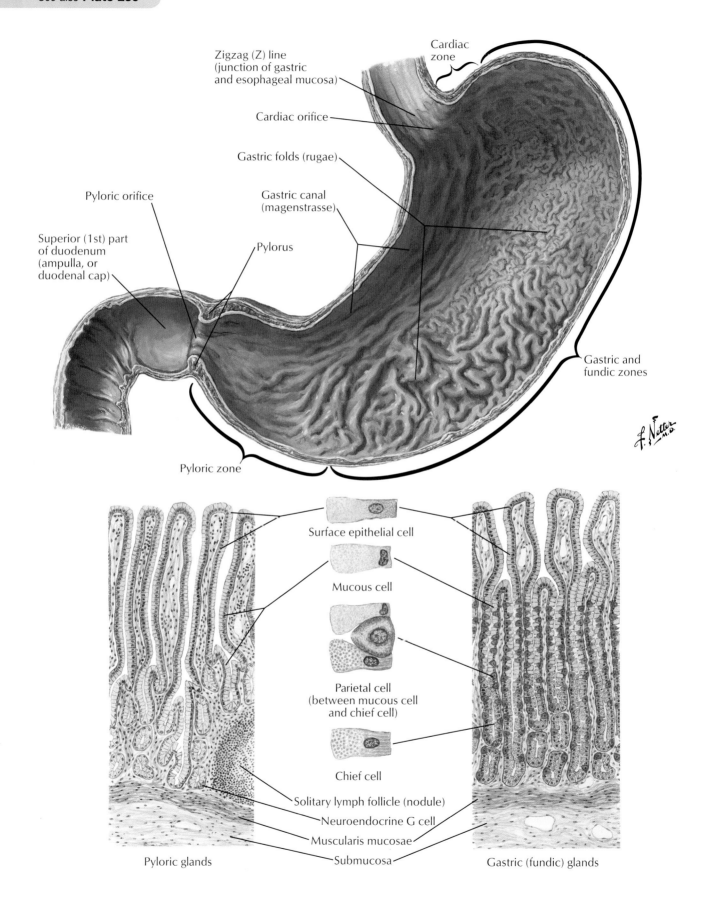

Zigzag (Z) line
(junction of gastric
and esophageal mucosa)

Cardiac orifice

Gastric folds (rugae)

Pyloric orifice

Gastric canal
(magenstrasse)

Superior (1st) part
of duodenum
(ampulla, or
duodenal cap)

Pylorus

Cardiac zone

Gastric and
fundic zones

Pyloric zone

Surface epithelial cell

Mucous cell

Parietal cell
(between mucous cell
and chief cell)

Chief cell

Solitary lymph follicle (nodule)

Neuroendocrine G cell

Muscularis mucosae

Submucosa

Pyloric glands

Gastric (fundic) glands

Plate 276

Viscera (Gut)

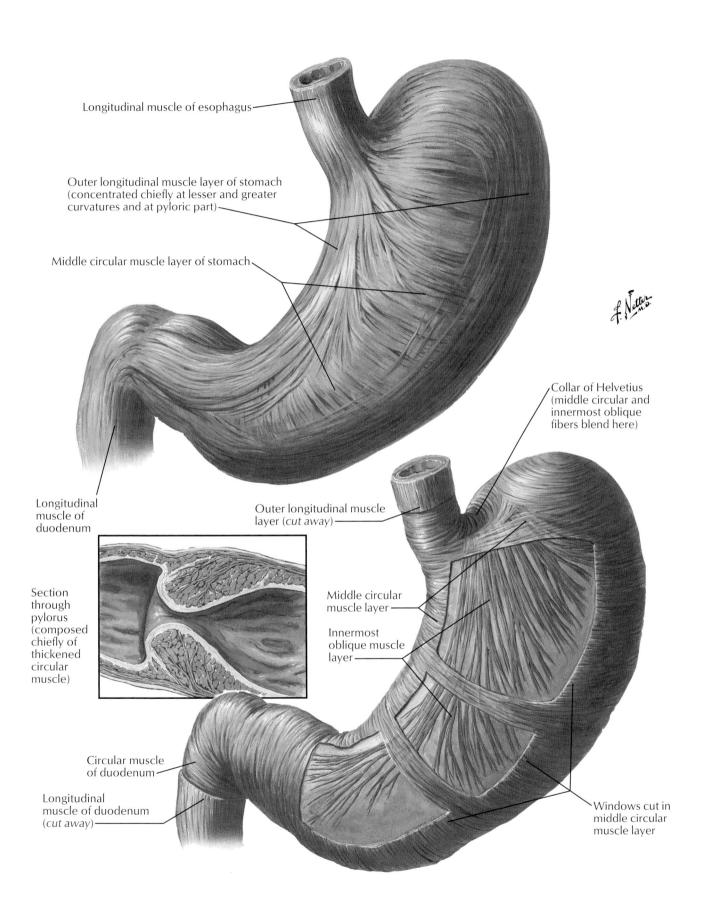

Longitudinal muscle of esophagus

Outer longitudinal muscle layer of stomach
(concentrated chiefly at lesser and greater
curvatures and at pyloric part)

Middle circular muscle layer of stomach

Longitudinal
muscle of
duodenum

Section
through
pylorus
(composed
chiefly of
thickened
circular
muscle)

Circular muscle
of duodenum

Longitudinal
muscle of duodenum
(*cut away*)

Collar of Helvetius
(middle circular and
innermost oblique
fibers blend here)

Outer longitudinal muscle
layer (*cut away*)

Middle circular
muscle layer

Innermost
oblique muscle
layer

Windows cut in
middle circular
muscle layer

F. Netter M.D.

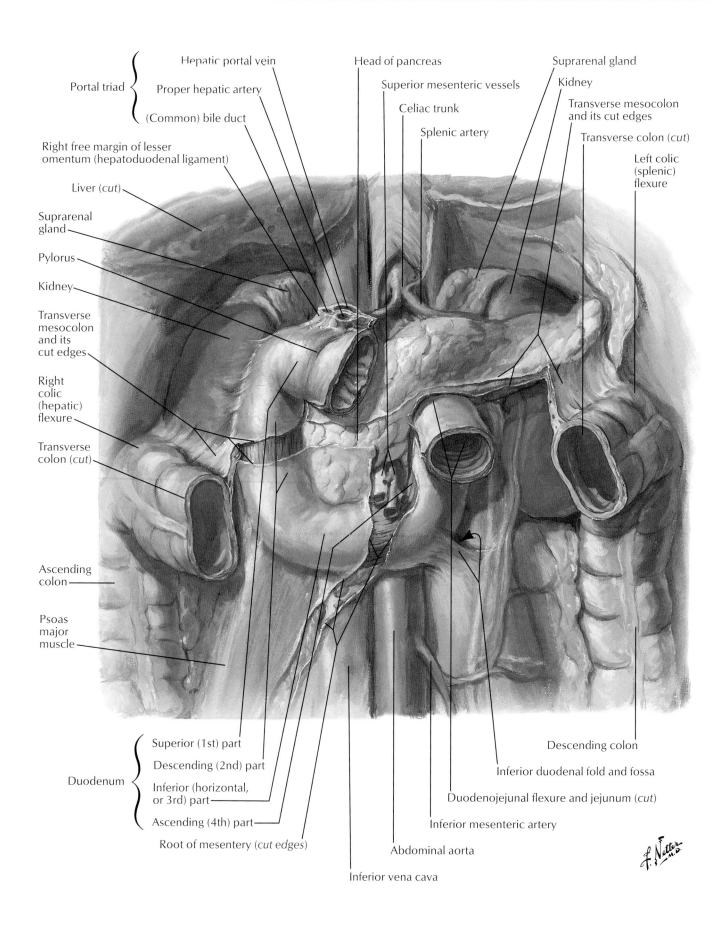

Portal triad {
Hepatic portal vein
Proper hepatic artery
(Common) bile duct

Head of pancreas
Superior mesenteric vessels
Celiac trunk
Splenic artery

Suprarenal gland
Kidney
Transverse mesocolon and its cut edges
Transverse colon (cut)
Left colic (splenic) flexure

Right free margin of lesser omentum (hepatoduodenal ligament)

Liver (cut)

Suprarenal gland

Pylorus

Kidney

Transverse mesocolon and its cut edges

Right colic (hepatic) flexure

Transverse colon (cut)

Ascending colon

Psoas major muscle

Duodenum {
Superior (1st) part
Descending (2nd) part
Inferior (horizontal, or 3rd) part
Ascending (4th) part

Root of mesentery (cut edges)

Inferior vena cava

Abdominal aorta

Inferior mesenteric artery

Duodenojejunal flexure and jejunum (cut)

Inferior duodenal fold and fossa

Descending colon

f. Netter M.D.

Plate 278

Viscera (Gut)

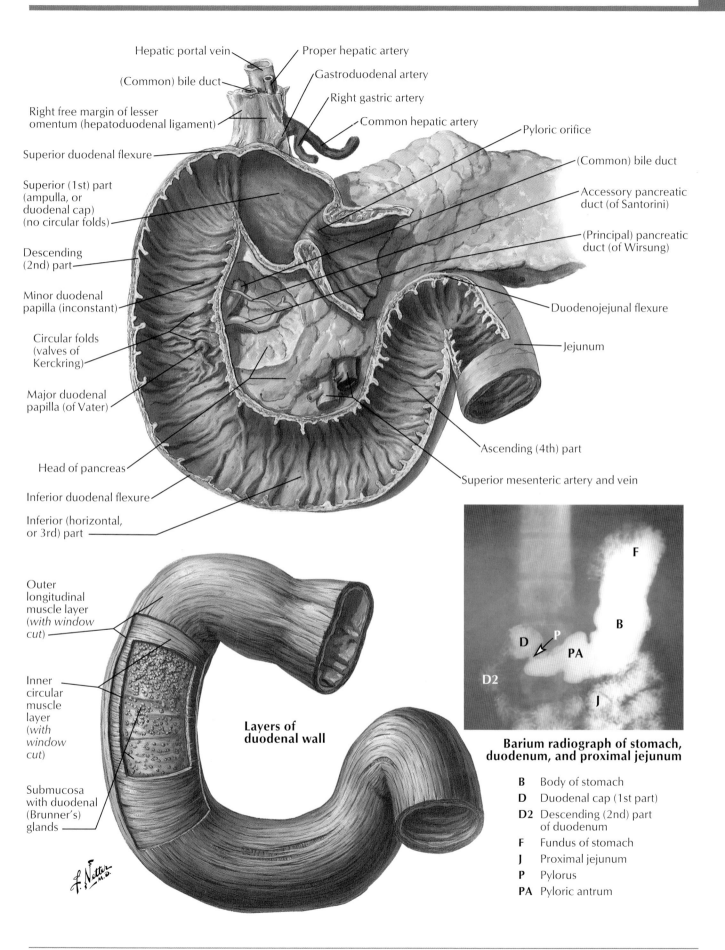

Hepatic portal vein

Proper hepatic artery

(Common) bile duct

Gastroduodenal artery

Right gastric artery

Right free margin of lesser omentum (hepatoduodenal ligament)

Common hepatic artery

Superior duodenal flexure

Pyloric orifice

(Common) bile duct

Superior (1st) part (ampulla, or duodenal cap) (no circular folds)

Accessory pancreatic duct (of Santorini)

(Principal) pancreatic duct (of Wirsung)

Descending (2nd) part

Minor duodenal papilla (inconstant)

Duodenojejunal flexure

Circular folds (valves of Kerckring)

Jejunum

Major duodenal papilla (of Vater)

Head of pancreas

Inferior duodenal flexure

Ascending (4th) part

Superior mesenteric artery and vein

Inferior (horizontal, or 3rd) part

Outer longitudinal muscle layer (*with window cut*)

Inner circular muscle layer (*with window cut*)

Submucosa with duodenal (Brunner's) glands

Layers of duodenal wall

Barium radiograph of stomach, duodenum, and proximal jejunum

B   Body of stomach
D   Duodenal cap (1st part)
D2 Descending (2nd) part of duodenum
F   Fundus of stomach
J   Proximal jejunum
P   Pylorus
PA Pyloric antrum

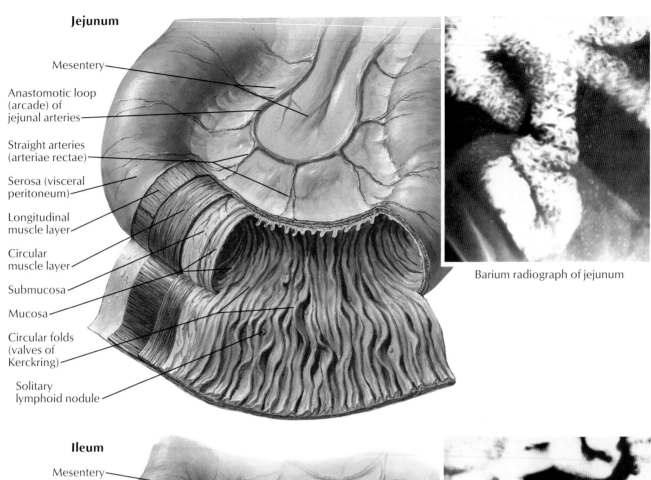

Jejunum

Mesentery

Anastomotic loop (arcade) of jejunal arteries

Straight arteries (arteriae rectae)

Serosa (visceral peritoneum)

Longitudinal muscle layer

Circular muscle layer

Submucosa

Mucosa

Circular folds (valves of Kerckring)

Solitary lymphoid nodule

Barium radiograph of jejunum

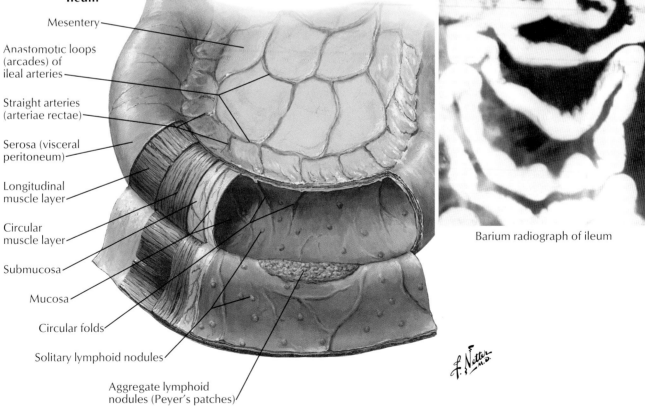

Ileum

Mesentery

Anastomotic loops (arcades) of ileal arteries

Straight arteries (arteriae rectae)

Serosa (visceral peritoneum)

Longitudinal muscle layer

Circular muscle layer

Submucosa

Mucosa

Circular folds

Solitary lymphoid nodules

Aggregate lymphoid nodules (Peyer's patches)

Barium radiograph of ileum

Plate 280 **Viscera (Gut)**

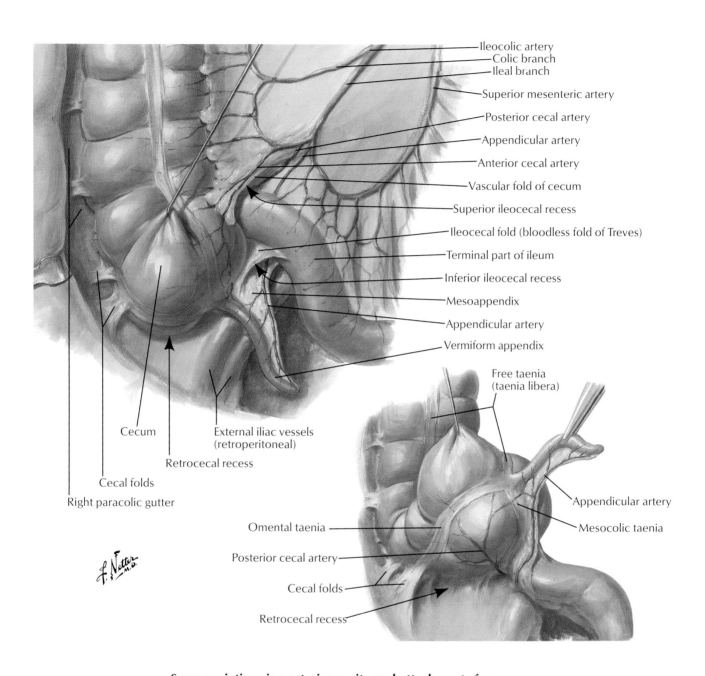

Ileocolic artery
Colic branch
Ileal branch
Superior mesenteric artery
Posterior cecal artery
Appendicular artery
Anterior cecal artery
Vascular fold of cecum
Superior ileocecal recess
Ileocecal fold (bloodless fold of Treves)
Terminal part of ileum
Inferior ileocecal recess
Mesoappendix
Appendicular artery
Vermiform appendix

Cecum
External iliac vessels (retroperitoneal)
Retrocecal recess
Cecal folds
Right paracolic gutter

Free taenia (taenia libera)
Appendicular artery
Mesocolic taenia
Omental taenia
Posterior cecal artery
Cecal folds
Retrocecal recess

Some variations in posterior peritoneal attachment of cecum

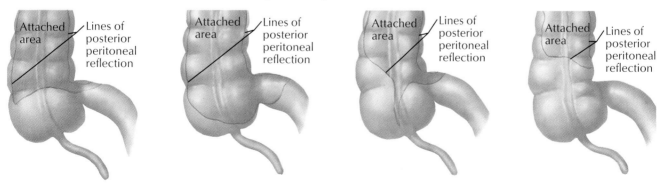

Attached area — Lines of posterior peritoneal reflection

Attached area — Lines of posterior peritoneal reflection

Attached area — Lines of posterior peritoneal reflection

Attached area — Lines of posterior peritoneal reflection

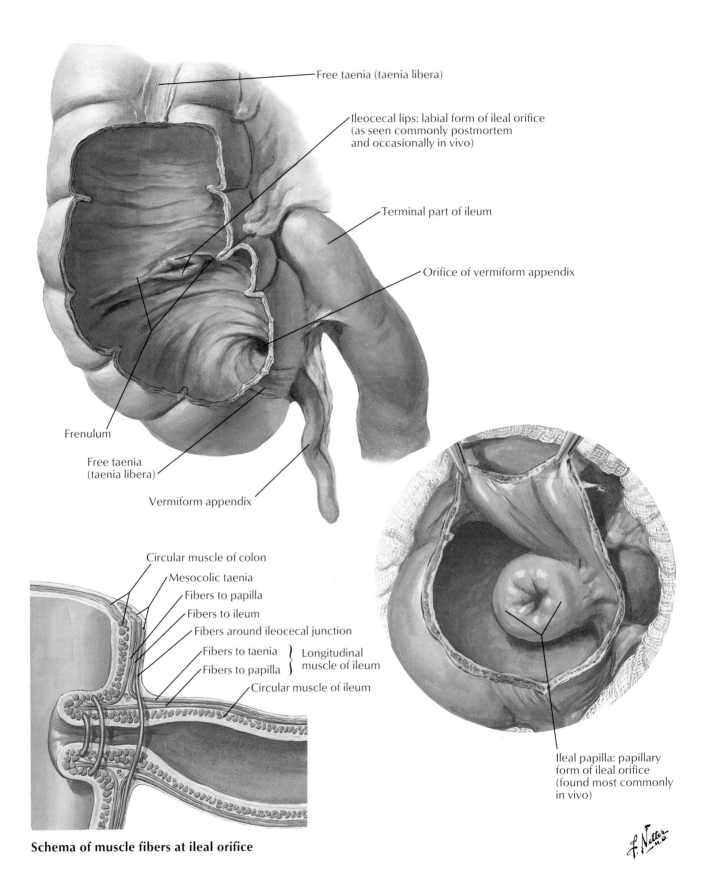

Free taenia (taenia libera)

Ileocecal lips: labial form of ileal orifice (as seen commonly postmortem and occasionally in vivo)

Terminal part of ileum

Orifice of vermiform appendix

Frenulum

Free taenia (taenia libera)

Vermiform appendix

Circular muscle of colon

Mesocolic taenia

Fibers to papilla

Fibers to ileum

Fibers around ileocecal junction

Fibers to taenia

Fibers to papilla

Longitudinal muscle of ileum

Circular muscle of ileum

Ileal papilla: papillary form of ileal orifice (found most commonly in vivo)

Schema of muscle fibers at ileal orifice

Plate 282   **Viscera (Gut)**

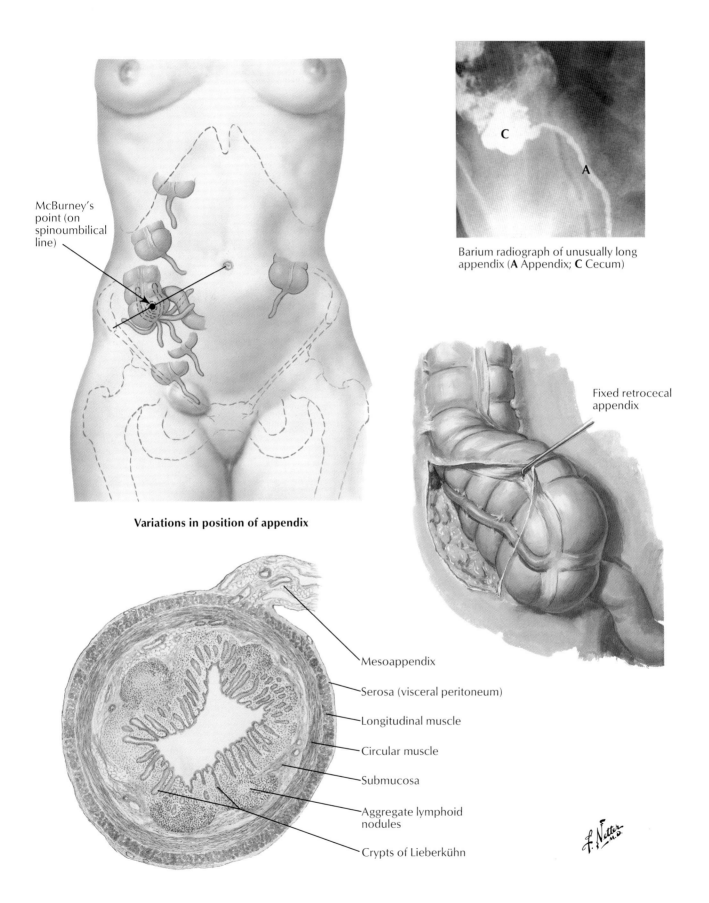

McBurney's point (on spinoumbilical line)

Variations in position of appendix

Barium radiograph of unusually long appendix (**A** Appendix; **C** Cecum)

Fixed retrocecal appendix

Mesoappendix

Serosa (visceral peritoneum)

Longitudinal muscle

Circular muscle

Submucosa

Aggregate lymphoid nodules

Crypts of Lieberkühn

For rectum and anal canal see **Plates 391–396**

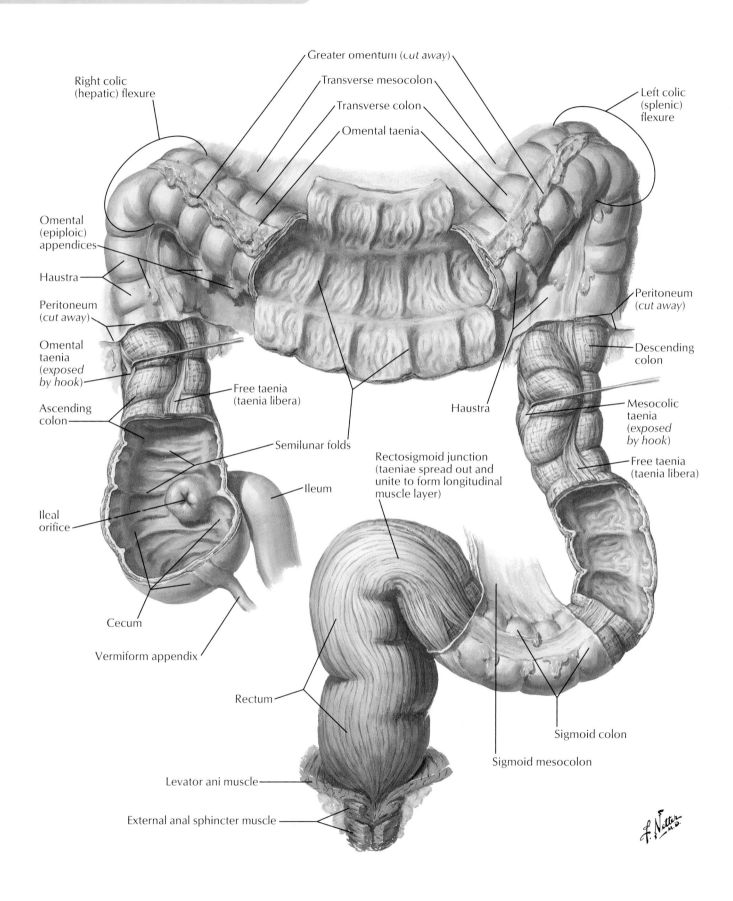

Greater omentum (*cut away*)

Transverse mesocolon

Transverse colon

Omental taenia

Right colic (hepatic) flexure

Left colic (splenic) flexure

Omental (epiploic) appendices

Haustra

Peritoneum (*cut away*)

Omental taenia (*exposed by hook*)

Ascending colon

Ileal orifice

Cecum

Vermiform appendix

Free taenia (taenia libera)

Semilunar folds

Ileum

Rectosigmoid junction (taeniae spread out and unite to form longitudinal muscle layer)

Haustra

Peritoneum (*cut away*)

Descending colon

Mesocolic taenia (*exposed by hook*)

Free taenia (taenia libera)

Rectum

Sigmoid colon

Sigmoid mesocolon

Levator ani muscle

External anal sphincter muscle

f. Netter M.D.

Plate 284 **Viscera (Gut)**

For rectum see **Plates 360, 361, 391–394**

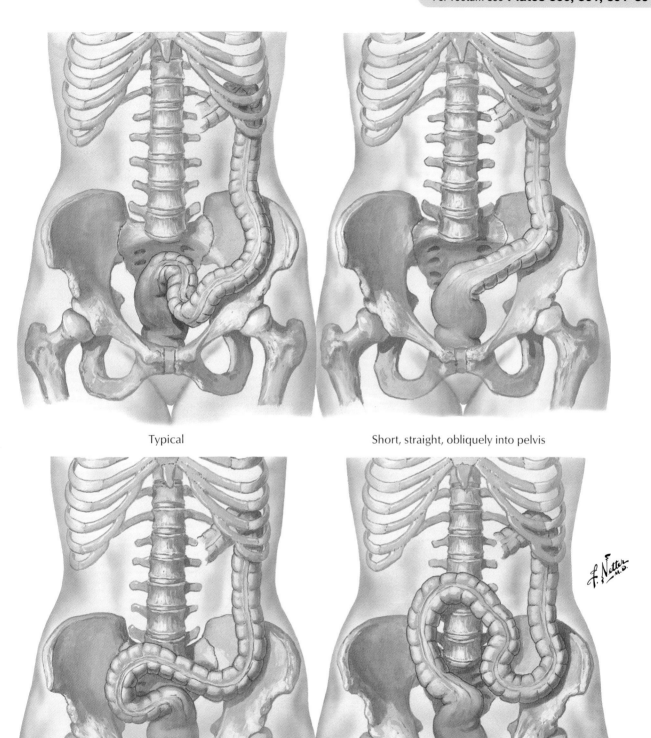

Typical

Short, straight, obliquely into pelvis

Looping to right side

Ascending high into abdomen

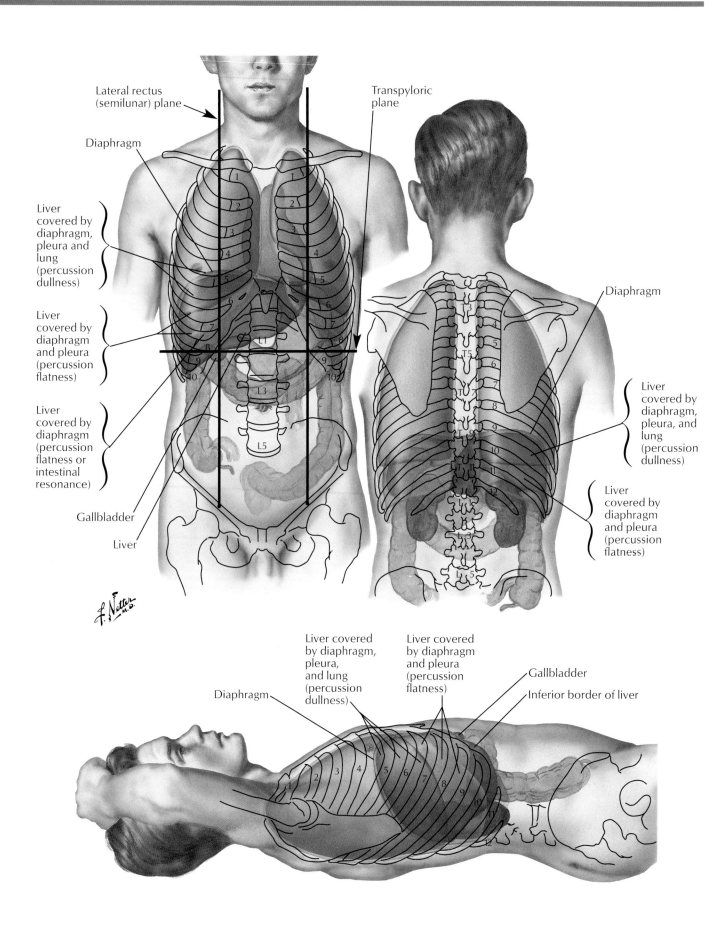

Lateral rectus (semilunar) plane

Transpyloric plane

Diaphragm

Liver covered by diaphragm, pleura and lung (percussion dullness)

Liver covered by diaphragm and pleura (percussion flatness)

Liver covered by diaphragm (percussion flatness or intestinal resonance)

Gallbladder

Liver

Diaphragm

Liver covered by diaphragm, pleura, and lung (percussion dullness)

Liver covered by diaphragm and pleura (percussion flatness)

Liver covered by diaphragm, pleura, and lung (percussion dullness)

Liver covered by diaphragm and pleura (percussion flatness)

Diaphragm

Gallbladder

Inferior border of liver

Plate 286

Viscera (Accessory Organs)

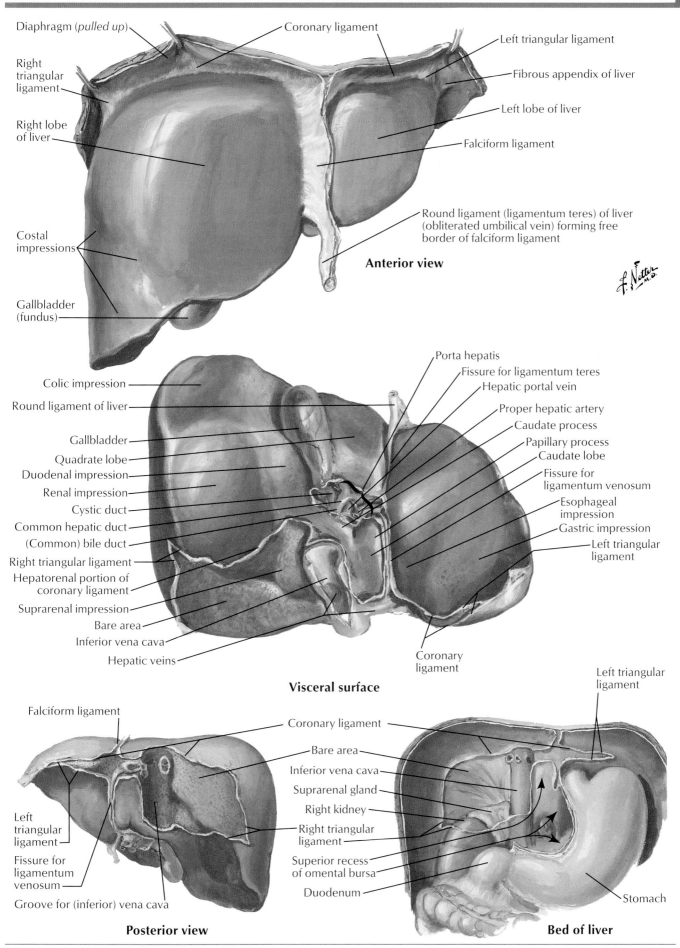

Diaphragm (*pulled up*)

Coronary ligament

Left triangular ligament

Right triangular ligament

Fibrous appendix of liver

Left lobe of liver

Right lobe of liver

Falciform ligament

Costal impressions

Gallbladder (fundus)

Round ligament (ligamentum teres) of liver (obliterated umbilical vein) forming free border of falciform ligament

Anterior view

Colic impression

Round ligament of liver

Gallbladder

Quadrate lobe

Duodenal impression

Renal impression

Cystic duct

Common hepatic duct

(Common) bile duct

Right triangular ligament

Hepatorenal portion of coronary ligament

Suprarenal impression

Bare area

Inferior vena cava

Hepatic veins

Porta hepatis

Fissure for ligamentum teres

Hepatic portal vein

Proper hepatic artery

Caudate process

Papillary process

Caudate lobe

Fissure for ligamentum venosum

Esophageal impression

Gastric impression

Left triangular ligament

Coronary ligament

Visceral surface

Falciform ligament

Coronary ligament

Bare area

Inferior vena cava

Suprarenal gland

Right kidney

Right triangular ligament

Superior recess of omental bursa

Duodenum

Left triangular ligament

Left triangular ligament

Fissure for ligamentum venosum

Groove for (inferior) vena cava

Stomach

Posterior view

Bed of liver

Viscera (Accessory Organs)

Plate 287

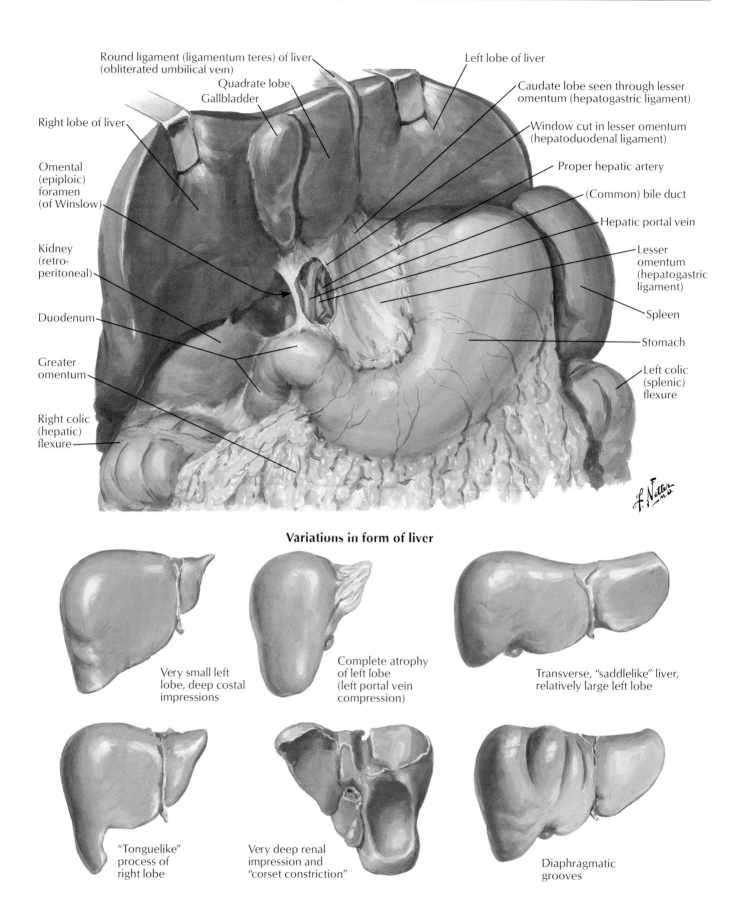

Round ligament (ligamentum teres) of liver (obliterated umbilical vein)

Quadrate lobe

Gallbladder

Left lobe of liver

Caudate lobe seen through lesser omentum (hepatogastric ligament)

Right lobe of liver

Window cut in lesser omentum (hepatoduodenal ligament)

Omental (epiploic) foramen (of Winslow)

Proper hepatic artery

(Common) bile duct

Hepatic portal vein

Kidney (retroperitoneal)

Lesser omentum (hepatogastric ligament)

Duodenum

Spleen

Stomach

Greater omentum

Left colic (splenic) flexure

Right colic (hepatic) flexure

Variations in form of liver

Very small left lobe, deep costal impressions

Complete atrophy of left lobe (left portal vein compression)

Transverse, "saddlelike" liver, relatively large left lobe

"Tonguelike" process of right lobe

Very deep renal impression and "corset constriction"

Diaphragmatic grooves

Plate 288   **Viscera (Accessory Organs)**

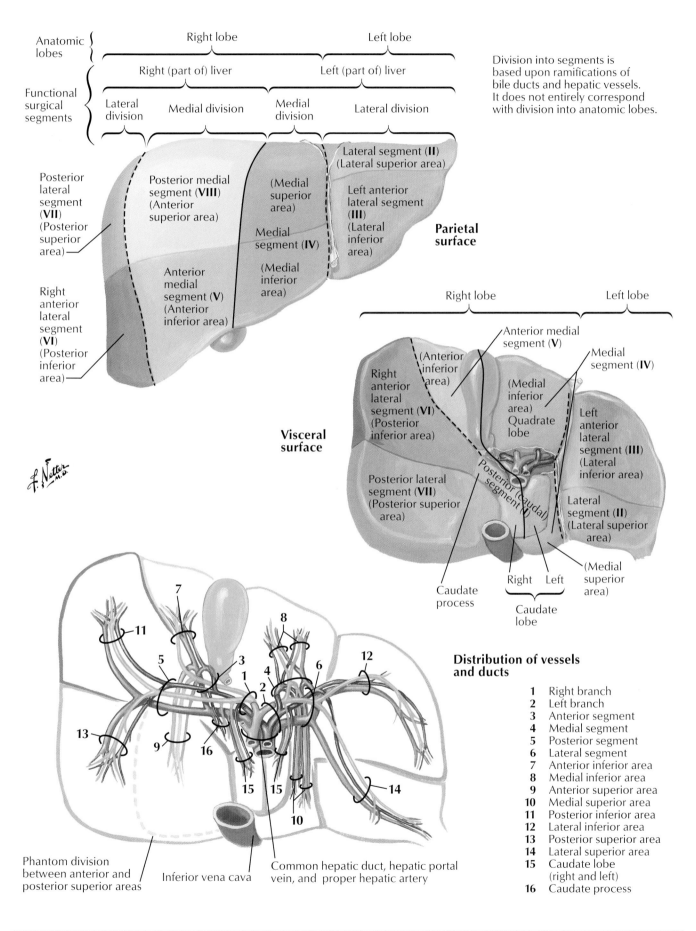

Anatomic lobes

Right lobe

Left lobe

Functional surgical segments

Right (part of) liver

Left (part of) liver

Lateral division

Medial division

Medial division

Lateral division

Division into segments is based upon ramifications of bile ducts and hepatic vessels. It does not entirely correspond with division into anatomic lobes.

Lateral segment (**II**) (Lateral superior area)

Posterior lateral segment (**VII**) (Posterior superior area)

Posterior medial segment (**VIII**) (Anterior superior area)

(Medial superior area)

Left anterior lateral segment (**III**) (Lateral inferior area)

Medial segment (**IV**)

Parietal surface

Right anterior lateral segment (**VI**) (Posterior inferior area)

Anterior medial segment (**V**) (Anterior inferior area)

(Medial inferior area)

Right lobe

Left lobe

Anterior medial segment (**V**)

(Anterior inferior area)

Medial segment (**IV**)

Right anterior lateral segment (**VI**) (Posterior inferior area)

(Medial inferior area) Quadrate lobe

Left anterior lateral segment (**III**) (Lateral inferior area)

Visceral surface

Posterior lateral segment (**VII**) (Posterior superior area)

Posterior (caudal) segment (I)

Lateral segment (**II**) (Lateral superior area)

(Medial superior area)

Caudate process

Right Left

Caudate lobe

Phantom division between anterior and posterior superior areas

Inferior vena cava

Common hepatic duct, hepatic portal vein, and proper hepatic artery

Distribution of vessels and ducts

1	Right branch
2	Left branch
3	Anterior segment
4	Medial segment
5	Posterior segment
6	Lateral segment
7	Anterior inferior area
8	Medial inferior area
9	Anterior superior area
10	Medial superior area
11	Posterior inferior area
12	Lateral inferior area
13	Posterior superior area
14	Lateral superior area
15	Caudate lobe (right and left)
16	Caudate process

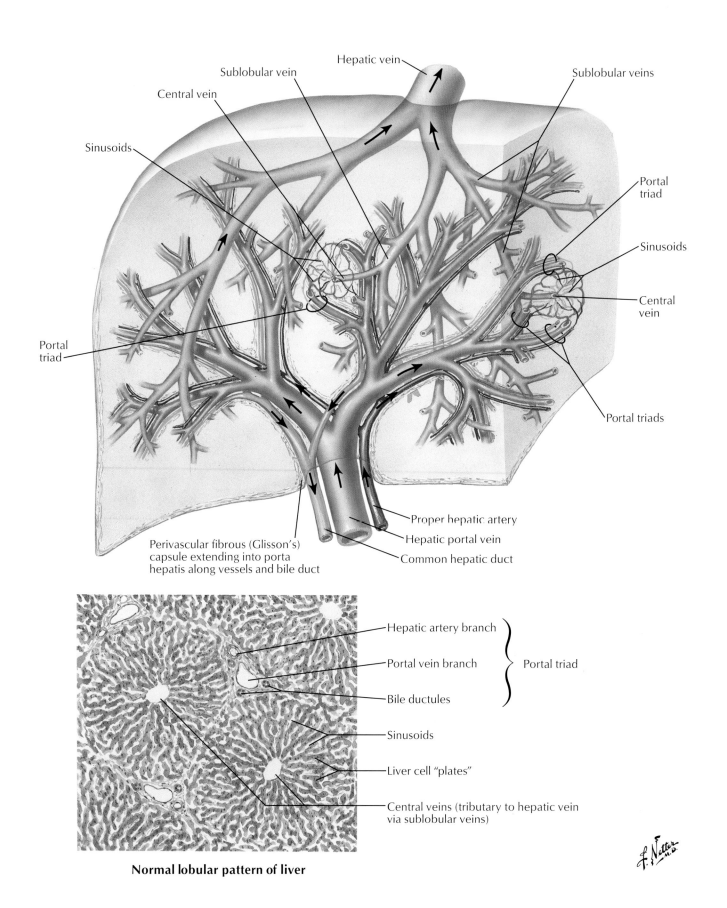

Hepatic vein

Sublobular vein

Central vein

Sinusoids

Sublobular veins

Portal triad

Sinusoids

Central vein

Portal triad

Portal triads

Proper hepatic artery

Hepatic portal vein

Common hepatic duct

Perivascular fibrous (Glisson's) capsule extending into porta hepatis along vessels and bile duct

Hepatic artery branch

Portal vein branch

Bile ductules

Portal triad

Sinusoids

Liver cell "plates"

Central veins (tributary to hepatic vein via sublobular veins)

Normal lobular pattern of liver

Plate 290

Viscera (Accessory Organs)

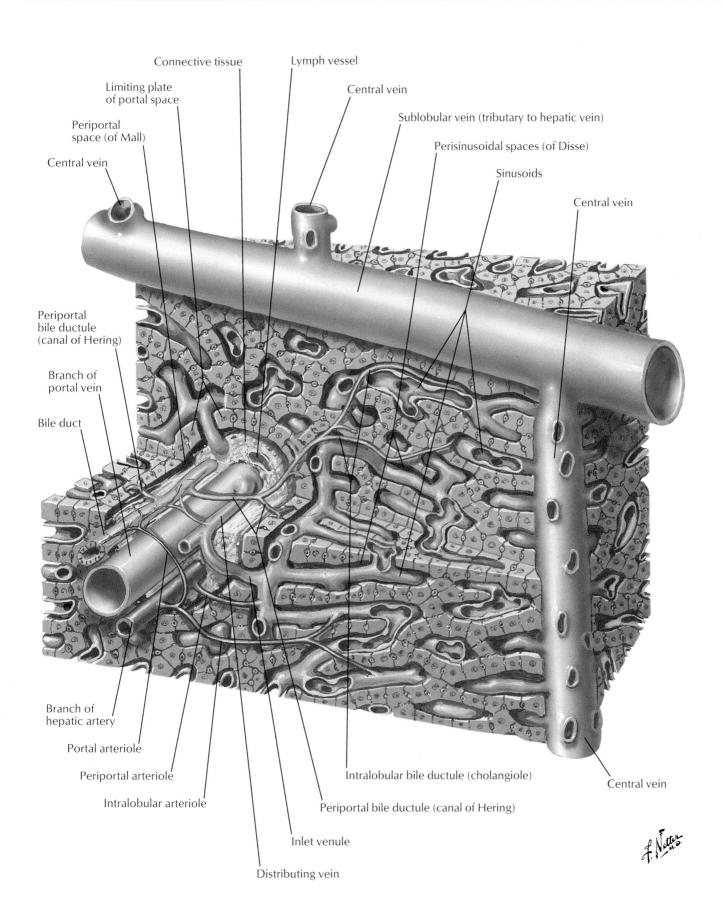

Connective tissue

Limiting plate
of portal space

Lymph vessel

Central vein

Periportal
space (of Mall)

Sublobular vein (tributary to hepatic vein)

Central vein

Perisinusoidal spaces (of Disse)

Sinusoids

Central vein

Periportal
bile ductule
(canal of Hering)

Branch of
portal vein

Bile duct

Branch of
hepatic artery

Portal arteriole

Periportal arteriole

Intralobular arteriole

Intralobular bile ductule (cholangiole)

Periportal bile ductule (canal of Hering)

Central vein

Inlet venule

Distributing vein

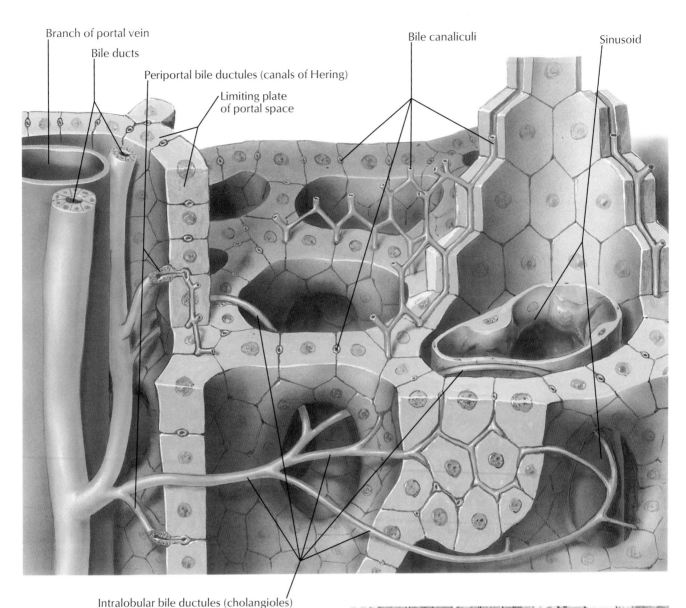

Branch of portal vein

Bile ducts

Periportal bile ductules (canals of Hering)

Limiting plate of portal space

Bile canaliculi

Sinusoid

Intralobular bile ductules (cholangioles)

Note: In the above illustration, bile canaliculi appear as structures with walls of their own. However, as shown in the histologic section at right, boundaries of canaliculi are actually a specialization of surface membranes of adjoining liver parenchymal cells.

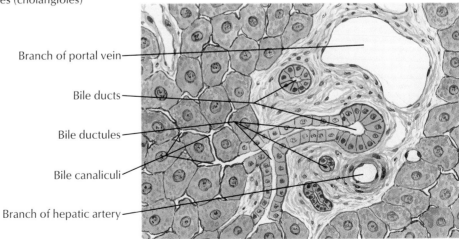

Branch of portal vein

Bile ducts

Bile ductules

Bile canaliculi

Branch of hepatic artery

Low-power section of liver

Plate 292 **Viscera (Accessory Organs)**

Transverse Section: Level of T10, Esophagogastric Junction

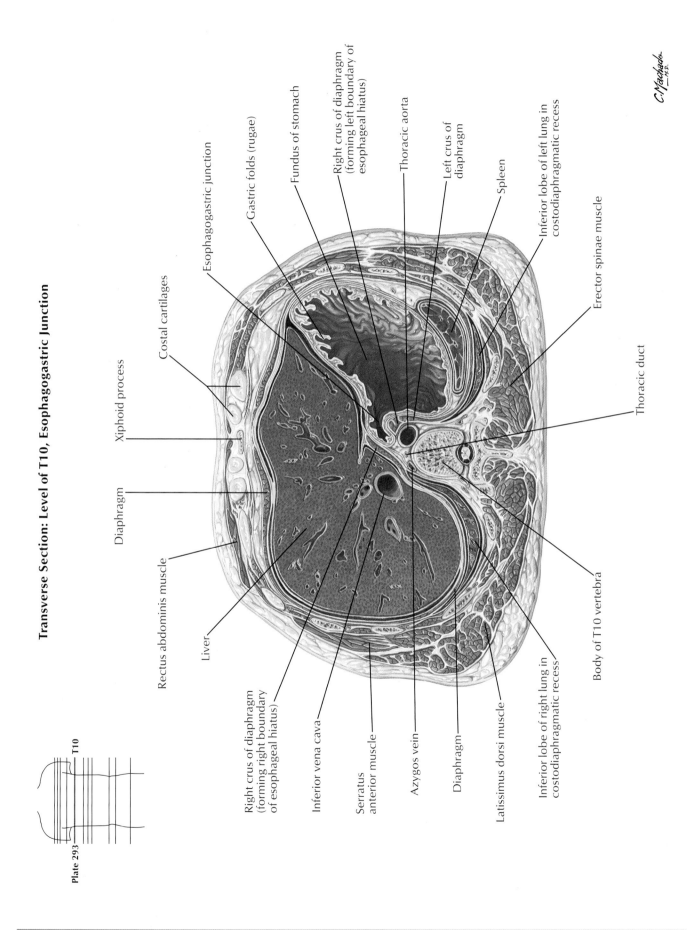

Esophagogastric junction

Gastric folds (rugae)

Fundus of stomach

Right crus of diaphragm (forming left boundary of esophageal hiatus)

Thoracic aorta

Left crus of diaphragm

Spleen

Inferior lobe of left lung in costodiaphragmatic recess

Erector spinae muscle

Costal cartilages

Xiphoid process

Diaphragm

Rectus abdominis muscle

Liver

Right crus of diaphragm (forming right boundary of esophageal hiatus)

Inferior vena cava

Serratus anterior muscle

Azygos vein

Diaphragm

Latissimus dorsi muscle

Inferior lobe of right lung in costodiaphragmatic recess

Body of T10 vertebra

Thoracic duct

T10

Plate 293

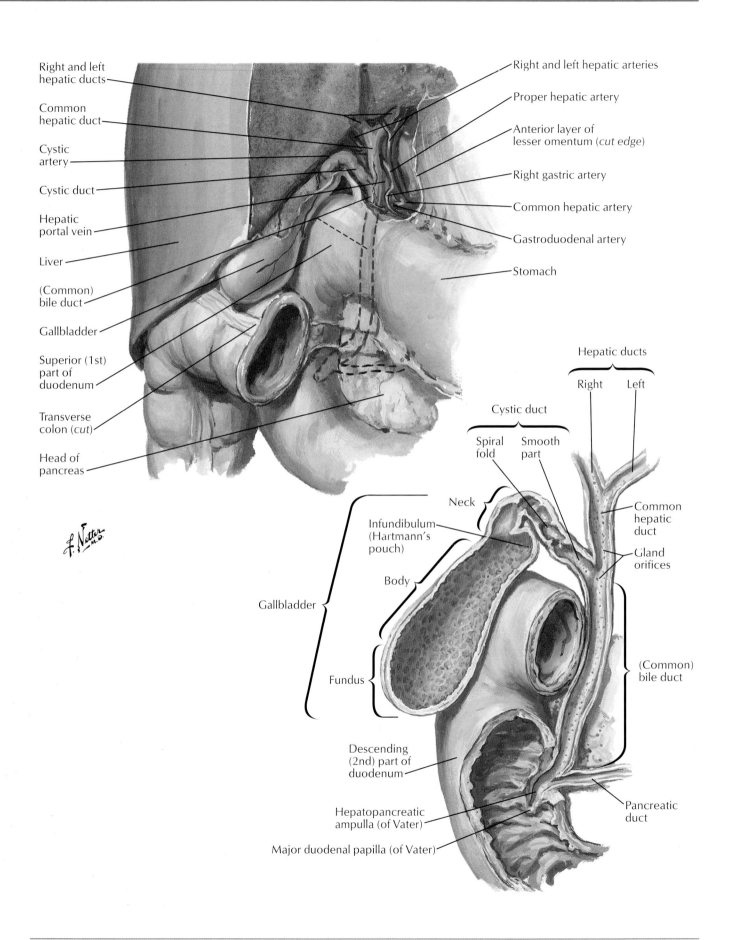

Right and left hepatic ducts

Common hepatic duct

Cystic artery

Cystic duct

Hepatic portal vein

Liver

(Common) bile duct

Gallbladder

Superior (1st) part of duodenum

Transverse colon (*cut*)

Head of pancreas

Right and left hepatic arteries

Proper hepatic artery

Anterior layer of lesser omentum (*cut edge*)

Right gastric artery

Common hepatic artery

Gastroduodenal artery

Stomach

Hepatic ducts

Right   Left

Cystic duct

Spiral fold   Smooth part

Neck

Infundibulum (Hartmann's pouch)

Body

Gallbladder

Fundus

Common hepatic duct

Gland orifices

(Common) bile duct

Descending (2nd) part of duodenum

Hepatopancreatic ampulla (of Vater)

Major duodenal papilla (of Vater)

Pancreatic duct

Plate 294   **Viscera (Accessory Organs)**

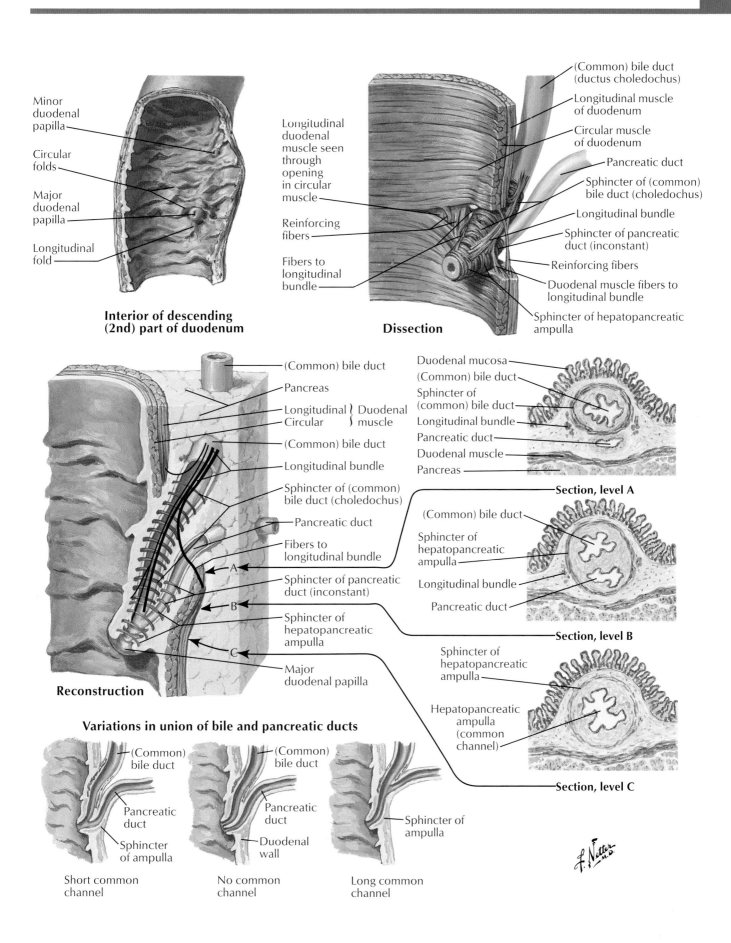

Minor duodenal papilla

Circular folds

Major duodenal papilla

Longitudinal fold

Interior of descending (2nd) part of duodenum

Longitudinal duodenal muscle seen through opening in circular muscle

Reinforcing fibers

Fibers to longitudinal bundle

(Common) bile duct (ductus choledochus)

Longitudinal muscle of duodenum

Circular muscle of duodenum

Pancreatic duct

Sphincter of (common) bile duct (choledochus)

Longitudinal bundle

Sphincter of pancreatic duct (inconstant)

Reinforcing fibers

Duodenal muscle fibers to longitudinal bundle

Sphincter of hepatopancreatic ampulla

Dissection

(Common) bile duct

Pancreas

Longitudinal / Duodenal
Circular / muscle

(Common) bile duct

Longitudinal bundle

Sphincter of (common) bile duct (choledochus)

Pancreatic duct

Fibers to longitudinal bundle

A

Sphincter of pancreatic duct (inconstant)

B

Sphincter of hepatopancreatic ampulla

C

Major duodenal papilla

Reconstruction

Duodenal mucosa

(Common) bile duct

Sphincter of (common) bile duct

Longitudinal bundle

Pancreatic duct

Duodenal muscle

Pancreas

Section, level A

(Common) bile duct

Sphincter of hepatopancreatic ampulla

Longitudinal bundle

Pancreatic duct

Section, level B

Sphincter of hepatopancreatic ampulla

Hepatopancreatic ampulla (common channel)

Section, level C

Variations in union of bile and pancreatic ducts

(Common) bile duct

Pancreatic duct

Sphincter of ampulla

Short common channel

(Common) bile duct

Pancreatic duct

Duodenal wall

No common channel

Sphincter of ampulla

Long common channel

Variations in cystic duct

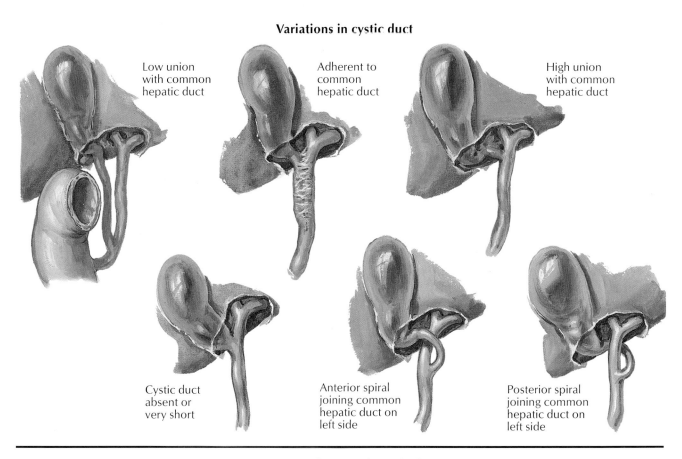

Low union with common hepatic duct

Adherent to common hepatic duct

High union with common hepatic duct

Cystic duct absent or very short

Anterior spiral joining common hepatic duct on left side

Posterior spiral joining common hepatic duct on left side

Accessory (aberrant) hepatic ducts

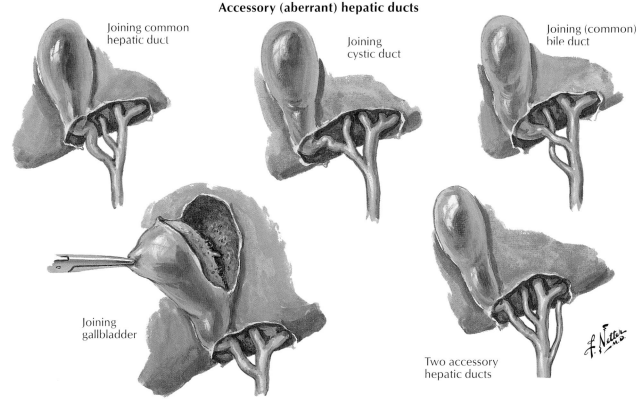

Joining common hepatic duct

Joining cystic duct

Joining (common) bile duct

Joining gallbladder

Two accessory hepatic ducts

Plate 296

Viscera (Accessory Organs)

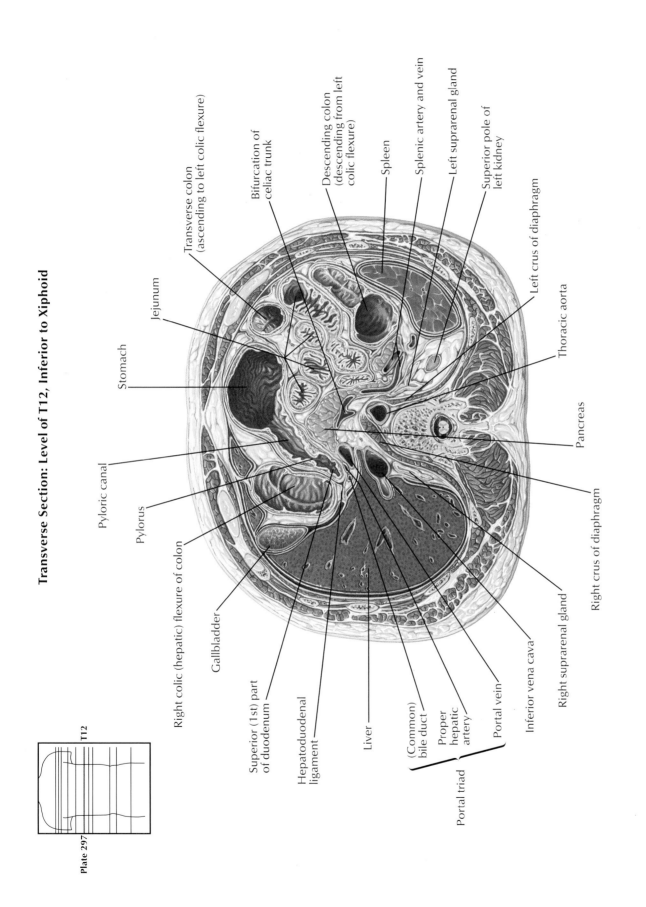

Transverse Section: Level of T12, Inferior to Xiphoid

Transverse colon
(ascending to left colic flexure)

Bifurcation of
celiac trunk

Descending colon
(descending from left
colic flexure)

Spleen

Splenic artery and vein

Left suprarenal gland

Superior pole of
left kidney

Left crus of diaphragm

Thoracic aorta

Jejunum

Stomach

Pancreas

Pyloric canal

Pylorus

Right colic (hepatic) flexure of colon

Gallbladder

Superior (1st) part
of duodenum

Hepatoduodenal
ligament

Liver

(Common)
bile duct

Proper
hepatic
artery

Portal vein

Portal triad

Inferior vena cava

Right suprarenal gland

Right crus of diaphragm

Plate 297

T12

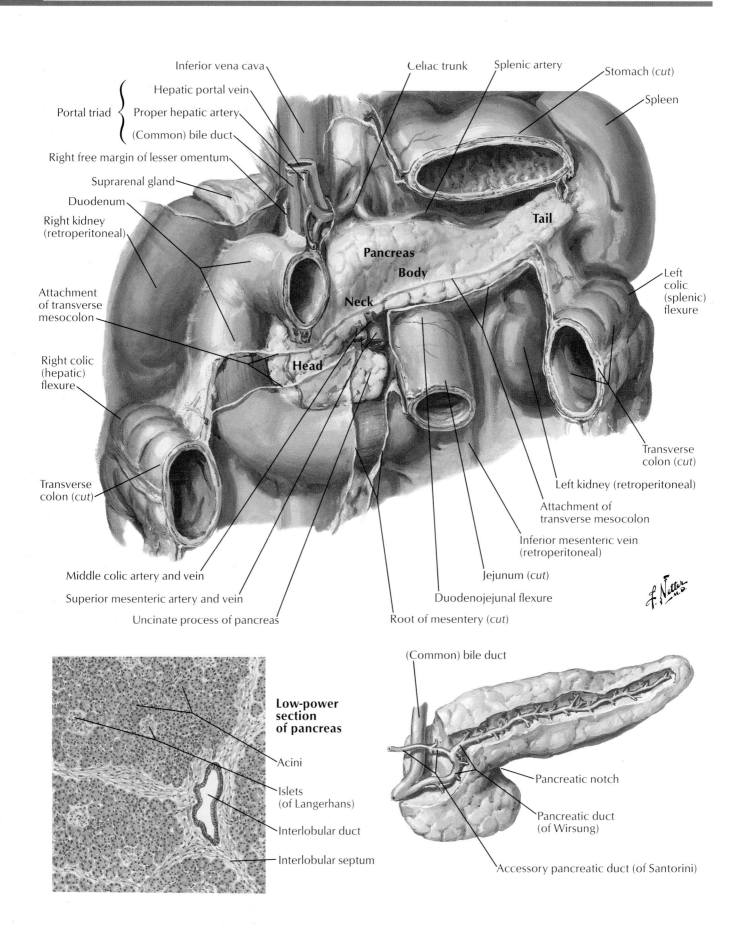

Inferior vena cava

Celiac trunk

Splenic artery

Stomach (cut)

Spleen

Portal triad
- Hepatic portal vein
- Proper hepatic artery
- (Common) bile duct

Right free margin of lesser omentum

Suprarenal gland

Duodenum

Right kidney (retroperitoneal)

Attachment of transverse mesocolon

Right colic (hepatic) flexure

Transverse colon (cut)

Middle colic artery and vein

Superior mesenteric artery and vein

Uncinate process of pancreas

Tail

Pancreas

Body

Neck

Head

Left colic (splenic) flexure

Transverse colon (cut)

Left kidney (retroperitoneal)

Attachment of transverse mesocolon

Inferior mesenteric vein (retroperitoneal)

Jejunum (cut)

Duodenojejunal flexure

Root of mesentery (cut)

Low-power section of pancreas

Acini

Islets (of Langerhans)

Interlobular duct

Interlobular septum

(Common) bile duct

Pancreatic notch

Pancreatic duct (of Wirsung)

Accessory pancreatic duct (of Santorini)

Plate 298

Viscera (Accessory Organs)

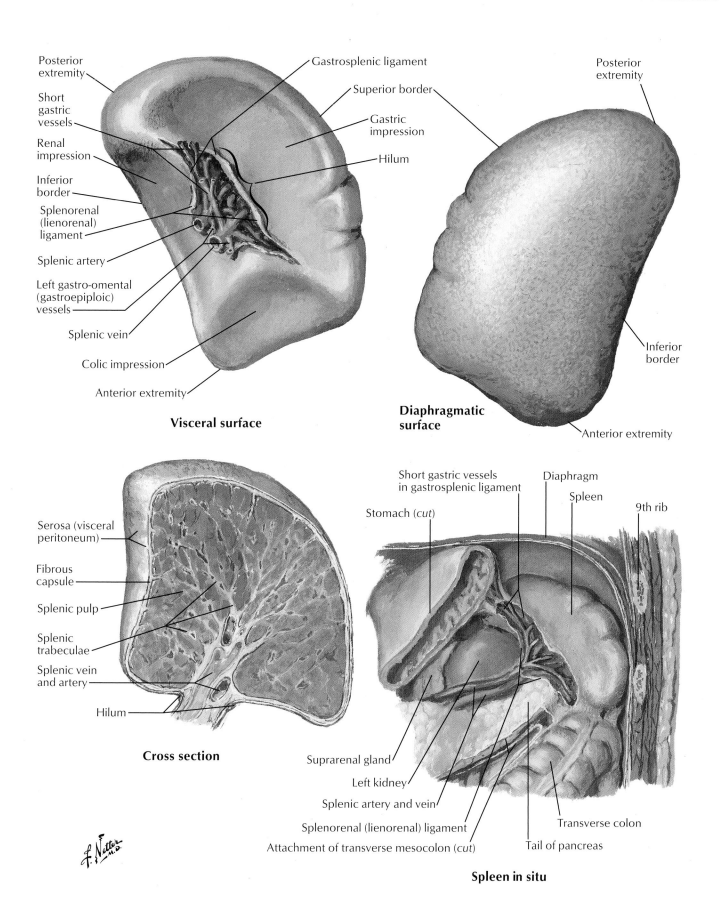

Posterior extremity

Short gastric vessels

Renal impression

Inferior border

Splenorenal (lienorenal) ligament

Splenic artery

Left gastro-omental (gastroepiploic) vessels

Splenic vein

Colic impression

Anterior extremity

Gastrosplenic ligament

Superior border

Gastric impression

Hilum

Visceral surface

Posterior extremity

Inferior border

Anterior extremity

Diaphragmatic surface

Serosa (visceral peritoneum)

Fibrous capsule

Splenic pulp

Splenic trabeculae

Splenic vein and artery

Hilum

Cross section

Short gastric vessels in gastrosplenic ligament

Diaphragm

Spleen

9th rib

Stomach (*cut*)

Suprarenal gland

Left kidney

Splenic artery and vein

Splenorenal (lienorenal) ligament

Attachment of transverse mesocolon (*cut*)

Transverse colon

Tail of pancreas

Spleen in situ

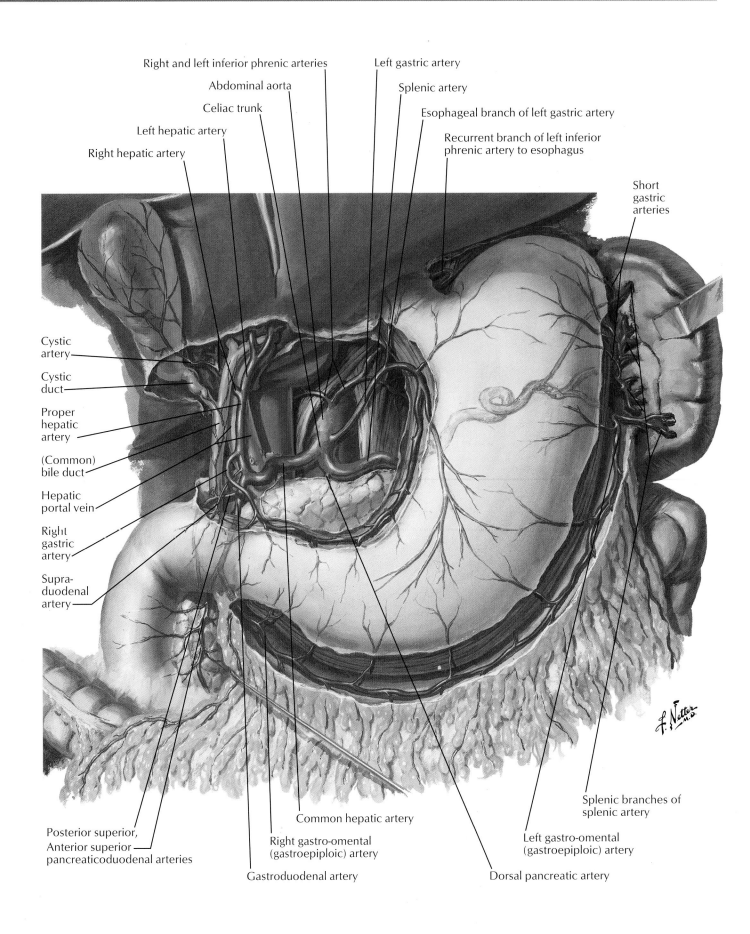

Right and left inferior phrenic arteries

Abdominal aorta

Celiac trunk

Left hepatic artery

Right hepatic artery

Left gastric artery

Splenic artery

Esophageal branch of left gastric artery

Recurrent branch of left inferior phrenic artery to esophagus

Short gastric arteries

Cystic artery

Cystic duct

Proper hepatic artery

(Common) bile duct

Hepatic portal vein

Right gastric artery

Supra-duodenal artery

Splenic branches of splenic artery

Left gastro-omental (gastroepiploic) artery

Dorsal pancreatic artery

Common hepatic artery

Right gastro-omental (gastroepiploic) artery

Gastroduodenal artery

Posterior superior, Anterior superior pancreaticoduodenal arteries

Plate 300

Visceral Vasculature

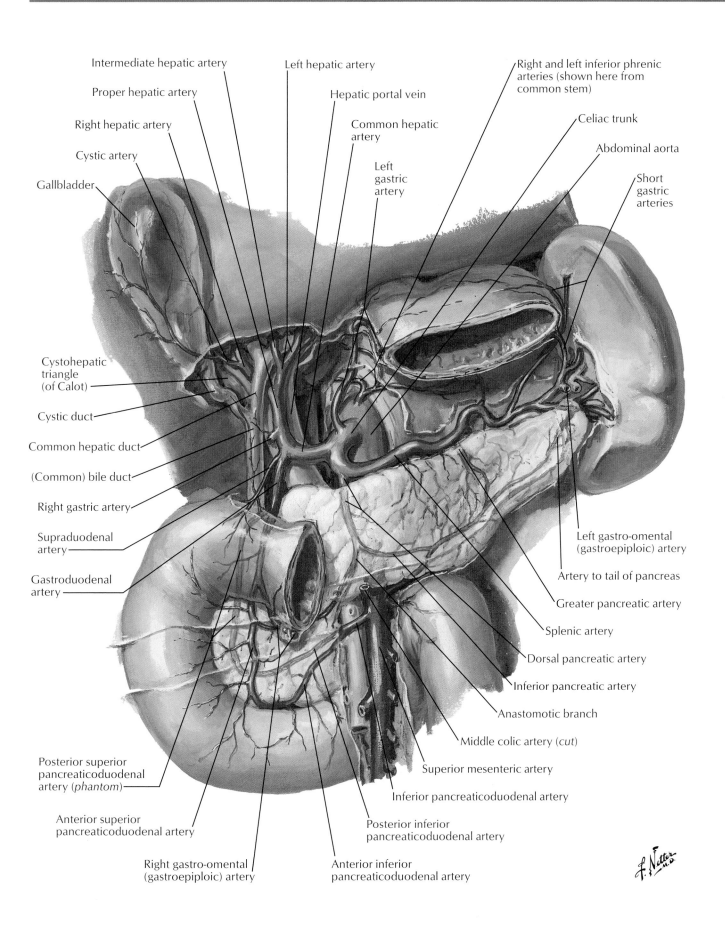

Intermediate hepatic artery

Proper hepatic artery

Right hepatic artery

Cystic artery

Gallbladder

Left hepatic artery

Hepatic portal vein

Common hepatic artery

Left gastric artery

Right and left inferior phrenic arteries (shown here from common stem)

Celiac trunk

Abdominal aorta

Short gastric arteries

Cystohepatic triangle (of Calot)

Cystic duct

Common hepatic duct

(Common) bile duct

Right gastric artery

Supraduodenal artery

Gastroduodenal artery

Posterior superior pancreaticoduodenal artery (*phantom*)

Anterior superior pancreaticoduodenal artery

Right gastro-omental (gastroepiploic) artery

Anterior inferior pancreaticoduodenal artery

Posterior inferior pancreaticoduodenal artery

Inferior pancreaticoduodenal artery

Superior mesenteric artery

Middle colic artery (*cut*)

Anastomotic branch

Inferior pancreatic artery

Dorsal pancreatic artery

Splenic artery

Greater pancreatic artery

Artery to tail of pancreas

Left gastro-omental (gastroepiploic) artery

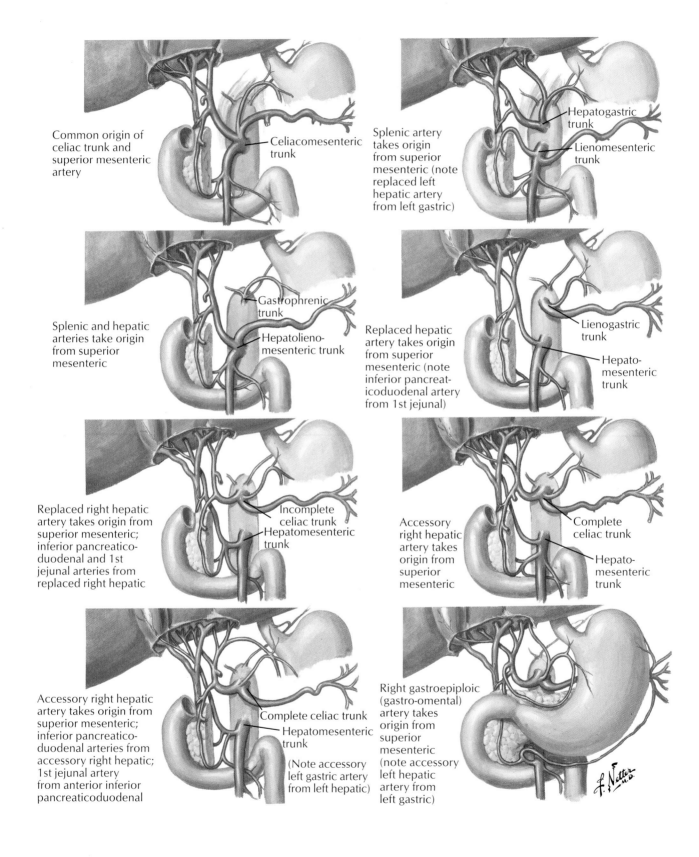

Plate 302   **Visceral Vasculature**

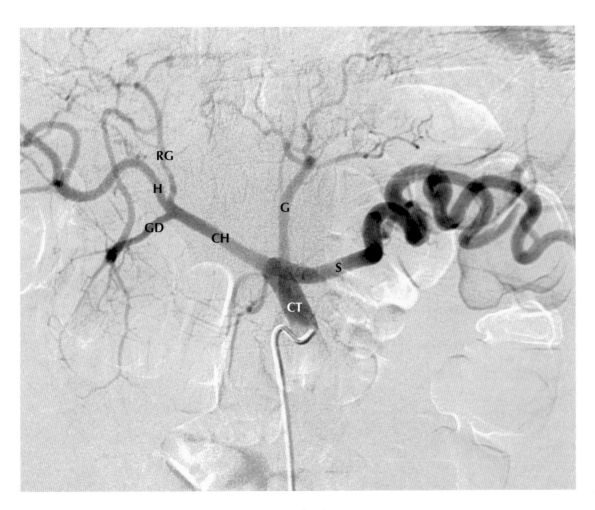

CH	Common hepatic artery
CT	Celiac trunk
G	Left gastric artery
GD	Gastroduodenal artery
H	Proper hepatic artery
RG	Right gastric artery
S	Splenic artery

Duodenum and head of pancreas reflected to left

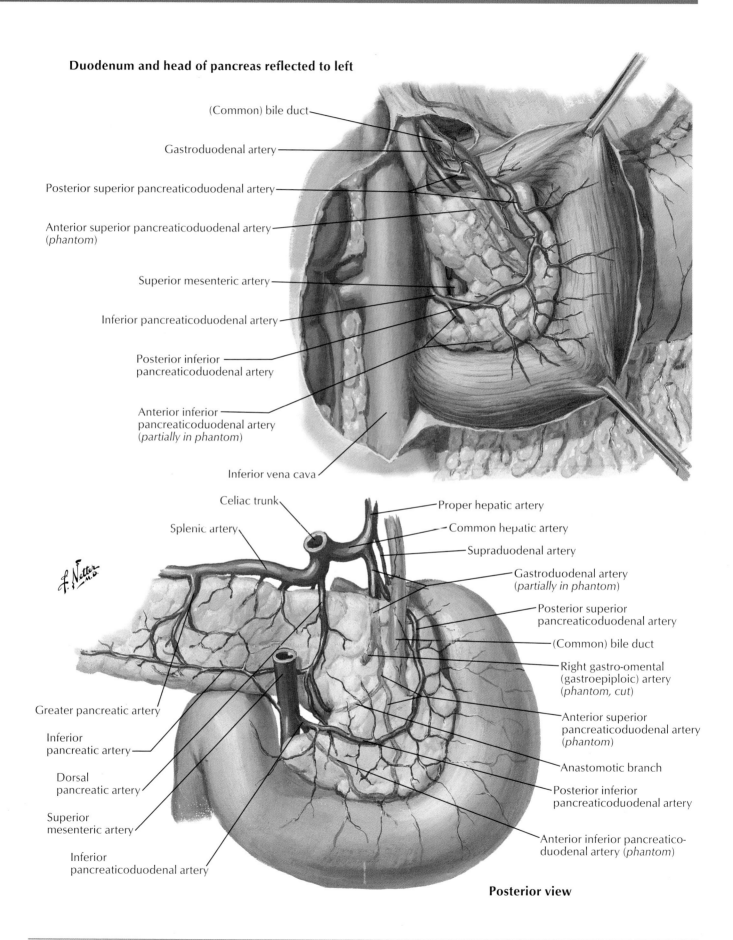

(Common) bile duct

Gastroduodenal artery

Posterior superior pancreaticoduodenal artery

Anterior superior pancreaticoduodenal artery
(*phantom*)

Superior mesenteric artery

Inferior pancreaticoduodenal artery

Posterior inferior
pancreaticoduodenal artery

Anterior inferior
pancreaticoduodenal artery
(*partially in phantom*)

Inferior vena cava

Celiac trunk

Splenic artery

Greater pancreatic artery

Inferior
pancreatic artery

Dorsal
pancreatic artery

Superior
mesenteric artery

Inferior
pancreaticoduodenal artery

Proper hepatic artery

Common hepatic artery

Supraduodenal artery

Gastroduodenal artery
(*partially in phantom*)

Posterior superior
pancreaticoduodenal artery

(Common) bile duct

Right gastro-omental
(gastroepiploic) artery
(*phantom, cut*)

Anterior superior
pancreaticoduodenal artery
(*phantom*)

Anastomotic branch

Posterior inferior
pancreaticoduodenal artery

Anterior inferior pancreaticoduodenal artery (*phantom*)

Posterior view

Plate 304   **Visceral Vasculature**

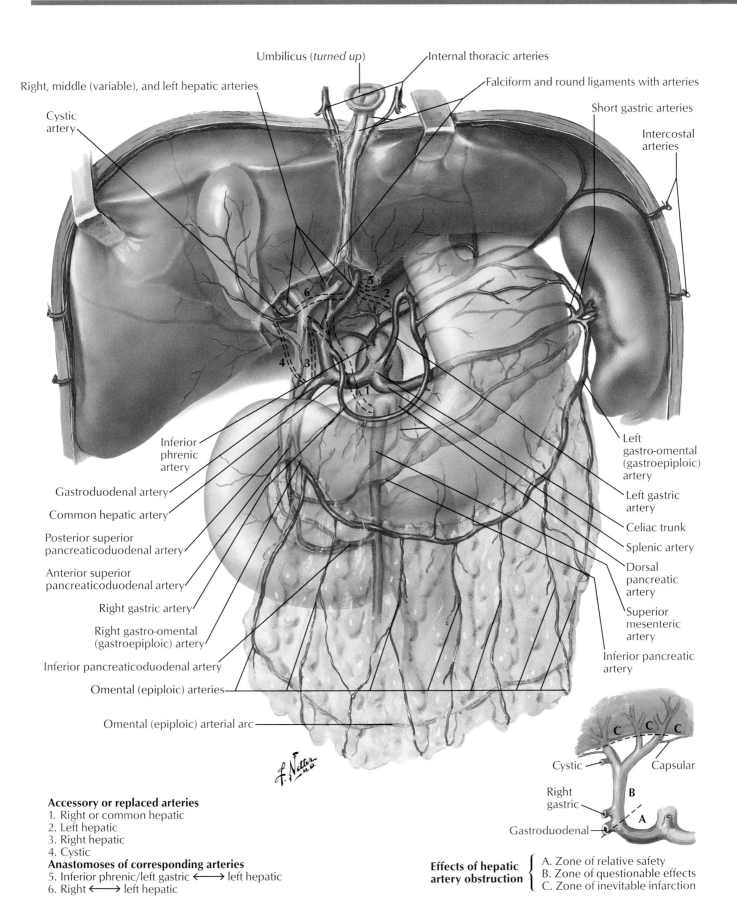

Umbilicus (*turned up*)

Internal thoracic arteries

Right, middle (variable), and left hepatic arteries

Falciform and round ligaments with arteries

Short gastric arteries

Cystic artery

Intercostal arteries

Inferior phrenic artery

Gastroduodenal artery

Common hepatic artery

Posterior superior pancreaticoduodenal artery

Anterior superior pancreaticoduodenal artery

Right gastric artery

Right gastro-omental (gastroepiploic) artery

Inferior pancreaticoduodenal artery

Omental (epiploic) arteries

Omental (epiploic) arterial arc

Left gastro-omental (gastroepiploic) artery

Left gastric artery

Celiac trunk

Splenic artery

Dorsal pancreatic artery

Superior mesenteric artery

Inferior pancreatic artery

Cystic

Capsular

Right gastric

Gastroduodenal

Accessory or replaced arteries
1. Right or common hepatic
2. Left hepatic
3. Right hepatic
4. Cystic

Anastomoses of corresponding arteries
5. Inferior phrenic/left gastric ⟷ left hepatic
6. Right ⟷ left hepatic

Effects of hepatic artery obstruction { A. Zone of relative safety
B. Zone of questionable effects
C. Zone of inevitable infarction

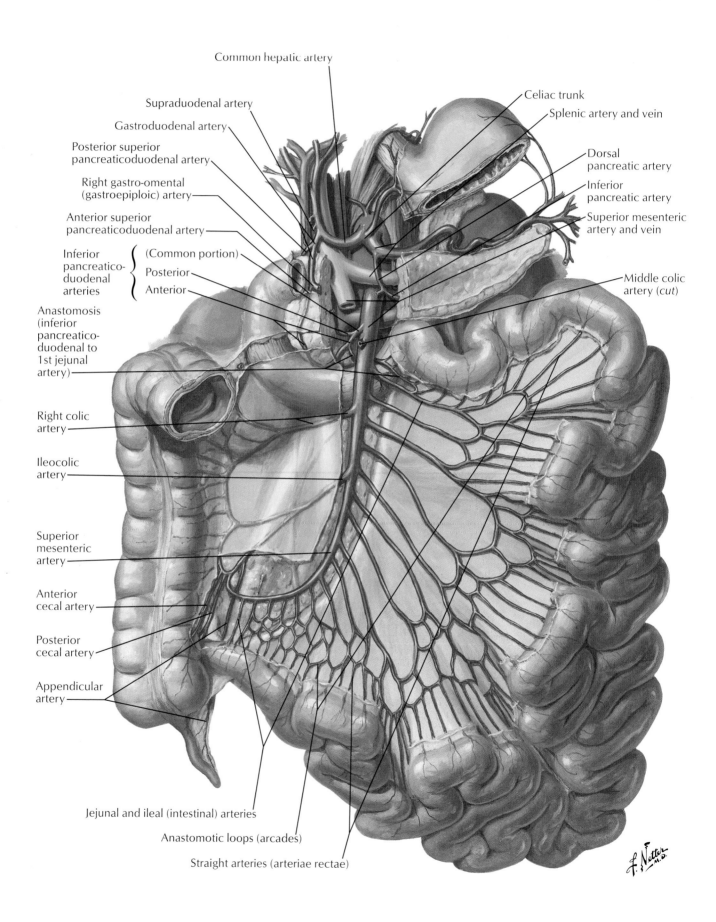

Common hepatic artery

Supraduodenal artery

Gastroduodenal artery

Posterior superior
pancreaticoduodenal artery

Right gastro-omental
(gastroepiploic) artery

Anterior superior
pancreaticoduodenal artery

Inferior
pancreatico-
duodenal
arteries
{ (Common portion)
Posterior
Anterior

Anastomosis
(inferior
pancreatico-
duodenal to
1st jejunal
artery)

Right colic
artery

Ileocolic
artery

Superior
mesenteric
artery

Anterior
cecal artery

Posterior
cecal artery

Appendicular
artery

Celiac trunk

Splenic artery and vein

Dorsal
pancreatic artery

Inferior
pancreatic artery

Superior mesenteric
artery and vein

Middle colic
artery (cut)

Jejunal and ileal (intestinal) arteries

Anastomotic loops (arcades)

Straight arteries (arteriae rectae)

Plate 306   **Visceral Vasculature**

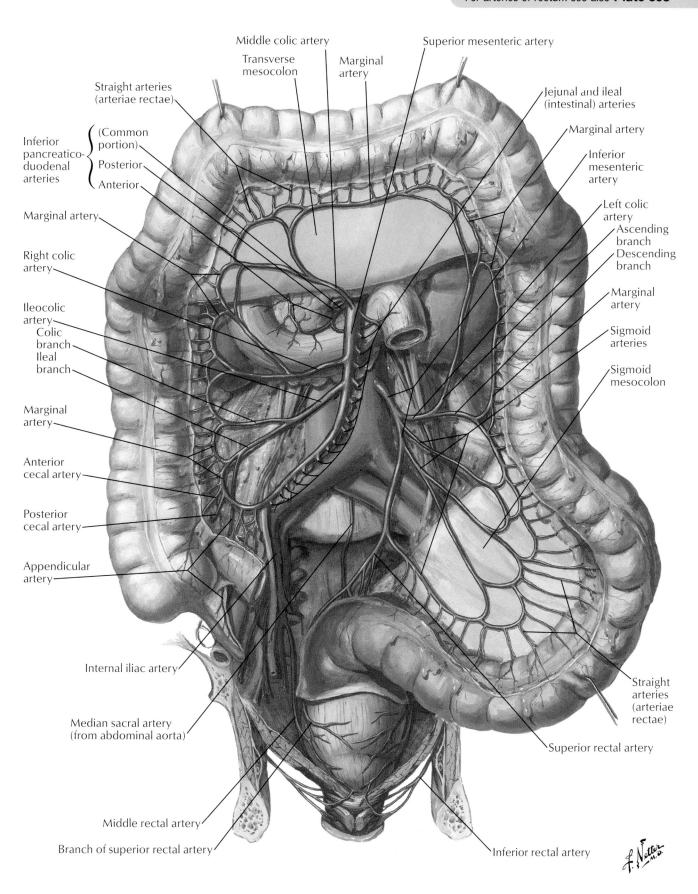

Middle colic artery

Transverse mesocolon

Marginal artery

Superior mesenteric artery

Jejunal and ileal (intestinal) arteries

Straight arteries (arteriae rectae)

(Common portion)

Posterior

Anterior

Inferior pancreaticoduodenal arteries

Marginal artery

Right colic artery

Ileocolic artery

Colic branch

Ileal branch

Marginal artery

Anterior cecal artery

Posterior cecal artery

Appendicular artery

Internal iliac artery

Median sacral artery (from abdominal aorta)

Middle rectal artery

Branch of superior rectal artery

Marginal artery

Inferior mesenteric artery

Left colic artery

Ascending branch

Descending branch

Marginal artery

Sigmoid arteries

Sigmoid mesocolon

Straight arteries (arteriae rectae)

Superior rectal artery

Inferior rectal artery

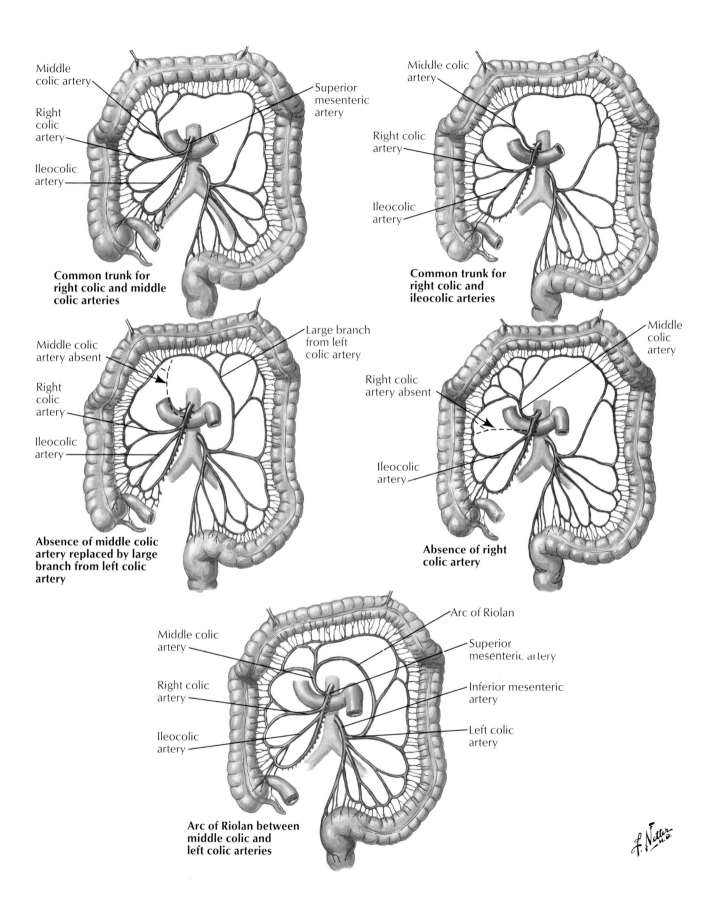

Middle colic artery

Right colic artery

Ileocolic artery

Superior mesenteric artery

Common trunk for right colic and middle colic arteries

Middle colic artery

Right colic artery

Ileocolic artery

Common trunk for right colic and ileocolic arteries

Middle colic artery absent

Right colic artery

Ileocolic artery

Large branch from left colic artery

Absence of middle colic artery replaced by large branch from left colic artery

Right colic artery absent

Ileocolic artery

Middle colic artery

Absence of right colic artery

Middle colic artery

Right colic artery

Ileocolic artery

Arc of Riolan

Superior mesenteric artery

Inferior mesenteric artery

Left colic artery

Arc of Riolan between middle colic and left colic arteries

Plate 308   **Visceral Vasculature**

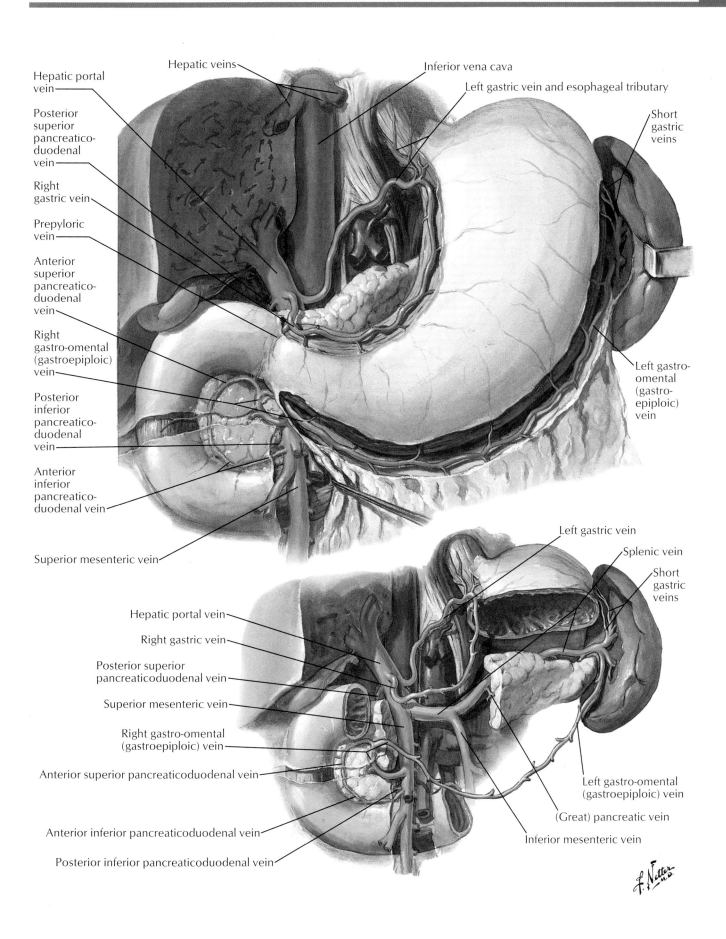

Hepatic veins

Inferior vena cava

Left gastric vein and esophageal tributary

Hepatic portal vein

Posterior superior pancreatico-duodenal vein

Right gastric vein

Prepyloric vein

Anterior superior pancreatico-duodenal vein

Right gastro-omental (gastroepiploic) vein

Posterior inferior pancreatico-duodenal vein

Anterior inferior pancreatico-duodenal vein

Superior mesenteric vein

Short gastric veins

Left gastro-omental (gastro-epiploic) vein

Left gastric vein

Splenic vein

Short gastric veins

Hepatic portal vein

Right gastric vein

Posterior superior pancreaticoduodenal vein

Superior mesenteric vein

Right gastro-omental (gastroepiploic) vein

Anterior superior pancreaticoduodenal vein

Anterior inferior pancreaticoduodenal vein

Posterior inferior pancreaticoduodenal vein

Left gastro-omental (gastroepiploic) vein

(Great) pancreatic vein

Inferior mesenteric vein

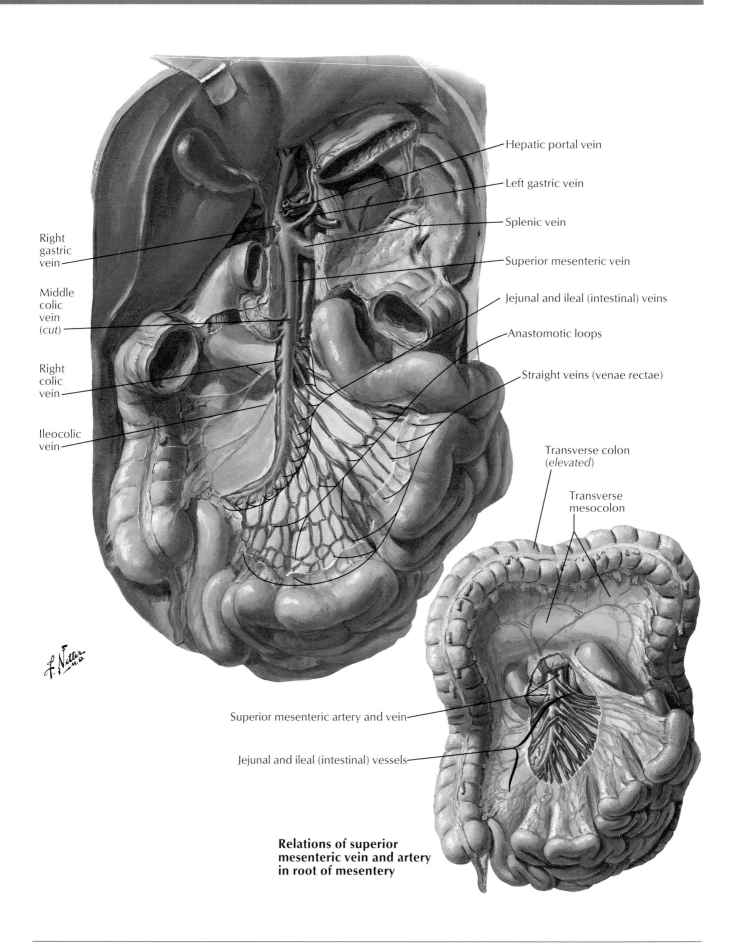

Hepatic portal vein

Left gastric vein

Splenic vein

Superior mesenteric vein

Jejunal and ileal (intestinal) veins

Anastomotic loops

Straight veins (venae rectae)

Right
gastric
vein

Middle
colic
vein
(*cut*)

Right
colic
vein

Ileocolic
vein

Transverse colon
(*elevated*)

Transverse
mesocolon

Superior mesenteric artery and vein

Jejunal and ileal (intestinal) vessels

**Relations of superior
mesenteric vein and artery
in root of mesentery**

Plate 310   **Visceral Vasculature**

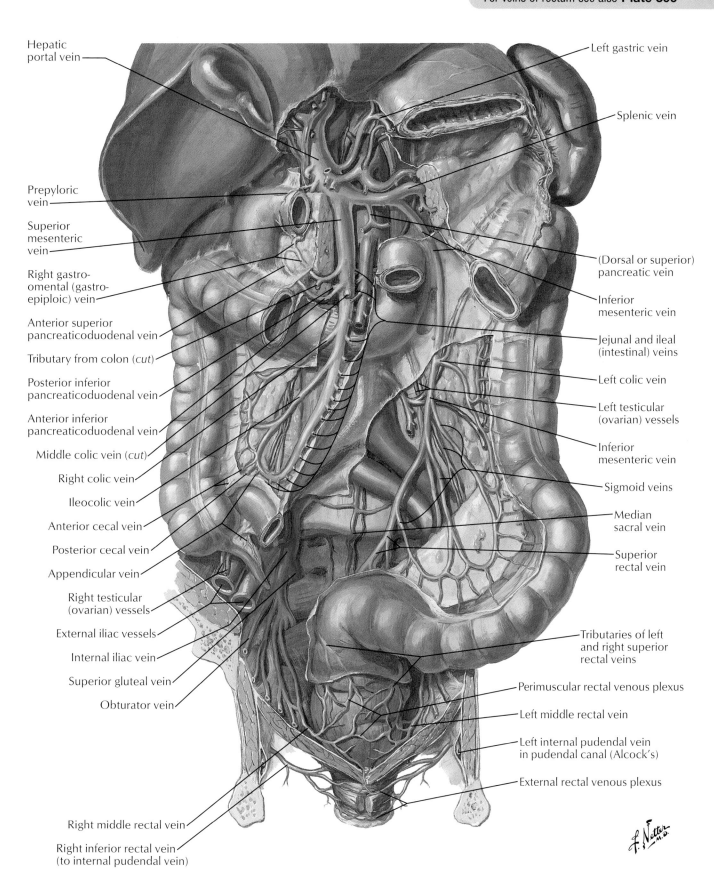

Hepatic portal vein

Left gastric vein

Prepyloric vein

Splenic vein

Superior mesenteric vein

(Dorsal or superior) pancreatic vein

Right gastro-omental (gastro-epiploic) vein

Inferior mesenteric vein

Anterior superior pancreaticoduodenal vein

Jejunal and ileal (intestinal) veins

Tributary from colon (cut)

Left colic vein

Posterior inferior pancreaticoduodenal vein

Left testicular (ovarian) vessels

Anterior inferior pancreaticoduodenal vein

Inferior mesenteric vein

Middle colic vein (cut)

Right colic vein

Sigmoid veins

Ileocolic vein

Median sacral vein

Anterior cecal vein

Posterior cecal vein

Superior rectal vein

Appendicular vein

Right testicular (ovarian) vessels

External iliac vessels

Tributaries of left and right superior rectal veins

Internal iliac vein

Perimuscular rectal venous plexus

Superior gluteal vein

Left middle rectal vein

Obturator vein

Left internal pudendal vein in pudendal canal (Alcock's)

External rectal venous plexus

Right middle rectal vein

Right inferior rectal vein (to internal pudendal vein)

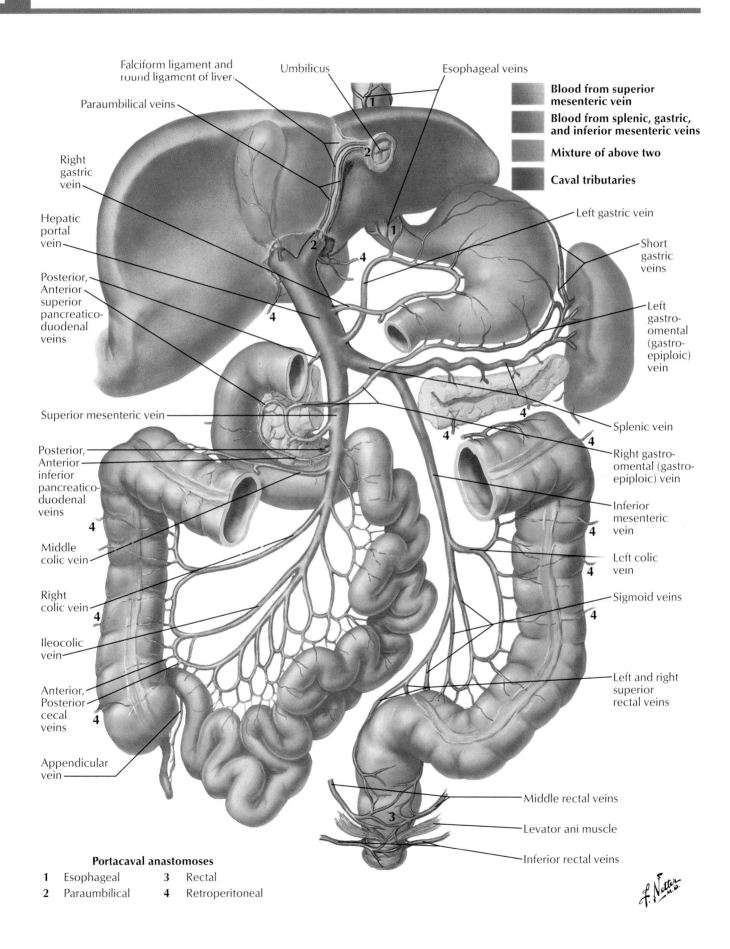

Falciform ligament and round ligament of liver

Umbilicus

Esophageal veins

Paraumbilical veins

Blood from superior mesenteric vein

Blood from splenic, gastric, and inferior mesenteric veins

Mixture of above two

Caval tributaries

Right gastric vein

Left gastric vein

Short gastric veins

Hepatic portal vein

Left gastro-omental (gastro-epiploic) vein

Posterior, Anterior superior pancreatico-duodenal veins

Superior mesenteric vein

Splenic vein

Posterior, Anterior inferior pancreatico-duodenal veins

Right gastro-omental (gastro-epiploic) vein

Inferior mesenteric vein

Middle colic vein

Left colic vein

Right colic vein

Sigmoid veins

Ileocolic vein

Left and right superior rectal veins

Anterior, Posterior cecal veins

Appendicular vein

Middle rectal veins

Levator ani muscle

Inferior rectal veins

Portacaval anastomoses

1	Esophageal	3	Rectal
2	Paraumbilical	4	Retroperitoneal

f. Netter m.d.

Plate 312

Visceral Vasculature

Typical arrangement

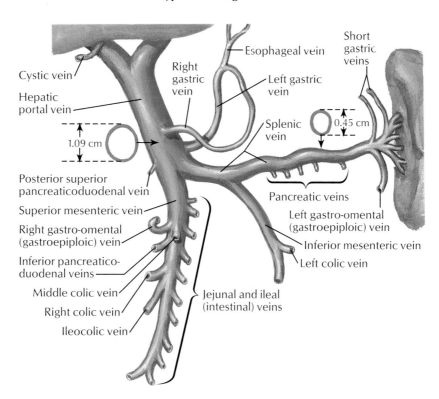

Cystic vein

Hepatic portal vein

1.09 cm

Posterior superior pancreaticoduodenal vein

Superior mesenteric vein

Right gastro-omental (gastroepiploic) vein

Inferior pancreaticoduodenal veins

Middle colic vein

Right colic vein

Ileocolic vein

Right gastric vein

Esophageal vein

Left gastric vein

Short gastric veins

Splenic vein

0.45 cm

Pancreatic veins

Left gastro-omental (gastroepiploic) vein

Inferior mesenteric vein

Left colic vein

Jejunal and ileal (intestinal) veins

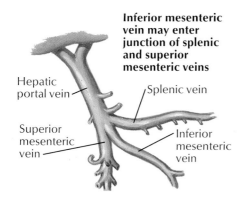

Inferior mesenteric vein may enter junction of splenic and superior mesenteric veins

Hepatic portal vein

Superior mesenteric vein

Splenic vein

Inferior mesenteric vein

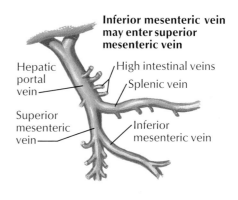

Inferior mesenteric vein may enter superior mesenteric vein

Hepatic portal vein

Superior mesenteric vein

High intestinal veins

Splenic vein

Inferior mesenteric vein

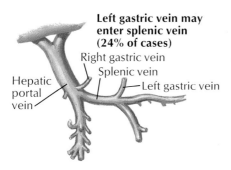

Left gastric vein may enter splenic vein (24% of cases)

Hepatic portal vein

Right gastric vein

Splenic vein

Left gastric vein

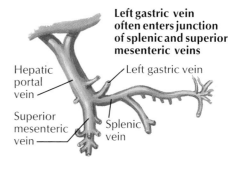

Left gastric vein often enters junction of splenic and superior mesenteric veins

Hepatic portal vein

Superior mesenteric vein

Left gastric vein

Splenic vein

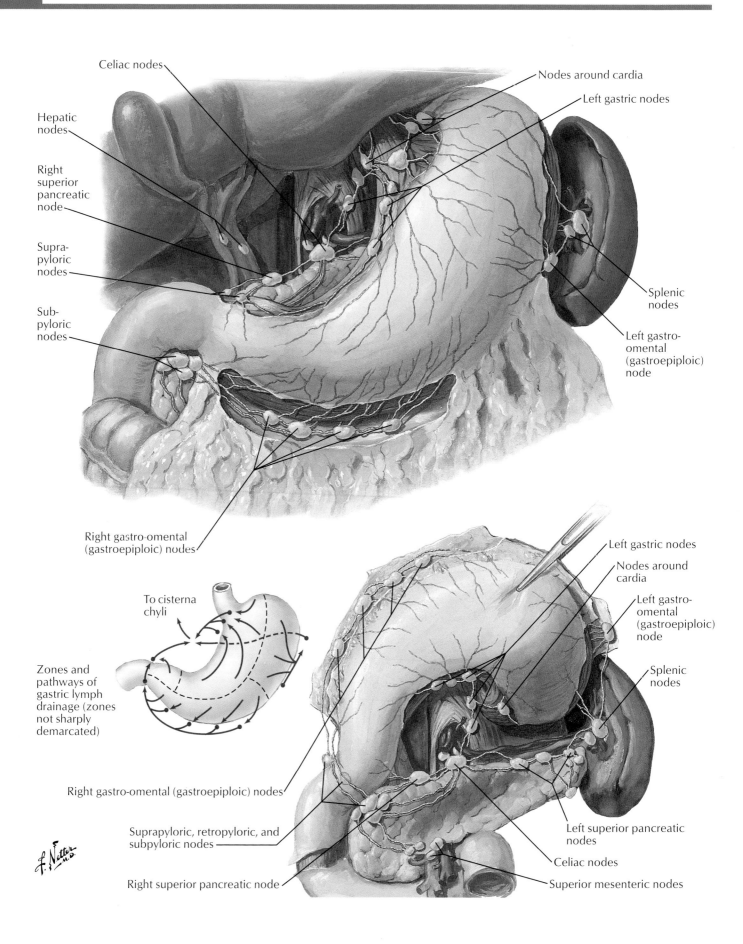

Celiac nodes

Hepatic nodes

Right superior pancreatic node

Supra-pyloric nodes

Sub-pyloric nodes

Nodes around cardia

Left gastric nodes

Splenic nodes

Left gastro-omental (gastroepiploic) node

Right gastro-omental (gastroepiploic) nodes

To cisterna chyli

Zones and pathways of gastric lymph drainage (zones not sharply demarcated)

Right gastro-omental (gastroepiploic) nodes

Suprapyloric, retropyloric, and subpyloric nodes

Right superior pancreatic node

Left gastric nodes

Nodes around cardia

Left gastro-omental (gastroepiploic) node

Splenic nodes

Left superior pancreatic nodes

Celiac nodes

Superior mesenteric nodes

Plate 314 **Visceral Vasculature**

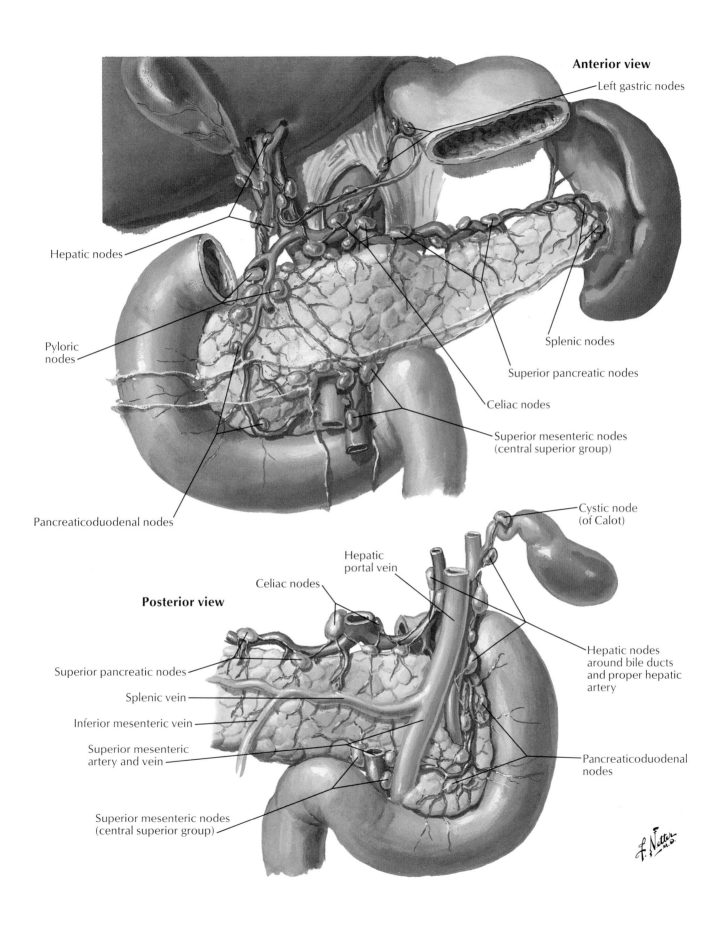

Anterior view

Left gastric nodes

Hepatic nodes

Pyloric nodes

Pancreaticoduodenal nodes

Splenic nodes

Superior pancreatic nodes

Celiac nodes

Superior mesenteric nodes
(central superior group)

Cystic node
(of Calot)

Hepatic portal vein

Celiac nodes

Posterior view

Hepatic nodes around bile ducts and proper hepatic artery

Superior pancreatic nodes

Splenic vein

Inferior mesenteric vein

Superior mesenteric artery and vein

Pancreaticoduodenal nodes

Superior mesenteric nodes
(central superior group)

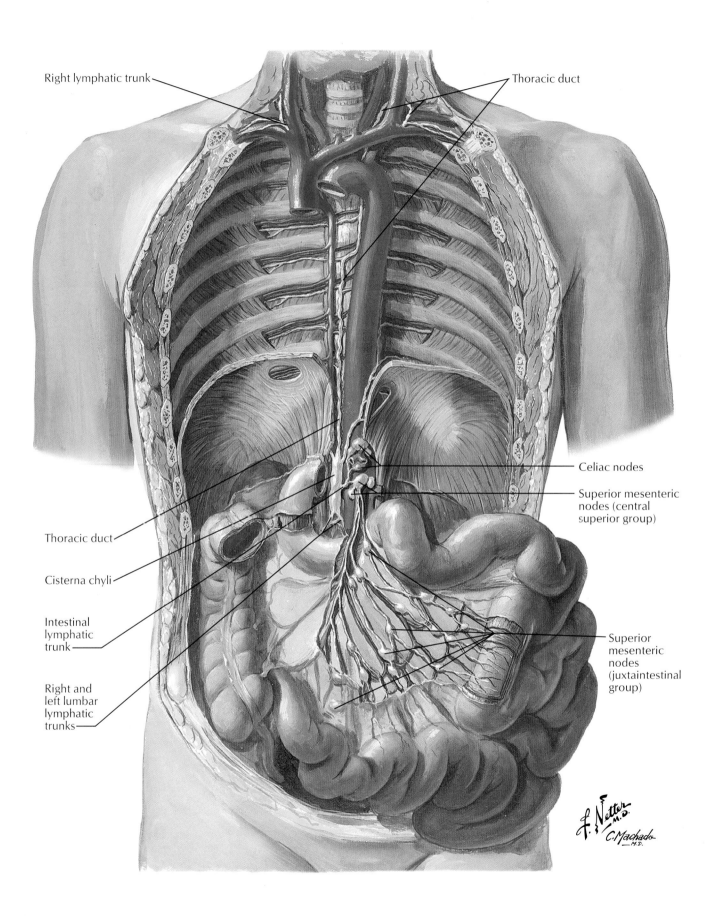

Right lymphatic trunk

Thoracic duct

Celiac nodes

Superior mesenteric nodes (central superior group)

Thoracic duct

Cisterna chyli

Intestinal lymphatic trunk

Superior mesenteric nodes (juxtaintestinal group)

Right and left lumbar lymphatic trunks

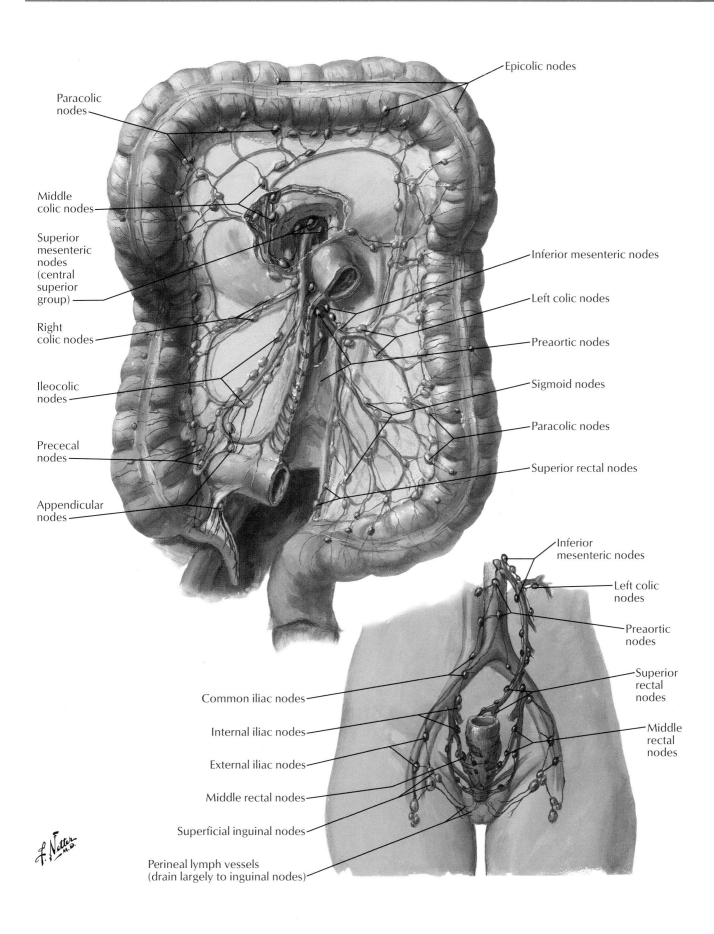

Epicolic nodes

Paracolic nodes

Middle colic nodes

Superior mesenteric nodes (central superior group)

Right colic nodes

Ileocolic nodes

Prececal nodes

Appendicular nodes

Inferior mesenteric nodes

Left colic nodes

Preaortic nodes

Sigmoid nodes

Paracolic nodes

Superior rectal nodes

Inferior mesenteric nodes

Left colic nodes

Preaortic nodes

Superior rectal nodes

Middle rectal nodes

Common iliac nodes

Internal iliac nodes

External iliac nodes

Middle rectal nodes

Superficial inguinal nodes

Perineal lymph vessels (drain largely to inguinal nodes)

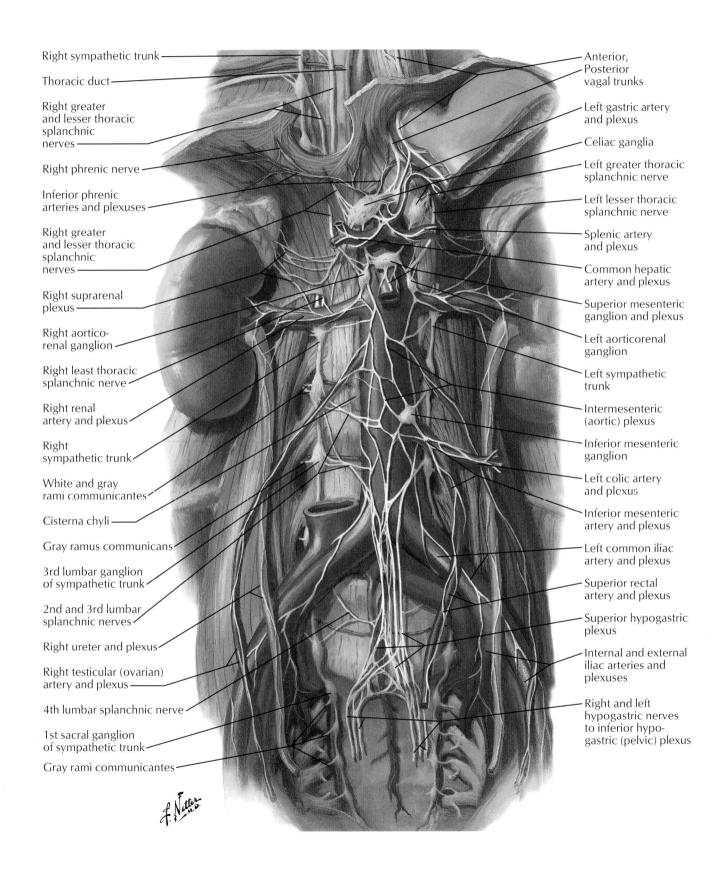

Right sympathetic trunk

Thoracic duct

Right greater and lesser thoracic splanchnic nerves

Right phrenic nerve

Inferior phrenic arteries and plexuses

Right greater and lesser thoracic splanchnic nerves

Right suprarenal plexus

Right aortico-renal ganglion

Right least thoracic splanchnic nerve

Right renal artery and plexus

Right sympathetic trunk

White and gray rami communicantes

Cisterna chyli

Gray ramus communicans

3rd lumbar ganglion of sympathetic trunk

2nd and 3rd lumbar splanchnic nerves

Right ureter and plexus

Right testicular (ovarian) artery and plexus

4th lumbar splanchnic nerve

1st sacral ganglion of sympathetic trunk

Gray rami communicantes

Anterior, Posterior vagal trunks

Left gastric artery and plexus

Celiac ganglia

Left greater thoracic splanchnic nerve

Left lesser thoracic splanchnic nerve

Splenic artery and plexus

Common hepatic artery and plexus

Superior mesenteric ganglion and plexus

Left aorticorenal ganglion

Left sympathetic trunk

Intermesenteric (aortic) plexus

Inferior mesenteric ganglion

Left colic artery and plexus

Inferior mesenteric artery and plexus

Left common iliac artery and plexus

Superior rectal artery and plexus

Superior hypogastric plexus

Internal and external iliac arteries and plexuses

Right and left hypogastric nerves to inferior hypo-gastric (pelvic) plexus

Plate 318

Innervation

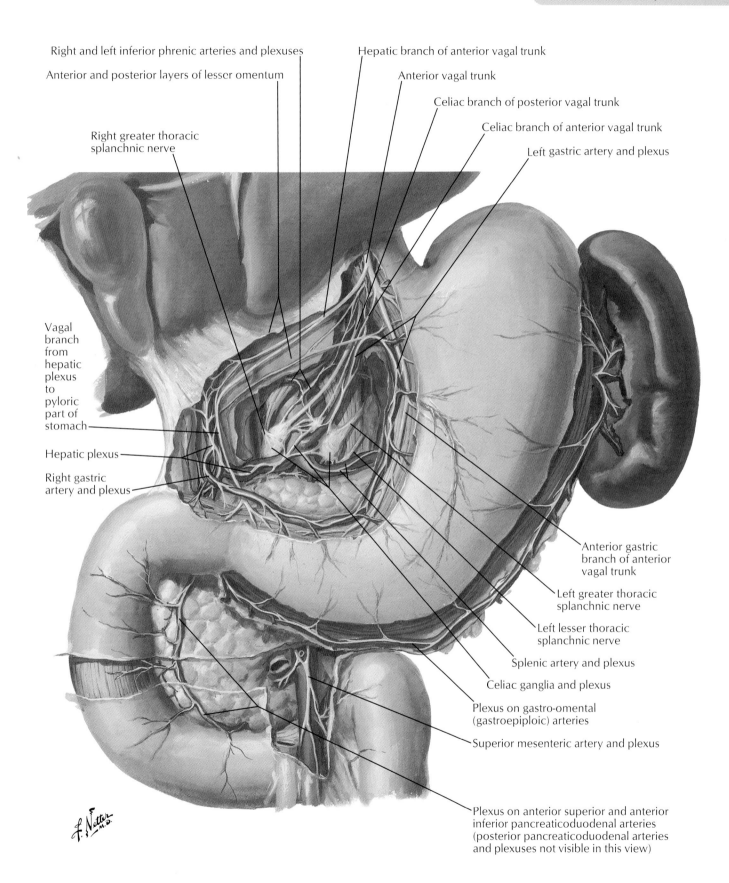

Right and left inferior phrenic arteries and plexuses

Anterior and posterior layers of lesser omentum

Right greater thoracic splanchnic nerve

Hepatic branch of anterior vagal trunk

Anterior vagal trunk

Celiac branch of posterior vagal trunk

Celiac branch of anterior vagal trunk

Left gastric artery and plexus

Vagal branch from hepatic plexus to pyloric part of stomach

Hepatic plexus

Right gastric artery and plexus

Anterior gastric branch of anterior vagal trunk

Left greater thoracic splanchnic nerve

Left lesser thoracic splanchnic nerve

Splenic artery and plexus

Celiac ganglia and plexus

Plexus on gastro-omental (gastroepiploic) arteries

Superior mesenteric artery and plexus

Plexus on anterior superior and anterior inferior pancreaticoduodenal arteries (posterior pancreaticoduodenal arteries and plexuses not visible in this view)

Innervation

Plate 319

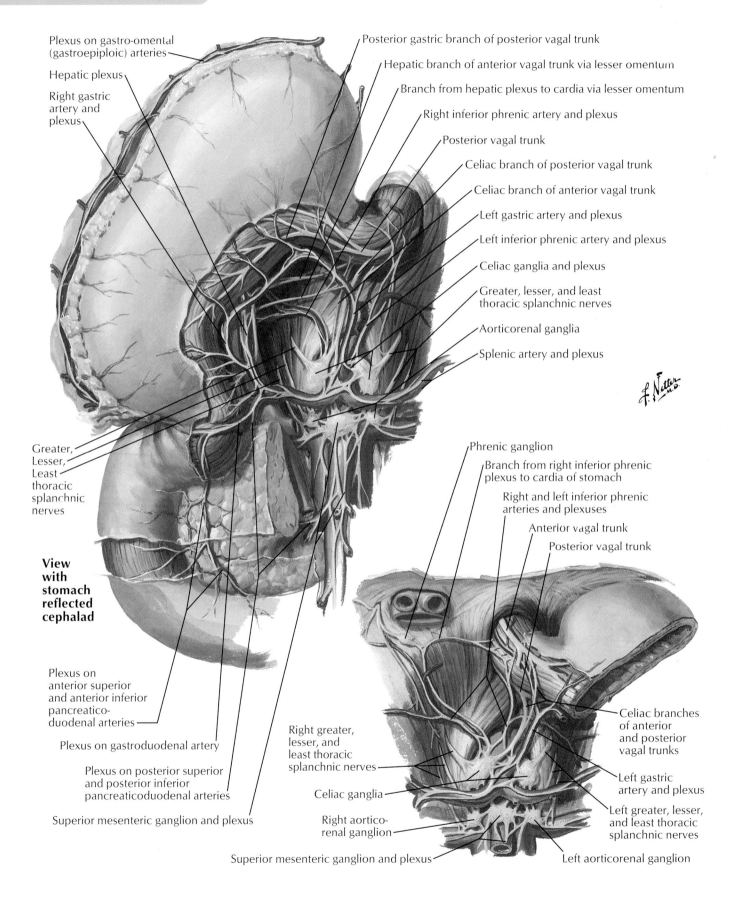

Plexus on gastro-omental (gastroepiploic) arteries

Hepatic plexus

Right gastric artery and plexus

Posterior gastric branch of posterior vagal trunk

Hepatic branch of anterior vagal trunk via lesser omentum

Branch from hepatic plexus to cardia via lesser omentum

Right inferior phrenic artery and plexus

Posterior vagal trunk

Celiac branch of posterior vagal trunk

Celiac branch of anterior vagal trunk

Left gastric artery and plexus

Left inferior phrenic artery and plexus

Celiac ganglia and plexus

Greater, lesser, and least thoracic splanchnic nerves

Aorticorenal ganglia

Splenic artery and plexus

Greater, Lesser, Least thoracic splanchnic nerves

View with stomach reflected cephalad

Plexus on anterior superior and anterior inferior pancreatico-duodenal arteries

Plexus on gastroduodenal artery

Plexus on posterior superior and posterior inferior pancreaticoduodenal arteries

Superior mesenteric ganglion and plexus

Right greater, lesser, and least thoracic splanchnic nerves

Celiac ganglia

Right aortico-renal ganglion

Superior mesenteric ganglion and plexus

Phrenic ganglion

Branch from right inferior phrenic plexus to cardia of stomach

Right and left inferior phrenic arteries and plexuses

Anterior vagal trunk

Posterior vagal trunk

Celiac branches of anterior and posterior vagal trunks

Left gastric artery and plexus

Left greater, lesser, and least thoracic splanchnic nerves

Left aorticorenal ganglion

Plate 320

Innervation

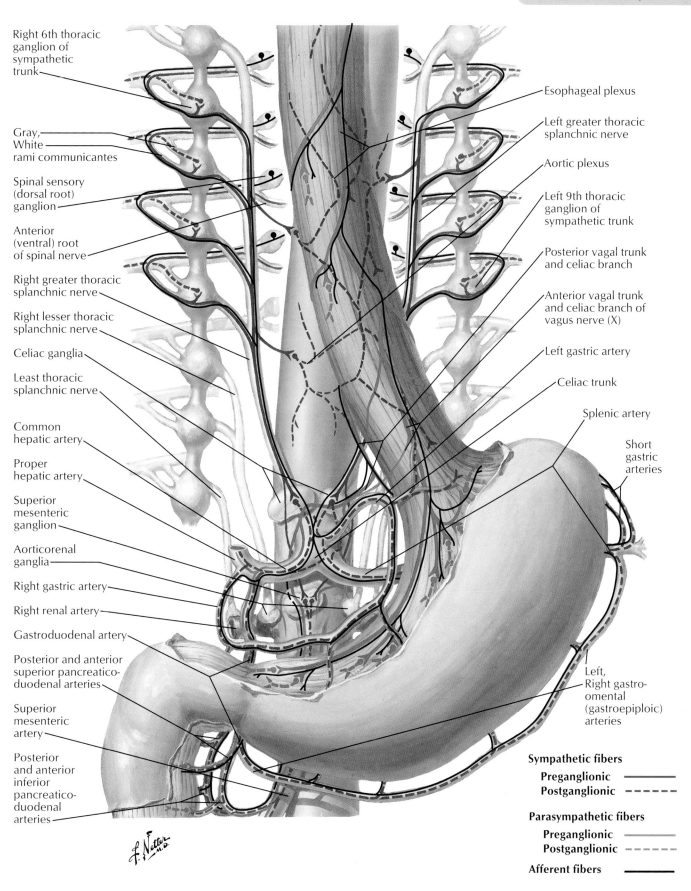

Right 6th thoracic ganglion of sympathetic trunk

Gray, White rami communicantes

Spinal sensory (dorsal root) ganglion

Anterior (ventral) root of spinal nerve

Right greater thoracic splanchnic nerve

Right lesser thoracic splanchnic nerve

Celiac ganglia

Least thoracic splanchnic nerve

Common hepatic artery

Proper hepatic artery

Superior mesenteric ganglion

Aorticorenal ganglia

Right gastric artery

Right renal artery

Gastroduodenal artery

Posterior and anterior superior pancreatico-duodenal arteries

Superior mesenteric artery

Posterior and anterior inferior pancreatico-duodenal arteries

Esophageal plexus

Left greater thoracic splanchnic nerve

Aortic plexus

Left 9th thoracic ganglion of sympathetic trunk

Posterior vagal trunk and celiac branch

Anterior vagal trunk and celiac branch of vagus nerve (X)

Left gastric artery

Celiac trunk

Splenic artery

Short gastric arteries

Left, Right gastro-omental (gastroepiploic) arteries

Sympathetic fibers
Preganglionic ————
Postganglionic — — — —

Parasympathetic fibers
Preganglionic ————
Postganglionic — — — —

Afferent fibers ————

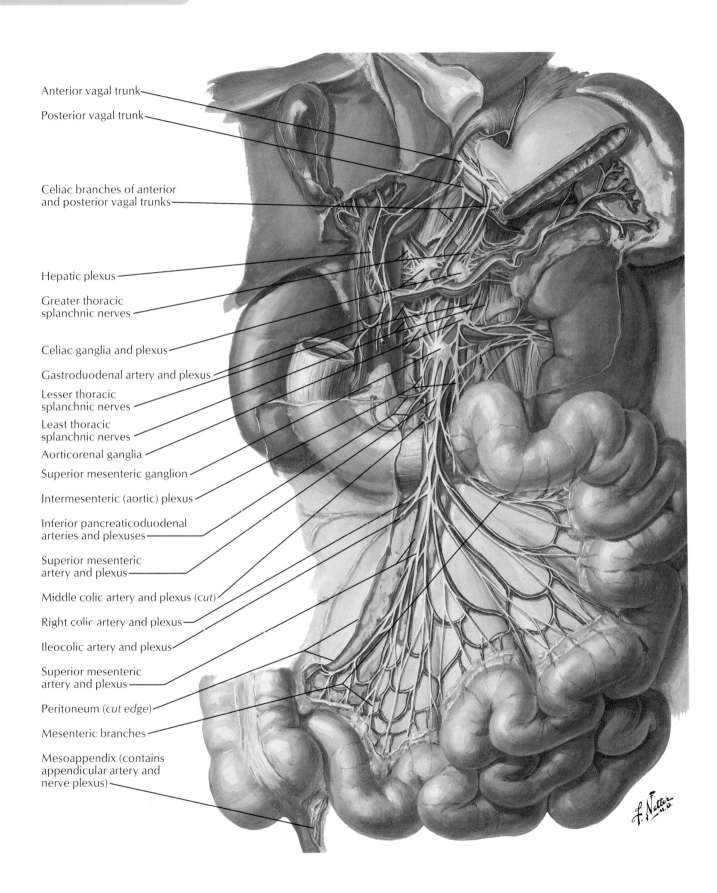

Anterior vagal trunk

Posterior vagal trunk

Celiac branches of anterior and posterior vagal trunks

Hepatic plexus

Greater thoracic splanchnic nerves

Celiac ganglia and plexus

Gastroduodenal artery and plexus

Lesser thoracic splanchnic nerves

Least thoracic splanchnic nerves

Aorticorenal ganglia

Superior mesenteric ganglion

Intermesenteric (aortic) plexus

Inferior pancreaticoduodenal arteries and plexuses

Superior mesenteric artery and plexus

Middle colic artery and plexus (cut)

Right colic artery and plexus

Ileocolic artery and plexus

Superior mesenteric artery and plexus

Peritoneum (cut edge)

Mesenteric branches

Mesoappendix (contains appendicular artery and nerve plexus)

Plate 322

Innervation

For nerves of rectum see **Plates 165, 166, 410–413**

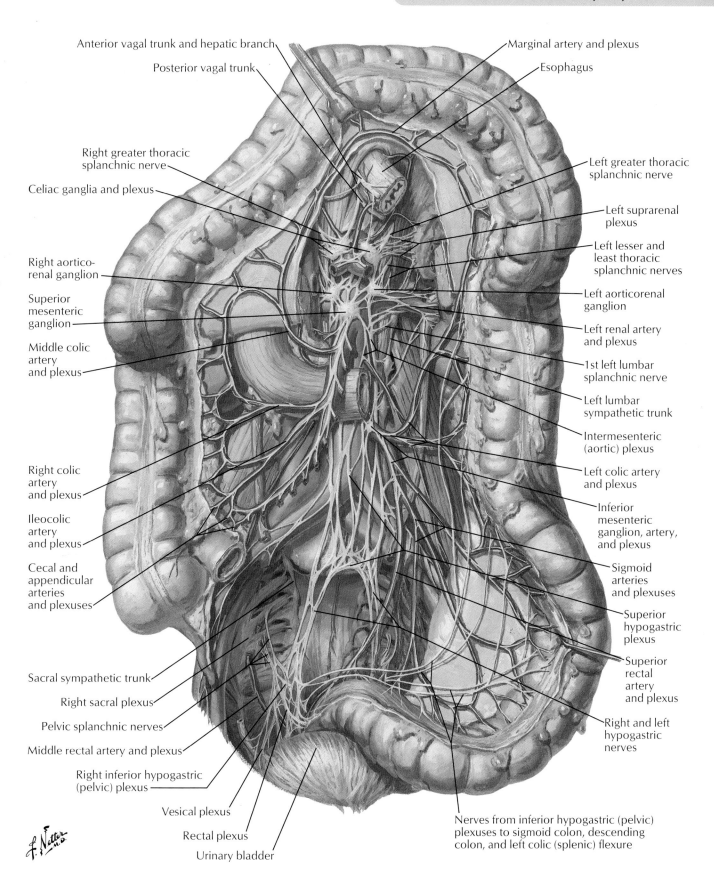

Anterior vagal trunk and hepatic branch

Posterior vagal trunk

Right greater thoracic splanchnic nerve

Celiac ganglia and plexus

Right aortico-renal ganglion

Superior mesenteric ganglion

Middle colic artery and plexus

Right colic artery and plexus

Ileocolic artery and plexus

Cecal and appendicular arteries and plexuses

Sacral sympathetic trunk

Right sacral plexus

Pelvic splanchnic nerves

Middle rectal artery and plexus

Right inferior hypogastric (pelvic) plexus

Vesical plexus

Rectal plexus

Urinary bladder

Marginal artery and plexus

Esophagus

Left greater thoracic splanchnic nerve

Left suprarenal plexus

Left lesser and least thoracic splanchnic nerves

Left aorticorenal ganglion

Left renal artery and plexus

1st left lumbar splanchnic nerve

Left lumbar sympathetic trunk

Intermesenteric (aortic) plexus

Left colic artery and plexus

Inferior mesenteric ganglion, artery, and plexus

Sigmoid arteries and plexuses

Superior hypogastric plexus

Superior rectal artery and plexus

Right and left hypogastric nerves

Nerves from inferior hypogastric (pelvic) plexuses to sigmoid colon, descending colon, and left colic (splenic) flexure

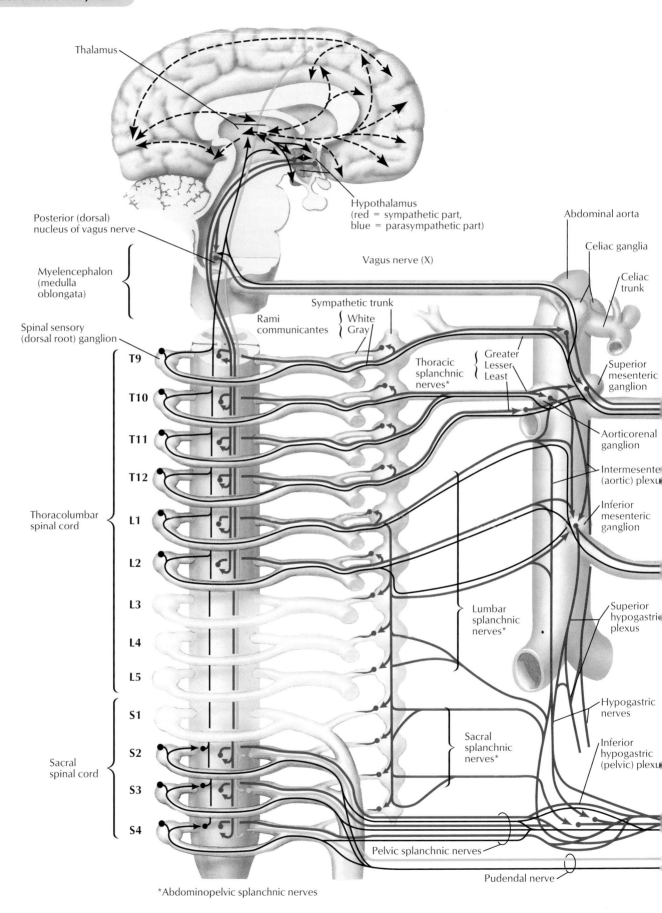

Thalamus

Posterior (dorsal) nucleus of vagus nerve

Myelencephalon (medulla oblongata)

Spinal sensory (dorsal root) ganglion

Thoracolumbar spinal cord

Sacral spinal cord

Hypothalamus (red = sympathetic part, blue = parasympathetic part)

Abdominal aorta

Celiac ganglia

Celiac trunk

Vagus nerve (X)

Sympathetic trunk

Rami communicantes {White Gray}

Thoracic splanchnic nerves* {Greater Lesser Least}

Superior mesenteric ganglion

Aorticorenal ganglion

Intermesenteric (aortic) plexus

Inferior mesenteric ganglion

Lumbar splanchnic nerves*

Superior hypogastric plexus

Hypogastric nerves

Inferior hypogastric (pelvic) plexus

Sacral splanchnic nerves*

Pelvic splanchnic nerves

Pudendal nerve

T9
T10
T11
T12
L1
L2
L3
L4
L5
S1
S2
S3
S4

*Abdominopelvic splanchnic nerves

Plate 324

Innervation

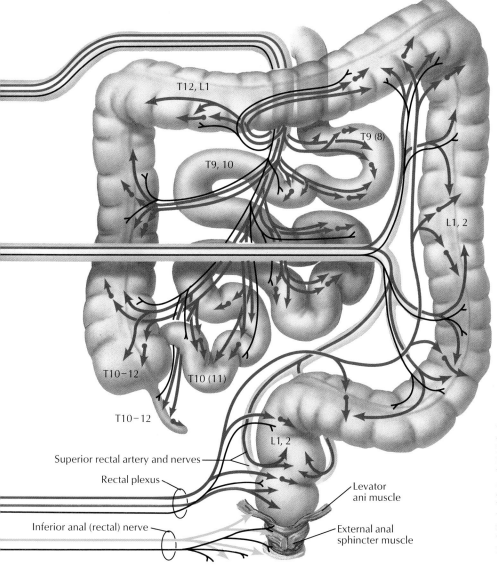

Sympathetic efferents
Parasympathetic efferents
Somatic efferents
Afferents and CNS connections
Indefinite paths

T12, L1

T9 (8)

T9, 10

L1, 2

T10–12

T10 (11)

T10–12

L1, 2

Superior rectal artery and nerves

Rectal plexus

Levator
ani muscle

Inferior anal (rectal) nerve

External anal
sphincter muscle

Chief segmental sources
of sympathetic fibers
innervating different
regions of intestinal
tract are indicated.
Numerous afferent fibers
are carried centripetally
through approximately
the same sympathetic
splanchnic nerves
that transmit
preganglionic fibers.

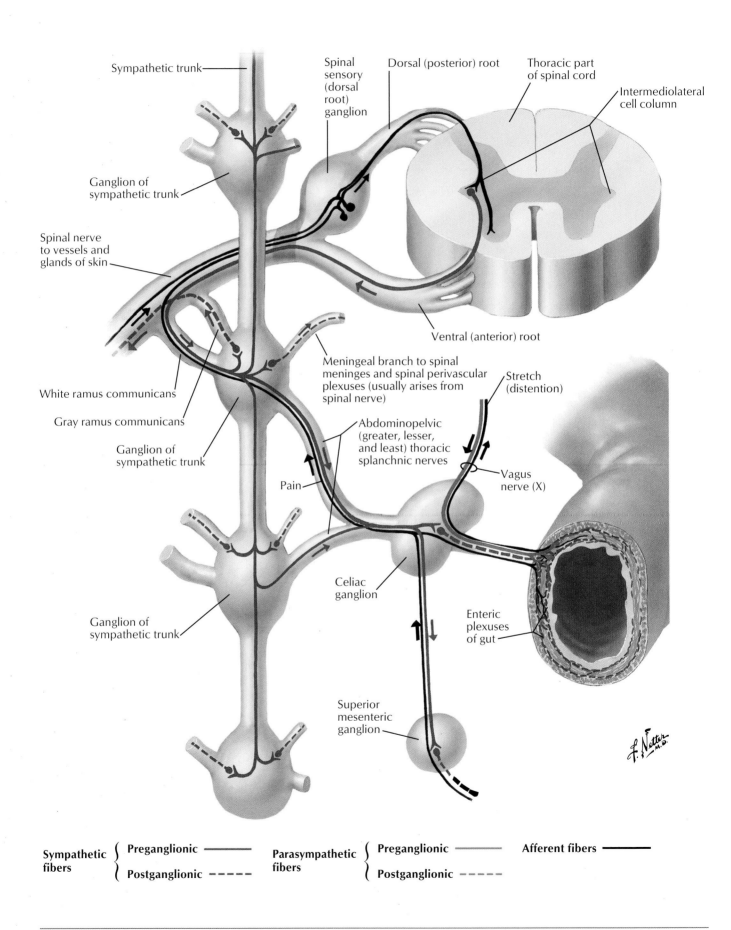

Sympathetic trunk

Spinal sensory (dorsal root) ganglion

Dorsal (posterior) root

Thoracic part of spinal cord

Intermediolateral cell column

Ganglion of sympathetic trunk

Spinal nerve to vessels and glands of skin

Ventral (anterior) root

Meningeal branch to spinal meninges and spinal perivascular plexuses (usually arises from spinal nerve)

Stretch (distention)

White ramus communicans

Gray ramus communicans

Ganglion of sympathetic trunk

Abdominopelvic (greater, lesser, and least) thoracic splanchnic nerves

Vagus nerve (X)

Pain

Celiac ganglion

Enteric plexuses of gut

Ganglion of sympathetic trunk

Superior mesenteric ganglion

Sympathetic fibers { Preganglionic ——— Postganglionic – – – –

Parasympathetic fibers { Preganglionic ——— Postganglionic – – – – –

Afferent fibers ———

Plate 325 **Innervation**

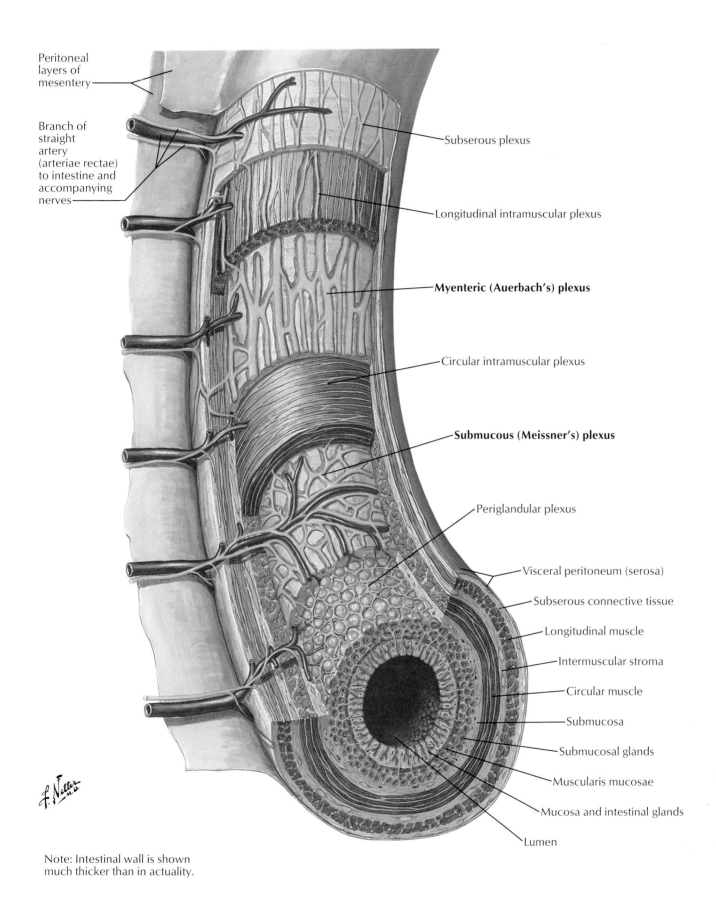

Peritoneal layers of mesentery

Branch of straight artery (arteriae rectae) to intestine and accompanying nerves

Subserous plexus

Longitudinal intramuscular plexus

Myenteric (Auerbach's) plexus

Circular intramuscular plexus

Submucous (Meissner's) plexus

Periglandular plexus

Visceral peritoneum (serosa)

Subserous connective tissue

Longitudinal muscle

Intermuscular stroma

Circular muscle

Submucosa

Submucosal glands

Muscularis mucosae

Mucosa and intestinal glands

Lumen

Note: Intestinal wall is shown much thicker than in actuality.

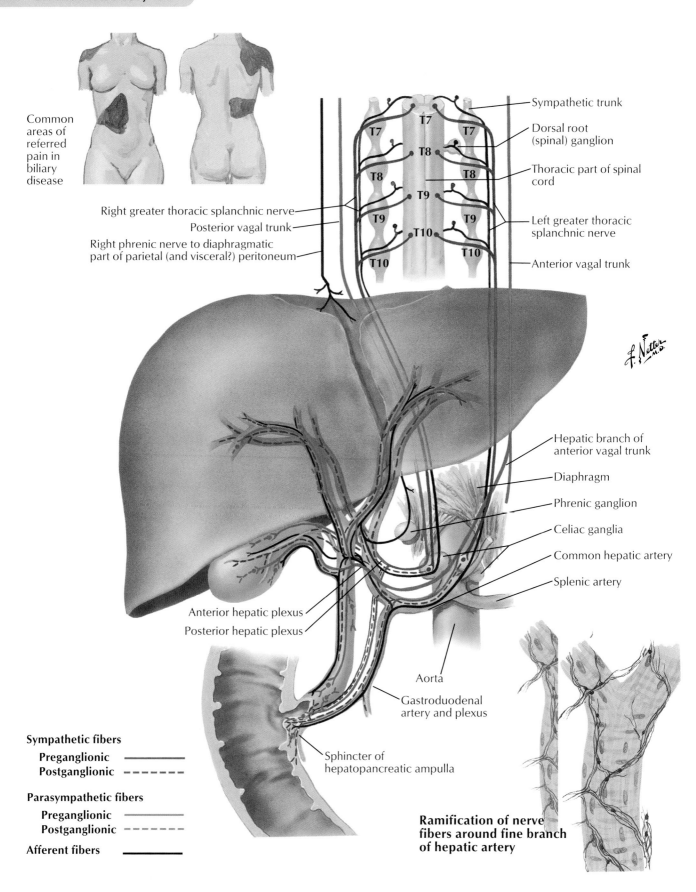

Common areas of referred pain in biliary disease

Sympathetic trunk

Dorsal root (spinal) ganglion

Thoracic part of spinal cord

Right greater thoracic splanchnic nerve

Posterior vagal trunk

Right phrenic nerve to diaphragmatic part of parietal (and visceral?) peritoneum

Left greater thoracic splanchnic nerve

Anterior vagal trunk

T7 T7 T7
T8 T8 T8
T9 T9 T9
T10 T10 T10

Hepatic branch of anterior vagal trunk

Diaphragm

Phrenic ganglion

Celiac ganglia

Common hepatic artery

Splenic artery

Anterior hepatic plexus

Posterior hepatic plexus

Aorta

Gastroduodenal artery and plexus

Sphincter of hepatopancreatic ampulla

Sympathetic fibers
Preganglionic ——————
Postganglionic – – – – – –

Parasympathetic fibers
Preganglionic ——————
Postganglionic – – – – – –

Afferent fibers ——————

Ramification of nerve fibers around fine branch of hepatic artery

Plate 327

Innervation

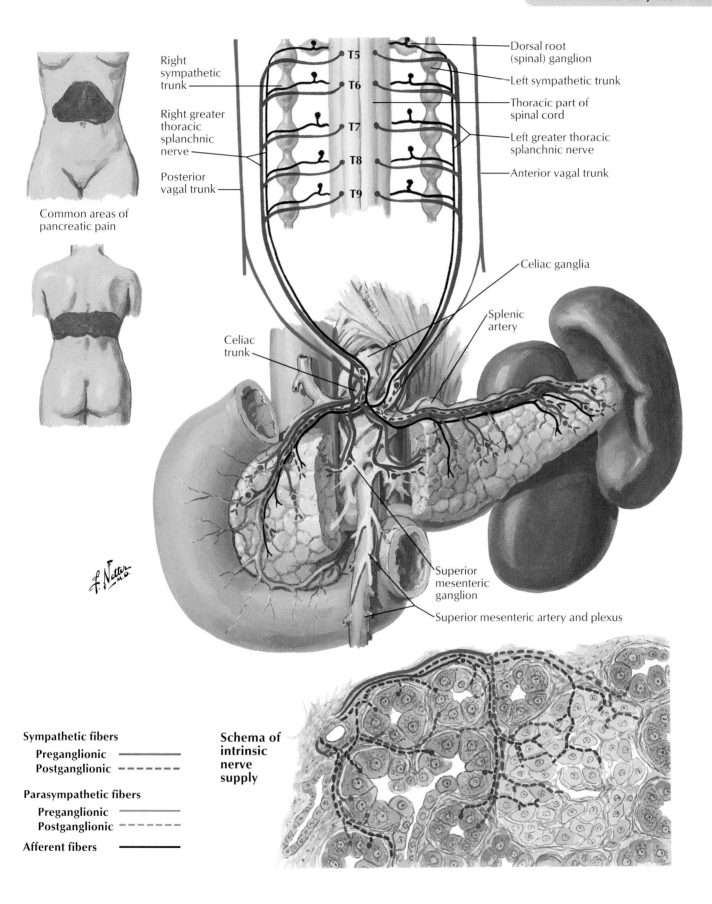

Common areas of pancreatic pain

Right sympathetic trunk

Right greater thoracic splanchnic nerve

Posterior vagal trunk

T5
T6
T7
T8
T9

Dorsal root (spinal) ganglion

Left sympathetic trunk

Thoracic part of spinal cord

Left greater thoracic splanchnic nerve

Anterior vagal trunk

Celiac ganglia

Splenic artery

Celiac trunk

Superior mesenteric ganglion

Superior mesenteric artery and plexus

Sympathetic fibers
Preganglionic ———
Postganglionic – – – –

Parasympathetic fibers
Preganglionic ———
Postganglionic – – – –

Afferent fibers ———

Schema of intrinsic nerve supply

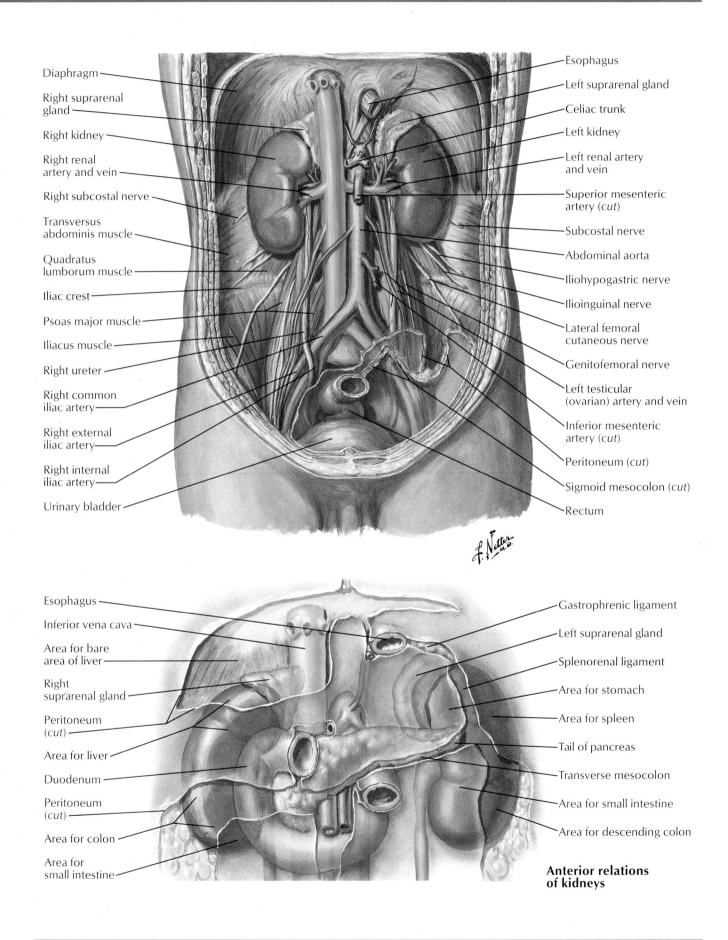

Diaphragm

Right suprarenal gland

Right kidney

Right renal artery and vein

Right subcostal nerve

Transversus abdominis muscle

Quadratus lumborum muscle

Iliac crest

Psoas major muscle

Iliacus muscle

Right ureter

Right common iliac artery

Right external iliac artery

Right internal iliac artery

Urinary bladder

Esophagus

Left suprarenal gland

Celiac trunk

Left kidney

Left renal artery and vein

Superior mesenteric artery (cut)

Subcostal nerve

Abdominal aorta

Iliohypogastric nerve

Ilioinguinal nerve

Lateral femoral cutaneous nerve

Genitofemoral nerve

Left testicular (ovarian) artery and vein

Inferior mesenteric artery (cut)

Peritoneum (cut)

Sigmoid mesocolon (cut)

Rectum

Esophagus

Inferior vena cava

Area for bare area of liver

Right suprarenal gland

Peritoneum (cut)

Area for liver

Duodenum

Peritoneum (cut)

Area for colon

Area for small intestine

Gastrophrenic ligament

Left suprarenal gland

Splenorenal ligament

Area for stomach

Area for spleen

Tail of pancreas

Transverse mesocolon

Area for small intestine

Area for descending colon

Anterior relations of kidneys

Plate 329   **Kidneys and Suprarenal Glands**

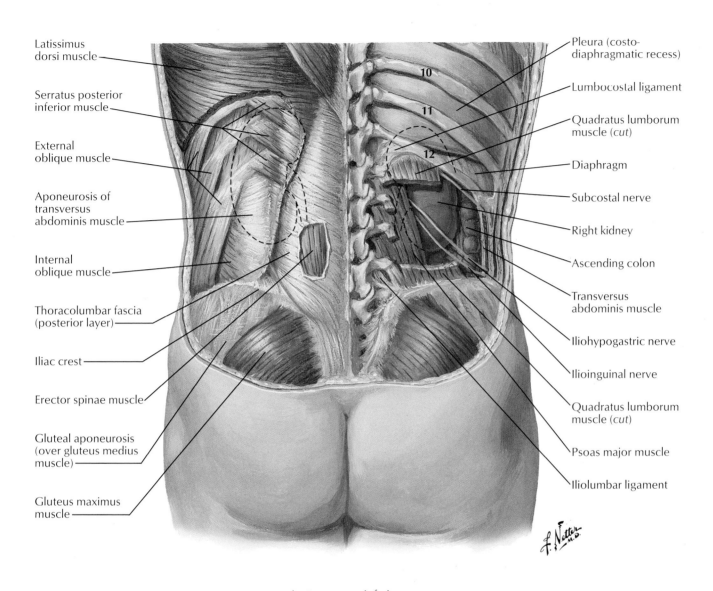

Latissimus dorsi muscle

Serratus posterior inferior muscle

External oblique muscle

Aponeurosis of transversus abdominis muscle

Internal oblique muscle

Thoracolumbar fascia (posterior layer)

Iliac crest

Erector spinae muscle

Gluteal aponeurosis (over gluteus medius muscle)

Gluteus maximus muscle

Pleura (costo-diaphragmatic recess)

Lumbocostal ligament

Quadratus lumborum muscle (cut)

Diaphragm

Subcostal nerve

Right kidney

Ascending colon

Transversus abdominis muscle

Iliohypogastric nerve

Ilioinguinal nerve

Quadratus lumborum muscle (cut)

Psoas major muscle

Iliolumbar ligament

10

11

12

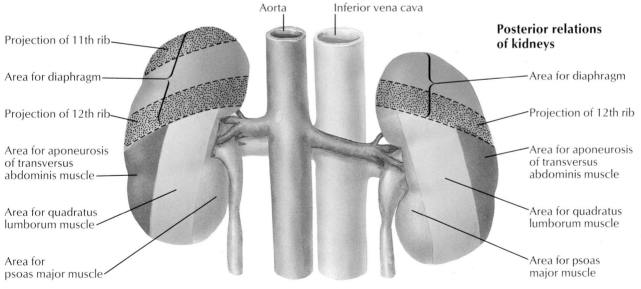

Aorta

Inferior vena cava

Posterior relations of kidneys

Projection of 11th rib

Area for diaphragm

Projection of 12th rib

Area for aponeurosis of transversus abdominis muscle

Area for quadratus lumborum muscle

Area for psoas major muscle

Area for diaphragm

Projection of 12th rib

Area for aponeurosis of transversus abdominis muscle

Area for quadratus lumborum muscle

Area for psoas major muscle

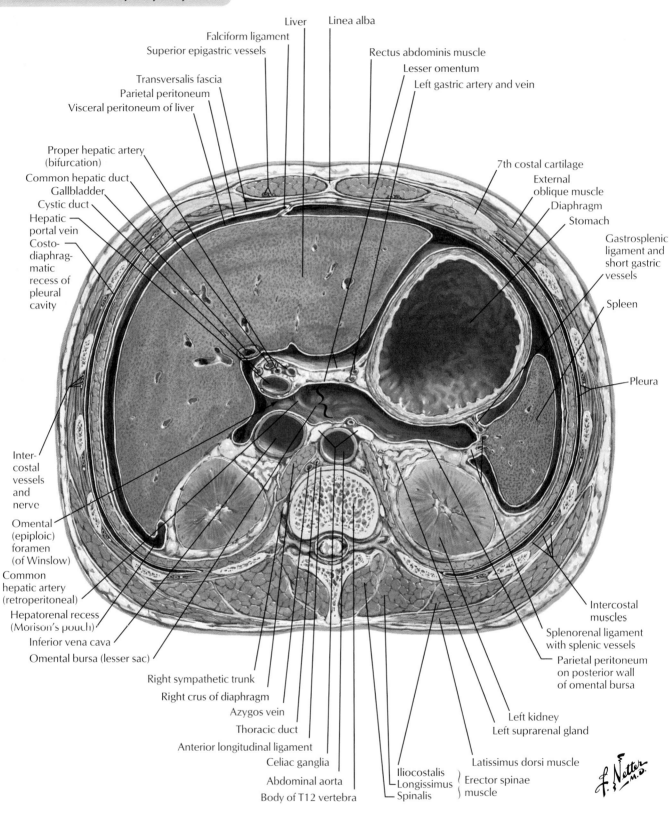

Liver

Linea alba

Falciform ligament

Superior epigastric vessels

Rectus abdominis muscle

Lesser omentum

Left gastric artery and vein

Transversalis fascia

Parietal peritoneum

Visceral peritoneum of liver

Proper hepatic artery (bifurcation)

Common hepatic duct

Gallbladder

Cystic duct

Hepatic portal vein

Costo-diaphrag-matic recess of pleural cavity

7th costal cartilage

External oblique muscle

Diaphragm

Stomach

Gastrosplenic ligament and short gastric vessels

Spleen

Pleura

Inter-costal vessels and nerve

Omental (epiploic) foramen (of Winslow)

Common hepatic artery (retroperitoneal)

Hepatorenal recess (Morison's pouch)

Inferior vena cava

Omental bursa (lesser sac)

Right sympathetic trunk

Right crus of diaphragm

Azygos vein

Thoracic duct

Anterior longitudinal ligament

Celiac ganglia

Abdominal aorta

Body of T12 vertebra

Iliocostalis

Longissimus

Spinalis

Erector spinae muscle

Latissimus dorsi muscle

Left kidney

Left suprarenal gland

Parietal peritoneum on posterior wall of omental bursa

Splenorenal ligament with splenic vessels

Intercostal muscles

Plate 331

Kidneys and Suprarenal Glands

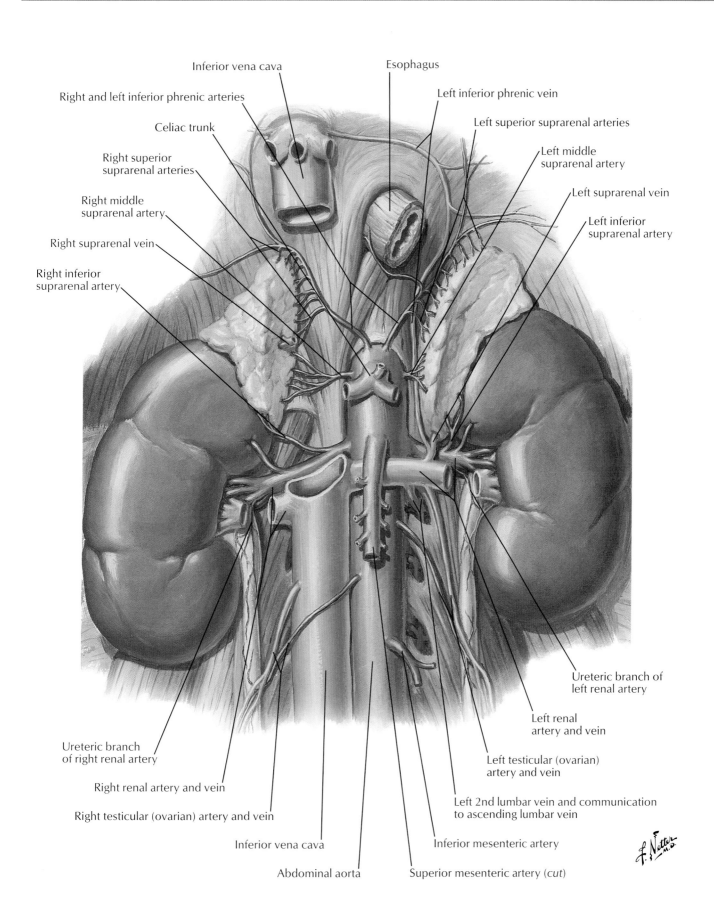

Inferior vena cava

Esophagus

Right and left inferior phrenic arteries

Left inferior phrenic vein

Celiac trunk

Left superior suprarenal arteries

Right superior suprarenal arteries

Left middle suprarenal artery

Right middle suprarenal artery

Left suprarenal vein

Right suprarenal vein

Left inferior suprarenal artery

Right inferior suprarenal artery

Ureteric branch of left renal artery

Left renal artery and vein

Ureteric branch of right renal artery

Left testicular (ovarian) artery and vein

Right renal artery and vein

Left 2nd lumbar vein and communication to ascending lumbar vein

Right testicular (ovarian) artery and vein

Inferior vena cava

Inferior mesenteric artery

Abdominal aorta

Superior mesenteric artery (cut)

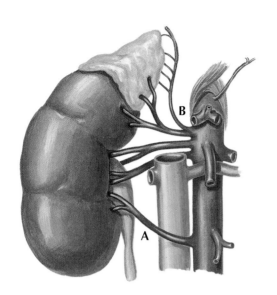

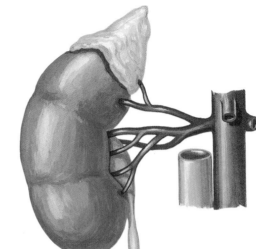

Proximal subdivision of renal artery

A Low accessory right renal artery may pass anterior to inferior vena cava instead of posterior to it

B Inferior phrenic artery with superior suprarenal arteries may arise from renal artery (middle suprarenal artery absent)

Double left renal vein may form ring around abdominal aorta

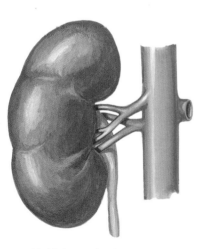

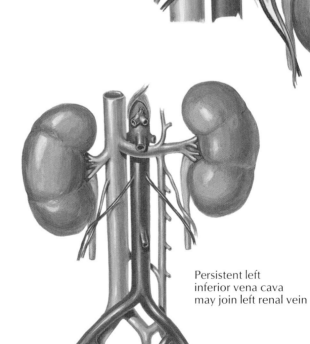

Multiple renal veins

Persistent left inferior vena cava may join left renal vein

Plate 333 **Kidneys and Suprarenal Glands**

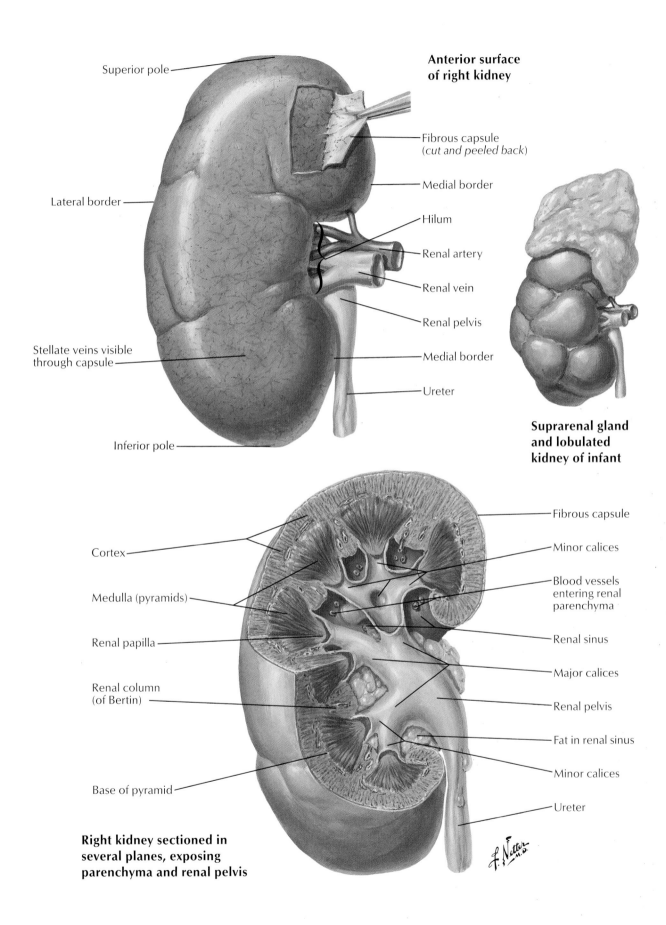

Superior pole

**Anterior surface
of right kidney**

Fibrous capsule
(*cut and peeled back*)

Medial border

Lateral border

Hilum

Renal artery

Renal vein

Renal pelvis

Stellate veins visible
through capsule

Medial border

Ureter

Inferior pole

**Suprarenal gland
and lobulated
kidney of infant**

Cortex

Fibrous capsule

Minor calices

Medulla (pyramids)

Blood vessels
entering renal
parenchyma

Renal papilla

Renal sinus

Major calices

Renal column
(of Bertin)

Renal pelvis

Fat in renal sinus

Base of pyramid

Minor calices

Ureter

**Right kidney sectioned in
several planes, exposing
parenchyma and renal pelvis**

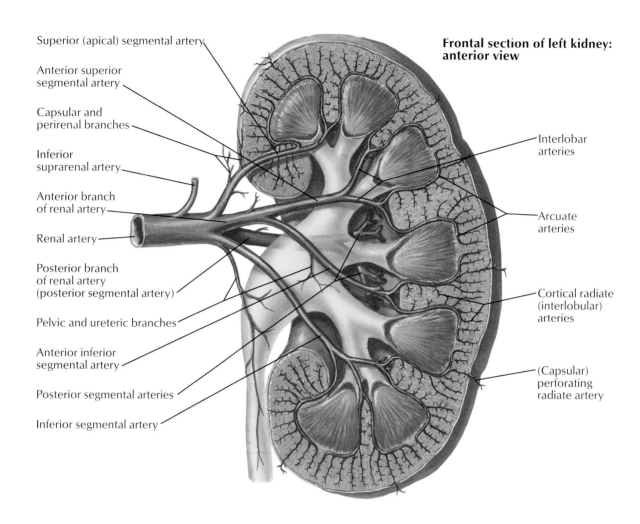

Superior (apical) segmental artery

Anterior superior segmental artery

Capsular and perirenal branches

Inferior suprarenal artery

Anterior branch of renal artery

Renal artery

Posterior branch of renal artery (posterior segmental artery)

Pelvic and ureteric branches

Anterior inferior segmental artery

Posterior segmental arteries

Inferior segmental artery

Frontal section of left kidney: anterior view

Interlobar arteries

Arcuate arteries

Cortical radiate (interlobular) arteries

(Capsular) perforating radiate artery

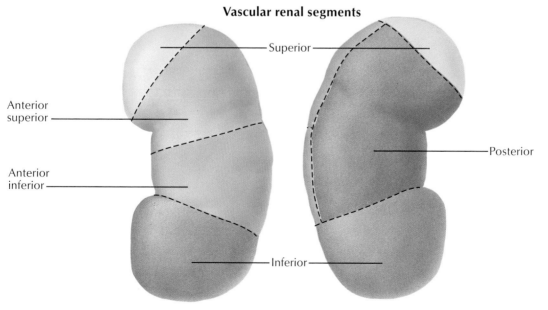

Vascular renal segments

Superior

Anterior superior

Anterior inferior

Posterior

Inferior

Anterior surface of left kidney

Posterior surface of left kidney

Plate 335

Kidneys and Suprarenal Glands

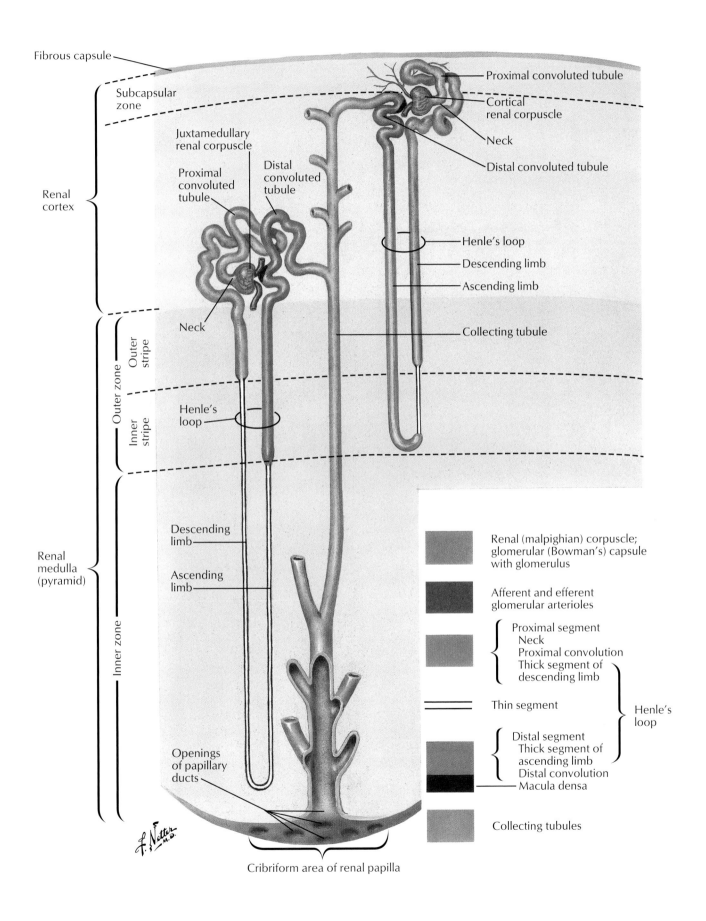

Fibrous capsule

Subcapsular zone

Renal cortex

Juxtamedullary renal corpuscle

Proximal convoluted tubule

Distal convoluted tubule

Proximal convoluted tubule

Cortical renal corpuscle

Neck

Distal convoluted tubule

Henle's loop

Descending limb

Ascending limb

Collecting tubule

Neck

Outer zone

Outer stripe

Inner stripe

Henle's loop

Renal medulla (pyramid)

Inner zone

Descending limb

Ascending limb

Openings of papillary ducts

Renal (malpighian) corpuscle; glomerular (Bowman's) capsule with glomerulus

Afferent and efferent glomerular arterioles

Proximal segment
Neck
Proximal convolution
Thick segment of descending limb

Thin segment

Henle's loop

Distal segment
Thick segment of ascending limb
Distal convolution
Macula densa

Collecting tubules

Cribriform area of renal papilla

F. Netter M.D.

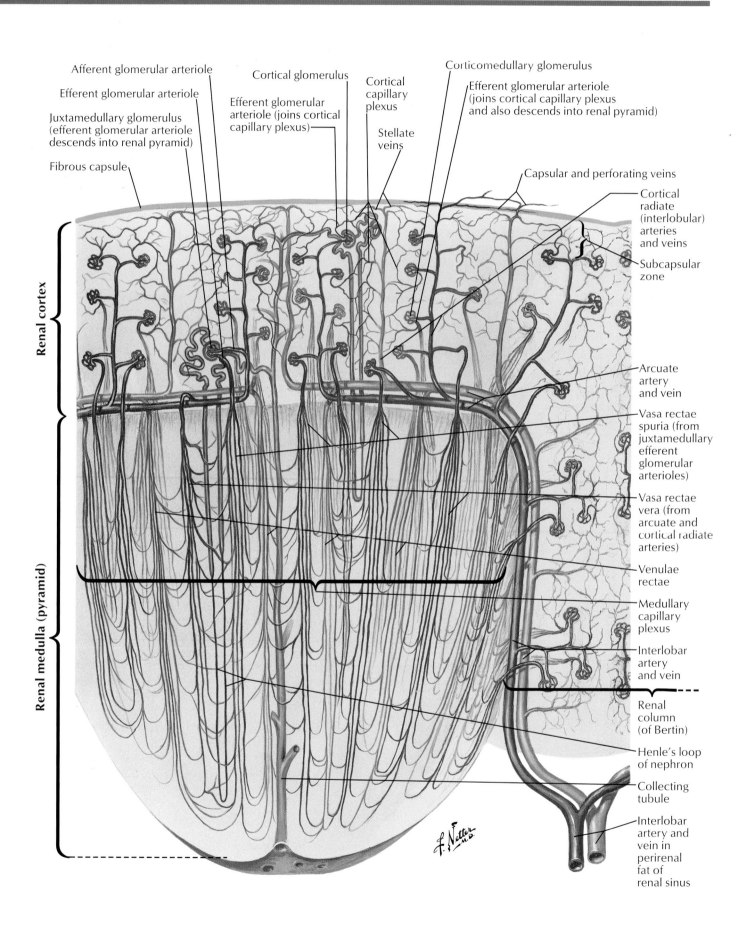

Afferent glomerular arteriole

Efferent glomerular arteriole

Juxtamedullary glomerulus (efferent glomerular arteriole descends into renal pyramid)

Fibrous capsule

Cortical glomerulus

Efferent glomerular arteriole (joins cortical capillary plexus)

Cortical capillary plexus

Stellate veins

Corticomedullary glomerulus

Efferent glomerular arteriole (joins cortical capillary plexus and also descends into renal pyramid)

Capsular and perforating veins

Cortical radiate (interlobular) arteries and veins

Subcapsular zone

Renal cortex

Arcuate artery and vein

Vasa rectae spuria (from juxtamedullary efferent glomerular arterioles)

Vasa rectae vera (from arcuate and cortical radiate arteries)

Venulae rectae

Medullary capillary plexus

Interlobar artery and vein

Renal medulla (pyramid)

Renal column (of Bertin)

Henle's loop of nephron

Collecting tubule

Interlobar artery and vein in perirenal fat of renal sinus

f. Netter
M.D.

Plate 337

Kidneys and Suprarenal Glands

Transverse Section: Level of T12–L1 Intervertebral Disc

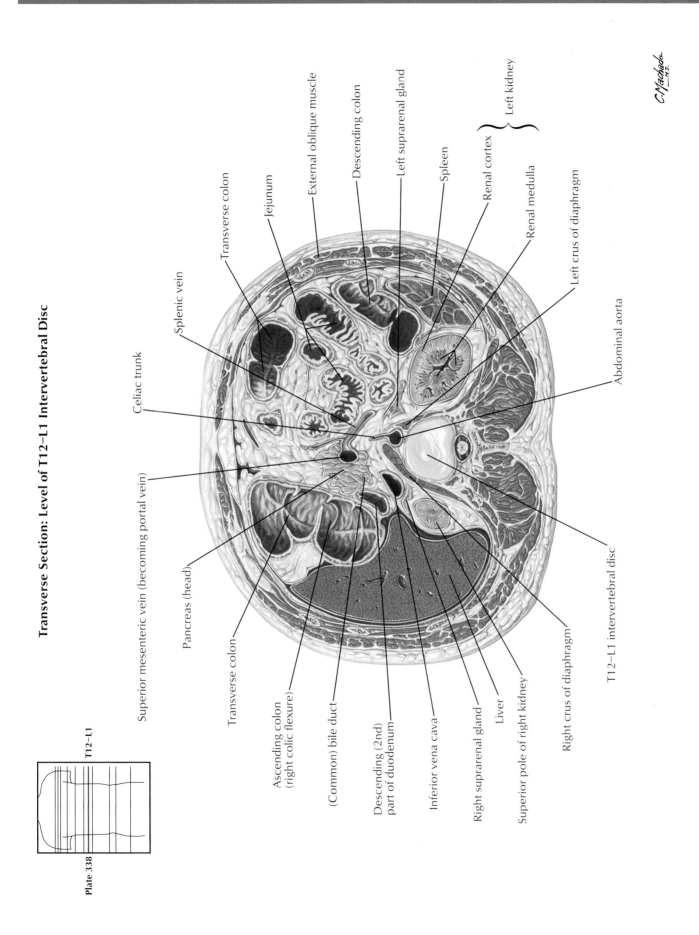

Transverse colon

Jejunum

External oblique muscle

Descending colon

Left suprarenal gland

Spleen

Renal cortex

Left kidney

Renal medulla

Left crus of diaphragm

Splenic vein

Celiac trunk

Abdominal aorta

Superior mesenteric vein (becoming portal vein)

Pancreas (head)

Transverse colon

Ascending colon (right colic flexure)

(Common) bile duct

Descending (2nd) part of duodenum

Inferior vena cava

Right suprarenal gland

Liver

Superior pole of right kidney

Right crus of diaphragm

T12–L1 intervertebral disc

T12–L1

Plate 338

Transverse Section: Level of L1–2 Intervertebral Disc

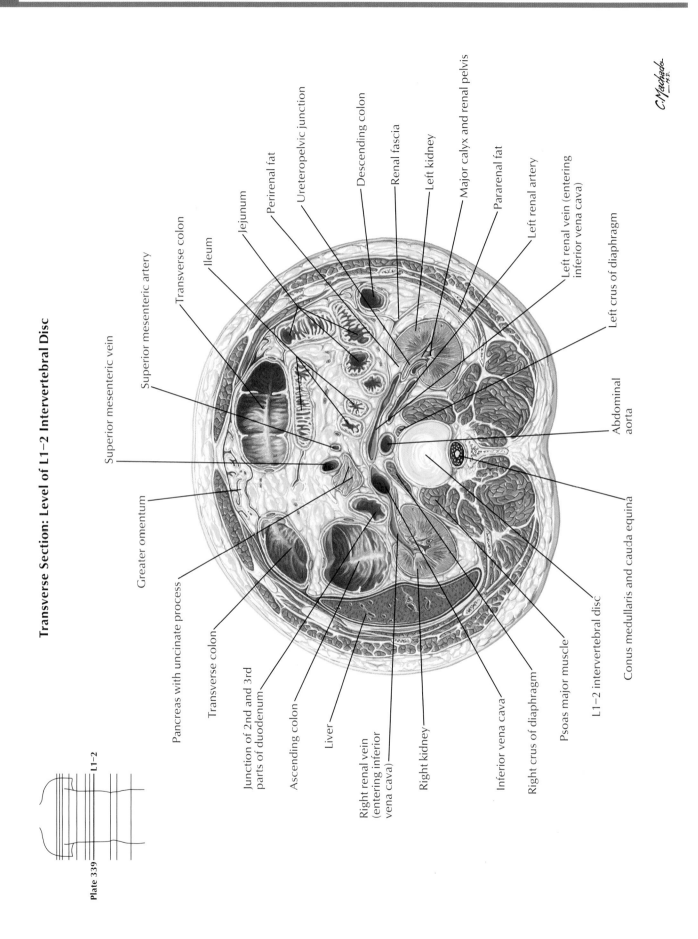

Superior mesenteric vein

Superior mesenteric artery

Transverse colon

Ileum

Jejunum

Perirenal fat

Ureteropelvic junction

Descending colon

Renal fascia

Left kidney

Major calyx and renal pelvis

Pararenal fat

Left renal artery

Left renal vein (entering inferior vena cava)

Left crus of diaphragm

Abdominal aorta

Conus medullaris and cauda equina

L1–2 intervertebral disc

Psoas major muscle

Right crus of diaphragm

Inferior vena cava

Right kidney

Right renal vein (entering inferior vena cava)

Liver

Ascending colon

Junction of 2nd and 3rd parts of duodenum

Transverse colon

Pancreas with uncinate process

Greater omentum

L1–2

Plate 339

Plate 339   **Kidneys and Suprarenal Glands**

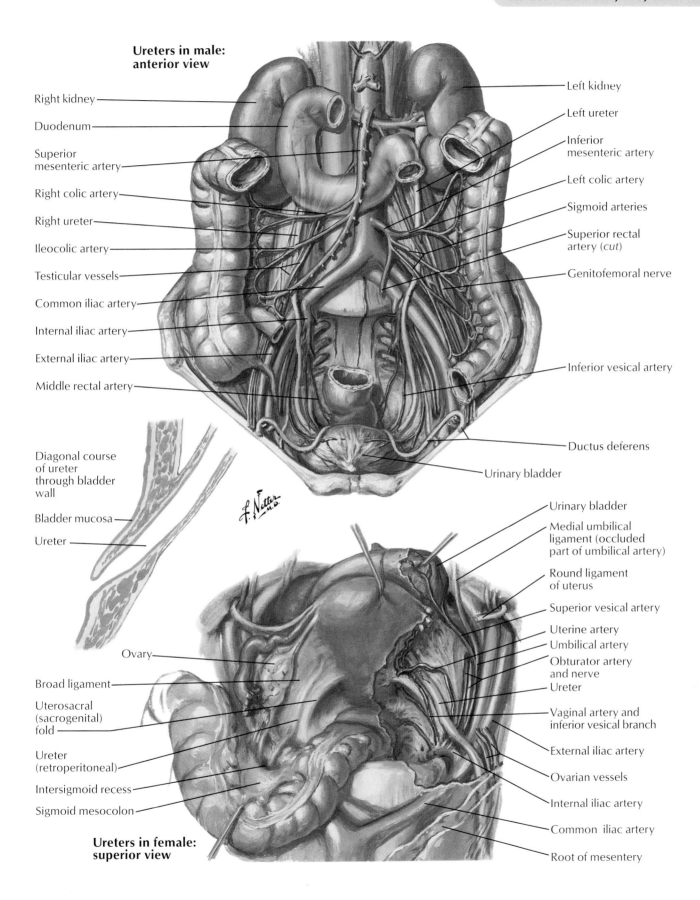

Ureters in male: anterior view

Right kidney

Duodenum

Superior mesenteric artery

Right colic artery

Right ureter

Ileocolic artery

Testicular vessels

Common iliac artery

Internal iliac artery

External iliac artery

Middle rectal artery

Left kidney

Left ureter

Inferior mesenteric artery

Left colic artery

Sigmoid arteries

Superior rectal artery (*cut*)

Genitofemoral nerve

Inferior vesical artery

Ductus deferens

Urinary bladder

Diagonal course of ureter through bladder wall

Bladder mucosa

Ureter

Urinary bladder

Medial umbilical ligament (occluded part of umbilical artery)

Round ligament of uterus

Superior vesical artery

Uterine artery

Umbilical artery

Obturator artery and nerve

Ureter

Vaginal artery and inferior vesical branch

External iliac artery

Ovarian vessels

Internal iliac artery

Common iliac artery

Root of mesentery

Ovary

Broad ligament

Uterosacral (sacrogenital) fold

Ureter (retroperitoneal)

Intersigmoid recess

Sigmoid mesocolon

Ureters in female: superior view

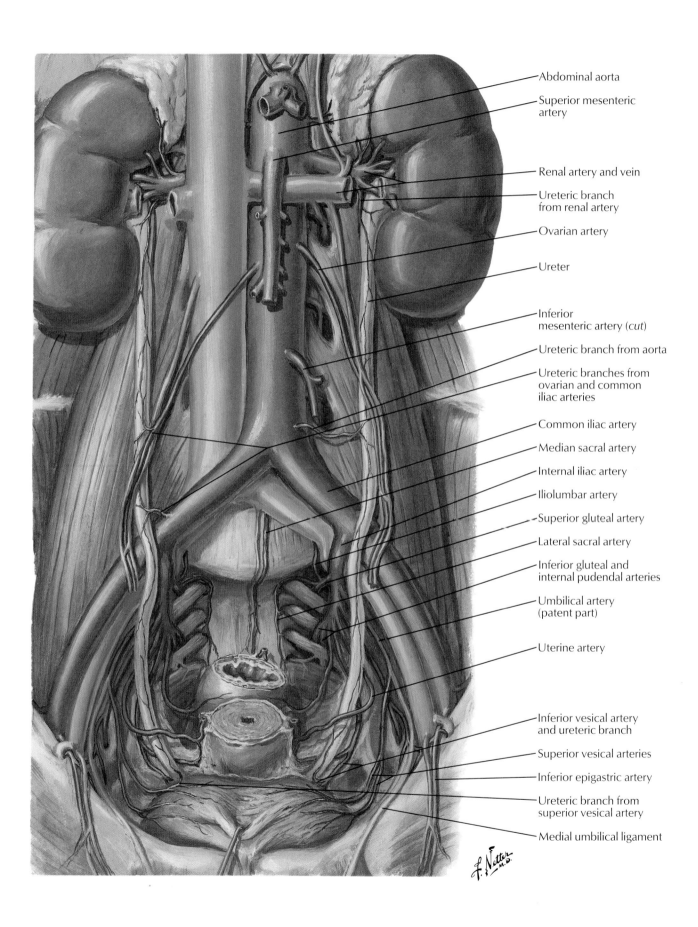

Abdominal aorta

Superior mesenteric artery

Renal artery and vein

Ureteric branch from renal artery

Ovarian artery

Ureter

Inferior mesenteric artery (*cut*)

Ureteric branch from aorta

Ureteric branches from ovarian and common iliac arteries

Common iliac artery

Median sacral artery

Internal iliac artery

Iliolumbar artery

Superior gluteal artery

Lateral sacral artery

Inferior gluteal and internal pudendal arteries

Umbilical artery (patent part)

Uterine artery

Inferior vesical artery and ureteric branch

Superior vesical arteries

Inferior epigastric artery

Ureteric branch from superior vesical artery

Medial umbilical ligament

Plate 341 **Kidneys and Suprarenal Glands**

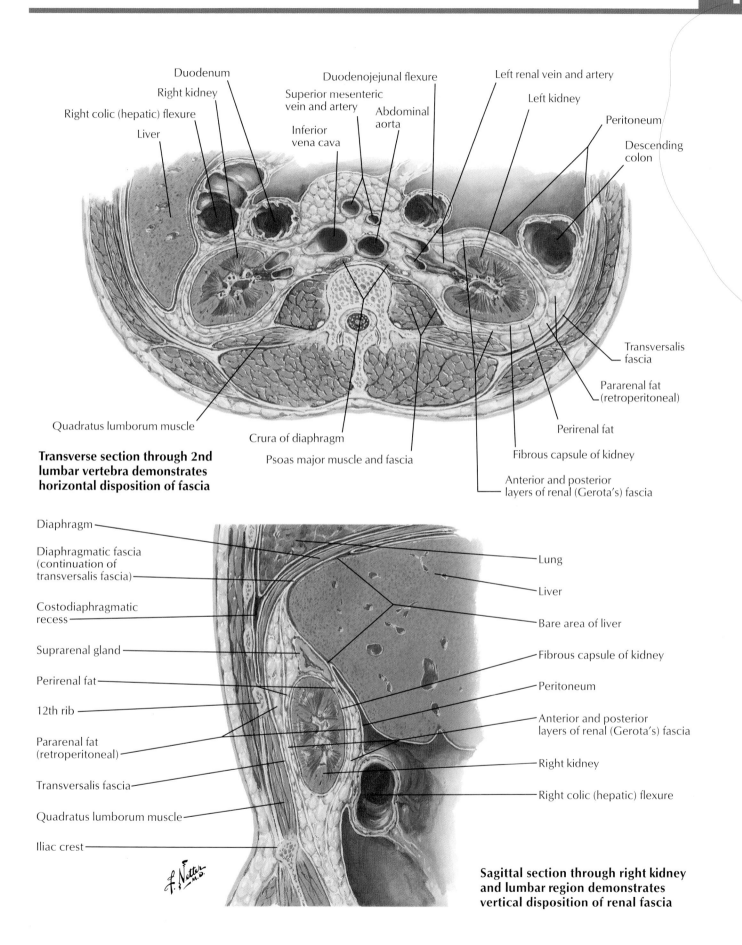

Duodenum

Right kidney

Right colic (hepatic) flexure

Liver

Duodenojejunal flexure

Superior mesenteric vein and artery

Abdominal aorta

Inferior vena cava

Left renal vein and artery

Left kidney

Peritoneum

Descending colon

Transversalis fascia

Pararenal fat (retroperitoneal)

Quadratus lumborum muscle

Crura of diaphragm

Psoas major muscle and fascia

Perirenal fat

Fibrous capsule of kidney

Anterior and posterior layers of renal (Gerota's) fascia

Transverse section through 2nd lumbar vertebra demonstrates horizontal disposition of fascia

Diaphragm

Diaphragmatic fascia (continuation of transversalis fascia)

Costodiaphragmatic recess

Suprarenal gland

Perirenal fat

12th rib

Pararenal fat (retroperitoneal)

Transversalis fascia

Quadratus lumborum muscle

Iliac crest

Lung

Liver

Bare area of liver

Fibrous capsule of kidney

Peritoneum

Anterior and posterior layers of renal (Gerota's) fascia

Right kidney

Right colic (hepatic) flexure

Sagittal section through right kidney and lumbar region demonstrates vertical disposition of renal fascia

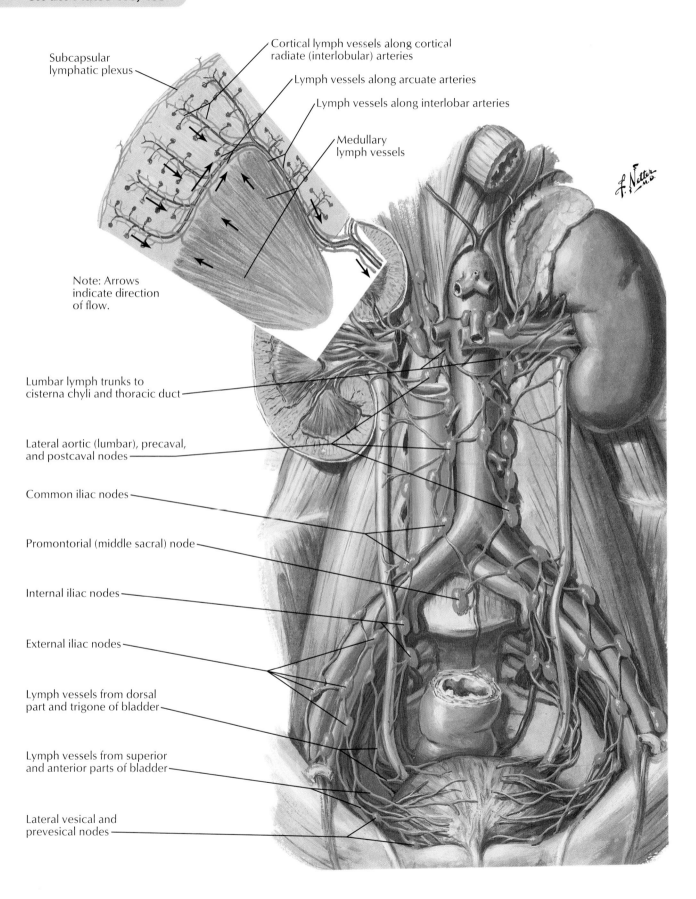

Subcapsular lymphatic plexus

Cortical lymph vessels along cortical radiate (interlobular) arteries

Lymph vessels along arcuate arteries

Lymph vessels along interlobar arteries

Medullary lymph vessels

Note: Arrows indicate direction of flow.

Lumbar lymph trunks to cisterna chyli and thoracic duct

Lateral aortic (lumbar), precaval, and postcaval nodes

Common iliac nodes

Promontorial (middle sacral) node

Internal iliac nodes

External iliac nodes

Lymph vessels from dorsal part and trigone of bladder

Lymph vessels from superior and anterior parts of bladder

Lateral vesical and prevesical nodes

Plate 343

Kidneys and Suprarenal Glands

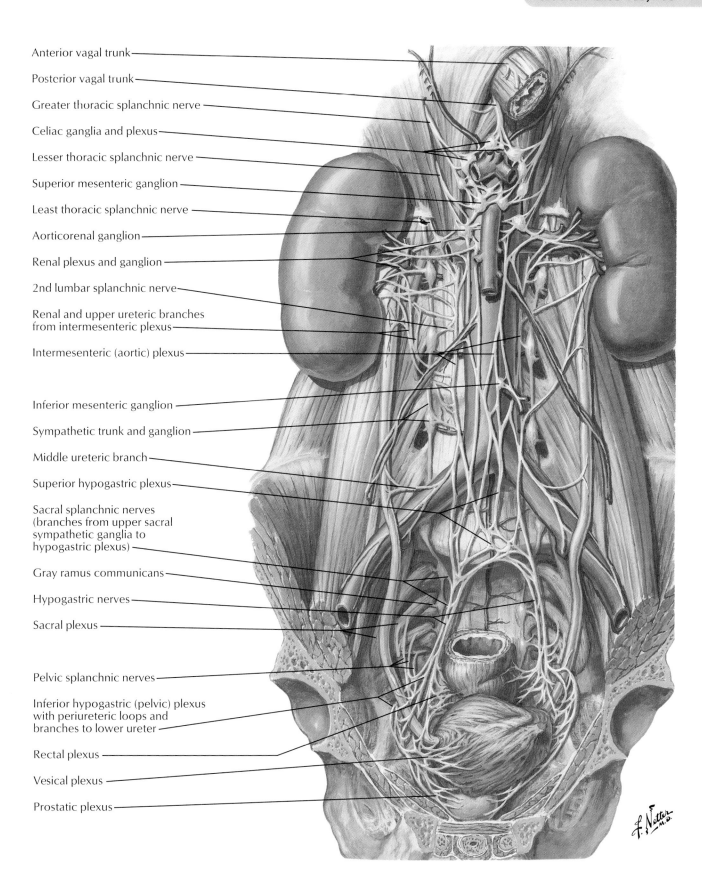

Anterior vagal trunk

Posterior vagal trunk

Greater thoracic splanchnic nerve

Celiac ganglia and plexus

Lesser thoracic splanchnic nerve

Superior mesenteric ganglion

Least thoracic splanchnic nerve

Aorticorenal ganglion

Renal plexus and ganglion

2nd lumbar splanchnic nerve

Renal and upper ureteric branches from intermesenteric plexus

Intermesenteric (aortic) plexus

Inferior mesenteric ganglion

Sympathetic trunk and ganglion

Middle ureteric branch

Superior hypogastric plexus

Sacral splanchnic nerves (branches from upper sacral sympathetic ganglia to hypogastric plexus)

Gray ramus communicans

Hypogastric nerves

Sacral plexus

Pelvic splanchnic nerves

Inferior hypogastric (pelvic) plexus with periureteric loops and branches to lower ureter

Rectal plexus

Vesical plexus

Prostatic plexus

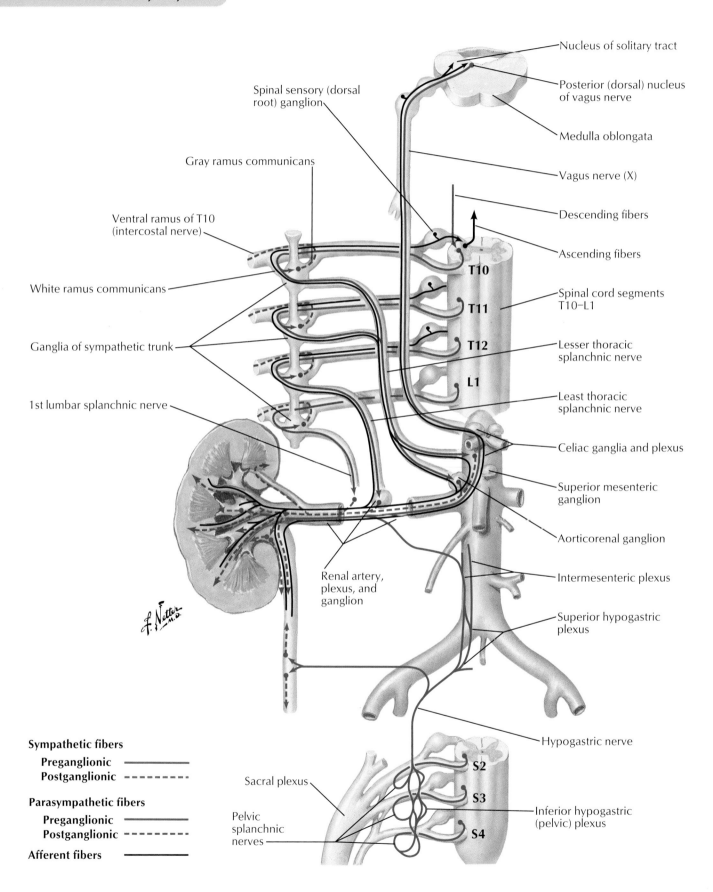

Nucleus of solitary tract

Posterior (dorsal) nucleus of vagus nerve

Medulla oblongata

Vagus nerve (X)

Descending fibers

Ascending fibers

Spinal cord segments T10–L1

Lesser thoracic splanchnic nerve

Least thoracic splanchnic nerve

Celiac ganglia and plexus

Superior mesenteric ganglion

Aorticorenal ganglion

Intermesenteric plexus

Superior hypogastric plexus

Hypogastric nerve

Inferior hypogastric (pelvic) plexus

Spinal sensory (dorsal root) ganglion

Gray ramus communicans

Ventral ramus of T10 (intercostal nerve)

White ramus communicans

Ganglia of sympathetic trunk

1st lumbar splanchnic nerve

Renal artery, plexus, and ganglion

Sacral plexus

Pelvic splanchnic nerves

T10

T11

T12

L1

S2

S3

S4

Sympathetic fibers
  Preganglionic ⎯⎯⎯
  Postganglionic - - - - -

Parasympathetic fibers
  Preganglionic ⎯⎯⎯
  Postganglionic - - - - -

Afferent fibers ⎯⎯⎯

Plate 345

Kidneys and Suprarenal Glands

See also **Plates 165–168**

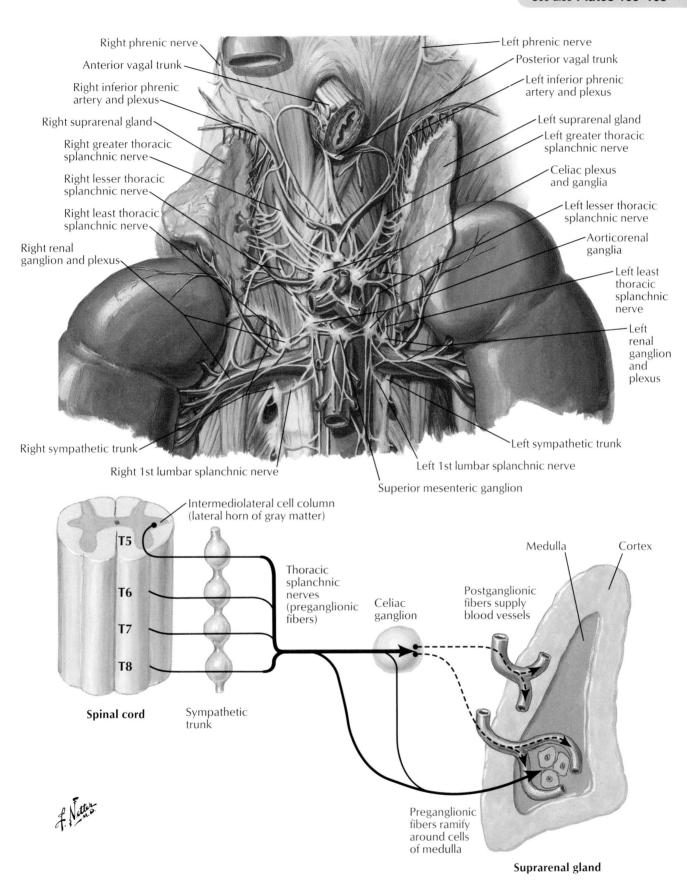

Right phrenic nerve

Anterior vagal trunk

Right inferior phrenic artery and plexus

Right suprarenal gland

Right greater thoracic splanchnic nerve

Right lesser thoracic splanchnic nerve

Right least thoracic splanchnic nerve

Right renal ganglion and plexus

Right sympathetic trunk

Right 1st lumbar splanchnic nerve

Left phrenic nerve

Posterior vagal trunk

Left inferior phrenic artery and plexus

Left suprarenal gland

Left greater thoracic splanchnic nerve

Celiac plexus and ganglia

Left lesser thoracic splanchnic nerve

Aorticorenal ganglia

Left least thoracic splanchnic nerve

Left renal ganglion and plexus

Left sympathetic trunk

Left 1st lumbar splanchnic nerve

Superior mesenteric ganglion

Intermediolateral cell column (lateral horn of gray matter)

T5

T6

T7

T8

Spinal cord

Sympathetic trunk

Thoracic splanchnic nerves (preganglionic fibers)

Celiac ganglion

Medulla   Cortex

Postganglionic fibers supply blood vessels

Preganglionic fibers ramify around cells of medulla

Suprarenal gland

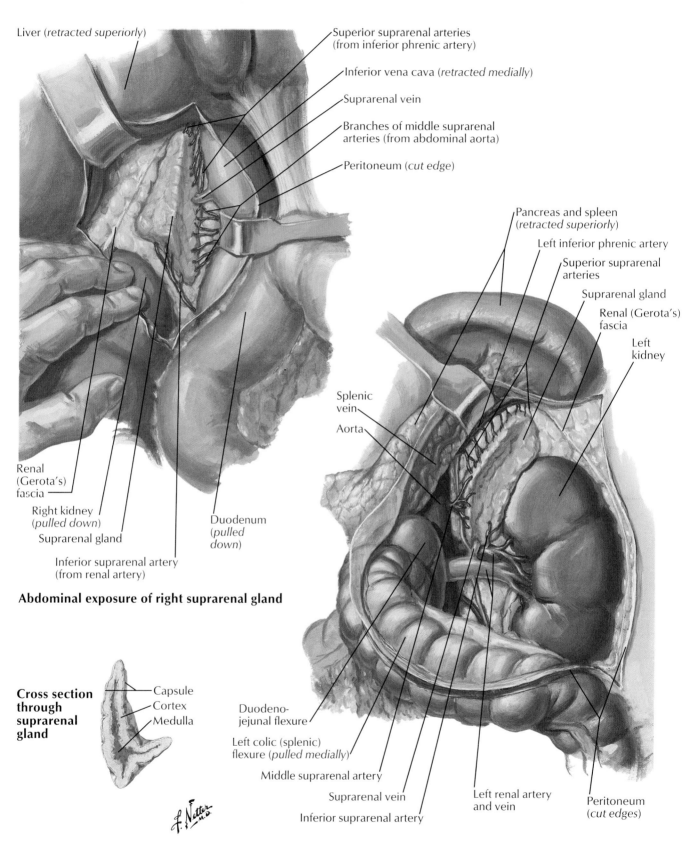

Liver (*retracted superiorly*)

Superior suprarenal arteries (from inferior phrenic artery)

Inferior vena cava (*retracted medially*)

Suprarenal vein

Branches of middle suprarenal arteries (from abdominal aorta)

Peritoneum (*cut edge*)

Pancreas and spleen (*retracted superiorly*)

Left inferior phrenic artery

Superior suprarenal arteries

Suprarenal gland

Renal (Gerota's) fascia

Left kidney

Splenic vein

Aorta

Renal (Gerota's) fascia

Right kidney (*pulled down*)

Suprarenal gland

Inferior suprarenal artery (from renal artery)

Duodenum (*pulled down*)

Abdominal exposure of right suprarenal gland

Cross section through suprarenal gland

Capsule

Cortex

Medulla

Duodeno-jejunal flexure

Left colic (splenic) flexure (*pulled medially*)

Middle suprarenal artery

Suprarenal vein

Inferior suprarenal artery

Left renal artery and vein

Peritoneum (*cut edges*)

Abdominal exposure of left suprarenal gland

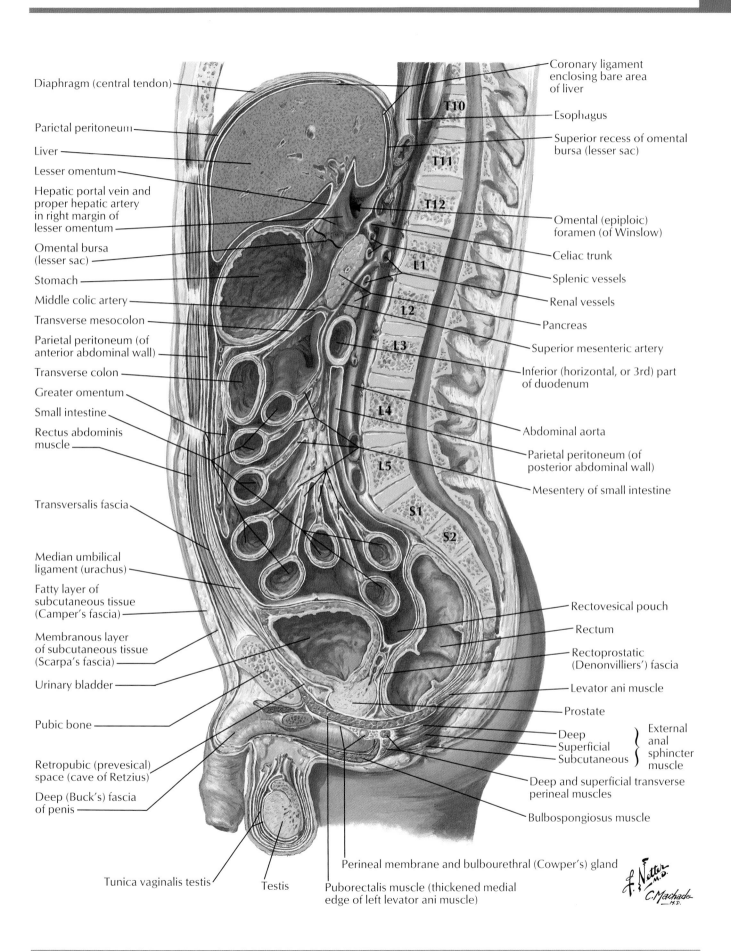

Diaphragm (central tendon)

Parietal peritoneum

Liver

Lesser omentum

Hepatic portal vein and proper hepatic artery in right margin of lesser omentum

Omental bursa (lesser sac)

Stomach

Middle colic artery

Transverse mesocolon

Parietal peritoneum (of anterior abdominal wall)

Transverse colon

Greater omentum

Small intestine

Rectus abdominis muscle

Transversalis fascia

Median umbilical ligament (urachus)

Fatty layer of subcutaneous tissue (Camper's fascia)

Membranous layer of subcutaneous tissue (Scarpa's fascia)

Urinary bladder

Pubic bone

Retropubic (prevesical) space (cave of Retzius)

Deep (Buck's) fascia of penis

Tunica vaginalis testis

Testis

Coronary ligament enclosing bare area of liver

Esophagus

Superior recess of omental bursa (lesser sac)

T10

T11

T12

L1

L2

L3

L4

L5

S1

S2

Omental (epiploic) foramen (of Winslow)

Celiac trunk

Splenic vessels

Renal vessels

Pancreas

Superior mesenteric artery

Inferior (horizontal, or 3rd) part of duodenum

Abdominal aorta

Parietal peritoneum (of posterior abdominal wall)

Mesentery of small intestine

Rectovesical pouch

Rectum

Rectoprostatic (Denonvilliers') fascia

Levator ani muscle

Prostate

Deep
Superficial
Subcutaneous

} External anal sphincter muscle

Deep and superficial transverse perineal muscles

Bulbospongiosus muscle

Perineal membrane and bulbourethral (Cowper's) gland

Puborectalis muscle (thickened medial edge of left levator ani muscle)

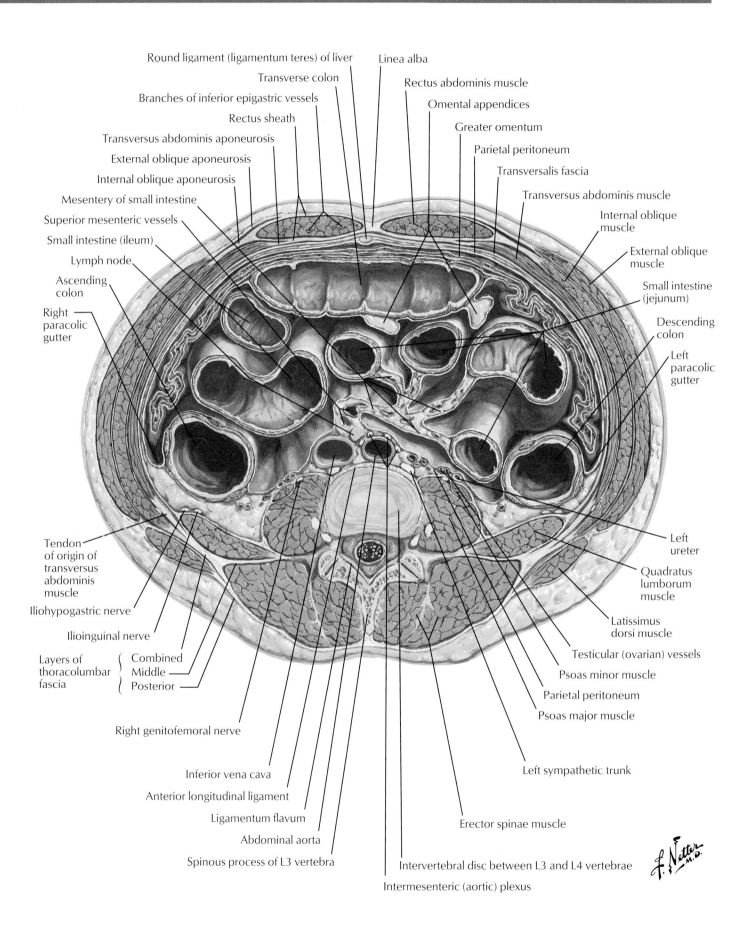

Round ligament (ligamentum teres) of liver

Transverse colon

Branches of inferior epigastric vessels

Rectus sheath

Transversus abdominis aponeurosis

External oblique aponeurosis

Internal oblique aponeurosis

Mesentery of small intestine

Superior mesenteric vessels

Small intestine (ileum)

Lymph node

Ascending colon

Right paracolic gutter

Linea alba

Rectus abdominis muscle

Omental appendices

Greater omentum

Parietal peritoneum

Transversalis fascia

Transversus abdominis muscle

Internal oblique muscle

External oblique muscle

Small intestine (jejunum)

Descending colon

Left paracolic gutter

Left ureter

Quadratus lumborum muscle

Latissimus dorsi muscle

Testicular (ovarian) vessels

Psoas minor muscle

Parietal peritoneum

Psoas major muscle

Left sympathetic trunk

Erector spinae muscle

Intervertebral disc between L3 and L4 vertebrae

Intermesenteric (aortic) plexus

Tendon of origin of transversus abdominis muscle

Iliohypogastric nerve

Ilioinguinal nerve

Layers of thoracolumbar fascia { Combined Middle Posterior

Right genitofemoral nerve

Inferior vena cava

Anterior longitudinal ligament

Ligamentum flavum

Abdominal aorta

Spinous process of L3 vertebra

Plate 349 **Abdominal Sections**

Series of abdominal axial CT images from superior (A) to inferior (D)

A

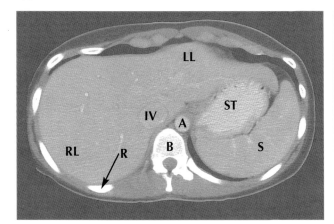

B

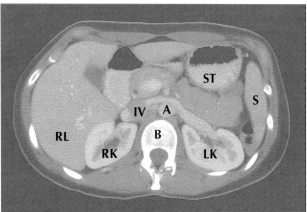

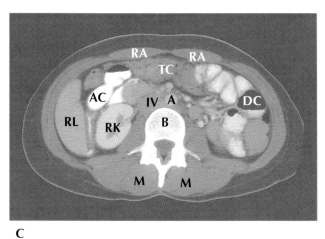

C

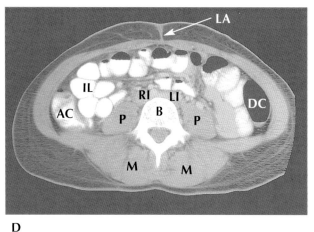

D

A	Aorta	**M**	Deep back muscles
AC	Ascending colon	**P**	Psoas muscle
B	Body of vertebra	**R**	Rib
DC	Descending colon	**RA**	Rectus abdominis muscle
IL	Ileum	**RI**	Right common iliac artery
IV	Inferior vena cava	**RL**	Right lobe of liver
LA	Linea alba	**S**	Spleen
LI	Left common iliac artery	**ST**	Stomach
LK	Left kidney	**TC**	Transverse colon
LL	Left lobe of liver		

Section 5 **Pelvis and Perineum**

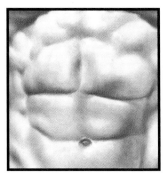
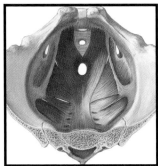
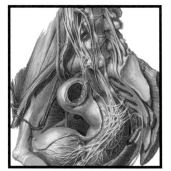
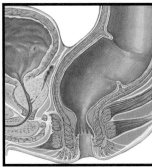

5 Pelvis and Perineum

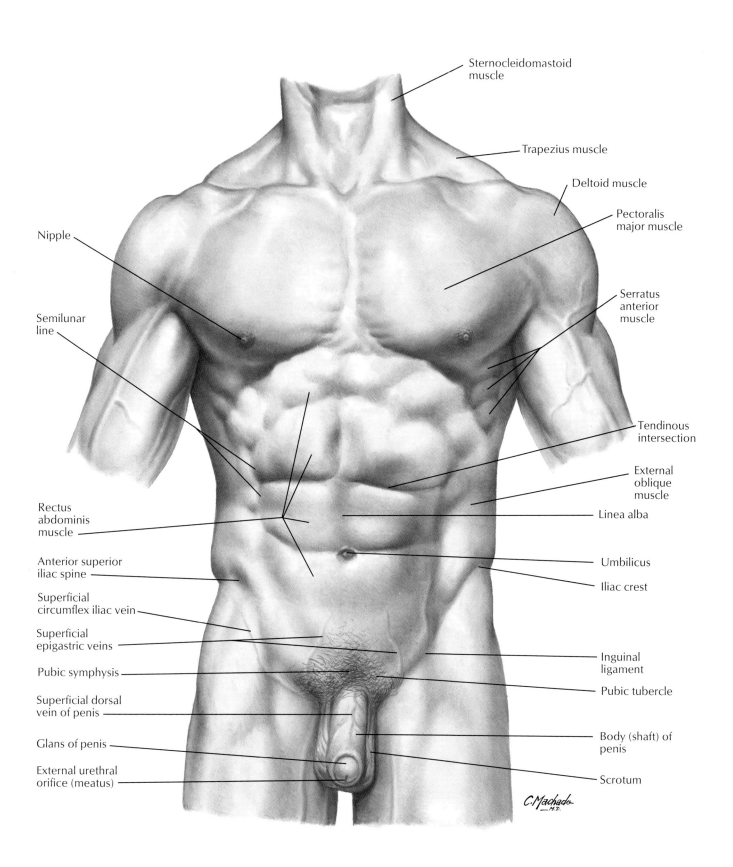

Sternocleidomastoid muscle

Trapezius muscle

Deltoid muscle

Pectoralis major muscle

Serratus anterior muscle

Nipple

Semilunar line

Tendinous intersection

External oblique muscle

Linea alba

Rectus abdominis muscle

Umbilicus

Anterior superior iliac spine

Iliac crest

Superficial circumflex iliac vein

Superficial epigastric veins

Inguinal ligament

Pubic symphysis

Pubic tubercle

Superficial dorsal vein of penis

Body (shaft) of penis

Glans of penis

External urethral orifice (meatus)

Scrotum

C.Machado M.D.

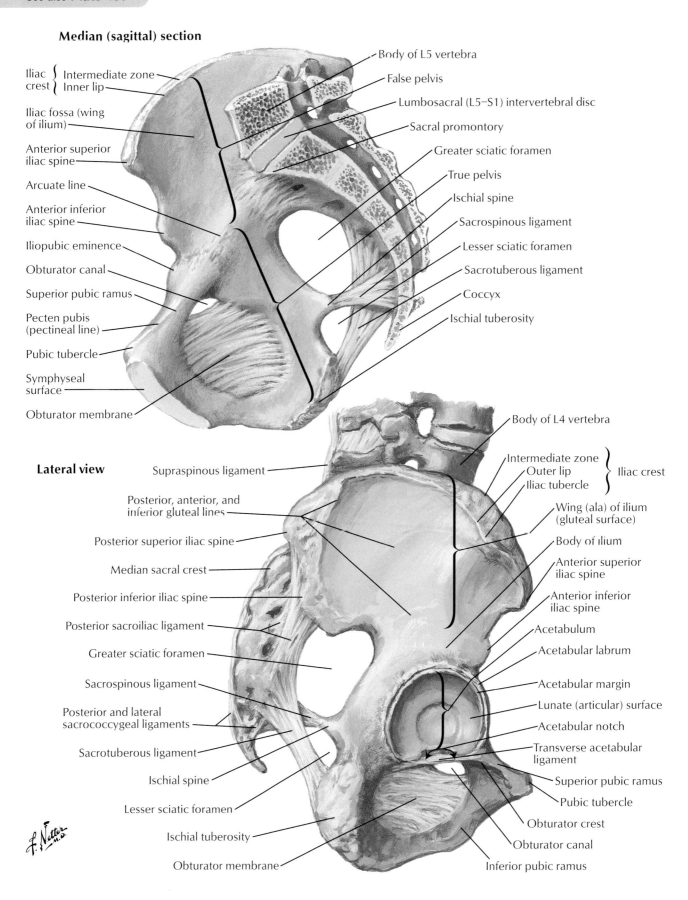

Median (sagittal) section

Iliac crest { Intermediate zone / Inner lip

Iliac fossa (wing of ilium)

Anterior superior iliac spine

Arcuate line

Anterior inferior iliac spine

Iliopubic eminence

Obturator canal

Superior pubic ramus

Pecten pubis (pectineal line)

Pubic tubercle

Symphyseal surface

Obturator membrane

Body of L5 vertebra

False pelvis

Lumbosacral (L5–S1) intervertebral disc

Sacral promontory

Greater sciatic foramen

True pelvis

Ischial spine

Sacrospinous ligament

Lesser sciatic foramen

Sacrotuberous ligament

Coccyx

Ischial tuberosity

Lateral view

Supraspinous ligament

Posterior, anterior, and inferior gluteal lines

Posterior superior iliac spine

Median sacral crest

Posterior inferior iliac spine

Posterior sacroiliac ligament

Greater sciatic foramen

Sacrospinous ligament

Posterior and lateral sacrococcygeal ligaments

Sacrotuberous ligament

Ischial spine

Lesser sciatic foramen

Ischial tuberosity

Obturator membrane

Body of L4 vertebra

Intermediate zone / Outer lip / Iliac tubercle } Iliac crest

Wing (ala) of ilium (gluteal surface)

Body of ilium

Anterior superior iliac spine

Anterior inferior iliac spine

Acetabulum

Acetabular labrum

Acetabular margin

Lunate (articular) surface

Acetabular notch

Transverse acetabular ligament

Superior pubic ramus

Pubic tubercle

Obturator crest

Obturator canal

Inferior pubic ramus

Plate 352 　　　　　　　　　　　　　　　**Bones and Ligaments**

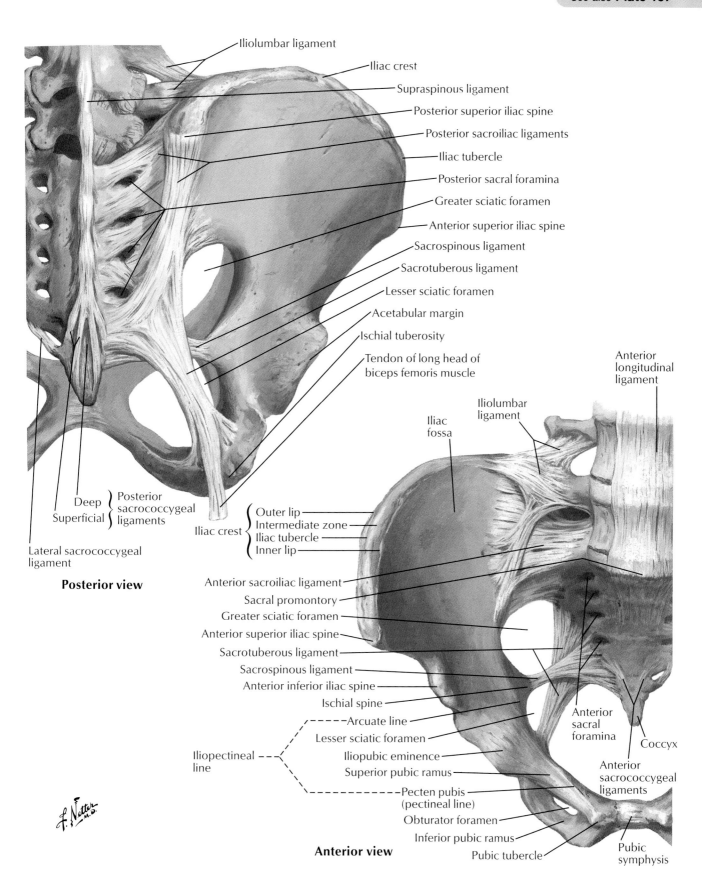

Iliolumbar ligament

Iliac crest

Supraspinous ligament

Posterior superior iliac spine

Posterior sacroiliac ligaments

Iliac tubercle

Posterior sacral foramina

Greater sciatic foramen

Anterior superior iliac spine

Sacrospinous ligament

Sacrotuberous ligament

Lesser sciatic foramen

Acetabular margin

Ischial tuberosity

Tendon of long head of biceps femoris muscle

Deep } Posterior
Superficial } sacrococcygeal ligaments

Iliac crest

Lateral sacrococcygeal ligament

Posterior view

Anterior longitudinal ligament

Iliac fossa

Iliolumbar ligament

Iliac crest
{ Outer lip
{ Intermediate zone
{ Iliac tubercle
{ Inner lip

Anterior sacroiliac ligament

Sacral promontory

Greater sciatic foramen

Anterior superior iliac spine

Sacrotuberous ligament

Sacrospinous ligament

Anterior inferior iliac spine

Ischial spine

Arcuate line

Lesser sciatic foramen

Iliopectineal line

Iliopubic eminence

Superior pubic ramus

Pecten pubis (pectineal line)

Obturator foramen

Inferior pubic ramus

Pubic tubercle

Anterior sacral foramina

Coccyx

Anterior sacrococcygeal ligaments

Pubic symphysis

Anterior view

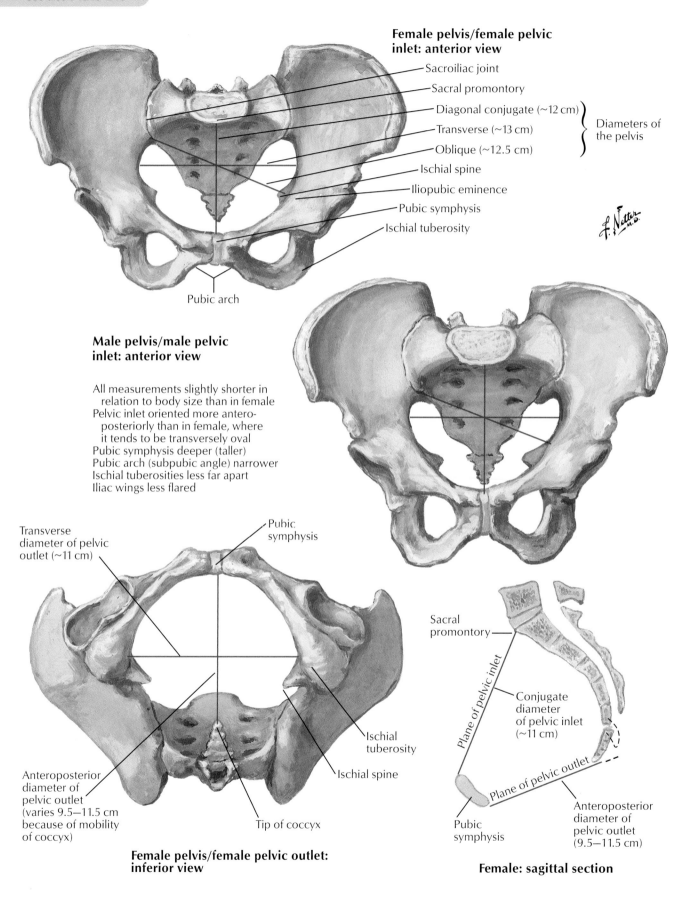

Female pelvis/female pelvic inlet: anterior view

Sacroiliac joint
Sacral promontory
Diagonal conjugate (~12 cm)
Transverse (~13 cm)
Oblique (~12.5 cm)
Ischial spine
Iliopubic eminence
Pubic symphysis
Ischial tuberosity

} Diameters of the pelvis

Pubic arch

Male pelvis/male pelvic inlet: anterior view

All measurements slightly shorter in relation to body size than in female
Pelvic inlet oriented more antero-posteriorly than in female, where it tends to be transversely oval
Pubic symphysis deeper (taller)
Pubic arch (subpubic angle) narrower
Ischial tuberosities less far apart
Iliac wings less flared

Transverse diameter of pelvic outlet (~11 cm)

Pubic symphysis

Ischial tuberosity
Ischial spine

Anteroposterior diameter of pelvic outlet (varies 9.5—11.5 cm because of mobility of coccyx)

Tip of coccyx

Female pelvis/female pelvic outlet: inferior view

Sacral promontory

Plane of pelvic inlet

Conjugate diameter of pelvic inlet (~11 cm)

Plane of pelvic outlet

Pubic symphysis

Anteroposterior diameter of pelvic outlet (9.5—11.5 cm)

Female: sagittal section

Plate 354

Bones and Ligaments

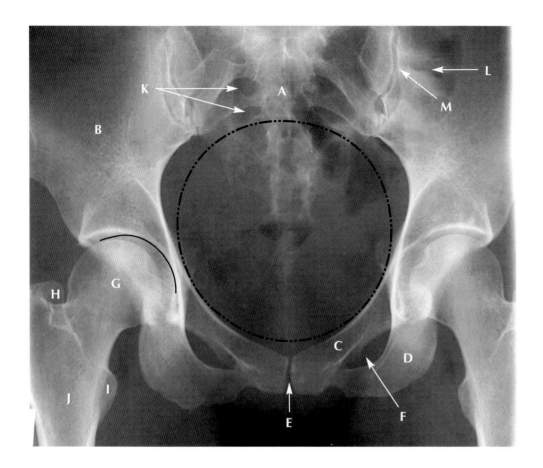

Female Pelvis

A   Sacrum
B   Ilium
C   Pubis
D   Ischium
E   Pubis symphysis
F   Obturator foramen
G   Head of femur
H   Greater trochanter
I   Lesser trochanter
J   Femur
K   Pelvic foramina
L   Air in colon
M   Sacroiliac joint
——   Acetabulum
·—··—··—·   Pelvic inlet

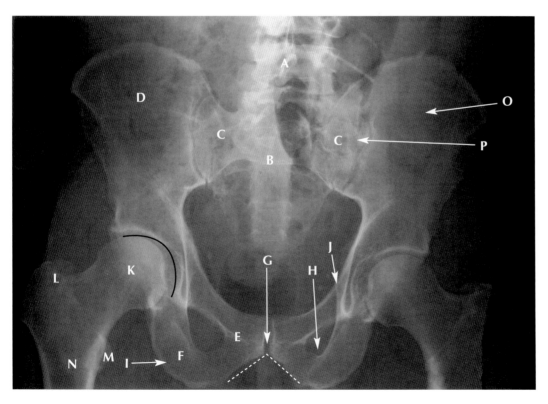

Male Pelvis

A   L5
B   Sacrum
C   Ala of sacrum
D   Ilium
E   Pubis
F   Ischium
G   Pubic symphysis
H   Obturator foramen
I   Ischial tuberosity
J   Ischial spine
K   Head of femur
L   Greater trochanter
M   Lesser trochanter
N   Femur
O   Air in colon
P   Sacroiliac joint
——   Acetabulum
--------   Subpubic angle

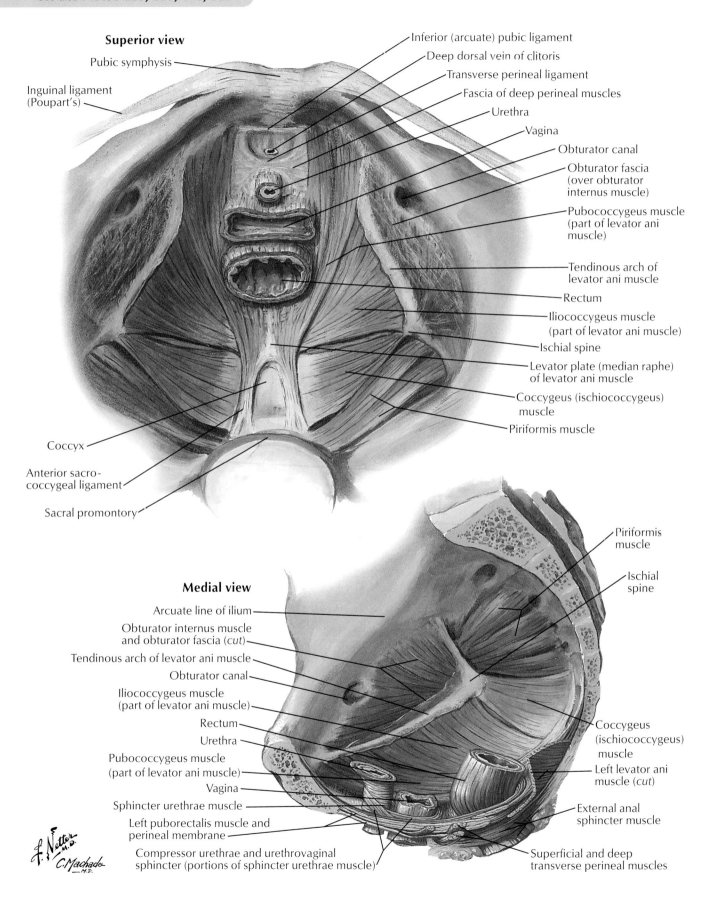

Superior view

Pubic symphysis

Inguinal ligament (Poupart's)

Inferior (arcuate) pubic ligament

Deep dorsal vein of clitoris

Transverse perineal ligament

Fascia of deep perineal muscles

Urethra

Vagina

Obturator canal

Obturator fascia (over obturator internus muscle)

Pubococcygeus muscle (part of levator ani muscle)

Tendinous arch of levator ani muscle

Rectum

Iliococcygeus muscle (part of levator ani muscle)

Ischial spine

Levator plate (median raphe) of levator ani muscle

Coccygeus (ischiococcygeus) muscle

Piriformis muscle

Coccyx

Anterior sacro-coccygeal ligament

Sacral promontory

Medial view

Arcuate line of ilium

Obturator internus muscle and obturator fascia (cut)

Tendinous arch of levator ani muscle

Obturator canal

Iliococcygeus muscle (part of levator ani muscle)

Rectum

Urethra

Pubococcygeus muscle (part of levator ani muscle)

Vagina

Sphincter urethrae muscle

Left puborectalis muscle and perineal membrane

Compressor urethrae and urethrovaginal sphincter (portions of sphincter urethrae muscle)

Piriformis muscle

Ischial spine

Coccygeus (ischiococcygeus) muscle

Left levator ani muscle (cut)

External anal sphincter muscle

Superficial and deep transverse perineal muscles

Plate 356

Pelvis Floor and Contents

For urogenital diaphragm see **Plate 379**

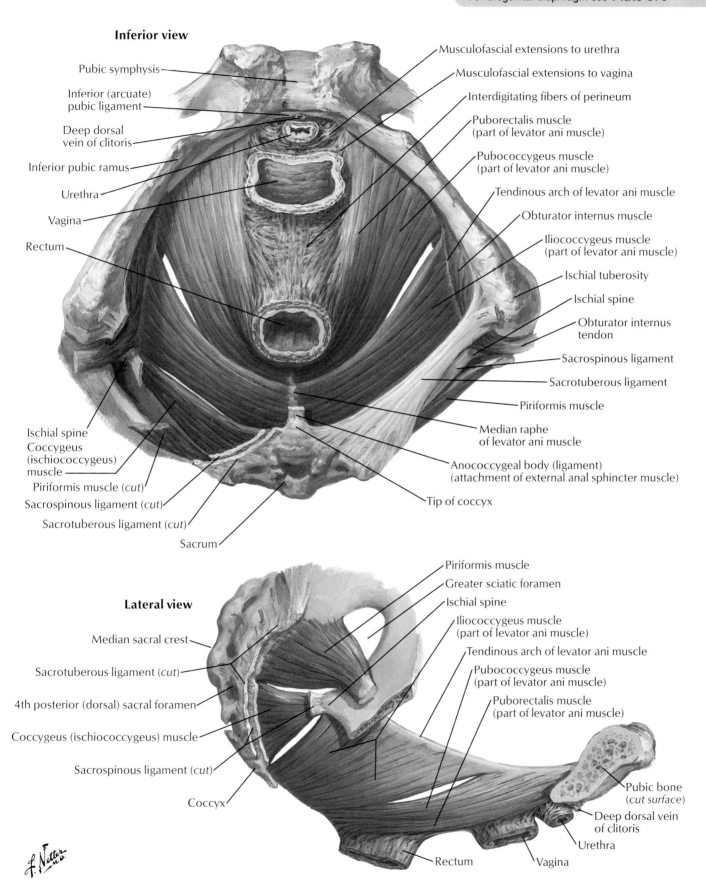

Inferior view

Pubic symphysis

Inferior (arcuate) pubic ligament

Deep dorsal vein of clitoris

Inferior pubic ramus

Urethra

Vagina

Rectum

Ischial spine

Coccygeus (ischiococcygeus) muscle

Piriformis muscle (*cut*)

Sacrospinous ligament (*cut*)

Sacrotuberous ligament (*cut*)

Sacrum

Musculofascial extensions to urethra

Musculofascial extensions to vagina

Interdigitating fibers of perineum

Puborectalis muscle (part of levator ani muscle)

Pubococcygeus muscle (part of levator ani muscle)

Tendinous arch of levator ani muscle

Obturator internus muscle

Iliococcygeus muscle (part of levator ani muscle)

Ischial tuberosity

Ischial spine

Obturator internus tendon

Sacrospinous ligament

Sacrotuberous ligament

Piriformis muscle

Median raphe of levator ani muscle

Anococcygeal body (ligament) (attachment of external anal sphincter muscle)

Tip of coccyx

Lateral view

Median sacral crest

Sacrotuberous ligament (*cut*)

4th posterior (dorsal) sacral foramen

Coccygeus (ischiococcygeus) muscle

Sacrospinous ligament (*cut*)

Coccyx

Piriformis muscle

Greater sciatic foramen

Ischial spine

Iliococcygeus muscle (part of levator ani muscle)

Tendinous arch of levator ani muscle

Pubococcygeus muscle (part of levator ani muscle)

Puborectalis muscle (part of levator ani muscle)

Pubic bone (*cut surface*)

Deep dorsal vein of clitoris

Urethra

Rectum

Vagina

**Superior view
(*viscera removed*)**

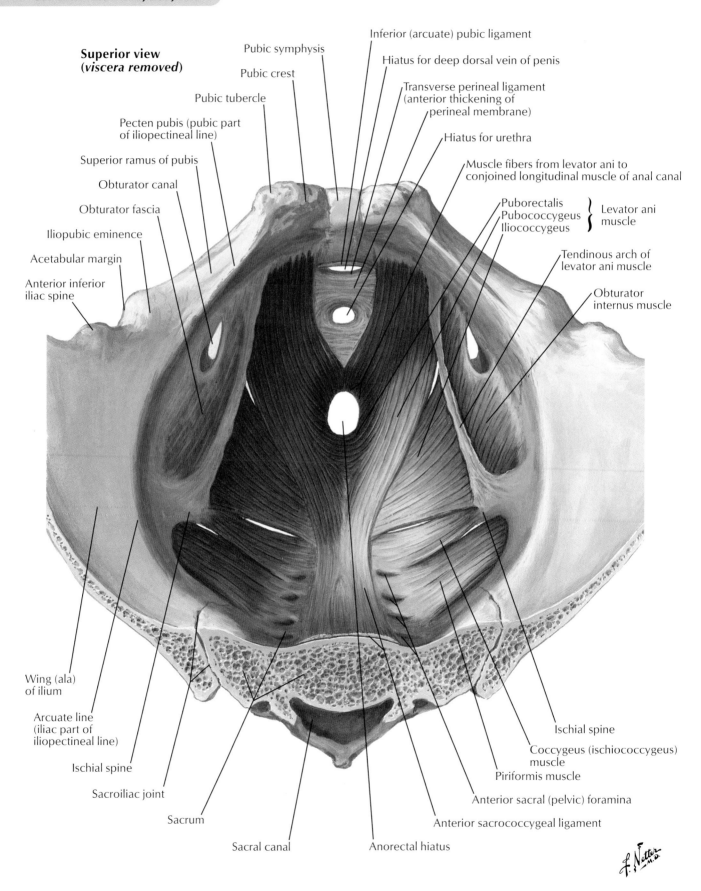

Pubic symphysis

Pubic crest

Pubic tubercle

Pecten pubis (pubic part
of iliopectineal line)

Superior ramus of pubis

Obturator canal

Obturator fascia

Iliopubic eminence

Acetabular margin

Anterior inferior
iliac spine

Inferior (arcuate) pubic ligament

Hiatus for deep dorsal vein of penis

Transverse perineal ligament
(anterior thickening of
perineal membrane)

Hiatus for urethra

Muscle fibers from levator ani to
conjoined longitudinal muscle of anal canal

Puborectalis ⎫
Pubococcygeus ⎬ Levator ani
Iliococcygeus ⎭ muscle

Tendinous arch of
levator ani muscle

Obturator
internus muscle

Wing (ala)
of ilium

Arcuate line
(iliac part of
iliopectineal line)

Ischial spine

Sacroiliac joint

Sacrum

Sacral canal

Anorectal hiatus

Ischial spine

Coccygeus (ischiococcygeus)
muscle

Piriformis muscle

Anterior sacral (pelvic) foramina

Anterior sacrococcygeal ligament

Plate 358

Pelvic Floor and Contents

Inferior view

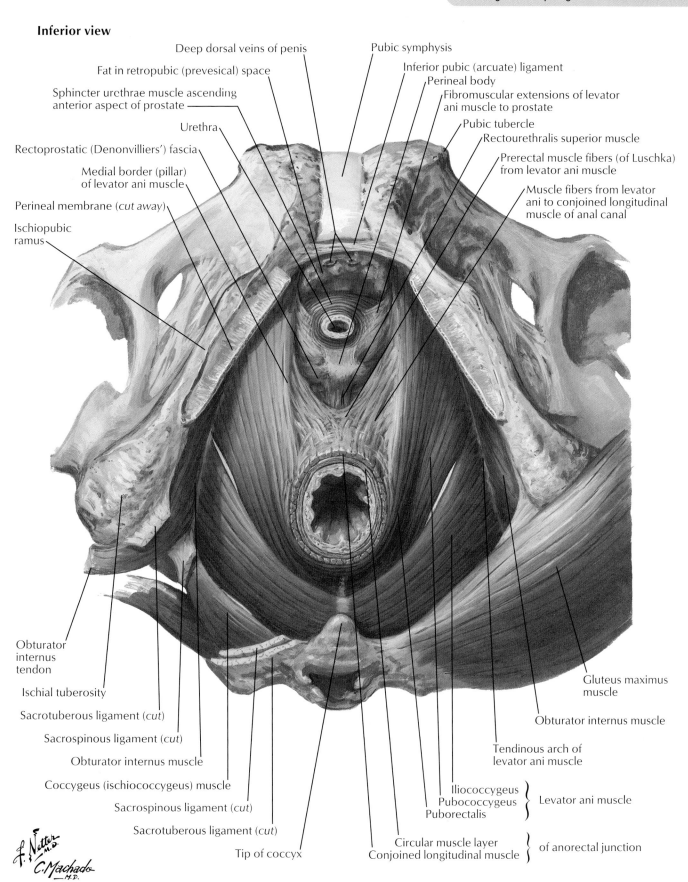

Deep dorsal veins of penis

Fat in retropubic (prevesical) space

Sphincter urethrae muscle ascending
anterior aspect of prostate

Urethra

Rectoprostatic (Denonvilliers') fascia

Medial border (pillar)
of levator ani muscle

Perineal membrane (cut away)

Ischiopubic
ramus

Pubic symphysis

Inferior pubic (arcuate) ligament

Perineal body

Fibromuscular extensions of levator
ani muscle to prostate

Pubic tubercle

Rectourethralis superior muscle

Prerectal muscle fibers (of Luschka)
from levator ani muscle

Muscle fibers from levator
ani to conjoined longitudinal
muscle of anal canal

Obturator
internus
tendon

Ischial tuberosity

Sacrotuberous ligament (cut)

Sacrospinous ligament (cut)

Obturator internus muscle

Coccygeus (ischiococcygeus) muscle

Sacrospinous ligament (cut)

Sacrotuberous ligament (cut)

Tip of coccyx

Circular muscle layer
Conjoined longitudinal muscle

Iliococcygeus
Pubococcygeus
Puborectalis

Levator ani muscle

of anorectal junction

Tendinous arch of
levator ani muscle

Obturator internus muscle

Gluteus maximus
muscle

Paramedian (sagittal) dissection

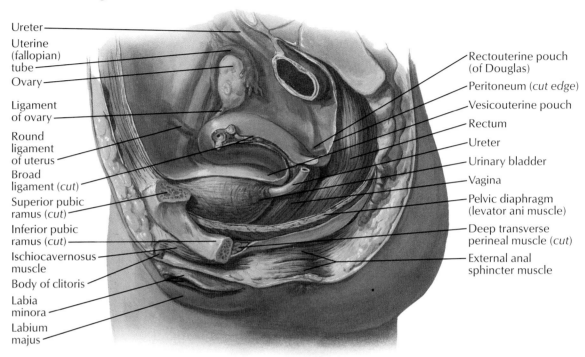

Ureter

Uterine (fallopian) tube

Ovary

Ligament of ovary

Round ligament of uterus

Broad ligament (*cut*)

Superior pubic ramus (*cut*)

Inferior pubic ramus (*cut*)

Ischiocavernosus muscle

Body of clitoris

Labia minora

Labium majus

Rectouterine pouch (of Douglas)

Peritoneum (*cut edge*)

Vesicouterine pouch

Rectum

Ureter

Urinary bladder

Vagina

Pelvic diaphragm (levator ani muscle)

Deep transverse perineal muscle (*cut*)

External anal sphincter muscle

Median (sagittal) section

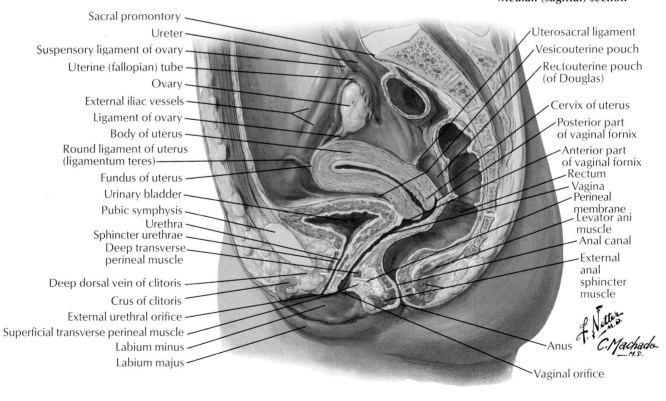

Sacral promontory

Ureter

Suspensory ligament of ovary

Uterine (fallopian) tube

Ovary

External iliac vessels

Ligament of ovary

Body of uterus

Round ligament of uterus (ligamentum teres)

Fundus of uterus

Urinary bladder

Pubic symphysis

Urethra

Sphincter urethrae

Deep transverse perineal muscle

Deep dorsal vein of clitoris

Crus of clitoris

External urethral orifice

Superficial transverse perineal muscle

Labium minus

Labium majus

Uterosacral ligament

Vesicouterine pouch

Rectouterine pouch (of Douglas)

Cervix of uterus

Posterior part of vaginal fornix

Anterior part of vaginal fornix

Rectum

Vagina

Perineal membrane

Levator ani muscle

Anal canal

External anal sphincter muscle

Anus

Vaginal orifice

Plate 360   **Pelvic Floor and Contents**

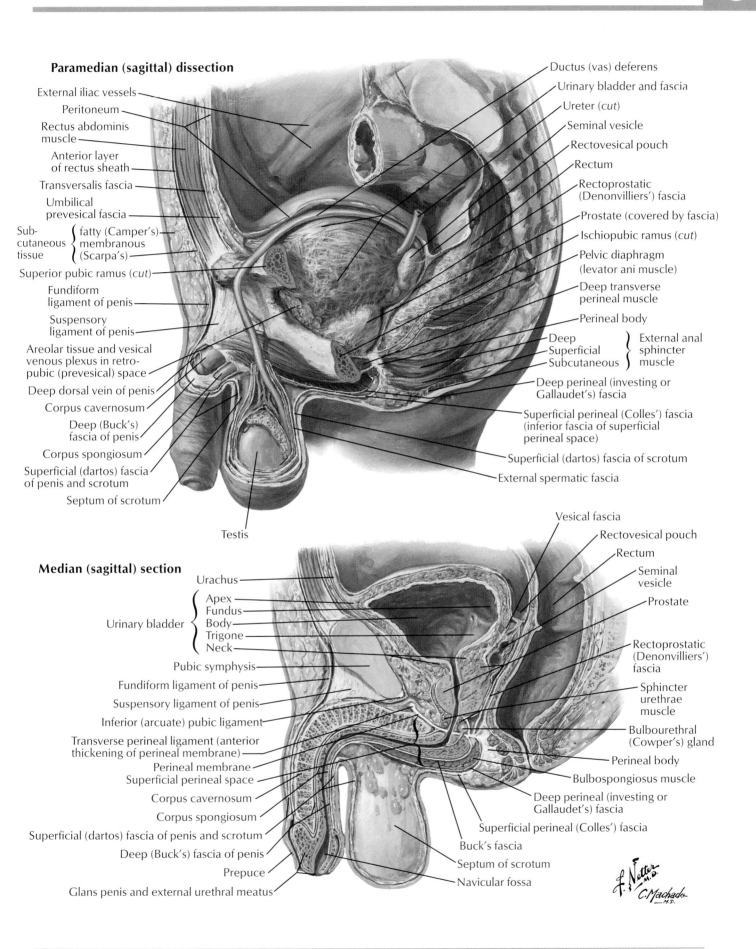

Paramedian (sagittal) dissection

External iliac vessels

Peritoneum

Rectus abdominis muscle

Anterior layer of rectus sheath

Transversalis fascia

Umbilical prevesical fascia

Subcutaneous tissue { fatty (Camper's) / membranous (Scarpa's) }

Superior pubic ramus (cut)

Fundiform ligament of penis

Suspensory ligament of penis

Areolar tissue and vesical venous plexus in retropubic (prevesical) space

Deep dorsal vein of penis

Corpus cavernosum

Deep (Buck's) fascia of penis

Corpus spongiosum

Superficial (dartos) fascia of penis and scrotum

Septum of scrotum

Testis

Ductus (vas) deferens

Urinary bladder and fascia

Ureter (cut)

Seminal vesicle

Rectovesical pouch

Rectum

Rectoprostatic (Denonvilliers') fascia

Prostate (covered by fascia)

Ischiopubic ramus (cut)

Pelvic diaphragm (levator ani muscle)

Deep transverse perineal muscle

Perineal body

Deep / Superficial / Subcutaneous } External anal sphincter muscle

Deep perineal (investing or Gallaudet's) fascia

Superficial perineal (Colles') fascia (inferior fascia of superficial perineal space)

Superficial (dartos) fascia of scrotum

External spermatic fascia

Median (sagittal) section

Urachus

Urinary bladder { Apex / Fundus / Body / Trigone / Neck }

Pubic symphysis

Fundiform ligament of penis

Suspensory ligament of penis

Inferior (arcuate) pubic ligament

Transverse perineal ligament (anterior thickening of perineal membrane)

Perineal membrane

Superficial perineal space

Corpus cavernosum

Corpus spongiosum

Superficial (dartos) fascia of penis and scrotum

Deep (Buck's) fascia of penis

Prepuce

Glans penis and external urethral meatus

Vesical fascia

Rectovesical pouch

Rectum

Seminal vesicle

Prostate

Rectoprostatic (Denonvilliers') fascia

Sphincter urethrae muscle

Bulbourethral (Cowper's) gland

Perineal body

Bulbospongiosus muscle

Deep perineal (investing or Gallaudet's) fascia

Superficial perineal (Colles') fascia

Buck's fascia

Septum of scrotum

Navicular fossa

Superior view

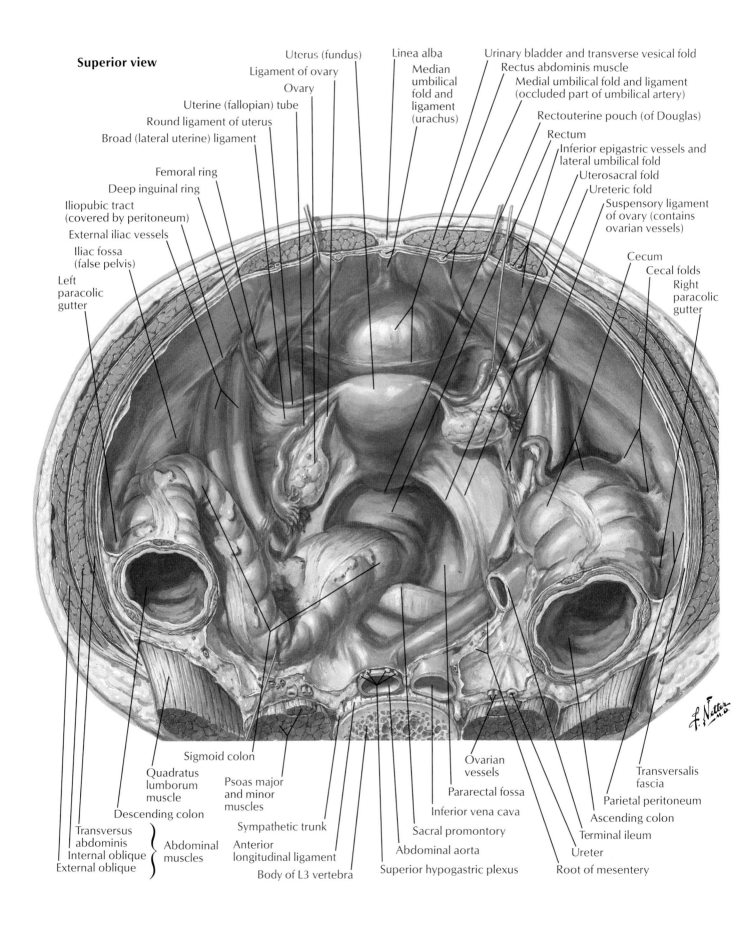

Uterus (fundus)

Ligament of ovary

Ovary

Uterine (fallopian) tube

Round ligament of uterus

Broad (lateral uterine) ligament

Femoral ring

Deep inguinal ring

Iliopubic tract
(covered by peritoneum)

External iliac vessels

Iliac fossa
(false pelvis)

Left
paracolic
gutter

Linea alba

Median
umbilical
fold and
ligament
(urachus)

Urinary bladder and transverse vesical fold

Rectus abdominis muscle

Medial umbilical fold and ligament
(occluded part of umbilical artery)

Rectouterine pouch (of Douglas)

Rectum

Inferior epigastric vessels and
lateral umbilical fold

Uterosacral fold

Ureteric fold

Suspensory ligament
of ovary (contains
ovarian vessels)

Cecum

Cecal folds

Right
paracolic
gutter

Sigmoid colon

Quadratus
lumborum
muscle

Descending colon

Transversus
abdominis

Internal oblique

External oblique
⎫
⎬
⎭
Abdominal
muscles

Psoas major
and minor
muscles

Sympathetic trunk

Anterior
longitudinal ligament

Body of L3 vertebra

Inferior vena cava

Sacral promontory

Abdominal aorta

Superior hypogastric plexus

Ovarian
vessels

Pararectal fossa

Transversalis
fascia

Parietal peritoneum

Ascending colon

Terminal ileum

Ureter

Root of mesentery

Plate 362

Pelvic Floor and Contents

Superior view

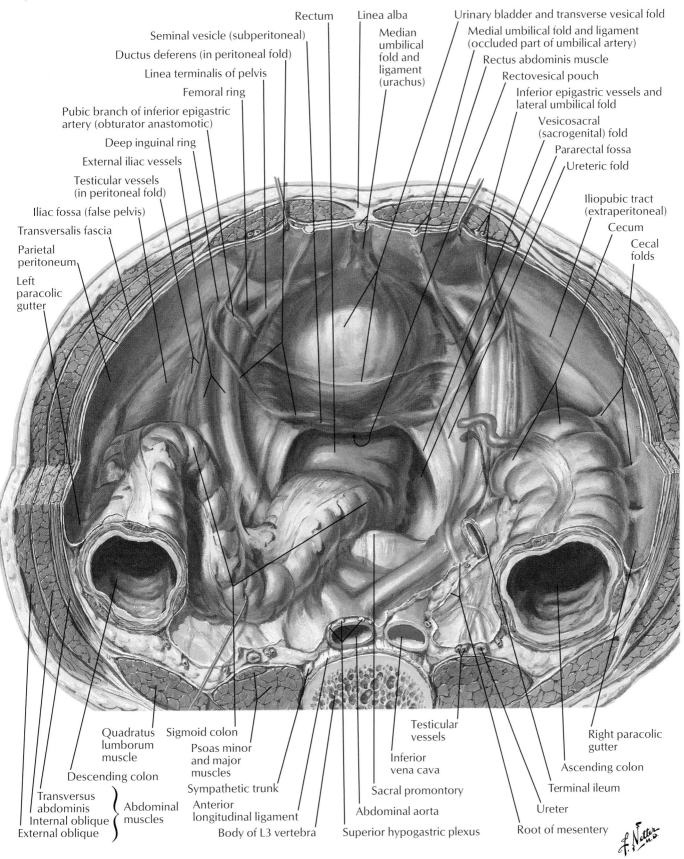

Rectum

Seminal vesicle (subperitoneal)

Ductus deferens (in peritoneal fold)

Linea terminalis of pelvis

Femoral ring

Pubic branch of inferior epigastric artery (obturator anastomotic)

Deep inguinal ring

External iliac vessels

Testicular vessels (in peritoneal fold)

Iliac fossa (false pelvis)

Transversalis fascia

Parietal peritoneum

Left paracolic gutter

Linea alba

Median umbilical fold and ligament (urachus)

Urinary bladder and transverse vesical fold

Medial umbilical fold and ligament (occluded part of umbilical artery)

Rectus abdominis muscle

Rectovesical pouch

Inferior epigastric vessels and lateral umbilical fold

Vesicosacral (sacrogenital) fold

Pararectal fossa

Ureteric fold

Iliopubic tract (extraperitoneal)

Cecum

Cecal folds

Quadratus lumborum muscle

Sigmoid colon

Psoas minor and major muscles

Anterior longitudinal ligament

Body of L3 vertebra

Descending colon

Transversus abdominis
Internal oblique
External oblique
} Abdominal muscles

Testicular vessels

Inferior vena cava

Sacral promontory

Abdominal aorta

Superior hypogastric plexus

Right paracolic gutter

Ascending colon

Terminal ileum

Ureter

Root of mesentery

F. Netter
M.D.

Female: superior view (peritoneum and loose areolar tissue removed)

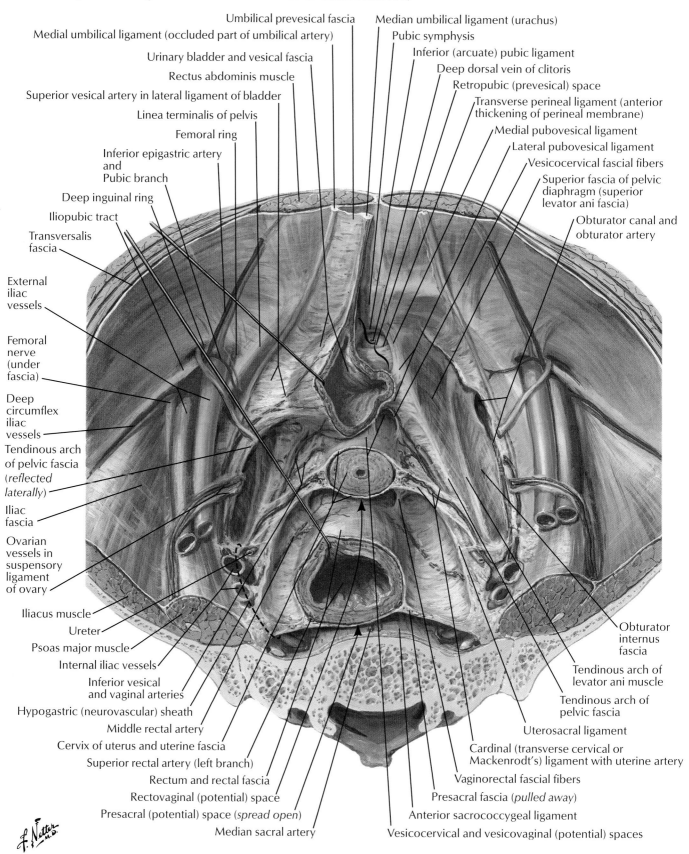

Umbilical prevesical fascia

Medial umbilical ligament (occluded part of umbilical artery)

Urinary bladder and vesical fascia

Rectus abdominis muscle

Superior vesical artery in lateral ligament of bladder

Linea terminalis of pelvis

Femoral ring

Inferior epigastric artery and Pubic branch

Deep inguinal ring

Iliopubic tract

Transversalis fascia

External iliac vessels

Femoral nerve (under fascia)

Deep circumflex iliac vessels

Tendinous arch of pelvic fascia (*reflected laterally*)

Iliac fascia

Ovarian vessels in suspensory ligament of ovary

Iliacus muscle

Ureter

Psoas major muscle

Internal iliac vessels

Inferior vesical and vaginal arteries

Hypogastric (neurovascular) sheath

Middle rectal artery

Cervix of uterus and uterine fascia

Superior rectal artery (left branch)

Rectum and rectal fascia

Rectovaginal (potential) space

Presacral (potential) space (*spread open*)

Median sacral artery

Median umbilical ligament (urachus)

Pubic symphysis

Inferior (arcuate) pubic ligament

Deep dorsal vein of clitoris

Retropubic (prevesical) space

Transverse perineal ligament (anterior thickening of perineal membrane)

Medial pubovesical ligament

Lateral pubovesical ligament

Vesicocervical fascial fibers

Superior fascia of pelvic diaphragm (superior levator ani fascia)

Obturator canal and obturator artery

Obturator internus fascia

Tendinous arch of levator ani muscle

Tendinous arch of pelvic fascia

Uterosacral ligament

Cardinal (transverse cervical or Mackenrodt's) ligament with uterine artery

Vaginorectal fascial fibers

Presacral fascia (*pulled away*)

Anterior sacrococcygeal ligament

Vesicocervical and vesicovaginal (potential) spaces

Plate 364 **Pelvic Floor and Contents**

Female: midsagittal section

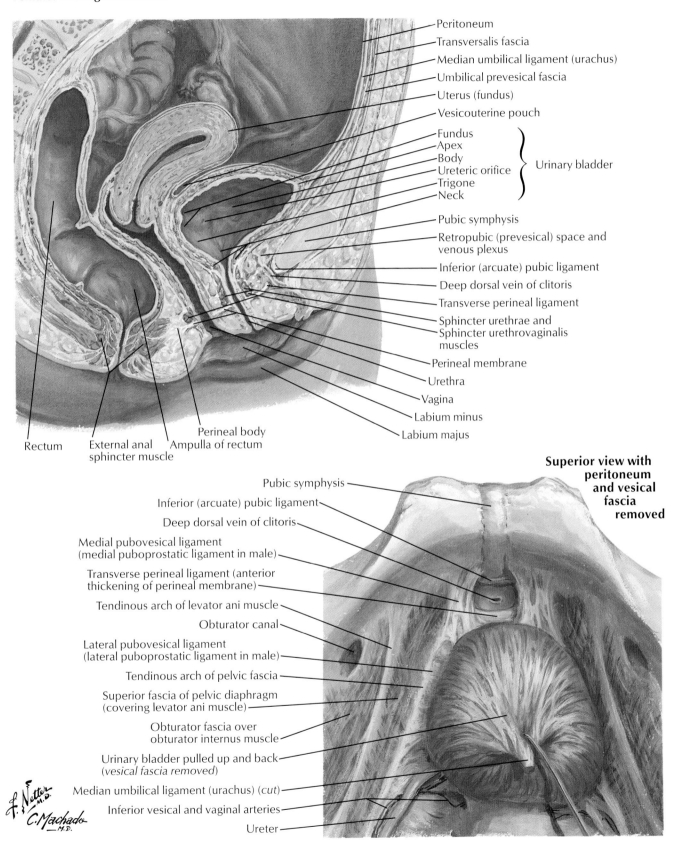

Peritoneum

Transversalis fascia

Median umbilical ligament (urachus)

Umbilical prevesical fascia

Uterus (fundus)

Vesicouterine pouch

Fundus
Apex
Body — Urinary bladder
Ureteric orifice
Trigone
Neck

Pubic symphysis

Retropubic (prevesical) space and venous plexus

Inferior (arcuate) pubic ligament

Deep dorsal vein of clitoris

Transverse perineal ligament

Sphincter urethrae and Sphincter urethrovaginalis muscles

Perineal membrane

Urethra

Vagina

Labium minus

Labium majus

Perineal body

Ampulla of rectum

External anal sphincter muscle

Rectum

Superior view with peritoneum and vesical fascia removed

Pubic symphysis

Inferior (arcuate) pubic ligament

Deep dorsal vein of clitoris

Medial pubovesical ligament (medial puboprostatic ligament in male)

Transverse perineal ligament (anterior thickening of perineal membrane)

Tendinous arch of levator ani muscle

Obturator canal

Lateral pubovesical ligament (lateral puboprostatic ligament in male)

Tendinous arch of pelvic fascia

Superior fascia of pelvic diaphragm (covering levator ani muscle)

Obturator fascia over obturator internus muscle

Urinary bladder pulled up and back (vesical fascia removed)

Median umbilical ligament (urachus) (cut)

Inferior vesical and vaginal arteries

Ureter

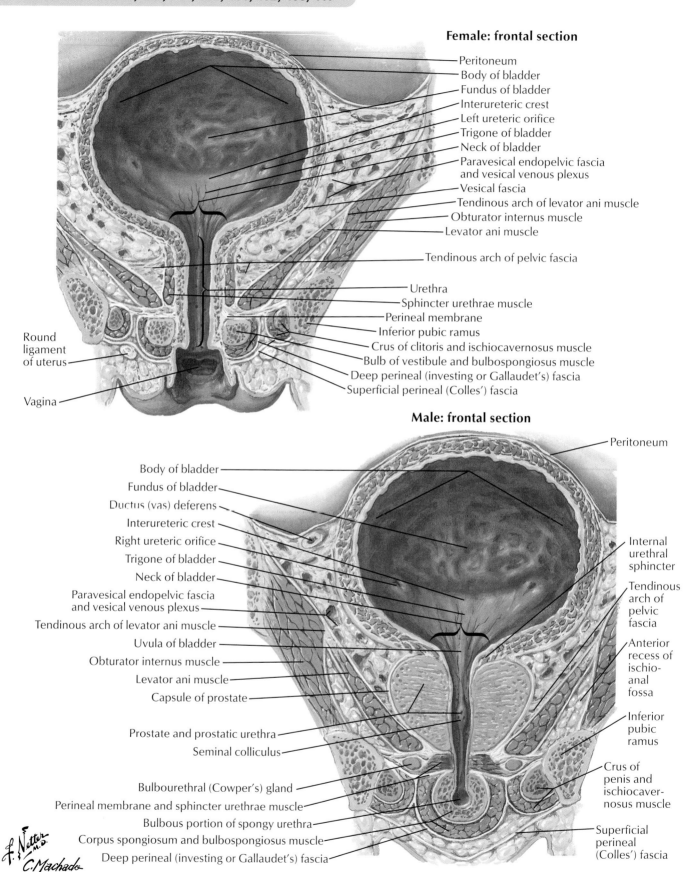

Female: frontal section

Peritoneum
Body of bladder
Fundus of bladder
Interureteric crest
Left ureteric orifice
Trigone of bladder
Neck of bladder
Paravesical endopelvic fascia and vesical venous plexus
Vesical fascia
Tendinous arch of levator ani muscle
Obturator internus muscle
Levator ani muscle

Tendinous arch of pelvic fascia

Urethra
Sphincter urethrae muscle
Perineal membrane
Inferior pubic ramus
Crus of clitoris and ischiocavernosus muscle
Bulb of vestibule and bulbospongiosus muscle
Deep perineal (investing or Gallaudet's) fascia
Superficial perineal (Colles') fascia

Round ligament of uterus

Vagina

Male: frontal section

Peritoneum

Body of bladder
Fundus of bladder
Ductus (vas) deferens
Interureteric crest
Right ureteric orifice
Trigone of bladder
Neck of bladder
Paravesical endopelvic fascia and vesical venous plexus
Tendinous arch of levator ani muscle
Uvula of bladder
Obturator internus muscle
Levator ani muscle
Capsule of prostate

Prostate and prostatic urethra
Seminal colliculus

Bulbourethral (Cowper's) gland
Perineal membrane and sphincter urethrae muscle
Bulbous portion of spongy urethra
Corpus spongiosum and bulbospongiosus muscle
Deep perineal (investing or Gallaudet's) fascia

Internal urethral sphincter

Tendinous arch of pelvic fascia

Anterior recess of ischio-anal fossa

Inferior pubic ramus

Crus of penis and ischiocavernosus muscle

Superficial perineal (Colles') fascia

Plate 366

Urinary Bladder

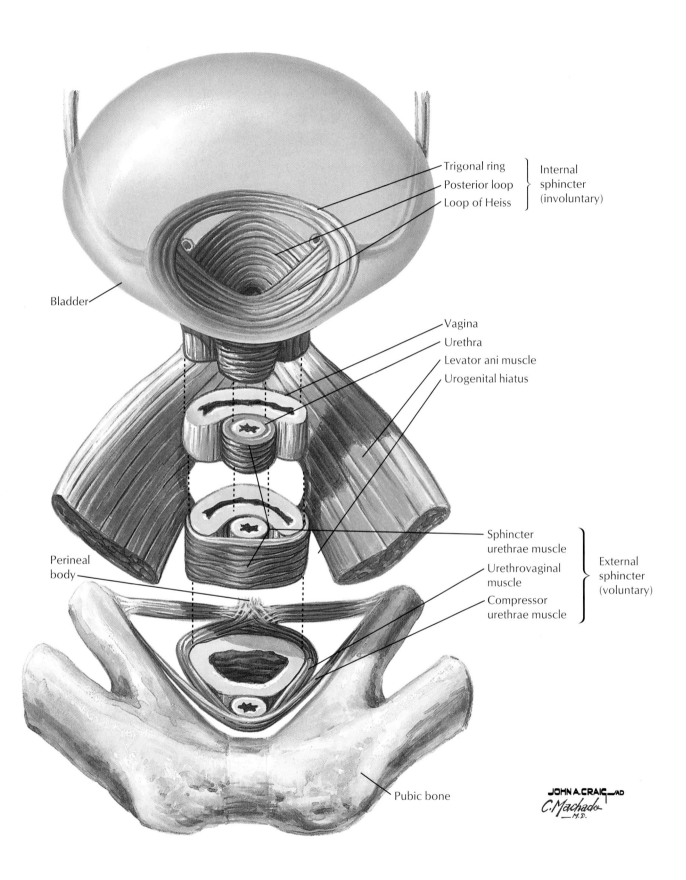

Trigonal ring
Posterior loop
Loop of Heiss
} Internal sphincter (involuntary)

Bladder

Vagina
Urethra
Levator ani muscle
Urogenital hiatus

Perineal body

Sphincter urethrae muscle
Urethrovaginal muscle
Compressor urethrae muscle
} External sphincter (voluntary)

Pubic bone

JOHN A. CRAIG—AD
C. Machado
—M.D.

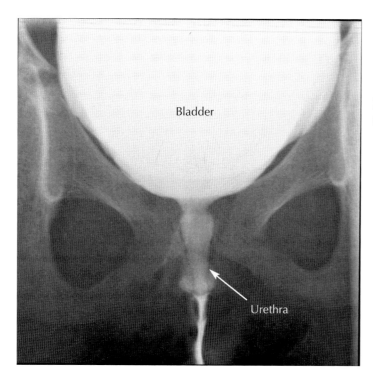

Female urethra,
8-year-old child

Voiding
cystourethrogram,
2-year-old male

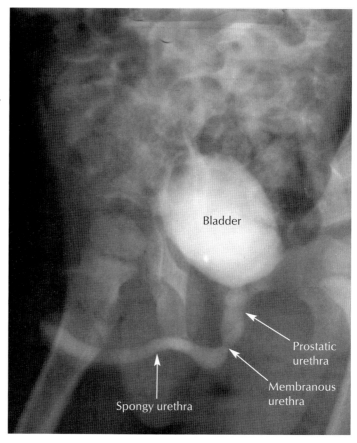

Plate 368

Urinary Bladder

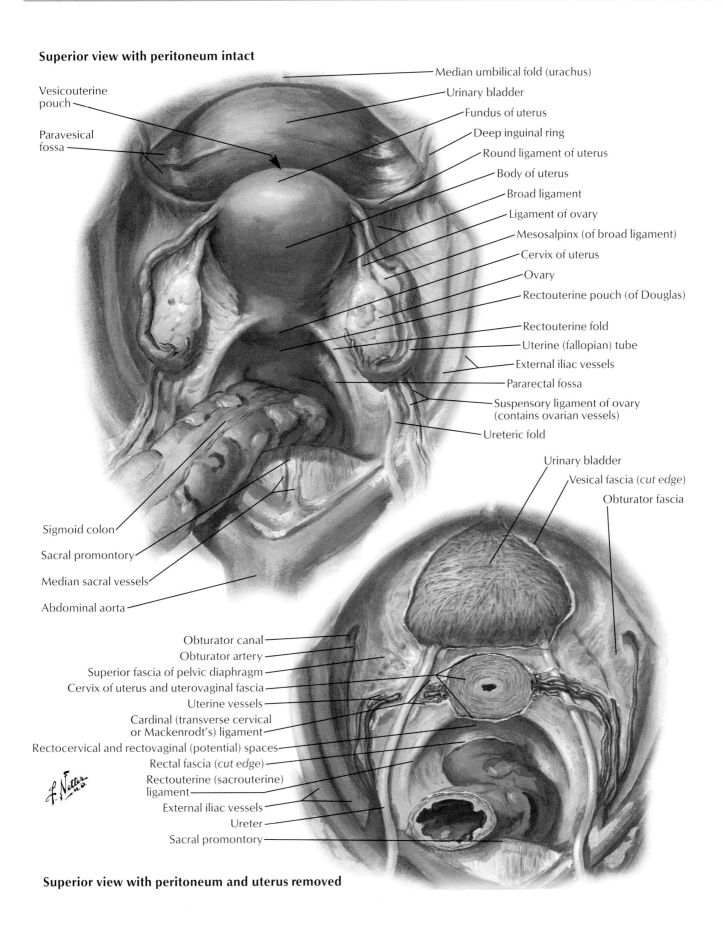

Superior view with peritoneum intact

Vesicouterine pouch

Paravesical fossa

Median umbilical fold (urachus)

Urinary bladder

Fundus of uterus

Deep inguinal ring

Round ligament of uterus

Body of uterus

Broad ligament

Ligament of ovary

Mesosalpinx (of broad ligament)

Cervix of uterus

Ovary

Rectouterine pouch (of Douglas)

Rectouterine fold

Uterine (fallopian) tube

External iliac vessels

Pararectal fossa

Suspensory ligament of ovary (contains ovarian vessels)

Ureteric fold

Sigmoid colon

Sacral promontory

Median sacral vessels

Abdominal aorta

Urinary bladder

Vesical fascia (cut edge)

Obturator fascia

Obturator canal

Obturator artery

Superior fascia of pelvic diaphragm

Cervix of uterus and uterovaginal fascia

Uterine vessels

Cardinal (transverse cervical or Mackenrodt's) ligament

Rectocervical and rectovaginal (potential) spaces

Rectal fascia (cut edge)

Rectouterine (sacrouterine) ligament

External iliac vessels

Ureter

Sacral promontory

Superior view with peritoneum and uterus removed

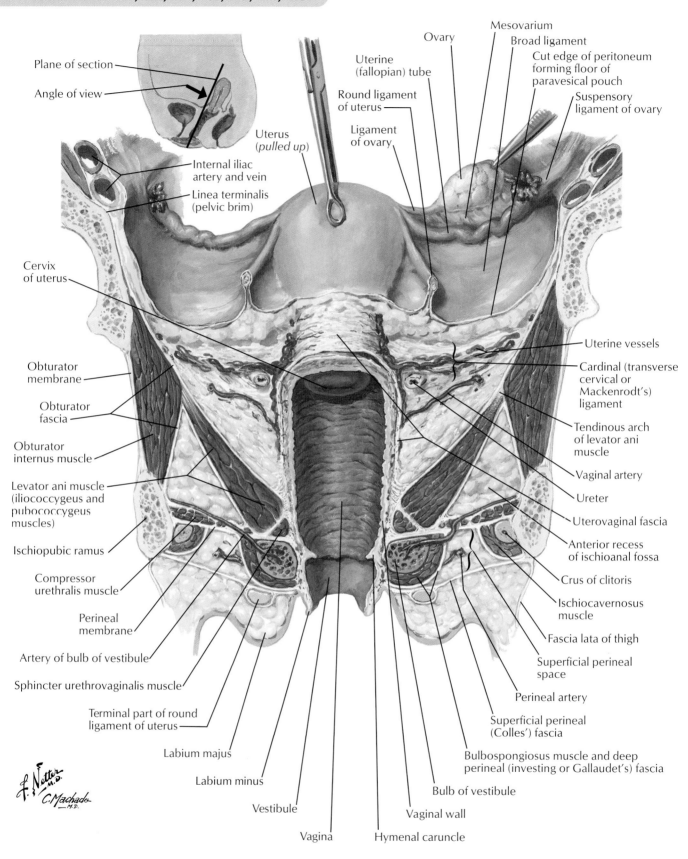

Plane of section

Angle of view

Mesovarium

Ovary

Broad ligament

Uterine (fallopian) tube

Cut edge of peritoneum forming floor of paravesical pouch

Round ligament of uterus

Suspensory ligament of ovary

Ligament of ovary

Uterus (*pulled up*)

Internal iliac artery and vein

Linea terminalis (pelvic brim)

Cervix of uterus

Uterine vessels

Cardinal (transverse cervical or Mackenrodt's) ligament

Obturator membrane

Obturator fascia

Obturator internus muscle

Tendinous arch of levator ani muscle

Vaginal artery

Ureter

Uterovaginal fascia

Levator ani muscle (iliococcygeus and pubococcygeus muscles)

Anterior recess of ischioanal fossa

Crus of clitoris

Ischiopubic ramus

Ischiocavernosus muscle

Compressor urethralis muscle

Fascia lata of thigh

Perineal membrane

Superficial perineal space

Artery of bulb of vestibule

Perineal artery

Sphincter urethrovaginalis muscle

Superficial perineal (Colles') fascia

Terminal part of round ligament of uterus

Bulbospongiosus muscle and deep perineal (investing or Gallaudet's) fascia

Labium majus

Labium minus

Bulb of vestibule

Vestibule

Vaginal wall

Vagina

Hymenal caruncle

Plate 370   **Uterus, Vagina, and Supporting Structures**

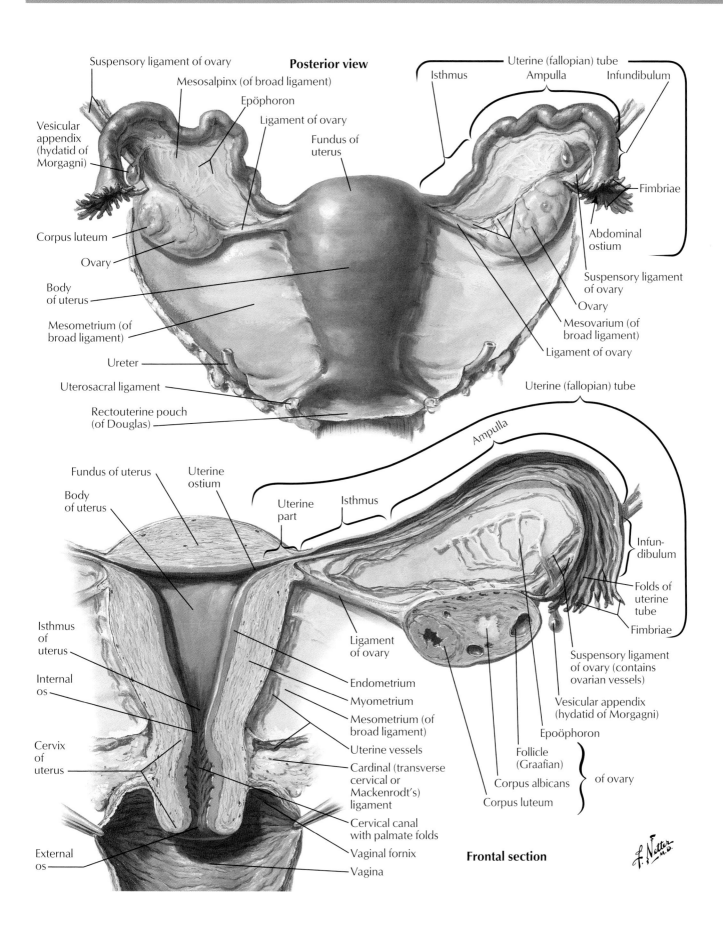

Posterior view

Suspensory ligament of ovary

Mesosalpinx (of broad ligament)

Epöphoron

Ligament of ovary

Fundus of uterus

Vesicular appendix (hydatid of Morgagni)

Corpus luteum

Ovary

Body of uterus

Mesometrium (of broad ligament)

Ureter

Uterosacral ligament

Rectouterine pouch (of Douglas)

Uterine (fallopian) tube

Isthmus   Ampulla   Infundibulum

Fimbriae

Abdominal ostium

Suspensory ligament of ovary

Ovary

Mesovarium (of broad ligament)

Ligament of ovary

Uterine (fallopian) tube

Ampulla

Fundus of uterus   Uterine ostium

Body of uterus

Uterine part   Isthmus

Isthmus of uterus

Internal os

Cervix of uterus

External os

Ligament of ovary

Endometrium

Myometrium

Mesometrium (of broad ligament)

Uterine vessels

Cardinal (transverse cervical or Mackenrodt's) ligament

Cervical canal with palmate folds

Vaginal fornix

Vagina

Infundibulum

Folds of uterine tube

Fimbriae

Suspensory ligament of ovary (contains ovarian vessels)

Vesicular appendix (hydatid of Morgagni)

Epoöphoron

Follicle (Graafian)

Corpus albicans

Corpus luteum

} of ovary

Frontal section

f. Netter M.D.

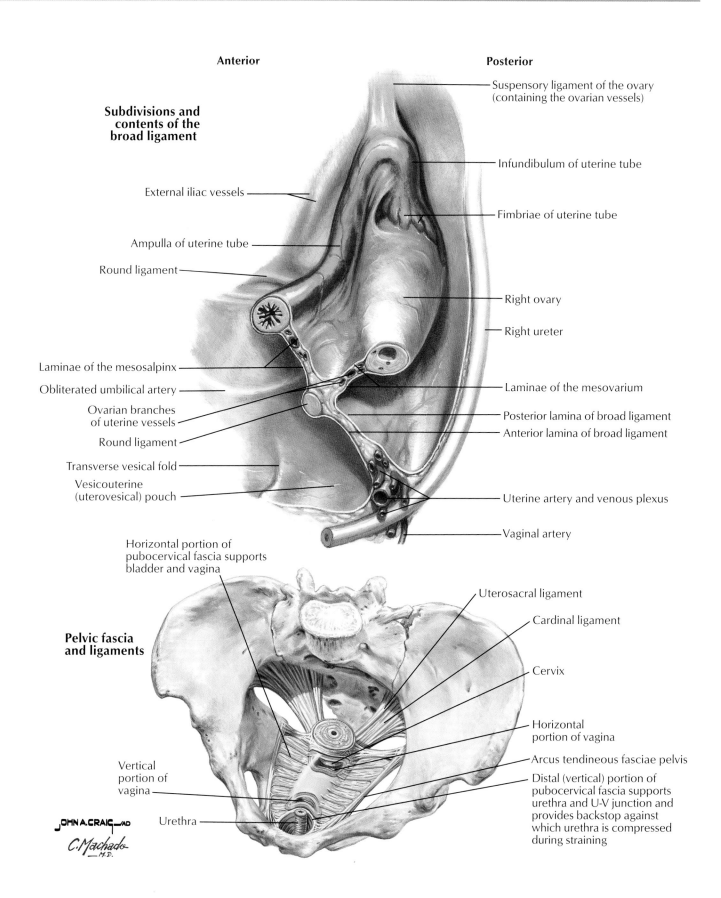

Anterior

Posterior

Subdivisions and
contents of the
broad ligament

Suspensory ligament of the ovary
(containing the ovarian vessels)

Infundibulum of uterine tube

External iliac vessels

Fimbriae of uterine tube

Ampulla of uterine tube

Round ligament

Right ovary

Right ureter

Laminae of the mesosalpinx

Obliterated umbilical artery

Ovarian branches
of uterine vessels

Laminae of the mesovarium

Round ligament

Posterior lamina of broad ligament

Anterior lamina of broad ligament

Transverse vesical fold

Vesicouterine
(uterovesical) pouch

Uterine artery and venous plexus

Vaginal artery

Horizontal portion of
pubocervical fascia supports
bladder and vagina

Uterosacral ligament

Cardinal ligament

**Pelvic fascia
and ligaments**

Cervix

Horizontal
portion of vagina

Vertical
portion of
vagina

Arcus tendineous fasciae pelvis

Distal (vertical) portion of
pubocervical fascia supports
urethra and U-V junction and
provides backstop against
which urethra is compressed
during straining

Urethra

JOHN A.CRAIG—MD
C.Machado
M.D.

Plate 372   **Uterus, Vagina, and Supporting Structures**

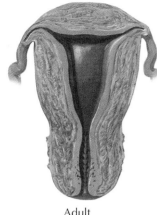
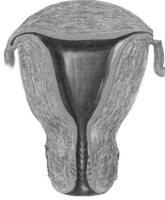
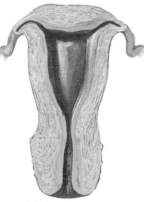

Adult
(nulliparous)

Adult
(parous)

Adult
(postmenopausal)

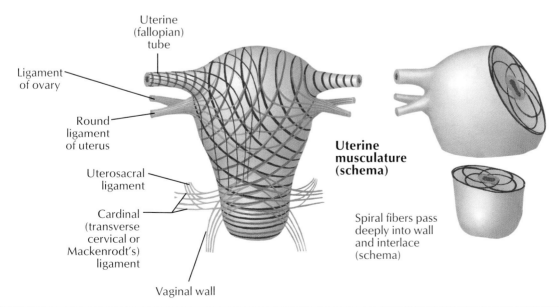

C Contrast medium in abdominal cavity

H Hysterosalpingogram uterus

R Right fallopian tube infection

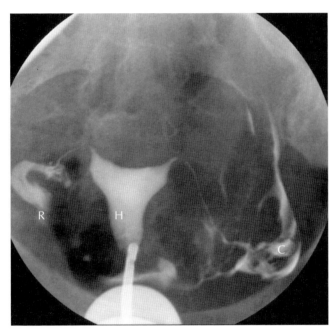

Uterine
(fallopian)
tube

Ligament
of ovary

Round
ligament
of uterus

Uterosacral
ligament

Cardinal
(transverse
cervical or
Mackenrodt's)
ligament

Vaginal wall

**Uterine
musculature
(schema)**

Spiral fibers pass
deeply into wall
and interlace
(schema)

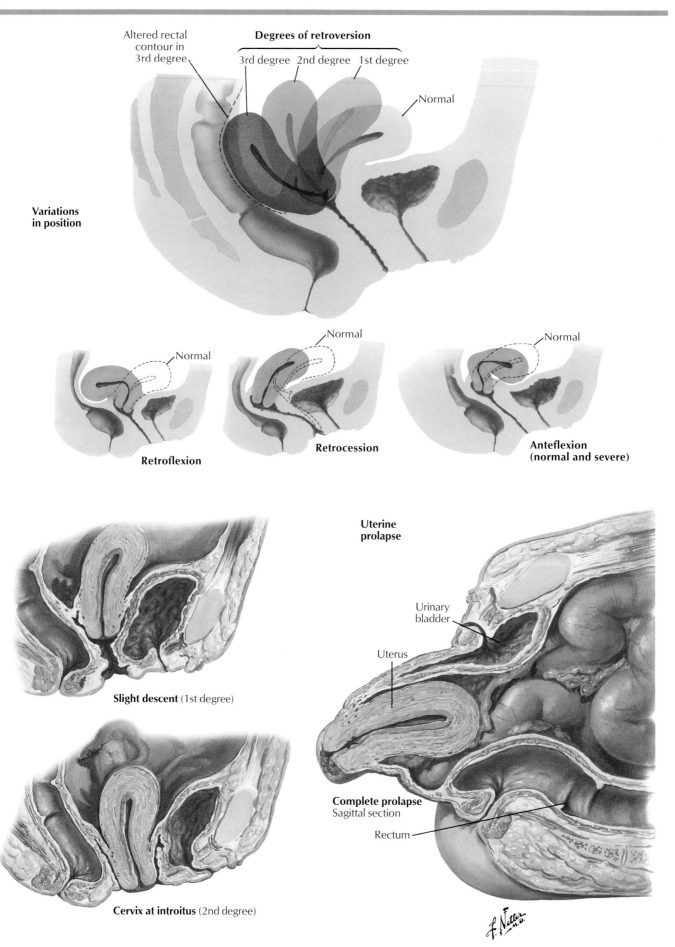

Variations in position

Altered rectal contour in 3rd degree

Degrees of retroversion

3rd degree 2nd degree 1st degree

Normal

Retroflexion

Normal

Retrocession

Normal

Anteflexion (normal and severe)

Normal

Slight descent (1st degree)

Cervix at introitus (2nd degree)

Uterine prolapse

Urinary bladder

Uterus

Complete prolapse
Sagittal section

Rectum

F. Netter M.D.

Plate 374

Uterus, Vagina, and Supporting Structures

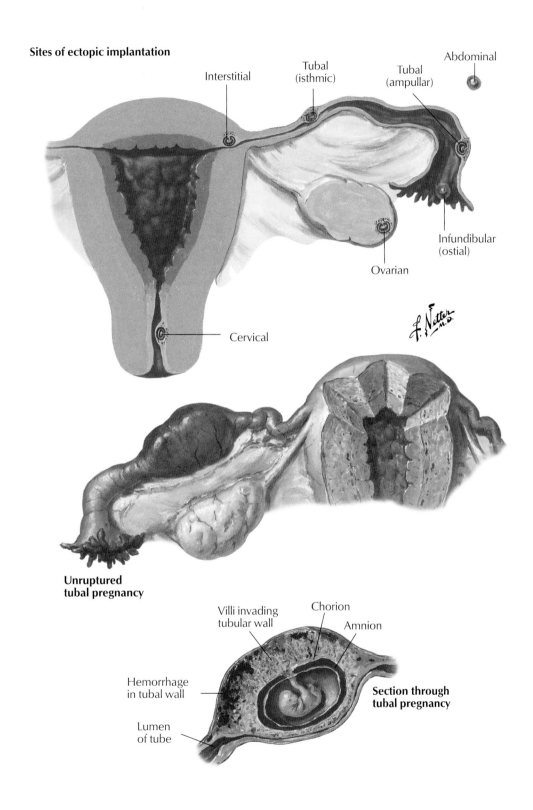

Sites of ectopic implantation

Interstitial

Tubal (isthmic)

Tubal (ampullar)

Abdominal

Infundibular (ostial)

Ovarian

Cervical

Unruptured tubal pregnancy

Villi invading tubular wall

Chorion

Amnion

Hemorrhage in tubal wall

Section through tubal pregnancy

Lumen of tube

Transverse Section: Pubic Crest, Femoral Heads, Coccyx

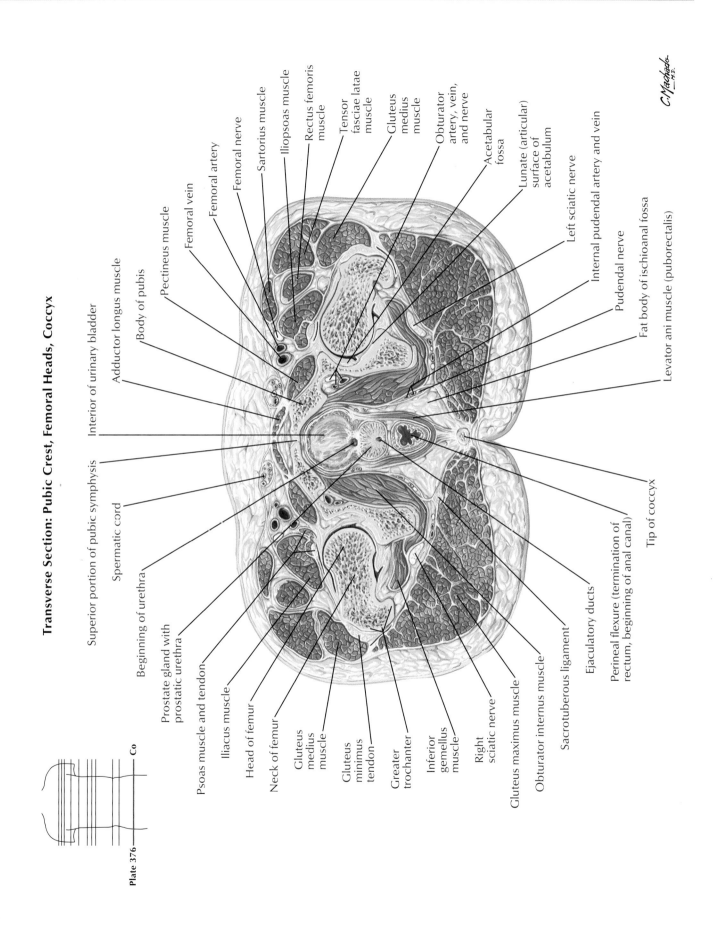

Interior of urinary bladder
Adductor longus muscle
Body of pubis
Pectineus muscle
Femoral vein
Femoral artery
Femoral nerve
Sartorius muscle
Iliopsoas muscle
Rectus femoris muscle
Tensor fasciae latae muscle
Gluteus medius muscle
Obturator artery, vein, and nerve
Acetabular fossa
Lunate (articular) surface of acetabulum
Left sciatic nerve
Internal pudendal artery and vein
Pudendal nerve
Fat body of ischioanal fossa
Levator ani muscle (puborectalis)

Superior portion of pubic symphysis
Spermatic cord
Beginning of urethra
Prostate gland with prostatic urethra
Iliacus muscle
Head of femur
Neck of femur
Gluteus medius muscle
Gluteus minimus tendon
Greater trochanter
Inferior gemellus muscle
Right sciatic nerve
Gluteus maximus muscle
Obturator internus muscle
Sacrotuberous ligament
Ejaculatory ducts
Perineal flexure (termination of rectum, beginning of anal canal)
Tip of coccyx

Psoas muscle and tendon

Co

Plate 376

Plate 376 **Regional Transverse Section**

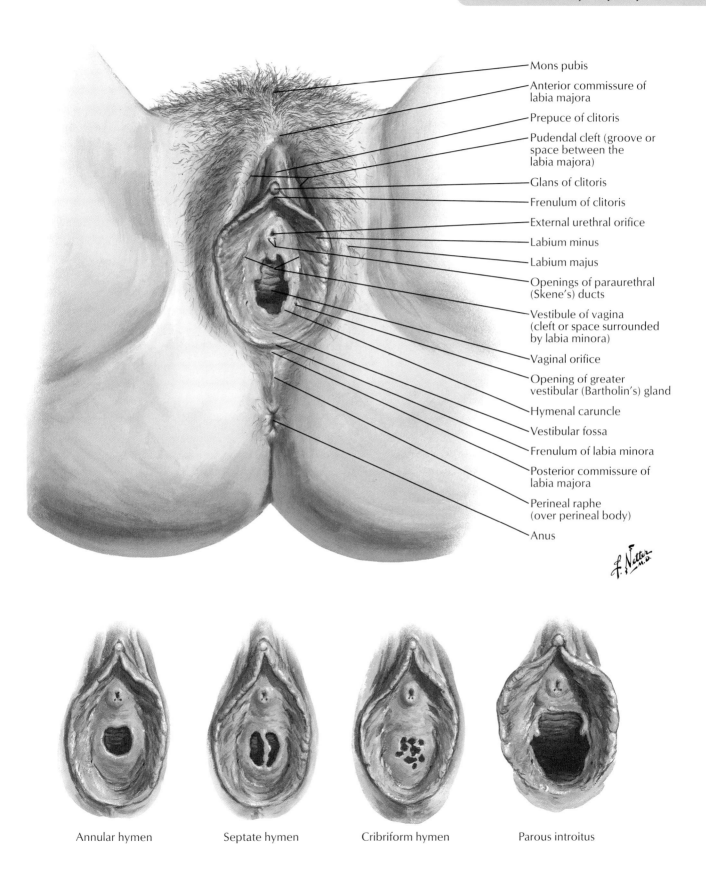

Mons pubis

Anterior commissure of labia majora

Prepuce of clitoris

Pudendal cleft (groove or space between the labia majora)

Glans of clitoris

Frenulum of clitoris

External urethral orifice

Labium minus

Labium majus

Openings of paraurethral (Skene's) ducts

Vestibule of vagina (cleft or space surrounded by labia minora)

Vaginal orifice

Opening of greater vestibular (Bartholin's) gland

Hymenal caruncle

Vestibular fossa

Frenulum of labia minora

Posterior commissure of labia majora

Perineal raphe (over perineal body)

Anus

Annular hymen

Septate hymen

Cribriform hymen

Parous introitus

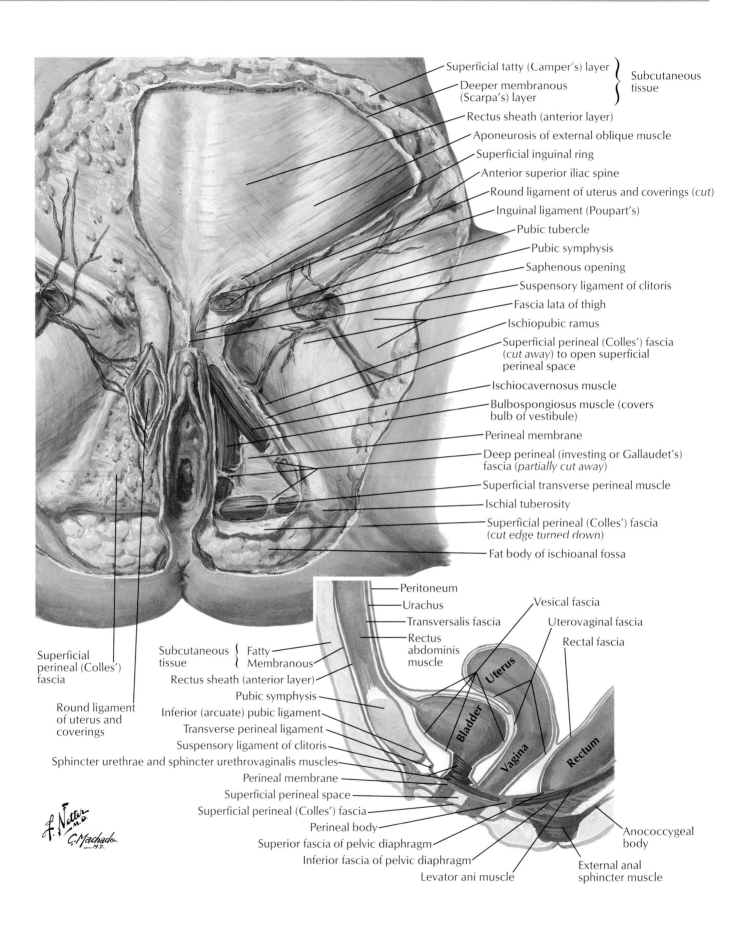

Superficial fatty (Camper's) layer
Deeper membranous (Scarpa's) layer
Subcutaneous tissue
Rectus sheath (anterior layer)
Aponeurosis of external oblique muscle
Superficial inguinal ring
Anterior superior iliac spine
Round ligament of uterus and coverings (cut)
Inguinal ligament (Poupart's)
Pubic tubercle
Pubic symphysis
Saphenous opening
Suspensory ligament of clitoris
Fascia lata of thigh
Ischiopubic ramus
Superficial perineal (Colles') fascia (cut away) to open superficial perineal space
Ischiocavernosus muscle
Bulbospongiosus muscle (covers bulb of vestibule)
Perineal membrane
Deep perineal (investing or Gallaudet's) fascia (partially cut away)
Superficial transverse perineal muscle
Ischial tuberosity
Superficial perineal (Colles') fascia (cut edge turned down)
Fat body of ischioanal fossa

Superficial perineal (Colles') fascia

Round ligament of uterus and coverings

Subcutaneous tissue { Fatty / Membranous }
Rectus sheath (anterior layer)
Pubic symphysis
Inferior (arcuate) pubic ligament
Transverse perineal ligament
Suspensory ligament of clitoris
Sphincter urethrae and sphincter urethrovaginalis muscles
Perineal membrane
Superficial perineal space
Superficial perineal (Colles') fascia
Perineal body
Superior fascia of pelvic diaphragm
Inferior fascia of pelvic diaphragm
Levator ani muscle

Peritoneum
Urachus
Transversalis fascia
Rectus abdominis muscle
Vesical fascia
Uterovaginal fascia
Rectal fascia
Uterus
Bladder
Vagina
Rectum
Anococcygeal body
External anal sphincter muscle

Plate 378   **Perineum and External Genitalia: Female**

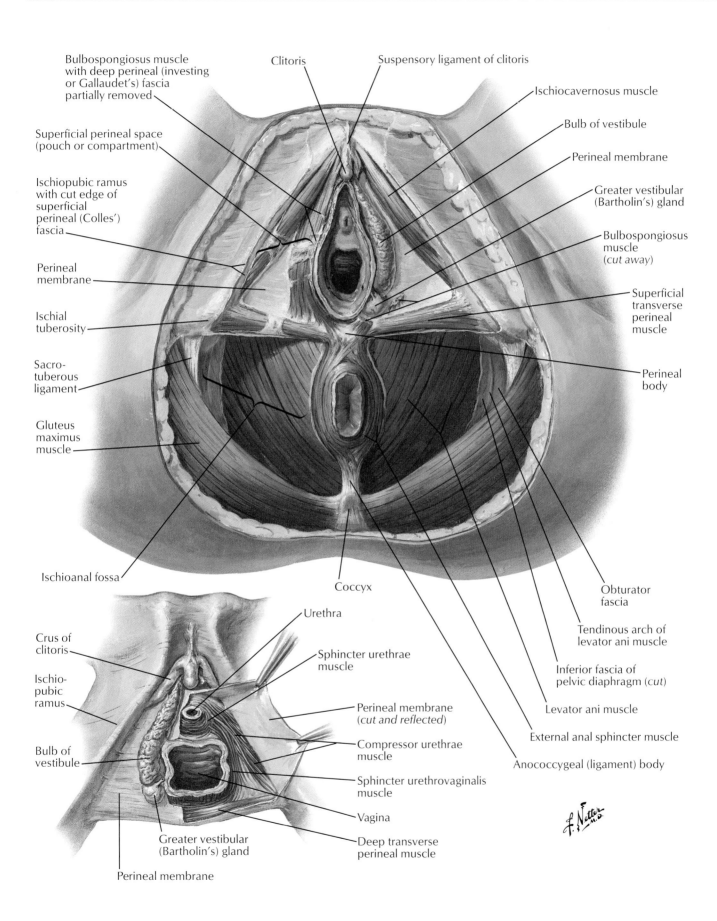

Bulbospongiosus muscle with deep perineal (investing or Gallaudet's) fascia partially removed

Clitoris

Suspensory ligament of clitoris

Ischiocavernosus muscle

Bulb of vestibule

Perineal membrane

Greater vestibular (Bartholin's) gland

Bulbospongiosus muscle (*cut away*)

Superficial perineal space (pouch or compartment)

Superficial transverse perineal muscle

Ischiopubic ramus with cut edge of superficial perineal (Colles') fascia

Perineal membrane

Perineal body

Ischial tuberosity

Sacro-tuberous ligament

Gluteus maximus muscle

Ischioanal fossa

Coccyx

Obturator fascia

Tendinous arch of levator ani muscle

Inferior fascia of pelvic diaphragm (*cut*)

Levator ani muscle

External anal sphincter muscle

Anococcygeal (ligament) body

Crus of clitoris

Ischio-pubic ramus

Bulb of vestibule

Urethra

Sphincter urethrae muscle

Perineal membrane (*cut and reflected*)

Compressor urethrae muscle

Sphincter urethrovaginalis muscle

Vagina

Greater vestibular (Bartholin's) gland

Deep transverse perineal muscle

Perineal membrane

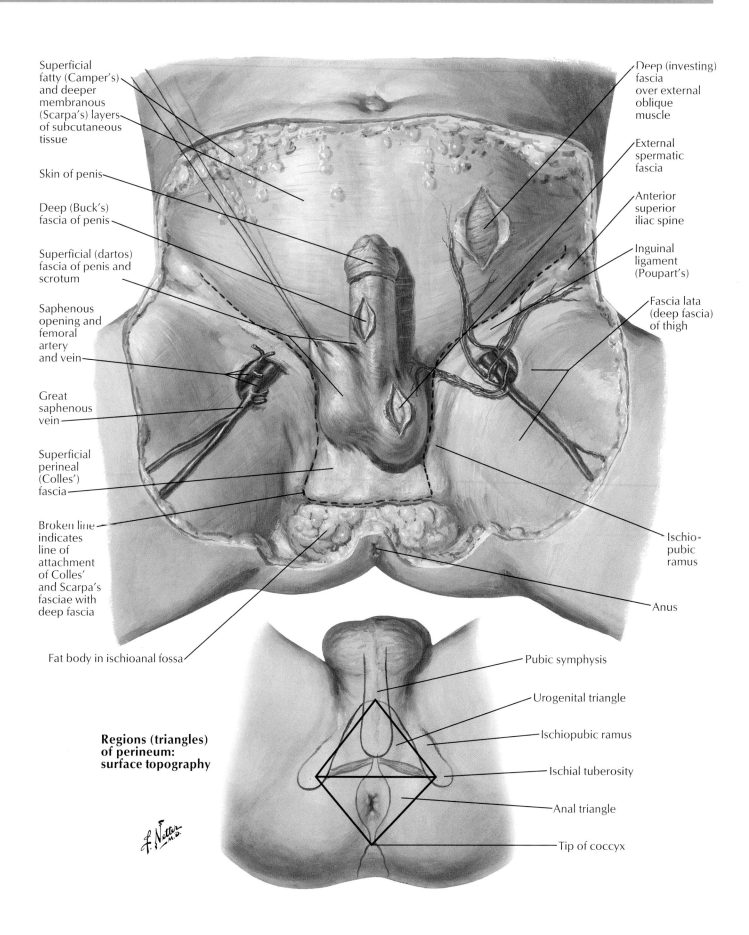

Superficial fatty (Camper's) and deeper membranous (Scarpa's) layers of subcutaneous tissue

Skin of penis

Deep (Buck's) fascia of penis

Superficial (dartos) fascia of penis and scrotum

Saphenous opening and femoral artery and vein

Great saphenous vein

Superficial perineal (Colles') fascia

Broken line indicates line of attachment of Colles' and Scarpa's fasciae with deep fascia

Fat body in ischioanal fossa

Deep (investing) fascia over external oblique muscle

External spermatic fascia

Anterior superior iliac spine

Inguinal ligament (Poupart's)

Fascia lata (deep fascia) of thigh

Ischio-pubic ramus

Anus

Regions (triangles) of perineum: surface topography

Pubic symphysis

Urogenital triangle

Ischiopubic ramus

Ischial tuberosity

Anal triangle

Tip of coccyx

Plate 380   **Perineum and External Genitalia: Male**

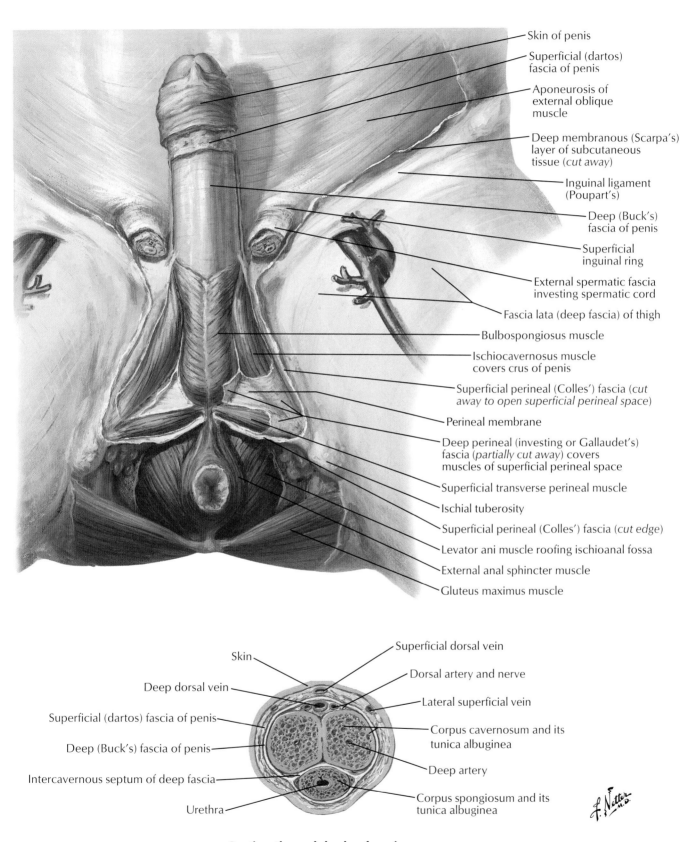

Skin of penis

Superficial (dartos)
fascia of penis

Aponeurosis of
external oblique
muscle

Deep membranous (Scarpa's)
layer of subcutaneous
tissue (*cut away*)

Inguinal ligament
(Poupart's)

Deep (Buck's)
fascia of penis

Superficial
inguinal ring

External spermatic fascia
investing spermatic cord

Fascia lata (deep fascia) of thigh

Bulbospongiosus muscle

Ischiocavernosus muscle
covers crus of penis

Superficial perineal (Colles') fascia (*cut
away to open superficial perineal space*)

Perineal membrane

Deep perineal (investing or Gallaudet's)
fascia (*partially cut away*) covers
muscles of superficial perineal space

Superficial transverse perineal muscle

Ischial tuberosity

Superficial perineal (Colles') fascia (*cut edge*)

Levator ani muscle roofing ischioanal fossa

External anal sphincter muscle

Gluteus maximus muscle

Superficial dorsal vein

Skin

Dorsal artery and nerve

Deep dorsal vein

Lateral superficial vein

Superficial (dartos) fascia of penis

Corpus cavernosum and its
tunica albuginea

Deep (Buck's) fascia of penis

Intercavernous septum of deep fascia

Deep artery

Corpus spongiosum and its
tunica albuginea

Urethra

Section through body of penis

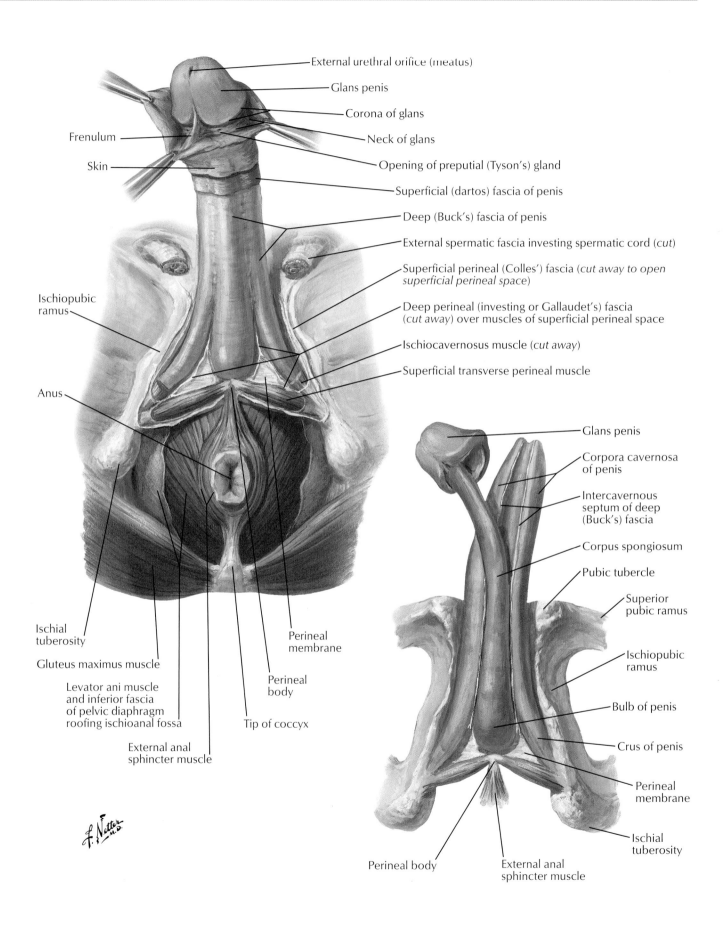

External urethral orifice (meatus)

Glans penis

Corona of glans

Neck of glans

Frenulum

Skin

Opening of preputial (Tyson's) gland

Superficial (dartos) fascia of penis

Deep (Buck's) fascia of penis

External spermatic fascia investing spermatic cord (*cut*)

Superficial perineal (Colles') fascia (*cut away to open superficial perineal space*)

Deep perineal (investing or Gallaudet's) fascia (*cut away*) over muscles of superficial perineal space

Ischiocavernosus muscle (*cut away*)

Superficial transverse perineal muscle

Ischiopubic ramus

Anus

Ischial tuberosity

Gluteus maximus muscle

Levator ani muscle and inferior fascia of pelvic diaphragm roofing ischioanal fossa

External anal sphincter muscle

Tip of coccyx

Perineal body

Perineal membrane

Glans penis

Corpora cavernosa of penis

Intercavernous septum of deep (Buck's) fascia

Corpus spongiosum

Pubic tubercle

Superior pubic ramus

Ischiopubic ramus

Bulb of penis

Crus of penis

Perineal membrane

Ischial tuberosity

Perineal body

External anal sphincter muscle

Plate 382   **Perineum and External Genitalia: Male**

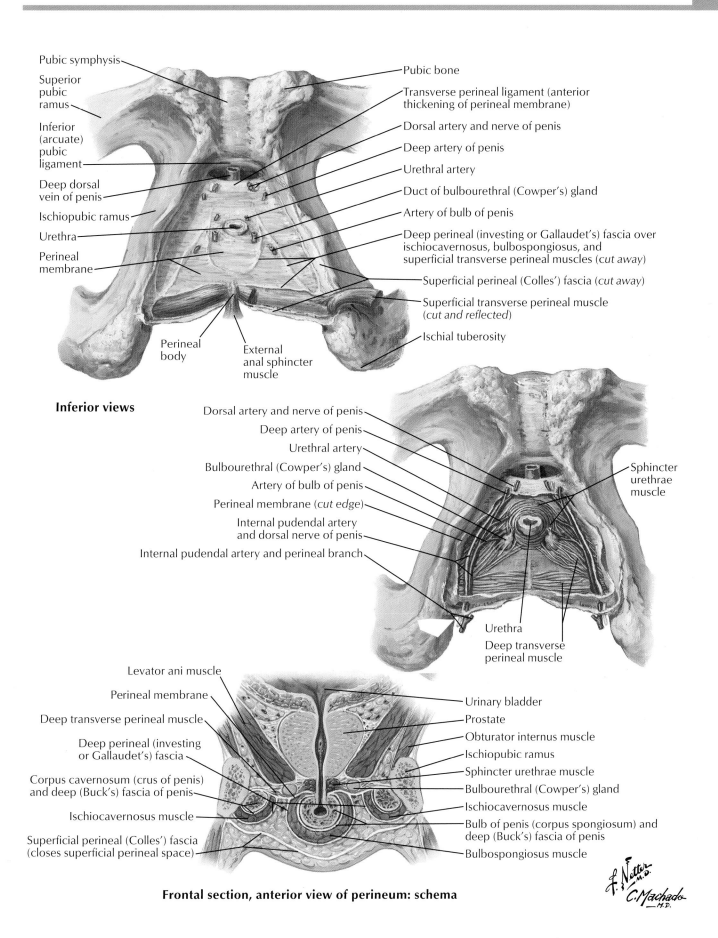

Pubic symphysis

Superior pubic ramus

Inferior (arcuate) pubic ligament

Deep dorsal vein of penis

Ischiopubic ramus

Urethra

Perineal membrane

Pubic bone

Transverse perineal ligament (anterior thickening of perineal membrane)

Dorsal artery and nerve of penis

Deep artery of penis

Urethral artery

Duct of bulbourethral (Cowper's) gland

Artery of bulb of penis

Deep perineal (investing or Gallaudet's) fascia over ischiocavernosus, bulbospongiosus, and superficial transverse perineal muscles (*cut away*)

Superficial perineal (Colles') fascia (*cut away*)

Superficial transverse perineal muscle (*cut and reflected*)

Ischial tuberosity

Perineal body

External anal sphincter muscle

Inferior views

Dorsal artery and nerve of penis

Deep artery of penis

Urethral artery

Bulbourethral (Cowper's) gland

Artery of bulb of penis

Perineal membrane (*cut edge*)

Internal pudendal artery and dorsal nerve of penis

Internal pudendal artery and perineal branch

Sphincter urethrae muscle

Urethra

Deep transverse perineal muscle

Levator ani muscle

Perineal membrane

Deep transverse perineal muscle

Deep perineal (investing or Gallaudet's) fascia

Corpus cavernosum (crus of penis) and deep (Buck's) fascia of penis

Ischiocavernosus muscle

Superficial perineal (Colles') fascia (closes superficial perineal space)

Urinary bladder

Prostate

Obturator internus muscle

Ischiopubic ramus

Sphincter urethrae muscle

Bulbourethral (Cowper's) gland

Ischiocavernosus muscle

Bulb of penis (corpus spongiosum) and deep (Buck's) fascia of penis

Bulbospongiosus muscle

Frontal section, anterior view of perineum: schema

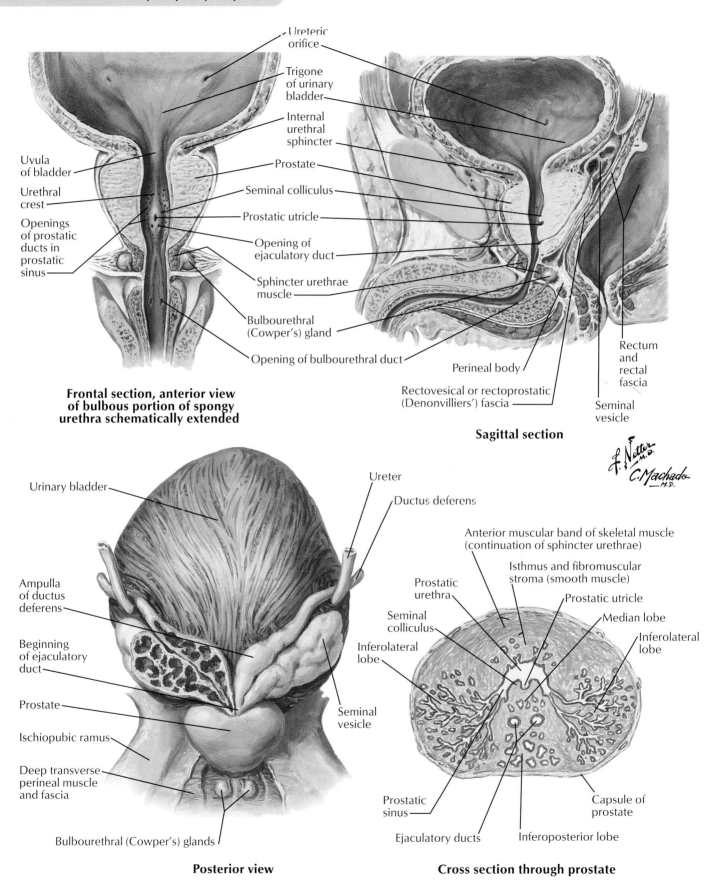

Ureteric orifice

Trigone of urinary bladder

Internal urethral sphincter

Prostate

Seminal colliculus

Prostatic utricle

Opening of ejaculatory duct

Sphincter urethrae muscle

Bulbourethral (Cowper's) gland

Opening of bulbourethral duct

Uvula of bladder

Urethral crest

Openings of prostatic ducts in prostatic sinus

Frontal section, anterior view of bulbous portion of spongy urethra schematically extended

Rectum and rectal fascia

Seminal vesicle

Perineal body

Rectovesical or rectoprostatic (Denonvilliers') fascia

Sagittal section

Urinary bladder

Ureter

Ductus deferens

Ampulla of ductus deferens

Beginning of ejaculatory duct

Prostate

Ischiopubic ramus

Deep transverse perineal muscle and fascia

Bulbourethral (Cowper's) glands

Seminal vesicle

Posterior view

Anterior muscular band of skeletal muscle (continuation of sphincter urethrae)

Isthmus and fibromuscular stroma (smooth muscle)

Prostatic utricle

Median lobe

Inferolateral lobe

Capsule of prostate

Inferoposterior lobe

Ejaculatory ducts

Prostatic sinus

Inferolateral lobe

Seminal colliculus

Prostatic urethra

Cross section through prostate

Plate 384

Perineum and External Genitalia: Male

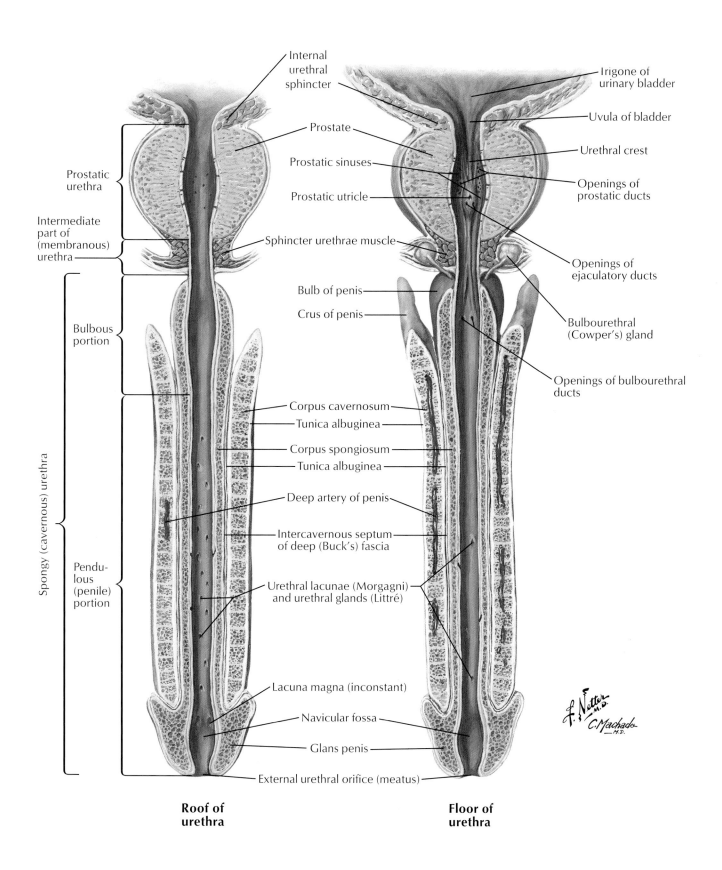

Internal urethral sphincter

Prostate

Prostatic sinuses

Prostatic utricle

Sphincter urethrae muscle

Bulb of penis

Crus of penis

Corpus cavernosum

Tunica albuginea

Corpus spongiosum

Tunica albuginea

Deep artery of penis

Intercavernous septum of deep (Buck's) fascia

Urethral lacunae (Morgagni) and urethral glands (Littré)

Lacuna magna (inconstant)

Navicular fossa

Glans penis

External urethral orifice (meatus)

Trigone of urinary bladder

Uvula of bladder

Urethral crest

Openings of prostatic ducts

Openings of ejaculatory ducts

Bulbourethral (Cowper's) gland

Openings of bulbourethral ducts

Prostatic urethra

Intermediate part of (membranous) urethra

Bulbous portion

Pendulous (penile) portion

Spongy (cavernous) urethra

Roof of urethra

Floor of urethra

Perineum and External Genitalia: Male

Plate 385

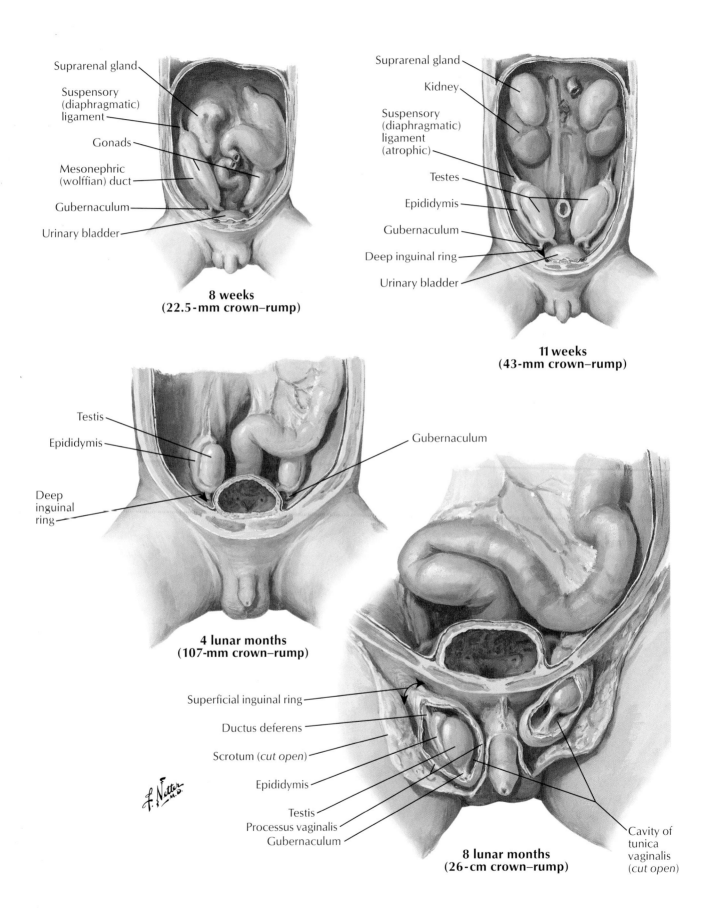

Suprarenal gland

Suspensory (diaphragmatic) ligament

Gonads

Mesonephric (wolffian) duct

Gubernaculum

Urinary bladder

8 weeks (22.5-mm crown–rump)

Suprarenal gland

Kidney

Suspensory (diaphragmatic) ligament (atrophic)

Testes

Epididymis

Gubernaculum

Deep inguinal ring

Urinary bladder

11 weeks (43-mm crown–rump)

Testis

Epididymis

Deep inguinal ring

Gubernaculum

4 lunar months (107-mm crown–rump)

Superficial inguinal ring

Ductus deferens

Scrotum (cut open)

Epididymis

Testis

Processus vaginalis

Gubernaculum

Cavity of tunica vaginalis (cut open)

8 lunar months (26-cm crown–rump)

Plate 386   **Perineum and External Genitalia: Male**

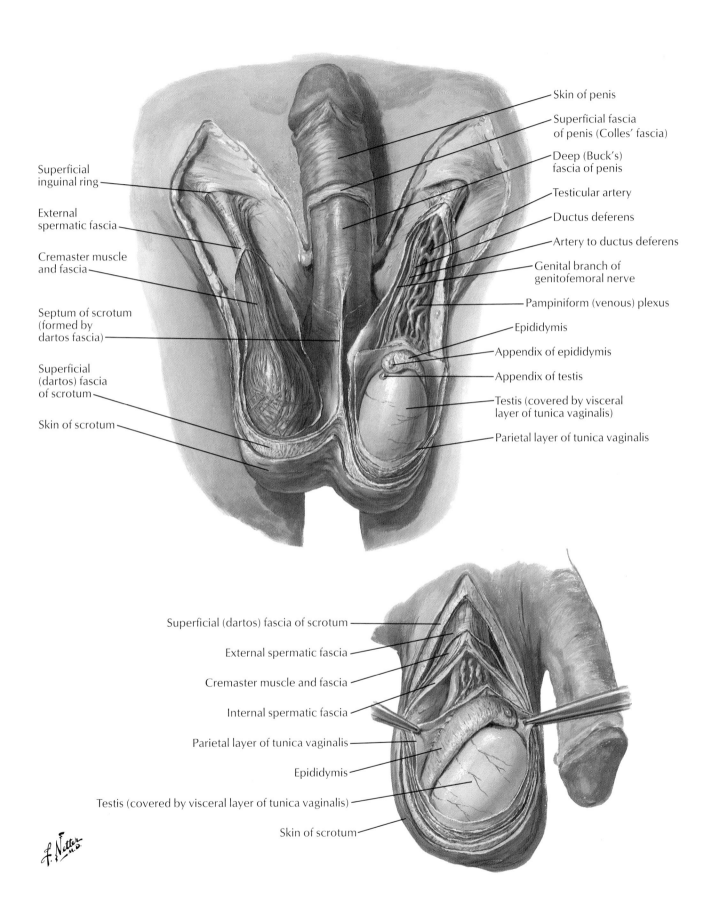

Skin of penis

Superficial fascia of penis (Colles' fascia)

Deep (Buck's) fascia of penis

Testicular artery

Ductus deferens

Artery to ductus deferens

Genital branch of genitofemoral nerve

Pampiniform (venous) plexus

Epididymis

Appendix of epididymis

Appendix of testis

Testis (covered by visceral layer of tunica vaginalis)

Parietal layer of tunica vaginalis

Superficial inguinal ring

External spermatic fascia

Cremaster muscle and fascia

Septum of scrotum (formed by dartos fascia)

Superficial (dartos) fascia of scrotum

Skin of scrotum

Superficial (dartos) fascia of scrotum

External spermatic fascia

Cremaster muscle and fascia

Internal spermatic fascia

Parietal layer of tunica vaginalis

Epididymis

Testis (covered by visceral layer of tunica vaginalis)

Skin of scrotum

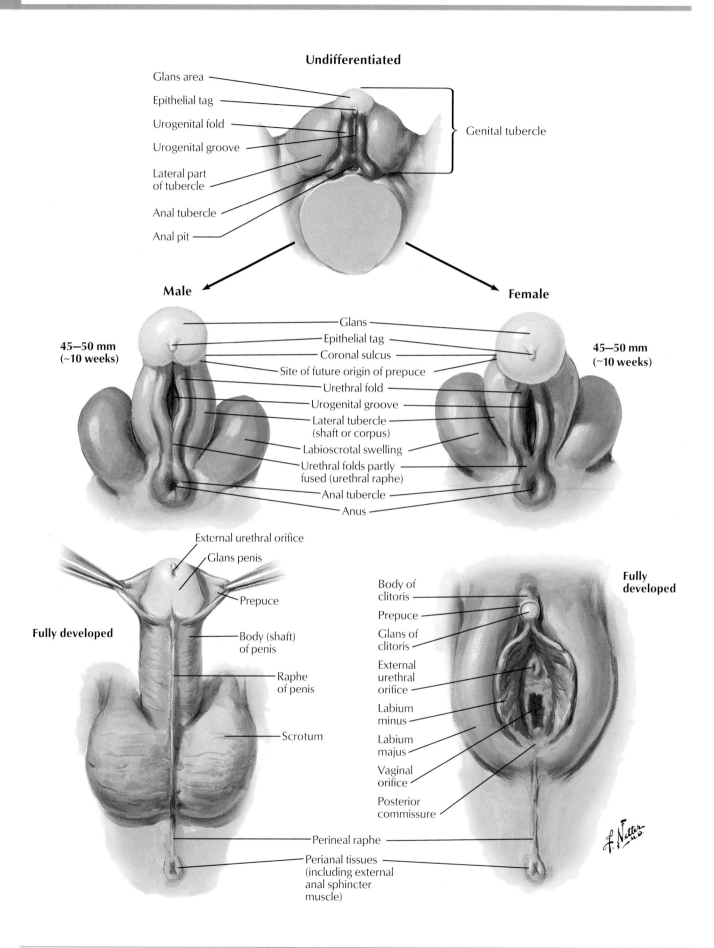

Undifferentiated

Glans area

Epithelial tag

Urogenital fold

Urogenital groove

Lateral part of tubercle

Anal tubercle

Anal pit

Genital tubercle

Male

Female

45—50 mm (~10 weeks)

45—50 mm (~10 weeks)

Glans

Epithelial tag

Coronal sulcus

Site of future origin of prepuce

Urethral fold

Urogenital groove

Lateral tubercle (shaft or corpus)

Labioscrotal swelling

Urethral folds partly fused (urethral raphe)

Anal tubercle

Anus

External urethral orifice

Glans penis

Prepuce

Body (shaft) of penis

Raphe of penis

Scrotum

Fully developed

Fully developed

Body of clitoris

Prepuce

Glans of clitoris

External urethral orifice

Labium minus

Labium majus

Vaginal orifice

Posterior commissure

Perineal raphe

Perianal tissues (including external anal sphincter muscle)

Plate 388   **Homologues of Genitalia**

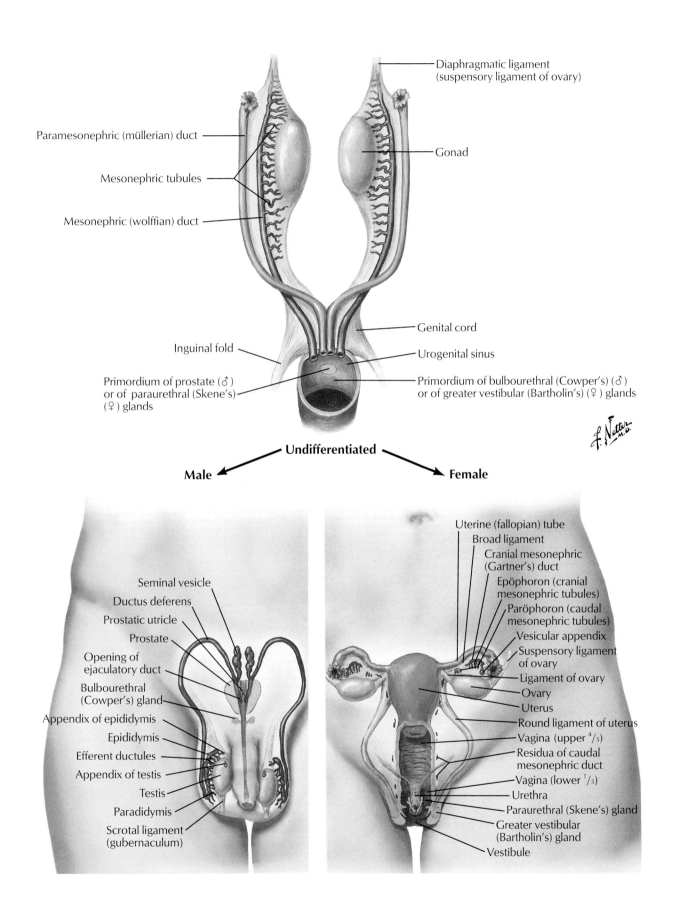

Diaphragmatic ligament (suspensory ligament of ovary)

Paramesonephric (müllerian) duct

Mesonephric tubules

Mesonephric (wolffian) duct

Gonad

Inguinal fold

Genital cord

Urogenital sinus

Primordium of prostate (♂) or of paraurethral (Skene's) (♀) glands

Primordium of bulbourethral (Cowper's) (♂) or of greater vestibular (Bartholin's) (♀) glands

Undifferentiated

Male

Female

Seminal vesicle

Ductus deferens

Prostatic utricle

Prostate

Opening of ejaculatory duct

Bulbourethral (Cowper's) gland

Appendix of epididymis

Epididymis

Efferent ductules

Appendix of testis

Testis

Paradidymis

Scrotal ligament (gubernaculum)

Uterine (fallopian) tube

Broad ligament

Cranial mesonephric (Gartner's) duct

Epöphoron (cranial mesonephric tubules)

Paröphoron (caudal mesonephric tubules)

Vesicular appendix

Suspensory ligament of ovary

Ligament of ovary

Ovary

Uterus

Round ligament of uterus

Vagina (upper $^4/_5$)

Residua of caudal mesonephric duct

Vagina (lower $^1/_5$)

Urethra

Paraurethral (Skene's) gland

Greater vestibular (Bartholin's) gland

Vestibule

Homologues of Genitalia

Plate 389

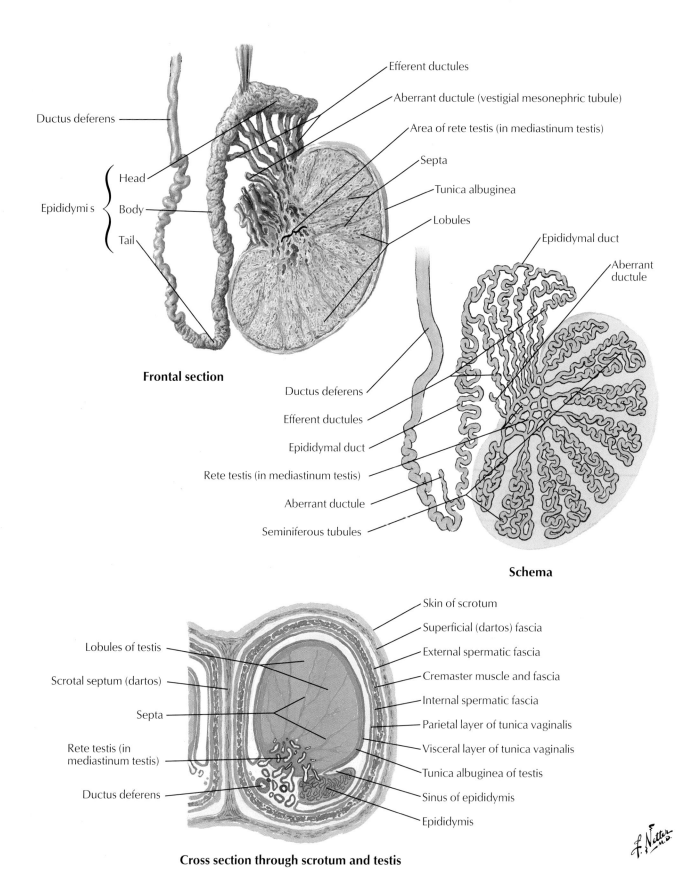

Frontal section

Ductus deferens

Epididymi s — Head / Body / Tail

Efferent ductules

Aberrant ductule (vestigial mesonephric tubule)

Area of rete testis (in mediastinum testis)

Septa

Tunica albuginea

Lobules

Epididymal duct

Aberrant ductule

Ductus deferens

Efferent ductules

Epididymal duct

Rete testis (in mediastinum testis)

Aberrant ductule

Seminiferous tubules

Schema

Lobules of testis

Scrotal septum (dartos)

Septa

Rete testis (in mediastinum testis)

Ductus deferens

Skin of scrotum

Superficial (dartos) fascia

External spermatic fascia

Cremaster muscle and fascia

Internal spermatic fascia

Parietal layer of tunica vaginalis

Visceral layer of tunica vaginalis

Tunica albuginea of testis

Sinus of epididymis

Epididymis

Cross section through scrotum and testis

Plate 390

Testis, Epididymis, and Ductus Deferens

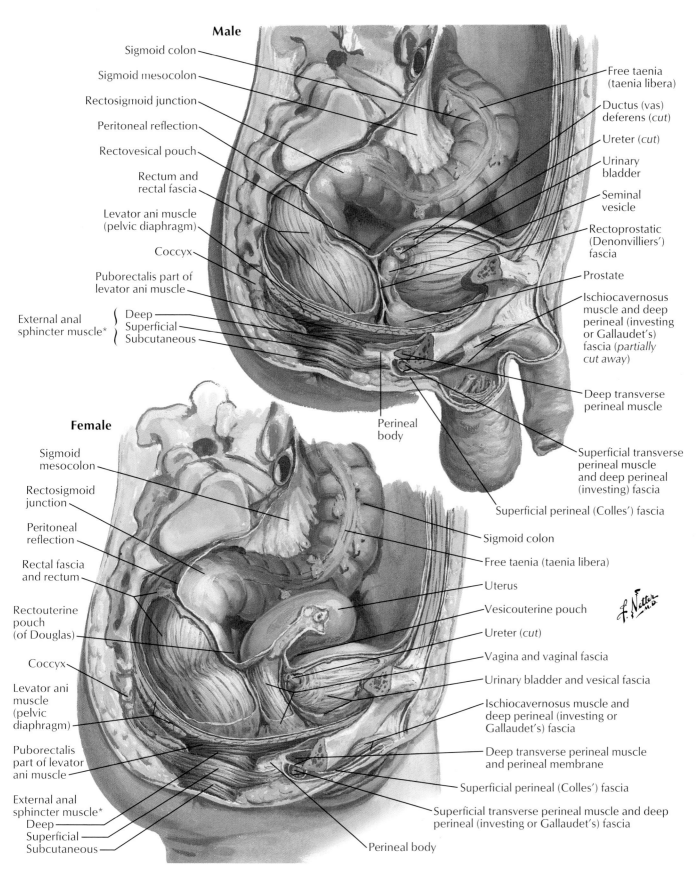

Male

Sigmoid colon

Sigmoid mesocolon

Rectosigmoid junction

Peritoneal reflection

Rectovesical pouch

Rectum and rectal fascia

Levator ani muscle (pelvic diaphragm)

Coccyx

Puborectalis part of levator ani muscle

External anal sphincter muscle* { Deep Superficial Subcutaneous

Free taenia (taenia libera)

Ductus (vas) deferens (cut)

Ureter (cut)

Urinary bladder

Seminal vesicle

Rectoprostatic (Denonvilliers') fascia

Prostate

Ischiocavernosus muscle and deep perineal (investing or Gallaudet's) fascia (partially cut away)

Deep transverse perineal muscle

Perineal body

Superficial transverse perineal muscle and deep perineal (investing) fascia

Superficial perineal (Colles') fascia

Female

Sigmoid mesocolon

Rectosigmoid junction

Peritoneal reflection

Rectal fascia and rectum

Rectouterine pouch (of Douglas)

Coccyx

Levator ani muscle (pelvic diaphragm)

Puborectalis part of levator ani muscle

External anal sphincter muscle* Deep Superficial Subcutaneous

Sigmoid colon

Free taenia (taenia libera)

Uterus

Vesicouterine pouch

Ureter (cut)

Vagina and vaginal fascia

Urinary bladder and vesical fascia

Ischiocavernosus muscle and deep perineal (investing or Gallaudet's) fascia

Deep transverse perineal muscle and perineal membrane

Superficial perineal (Colles') fascia

Superficial transverse perineal muscle and deep perineal (investing or Gallaudet's) fascia

Perineal body

*Parts variable and often indistinct

f. Netter. M.D.

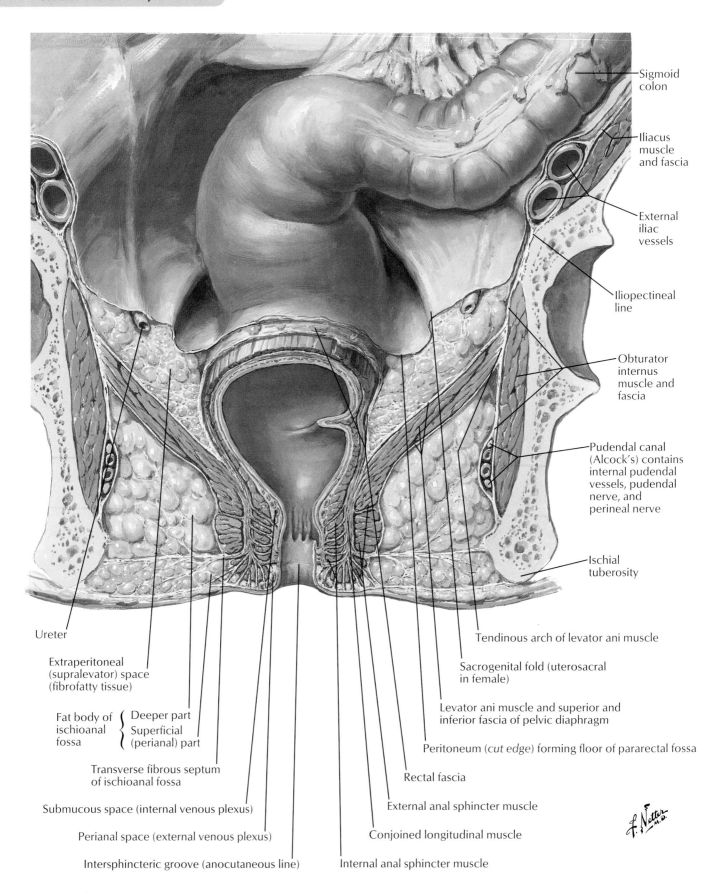

Sigmoid colon

Iliacus muscle and fascia

External iliac vessels

Iliopectineal line

Obturator internus muscle and fascia

Pudendal canal (Alcock's) contains internal pudendal vessels, pudendal nerve, and perineal nerve

Ischial tuberosity

Tendinous arch of levator ani muscle

Sacrogenital fold (uterosacral in female)

Levator ani muscle and superior and inferior fascia of pelvic diaphragm

Peritoneum (*cut edge*) forming floor of pararectal fossa

Rectal fascia

External anal sphincter muscle

Conjoined longitudinal muscle

Internal anal sphincter muscle

Ureter

Extraperitoneal (supralevator) space (fibrofatty tissue)

Fat body of ischioanal fossa { Deeper part / Superficial (perianal) part

Transverse fibrous septum of ischioanal fossa

Submucous space (internal venous plexus)

Perianal space (external venous plexus)

Intersphincteric groove (anocutaneous line)

Plate 392

Rectum

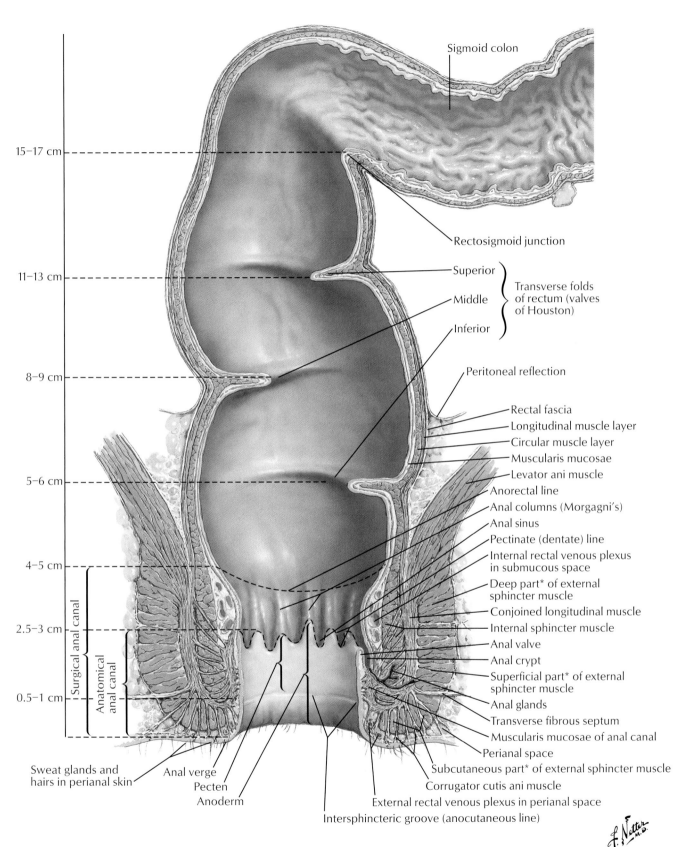

Sigmoid colon

15–17 cm

11–13 cm

8–9 cm

5–6 cm

4–5 cm

2.5–3 cm

0.5–1 cm

Surgical anal canal

Anatomical anal canal

Rectosigmoid junction

Superior
Middle
Inferior

Transverse folds of rectum (valves of Houston)

Peritoneal reflection

Rectal fascia
Longitudinal muscle layer
Circular muscle layer
Muscularis mucosae
Levator ani muscle
Anorectal line
Anal columns (Morgagni's)
Anal sinus
Pectinate (dentate) line
Internal rectal venous plexus in submucous space
Deep part* of external sphincter muscle
Conjoined longitudinal muscle
Internal sphincter muscle
Anal valve
Anal crypt
Superficial part* of external sphincter muscle
Anal glands
Transverse fibrous septum
Muscularis mucosae of anal canal
Perianal space
Subcutaneous part* of external sphincter muscle

Sweat glands and hairs in perianal skin
Anal verge
Pecten
Anoderm
Intersphincteric groove (anocutaneous line)
Corrugator cutis ani muscle
External rectal venous plexus in perianal space

*Parts variable and often indistinct

Rectum

Plate 393

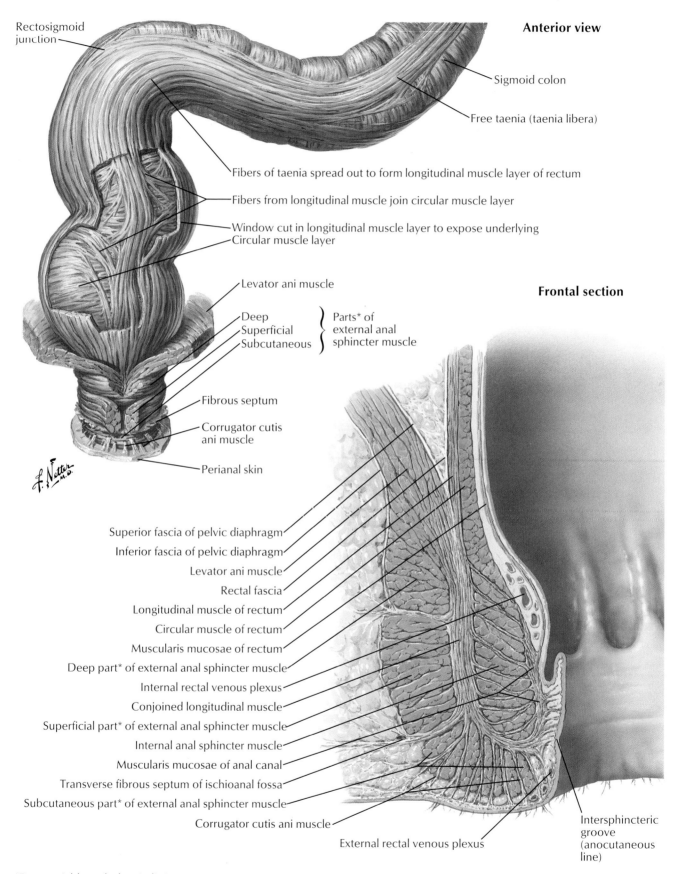

Rectosigmoid junction

Anterior view

Sigmoid colon

Free taenia (taenia libera)

Fibers of taenia spread out to form longitudinal muscle layer of rectum

Fibers from longitudinal muscle join circular muscle layer

Window cut in longitudinal muscle layer to expose underlying
Circular muscle layer

Levator ani muscle

Deep
Superficial
Subcutaneous

Parts* of
external anal
sphincter muscle

Frontal section

Fibrous septum

Corrugator cutis ani muscle

Perianal skin

Superior fascia of pelvic diaphragm
Inferior fascia of pelvic diaphragm
Levator ani muscle
Rectal fascia
Longitudinal muscle of rectum
Circular muscle of rectum
Muscularis mucosae of rectum
Deep part* of external anal sphincter muscle
Internal rectal venous plexus
Conjoined longitudinal muscle
Superficial part* of external anal sphincter muscle
Internal anal sphincter muscle
Muscularis mucosae of anal canal
Transverse fibrous septum of ischioanal fossa
Subcutaneous part* of external anal sphincter muscle
Corrugator cutis ani muscle

External rectal venous plexus

Intersphincteric groove (anocutaneous line)

*Parts variable and often indistinct

Plate 394 **Rectum**

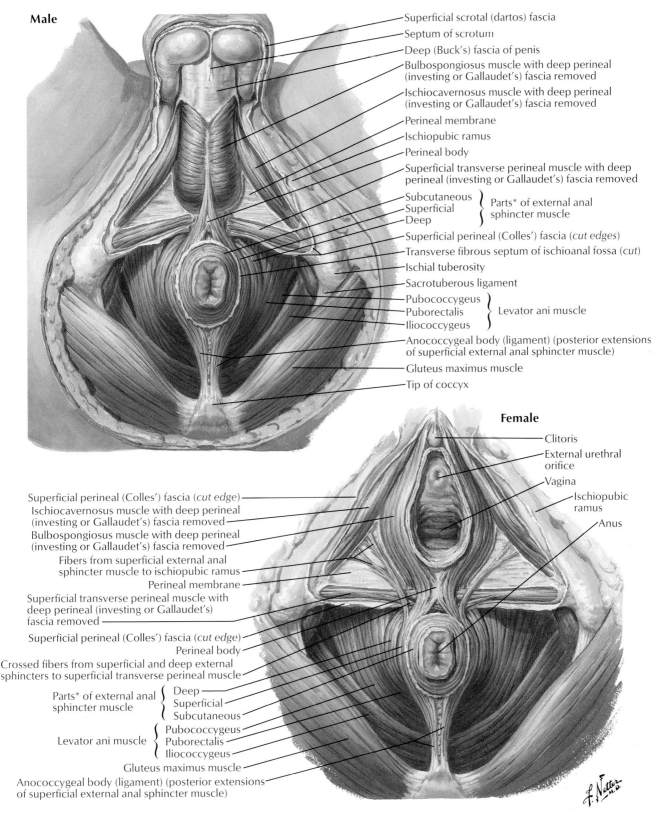

Male

Superficial scrotal (dartos) fascia
Septum of scrotum
Deep (Buck's) fascia of penis
Bulbospongiosus muscle with deep perineal (investing or Gallaudet's) fascia removed
Ischiocavernosus muscle with deep perineal (investing or Gallaudet's) fascia removed
Perineal membrane
Ischiopubic ramus
Perineal body
Superficial transverse perineal muscle with deep perineal (investing or Gallaudet's) fascia removed
Subcutaneous
Superficial
Deep
Parts* of external anal sphincter muscle
Superficial perineal (Colles') fascia (*cut edges*)
Transverse fibrous septum of ischioanal fossa (*cut*)
Ischial tuberosity
Sacrotuberous ligament
Pubococcygeus
Puborectalis
Iliococcygeus
Levator ani muscle
Anococcygeal body (ligament) (posterior extensions of superficial external anal sphincter muscle)
Gluteus maximus muscle
Tip of coccyx

Female

Clitoris
External urethral orifice
Vagina
Ischiopubic ramus
Anus

Superficial perineal (Colles') fascia (*cut edge*)
Ischiocavernosus muscle with deep perineal (investing or Gallaudet's) fascia removed
Bulbospongiosus muscle with deep perineal (investing or Gallaudet's) fascia removed
Fibers from superficial external anal sphincter muscle to ischiopubic ramus
Perineal membrane
Superficial transverse perineal muscle with deep perineal (investing or Gallaudet's) fascia removed
Superficial perineal (Colles') fascia (*cut edge*)
Perineal body
Crossed fibers from superficial and deep external sphincters to superficial transverse perineal muscle
Parts* of external anal sphincter muscle
Deep
Superficial
Subcutaneous
Levator ani muscle
Pubococcygeus
Puborectalis
Iliococcygeus
Gluteus maximus muscle
Anococcygeal body (ligament) (posterior extensions of superficial external anal sphincter muscle)

*Parts variable and often indistinct

Rectum

Plate 395

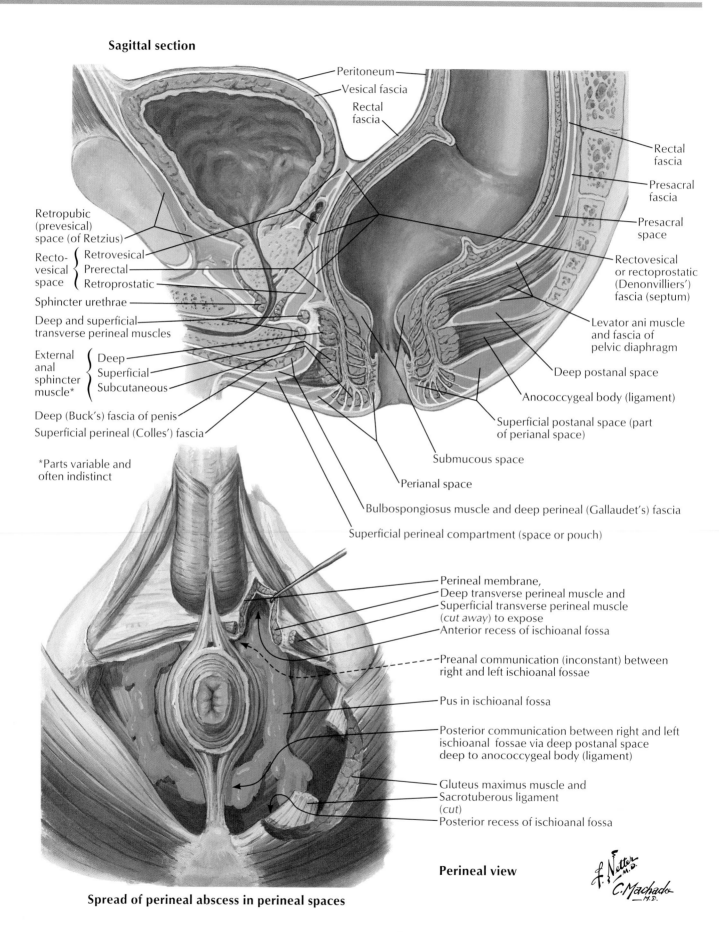

Sagittal section

Peritoneum

Vesical fascia

Rectal fascia

Rectal fascia

Presacral fascia

Presacral space

Rectovesical or rectoprostatic (Denonvilliers') fascia (septum)

Levator ani muscle and fascia of pelvic diaphragm

Deep postanal space

Anococcygeal body (ligament)

Superficial postanal space (part of perianal space)

Retropubic (prevesical) space (of Retzius)

Recto-vesical space { Retrovesical / Prerectal / Retroprostatic

Sphincter urethrae

Deep and superficial transverse perineal muscles

External anal sphincter muscle* { Deep / Superficial / Subcutaneous

Deep (Buck's) fascia of penis

Superficial perineal (Colles') fascia

*Parts variable and often indistinct

Submucous space

Perianal space

Bulbospongiosus muscle and deep perineal (Gallaudet's) fascia

Superficial perineal compartment (space or pouch)

Perineal membrane, Deep transverse perineal muscle and Superficial transverse perineal muscle (*cut away*) to expose Anterior recess of ischioanal fossa

Preanal communication (inconstant) between right and left ischioanal fossae

Pus in ischioanal fossa

Posterior communication between right and left ischioanal fossae via deep postanal space deep to anococcygeal body (ligament)

Gluteus maximus muscle and Sacrotuberous ligament (*cut*)

Posterior recess of ischioanal fossa

Spread of perineal abscess in perineal spaces

Perineal view

Plate 396 **Rectum**

Median (A) and paramedian (B) sagittal MR images of female pelvis

A
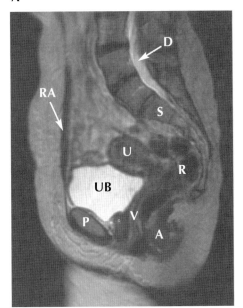

B
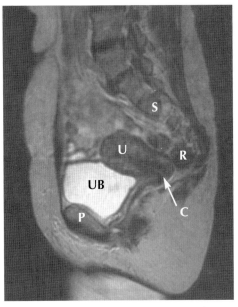

A	Anal canal	**RA**	Rectus abdominis muscle
C	External os of cervix	**S**	Sacrum
D	Dural (thecal) sac	**U**	Uterus
P	Pubic symphysis	**UB**	Urinary bladder
R	Rectum	**V**	Vagina

Median (C) and paramedian (D) sagittal MR images of male pelvis

C
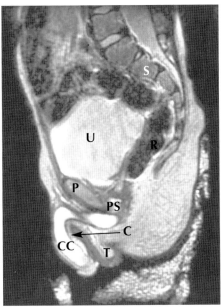

D
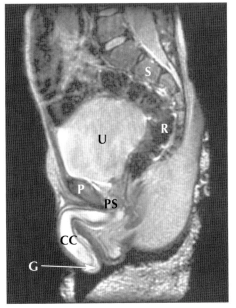

C	Corpus spongiosum	**R**	Rectum
CC	Corpus cavernosum	**S**	Sacrum
G	Glans penis	**T**	Testis
P	Pubic symphysis	**U**	Urinary bladder
PS	Prostate		

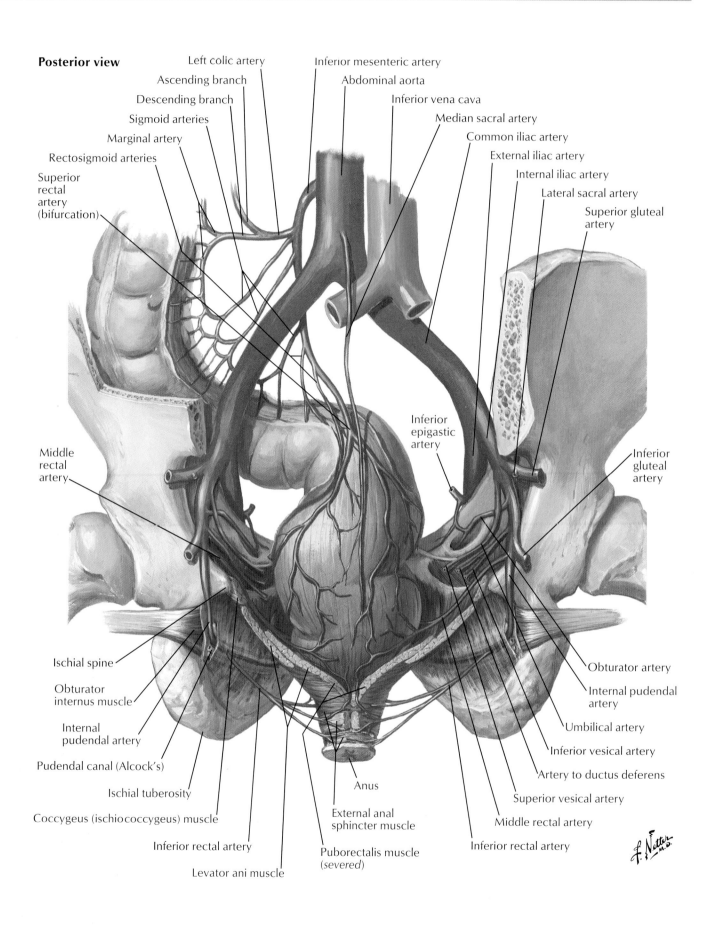

Posterior view

Left colic artery

Ascending branch

Descending branch

Sigmoid arteries

Marginal artery

Rectosigmoid arteries

Superior rectal artery (bifurcation)

Inferior mesenteric artery

Abdominal aorta

Inferior vena cava

Median sacral artery

Common iliac artery

External iliac artery

Internal iliac artery

Lateral sacral artery

Superior gluteal artery

Middle rectal artery

Inferior epigastic artery

Inferior gluteal artery

Ischial spine

Obturator internus muscle

Internal pudendal artery

Pudendal canal (Alcock's)

Ischial tuberosity

Coccygeus (ischiococcygeus) muscle

Inferior rectal artery

Levator ani muscle

Anus

External anal sphincter muscle

Puborectalis muscle (*severed*)

Obturator artery

Internal pudendal artery

Umbilical artery

Inferior vesical artery

Artery to ductus deferens

Superior vesical artery

Middle rectal artery

Inferior rectal artery

Plate 398   **Vasculature**

Anterior view

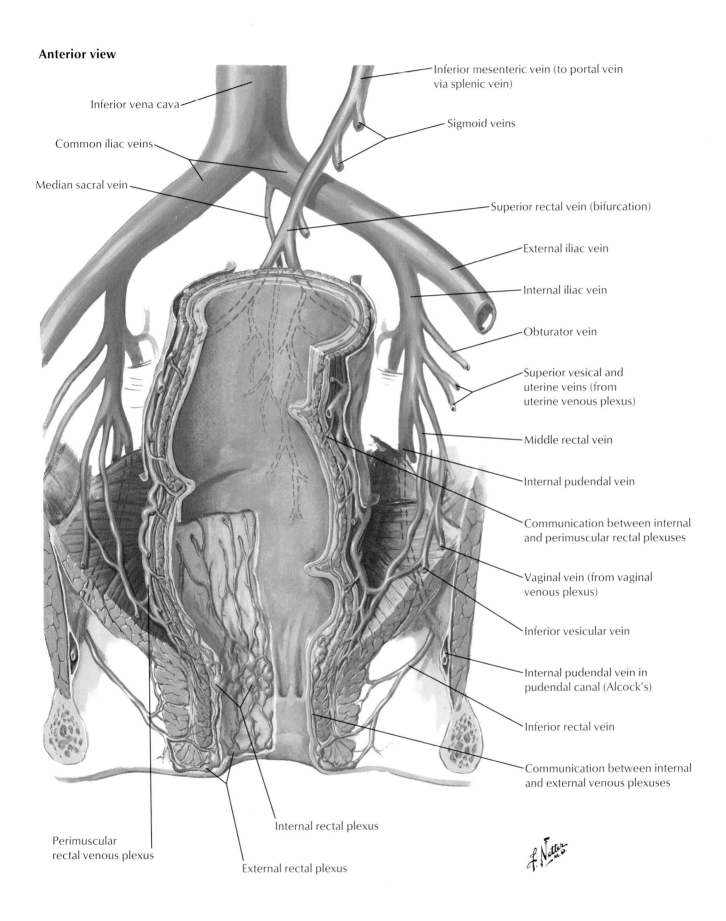

Inferior vena cava

Common iliac veins

Median sacral vein

Inferior mesenteric vein (to portal vein via splenic vein)

Sigmoid veins

Superior rectal vein (bifurcation)

External iliac vein

Internal iliac vein

Obturator vein

Superior vesical and uterine veins (from uterine venous plexus)

Middle rectal vein

Internal pudendal vein

Communication between internal and perimuscular rectal plexuses

Vaginal vein (from vaginal venous plexus)

Inferior vesicular vein

Internal pudendal vein in pudendal canal (Alcock's)

Inferior rectal vein

Communication between internal and external venous plexuses

Internal rectal plexus

Perimuscular rectal venous plexus

External rectal plexus

Anterior view

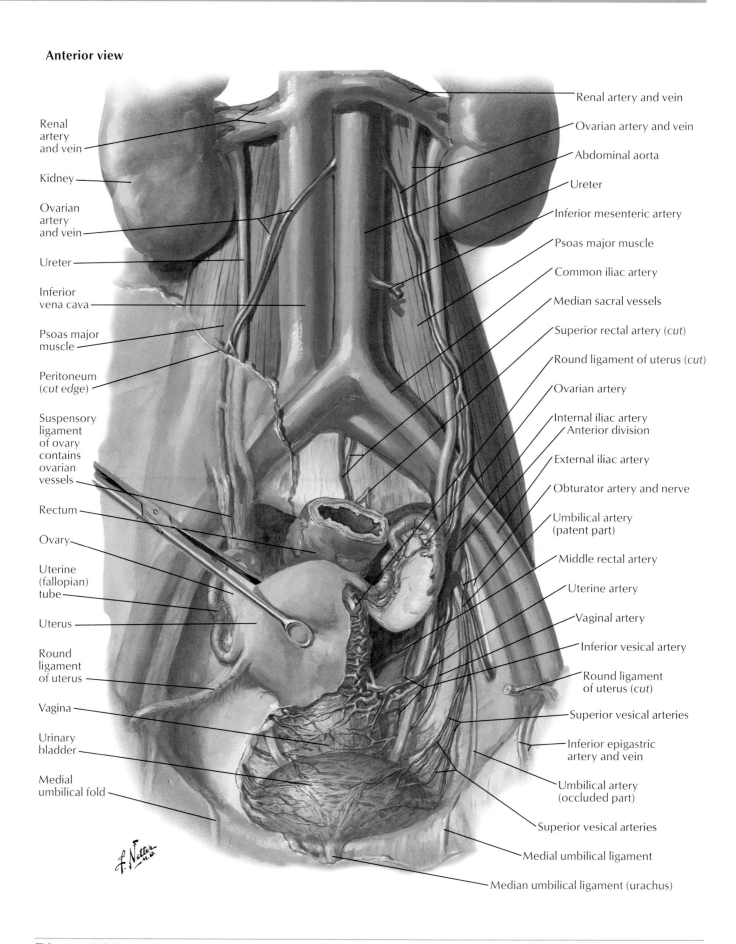

Renal artery and vein

Renal artery and vein

Ovarian artery and vein

Kidney

Abdominal aorta

Ovarian artery and vein

Ureter

Ureter

Inferior mesenteric artery

Inferior vena cava

Psoas major muscle

Psoas major muscle

Common iliac artery

Peritoneum (cut edge)

Median sacral vessels

Superior rectal artery (cut)

Suspensory ligament of ovary contains ovarian vessels

Round ligament of uterus (cut)

Ovarian artery

Internal iliac artery
Anterior division

Rectum

External iliac artery

Ovary

Obturator artery and nerve

Uterine (fallopian) tube

Umbilical artery (patent part)

Middle rectal artery

Uterus

Uterine artery

Round ligament of uterus

Vaginal artery

Vagina

Inferior vesical artery

Urinary bladder

Round ligament of uterus (cut)

Superior vesical arteries

Medial umbilical fold

Inferior epigastric artery and vein

Umbilical artery (occluded part)

Superior vesical arteries

Medial umbilical ligament

Median umbilical ligament (urachus)

Plate 400

Vasculature

Anterior view

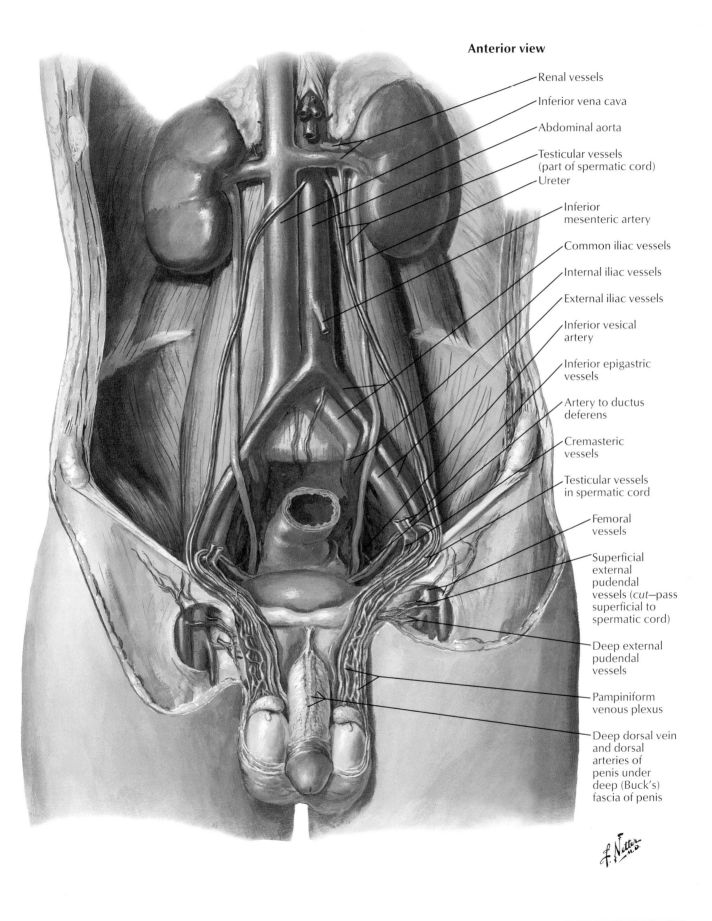

Renal vessels

Inferior vena cava

Abdominal aorta

Testicular vessels
(part of spermatic cord)

Ureter

Inferior
mesenteric artery

Common iliac vessels

Internal iliac vessels

External iliac vessels

Inferior vesical
artery

Inferior epigastric
vessels

Artery to ductus
deferens

Cremasteric
vessels

Testicular vessels
in spermatic cord

Femoral
vessels

Superficial
external
pudendal
vessels (cut–pass
superficial to
spermatic cord)

Deep external
pudendal
vessels

Pampiniform
venous plexus

Deep dorsal vein
and dorsal
arteries of
penis under
deep (Buck's)
fascia of penis

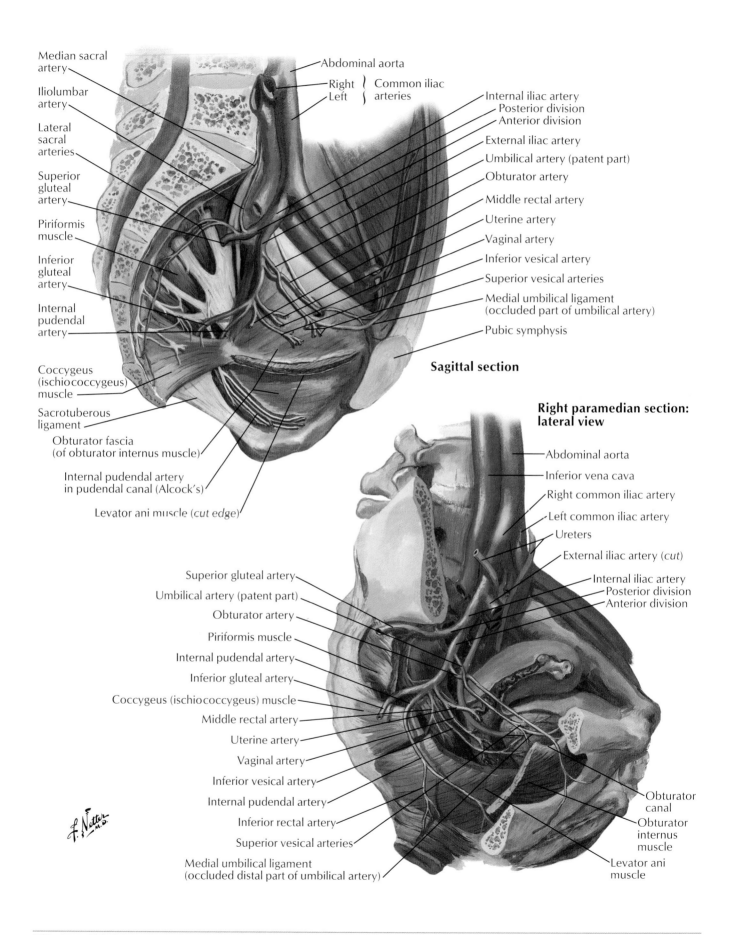

Median sacral artery

Iliolumbar artery

Lateral sacral arteries

Superior gluteal artery

Piriformis muscle

Inferior gluteal artery

Internal pudendal artery

Coccygeus (ischiococcygeus) muscle

Sacrotuberous ligament

Obturator fascia (of obturator internus muscle)

Internal pudendal artery in pudendal canal (Alcock's)

Levator ani muscle (cut edge)

Abdominal aorta

Right } Common iliac
Left } arteries

Internal iliac artery
Posterior division
Anterior division

External iliac artery

Umbilical artery (patent part)

Obturator artery

Middle rectal artery

Uterine artery

Vaginal artery

Inferior vesical artery

Superior vesical arteries

Medial umbilical ligament (occluded part of umbilical artery)

Pubic symphysis

Sagittal section

Right paramedian section: lateral view

Abdominal aorta

Inferior vena cava

Right common iliac artery

Left common iliac artery

Ureters

External iliac artery (cut)

Internal iliac artery
Posterior division
Anterior division

Superior gluteal artery

Umbilical artery (patent part)

Obturator artery

Piriformis muscle

Internal pudendal artery

Inferior gluteal artery

Coccygeus (ischiococcygeus) muscle

Middle rectal artery

Uterine artery

Vaginal artery

Inferior vesical artery

Internal pudendal artery

Inferior rectal artery

Superior vesical arteries

Medial umbilical ligament (occluded distal part of umbilical artery)

Obturator canal

Obturator internus muscle

Levator ani muscle

Plate 402   **Vasculature**

**Left paramedian section:
lateral view**

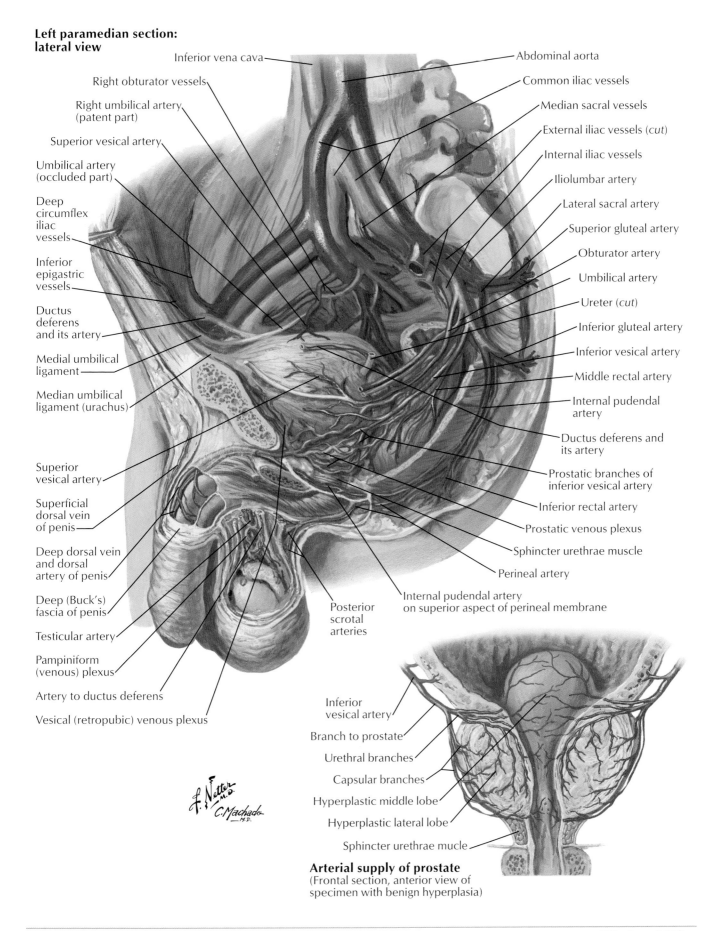

Inferior vena cava

Right obturator vessels

Right umbilical artery
(patent part)

Superior vesical artery

Umbilical artery
(occluded part)

Deep
circumflex
iliac
vessels

Inferior
epigastric
vessels

Ductus
deferens
and its artery

Medial umbilical
ligament

Median umbilical
ligament (urachus)

Superior
vesical artery

Superficial
dorsal vein
of penis

Deep dorsal vein
and dorsal
artery of penis

Deep (Buck's)
fascia of penis

Testicular artery

Pampiniform
(venous) plexus

Artery to ductus deferens

Vesical (retropubic) venous plexus

Abdominal aorta

Common iliac vessels

Median sacral vessels

External iliac vessels (*cut*)

Internal iliac vessels

Iliolumbar artery

Lateral sacral artery

Superior gluteal artery

Obturator artery

Umbilical artery

Ureter (*cut*)

Inferior gluteal artery

Inferior vesical artery

Middle rectal artery

Internal pudendal
artery

Ductus deferens and
its artery

Prostatic branches of
inferior vesical artery

Inferior rectal artery

Prostatic venous plexus

Sphincter urethrae muscle

Perineal artery

Posterior
scrotal
arteries

Internal pudendal artery
on superior aspect of perineal membrane

Inferior
vesical artery

Branch to prostate

Urethral branches

Capsular branches

Hyperplastic middle lobe

Hyperplastic lateral lobe

Sphincter urethrae mucle

Arterial supply of prostate
(Frontal section, anterior view of
specimen with benign hyperplasia)

Vasculature

Plate 403

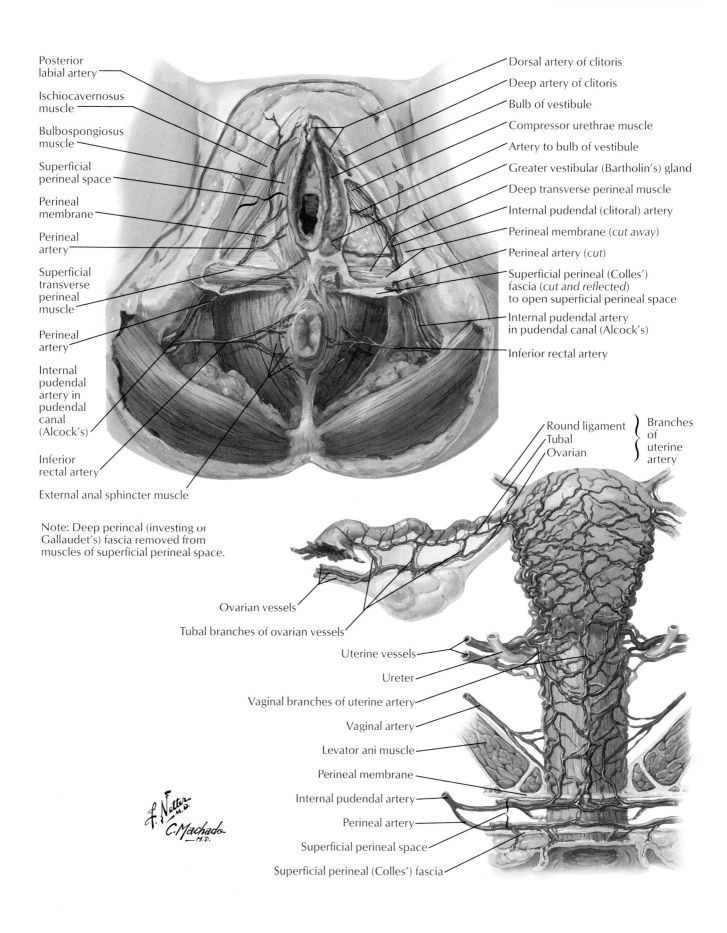

Posterior labial artery

Ischiocavernosus muscle

Bulbospongiosus muscle

Superficial perineal space

Perineal membrane

Perineal artery

Superficial transverse perineal muscle

Perineal artery

Internal pudendal artery in pudendal canal (Alcock's)

Inferior rectal artery

External anal sphincter muscle

Note: Deep perineal (investing or Gallaudet's) fascia removed from muscles of superficial perineal space.

Dorsal artery of clitoris

Deep artery of clitoris

Bulb of vestibule

Compressor urethrae muscle

Artery to bulb of vestibule

Greater vestibular (Bartholin's) gland

Deep transverse perineal muscle

Internal pudendal (clitoral) artery

Perineal membrane (*cut away*)

Perineal artery (*cut*)

Superficial perineal (Colles') fascia (*cut and reflected*) to open superficial perineal space

Internal pudendal artery in pudendal canal (Alcock's)

Inferior rectal artery

Round ligament
Tubal
Ovarian
} Branches of uterine artery

Ovarian vessels

Tubal branches of ovarian vessels

Uterine vessels

Ureter

Vaginal branches of uterine artery

Vaginal artery

Levator ani muscle

Perineal membrane

Internal pudendal artery

Perineal artery

Superficial perineal space

Superficial perineal (Colles') fascia

Plate 404　　　　　　　　　　　　　　　　　　　　　**Vasculature**

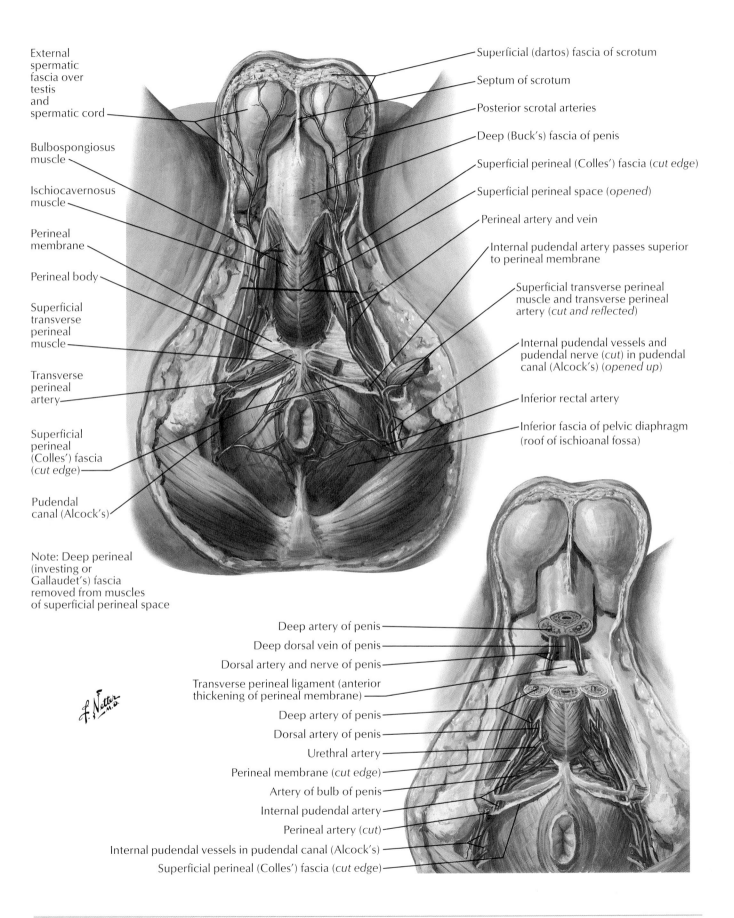

External spermatic fascia over testis and spermatic cord

Bulbospongiosus muscle

Ischiocavernosus muscle

Perineal membrane

Perineal body

Superficial transverse perineal muscle

Transverse perineal artery

Superficial perineal (Colles') fascia (cut edge)

Pudendal canal (Alcock's)

Note: Deep perineal (investing or Gallaudet's) fascia removed from muscles of superficial perineal space

Superficial (dartos) fascia of scrotum

Septum of scrotum

Posterior scrotal arteries

Deep (Buck's) fascia of penis

Superficial perineal (Colles') fascia (cut edge)

Superficial perineal space (opened)

Perineal artery and vein

Internal pudendal artery passes superior to perineal membrane

Superficial transverse perineal muscle and transverse perineal artery (cut and reflected)

Internal pudendal vessels and pudendal nerve (cut) in pudendal canal (Alcock's) (opened up)

Inferior rectal artery

Inferior fascia of pelvic diaphragm (roof of ischioanal fossa)

Deep artery of penis

Deep dorsal vein of penis

Dorsal artery and nerve of penis

Transverse perineal ligament (anterior thickening of perineal membrane)

Deep artery of penis

Dorsal artery of penis

Urethral artery

Perineal membrane (cut edge)

Artery of bulb of penis

Internal pudendal artery

Perineal artery (cut)

Internal pudendal vessels in pudendal canal (Alcock's)

Superficial perineal (Colles') fascia (cut edge)

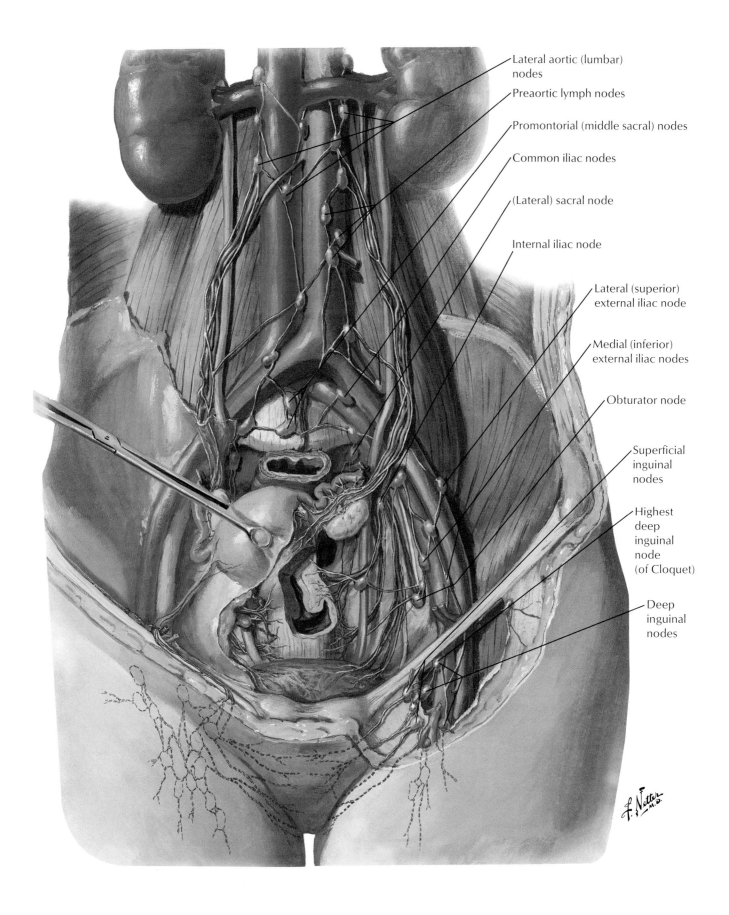

Lateral aortic (lumbar) nodes

Preaortic lymph nodes

Promontorial (middle sacral) nodes

Common iliac nodes

(Lateral) sacral node

Internal iliac node

Lateral (superior) external iliac node

Medial (inferior) external iliac nodes

Obturator node

Superficial inguinal nodes

Highest deep inguinal node (of Cloquet)

Deep inguinal nodes

Plate 406

Vasculature

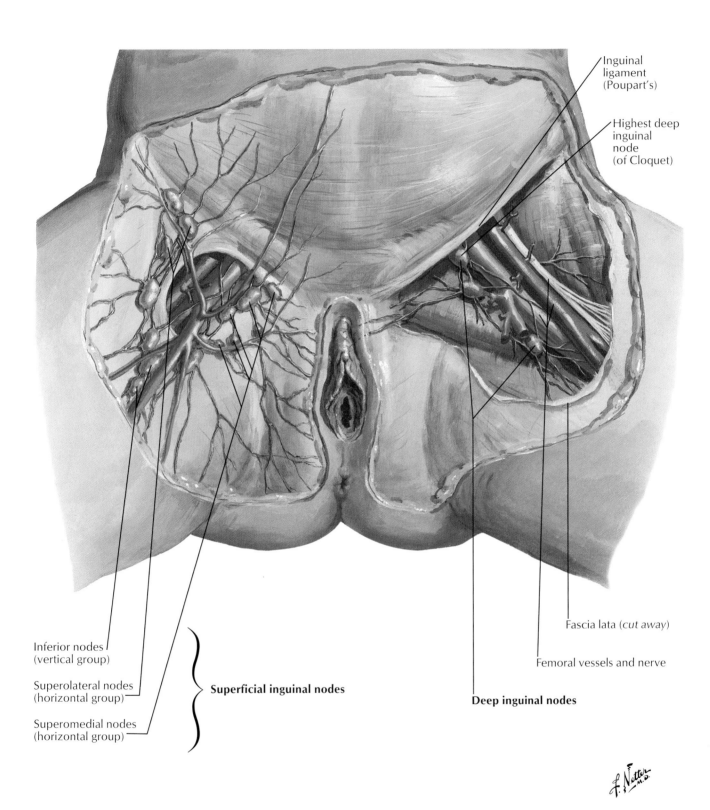

Inguinal
ligament
(Poupart's)

Highest deep
inguinal
node
(of Cloquet)

Fascia lata (*cut away*)

Femoral vessels and nerve

Deep inguinal nodes

Inferior nodes
(vertical group)

Superolateral nodes
(horizontal group)

Superomedial nodes
(horizontal group)

Superficial inguinal nodes

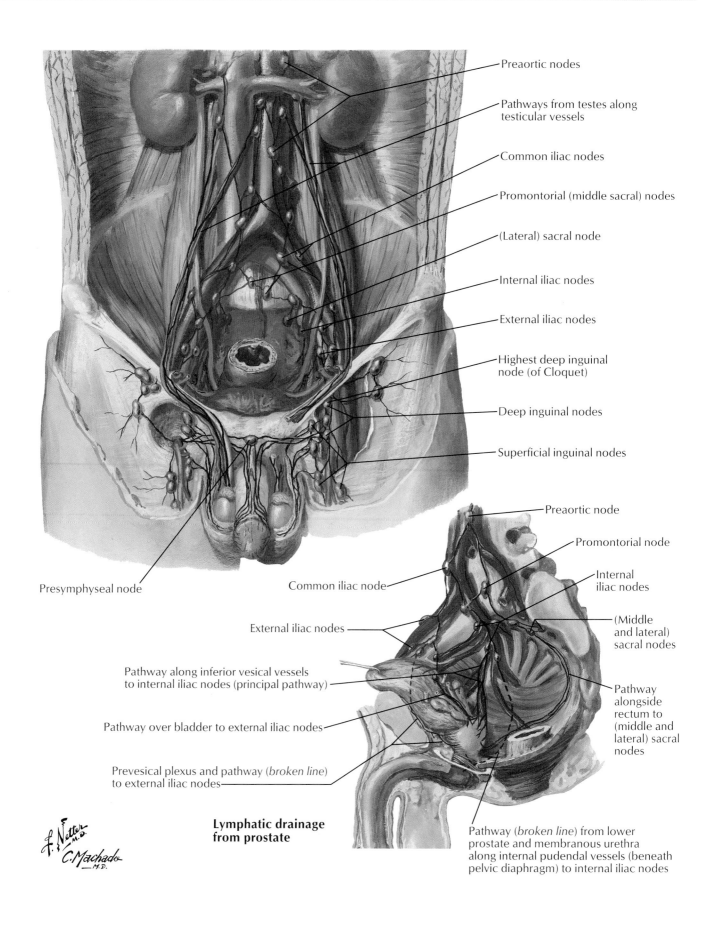

Preaortic nodes

Pathways from testes along testicular vessels

Common iliac nodes

Promontorial (middle sacral) nodes

(Lateral) sacral node

Internal iliac nodes

External iliac nodes

Highest deep inguinal node (of Cloquet)

Deep inguinal nodes

Superficial inguinal nodes

Presymphyseal node

Preaortic node

Promontorial node

Common iliac node

Internal iliac nodes

External iliac nodes

(Middle and lateral) sacral nodes

Pathway along inferior vesical vessels to internal iliac nodes (principal pathway)

Pathway over bladder to external iliac nodes

Pathway alongside rectum to (middle and lateral) sacral nodes

Prevesical plexus and pathway (*broken line*) to external iliac nodes

Lymphatic drainage from prostate

Pathway (*broken line*) from lower prostate and membranous urethra along internal pudendal vessels (beneath pelvic diaphragm) to internal iliac nodes

Plate 408 | **Vasculature**

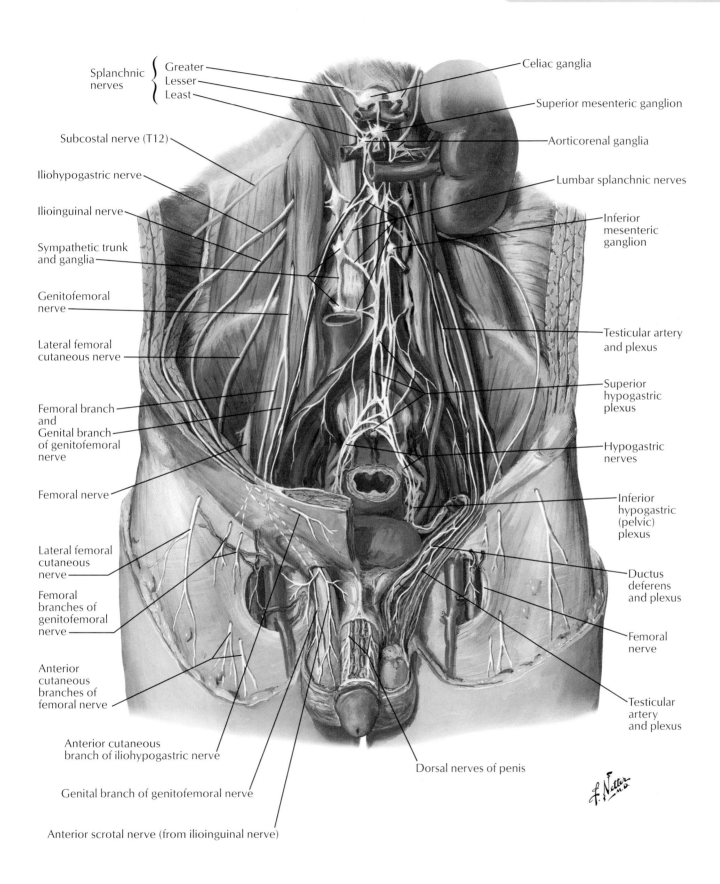

Splanchnic nerves
{ Greater
  Lesser
  Least

Subcostal nerve (T12)

Iliohypogastric nerve

Ilioinguinal nerve

Sympathetic trunk and ganglia

Genitofemoral nerve

Lateral femoral cutaneous nerve

Femoral branch and Genital branch of genitofemoral nerve

Femoral nerve

Lateral femoral cutaneous nerve

Femoral branches of genitofemoral nerve

Anterior cutaneous branches of femoral nerve

Anterior cutaneous branch of iliohypogastric nerve

Genital branch of genitofemoral nerve

Anterior scrotal nerve (from ilioinguinal nerve)

Celiac ganglia

Superior mesenteric ganglion

Aorticorenal ganglia

Lumbar splanchnic nerves

Inferior mesenteric ganglion

Testicular artery and plexus

Superior hypogastric plexus

Hypogastric nerves

Inferior hypogastric (pelvic) plexus

Ductus deferens and plexus

Femoral nerve

Testicular artery and plexus

Dorsal nerves of penis

f. Netter M.D.

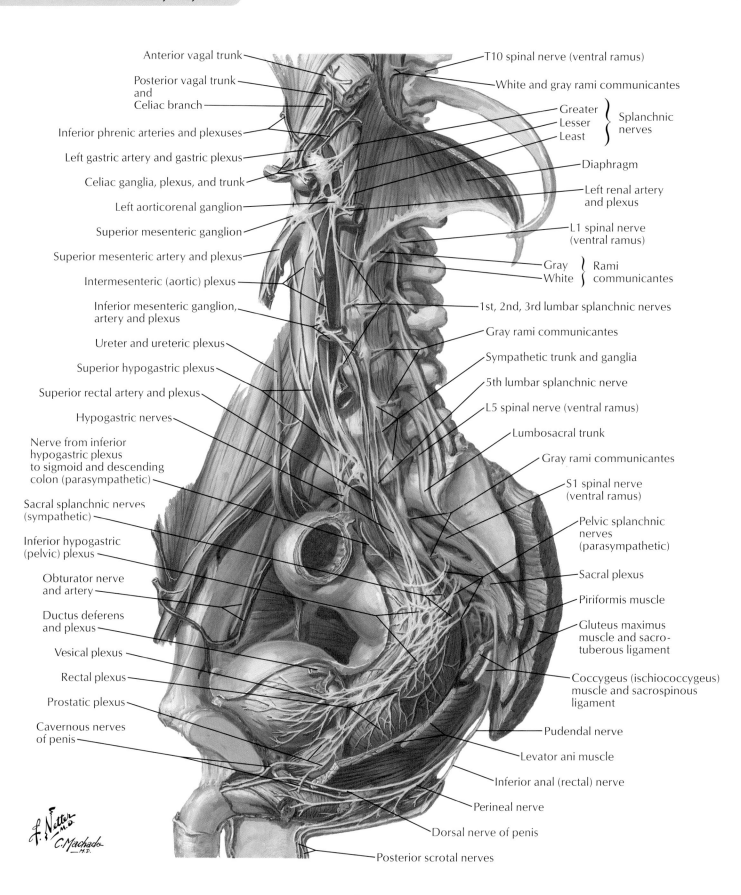

Anterior vagal trunk

Posterior vagal trunk and Celiac branch

Inferior phrenic arteries and plexuses

Left gastric artery and gastric plexus

Celiac ganglia, plexus, and trunk

Left aorticorenal ganglion

Superior mesenteric ganglion

Superior mesenteric artery and plexus

Intermesenteric (aortic) plexus

Inferior mesenteric ganglion, artery and plexus

Ureter and ureteric plexus

Superior hypogastric plexus

Superior rectal artery and plexus

Hypogastric nerves

Nerve from inferior hypogastric plexus to sigmoid and descending colon (parasympathetic)

Sacral splanchnic nerves (sympathetic)

Inferior hypogastric (pelvic) plexus

Obturator nerve and artery

Ductus deferens and plexus

Vesical plexus

Rectal plexus

Prostatic plexus

Cavernous nerves of penis

T10 spinal nerve (ventral ramus)

White and gray rami communicantes

Greater
Lesser } Splanchnic nerves
Least

Diaphragm

Left renal artery and plexus

L1 spinal nerve (ventral ramus)

Gray } Rami
White } communicantes

1st, 2nd, 3rd lumbar splanchnic nerves

Gray rami communicantes

Sympathetic trunk and ganglia

5th lumbar splanchnic nerve

L5 spinal nerve (ventral ramus)

Lumbosacral trunk

Gray rami communicantes

S1 spinal nerve (ventral ramus)

Pelvic splanchnic nerves (parasympathetic)

Sacral plexus

Piriformis muscle

Gluteus maximus muscle and sacro-tuberous ligament

Coccygeus (ischiococcygeus) muscle and sacrospinous ligament

Pudendal nerve

Levator ani muscle

Inferior anal (rectal) nerve

Perineal nerve

Dorsal nerve of penis

Posterior scrotal nerves

Plate 410   **Innervation**

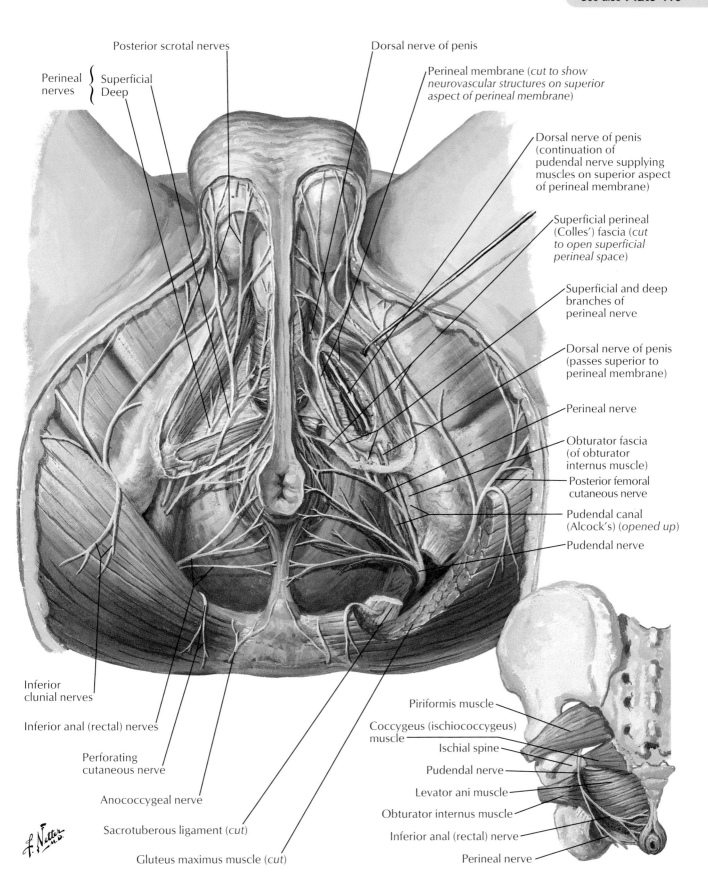

Posterior scrotal nerves

Dorsal nerve of penis

Perineal nerves { Superficial / Deep

Perineal membrane (cut to show neurovascular structures on superior aspect of perineal membrane)

Dorsal nerve of penis (continuation of pudendal nerve supplying muscles on superior aspect of perineal membrane)

Superficial perineal (Colles') fascia (cut to open superficial perineal space)

Superficial and deep branches of perineal nerve

Dorsal nerve of penis (passes superior to perineal membrane)

Perineal nerve

Obturator fascia (of obturator internus muscle)

Posterior femoral cutaneous nerve

Pudendal canal (Alcock's) (opened up)

Pudendal nerve

Inferior clunial nerves

Inferior anal (rectal) nerves

Perforating cutaneous nerve

Anococcygeal nerve

Sacrotuberous ligament (cut)

Gluteus maximus muscle (cut)

Piriformis muscle

Coccygeus (ischiococcygeus) muscle

Ischial spine

Pudendal nerve

Levator ani muscle

Obturator internus muscle

Inferior anal (rectal) nerve

Perineal nerve

Innervation

Plate 411

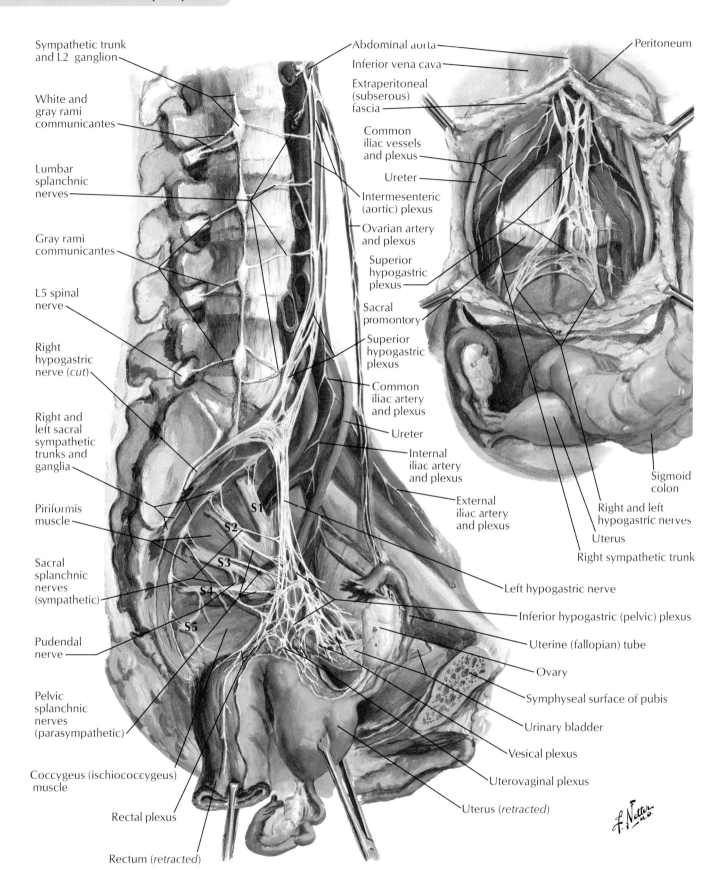

Sympathetic trunk and L2 ganglion

White and gray rami communicantes

Lumbar splanchnic nerves

Gray rami communicantes

L5 spinal nerve

Right hypogastric nerve (*cut*)

Right and left sacral sympathetic trunks and ganglia

Piriformis muscle

Sacral splanchnic nerves (sympathetic)

Pudendal nerve

Pelvic splanchnic nerves (parasympathetic)

Coccygeus (ischiococcygeus) muscle

Rectal plexus

Rectum (*retracted*)

Abdominal aorta

Inferior vena cava

Extraperitoneal (subserous) fascia

Common iliac vessels and plexus

Ureter

Intermesenteric (aortic) plexus

Ovarian artery and plexus

Superior hypogastric plexus

Sacral promontory

Superior hypogastric plexus

Common iliac artery and plexus

Ureter

Internal iliac artery and plexus

External iliac artery and plexus

Left hypogastric nerve

Inferior hypogastric (pelvic) plexus

Uterine (fallopian) tube

Ovary

Symphyseal surface of pubis

Urinary bladder

Vesical plexus

Uterovaginal plexus

Uterus (*retracted*)

Peritoneum

Sigmoid colon

Right and left hypogastric nerves

Uterus

Right sympathetic trunk

S1

S2

S3

S4

S5

Plate 412

Innervation

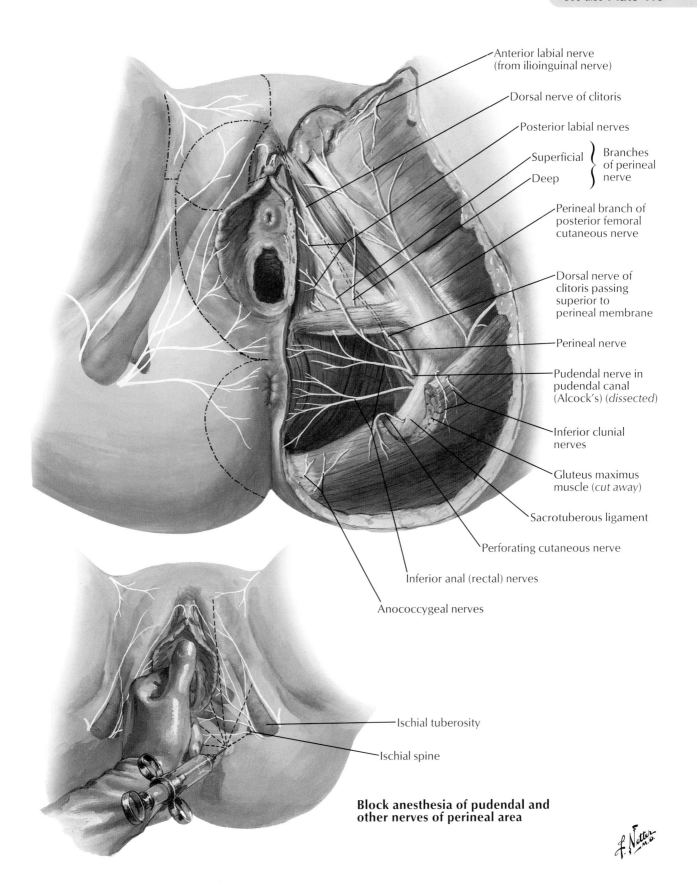

Anterior labial nerve
(from ilioinguinal nerve)

Dorsal nerve of clitoris

Posterior labial nerves

Superficial } Branches
of perineal
Deep } nerve

Perineal branch of
posterior femoral
cutaneous nerve

Dorsal nerve of
clitoris passing
superior to
perineal membrane

Perineal nerve

Pudendal nerve in
pudendal canal
(Alcock's) (*dissected*)

Inferior clunial
nerves

Gluteus maximus
muscle (*cut away*)

Sacrotuberous ligament

Perforating cutaneous nerve

Inferior anal (rectal) nerves

Anococcygeal nerves

Ischial tuberosity

Ischial spine

**Block anesthesia of pudendal and
other nerves of perineal area**

Innervation

Plate 413

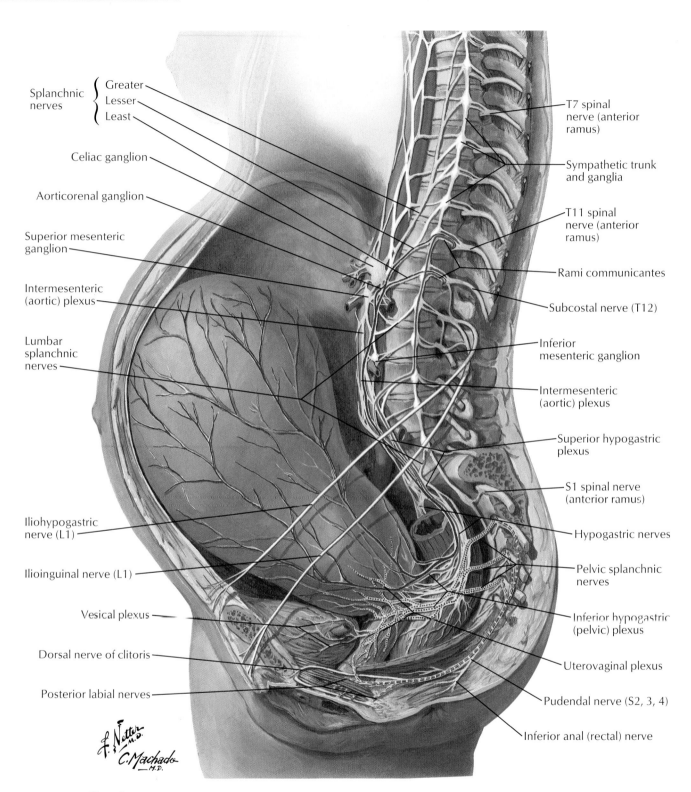

Splanchnic nerves
{ Greater
Lesser
Least

Celiac ganglion

Aorticorenal ganglion

Superior mesenteric ganglion

Intermesenteric (aortic) plexus

Lumbar splanchnic nerves

Iliohypogastric nerve (L1)

Ilioinguinal nerve (L1)

Vesical plexus

Dorsal nerve of clitoris

Posterior labial nerves

T7 spinal nerve (anterior ramus)

Sympathetic trunk and ganglia

T11 spinal nerve (anterior ramus)

Rami communicantes

Subcostal nerve (T12)

Inferior mesenteric ganglion

Intermesenteric (aortic) plexus

Superior hypogastric plexus

S1 spinal nerve (anterior ramus)

Hypogastric nerves

Pelvic splanchnic nerves

Inferior hypogastric (pelvic) plexus

Uterovaginal plexus

Pudendal nerve (S2, 3, 4)

Inferior anal (rectal) nerve

─────── Sensory fibers from uterine body and fundus accompany sympathetic fibers via hypogastric plexuses to T11, 12 (L1?)

─────── Motor fibers to uterine body and fundus (sympathetic)

············ Sensory fibers from cervix and upper vagina accompany pelvic splanchnic nerves (parasympathetic) to S2, 3, 4

············ Motor fibers to lower uterine segment, cervix, and upper vagina (parasympathetic)

─ ─ ─ ─ Sensory fibers from lower vagina and perineum accompany somatic fibers via pudendal nerve to S2, 3, 4

─ ─ ─ ─ Motor fibers to lower vagina and perineum via pudendal nerve (somatic)

Plate 414

Innervation

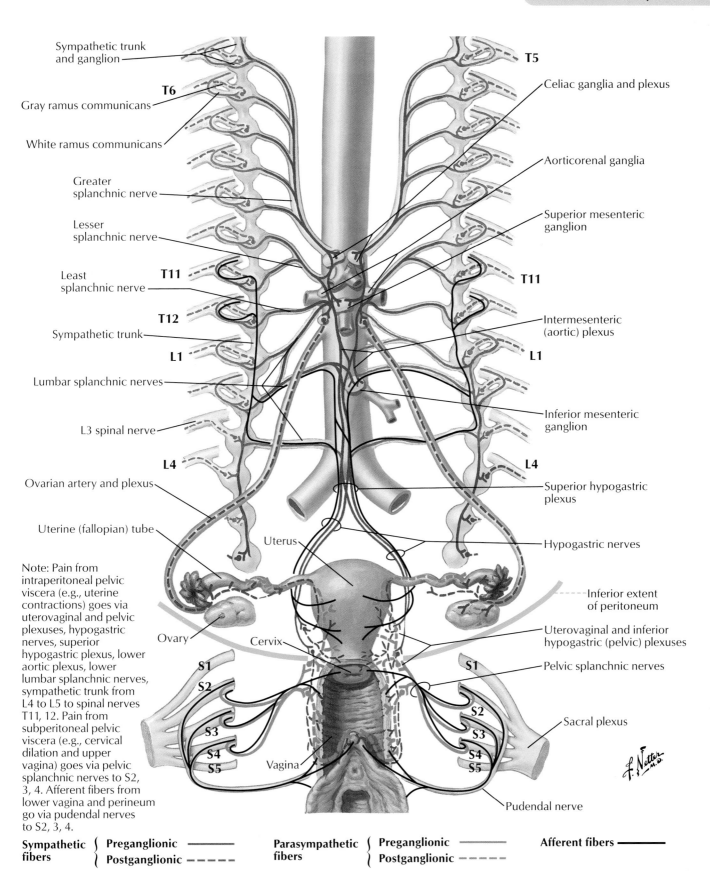

Sympathetic trunk and ganglion

T5

T6

Celiac ganglia and plexus

Gray ramus communicans

White ramus communicans

Aorticorenal ganglia

Greater splanchnic nerve

Superior mesenteric ganglion

Lesser splanchnic nerve

Least splanchnic nerve

T11

T11

T12

Intermesenteric (aortic) plexus

Sympathetic trunk

L1

L1

Lumbar splanchnic nerves

Inferior mesenteric ganglion

L3 spinal nerve

L4

L4

Ovarian artery and plexus

Superior hypogastric plexus

Uterine (fallopian) tube

Uterus

Hypogastric nerves

Note: Pain from intraperitoneal pelvic viscera (e.g., uterine contractions) goes via uterovaginal and pelvic plexuses, hypogastric nerves, superior hypogastric plexus, lower aortic plexus, lower lumbar splanchnic nerves, sympathetic trunk from L4 to L5 to spinal nerves T11, 12. Pain from subperitoneal pelvic viscera (e.g., cervical dilation and upper vagina) goes via pelvic splanchnic nerves to S2, 3, 4. Afferent fibers from lower vagina and perineum go via pudendal nerves to S2, 3, 4.

Ovary

Cervix

Vagina

Inferior extent of peritoneum

Uterovaginal and inferior hypogastric (pelvic) plexuses

Pelvic splanchnic nerves

S1

S1

S2

S2

S3

S3

Sacral plexus

S4

S4

S5

S5

Pudendal nerve

| Sympathetic fibers | Preganglionic ——— | Parasympathetic fibers | Preganglionic ——— | Afferent fibers ——— |
| | Postganglionic - - - | | Postganglionic - - - | |

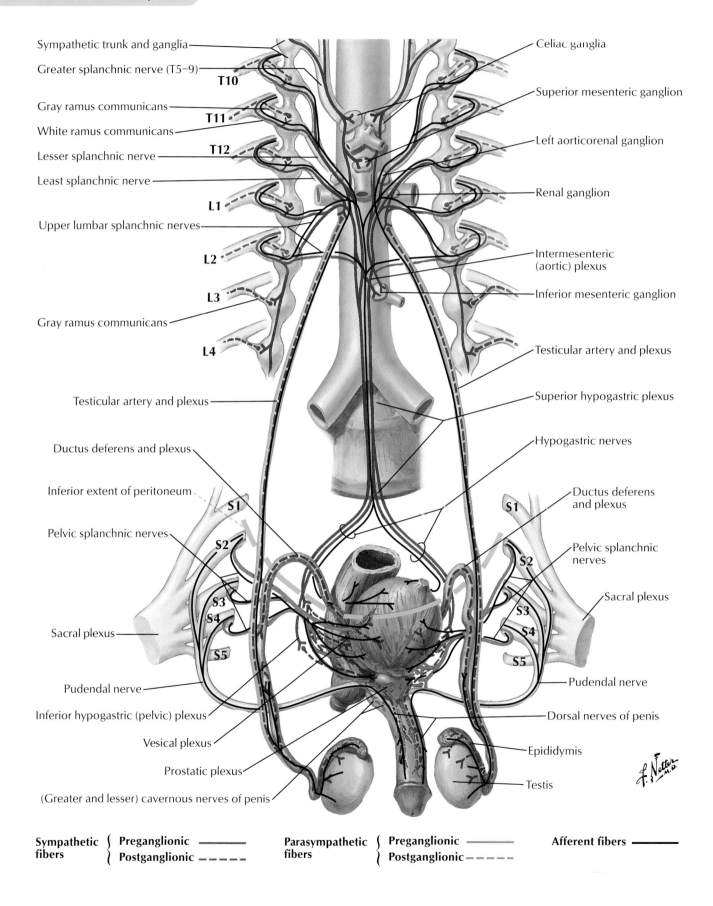

Sympathetic trunk and ganglia

Greater splanchnic nerve (T5–9)

T10

Gray ramus communicans

T11

White ramus communicans

Lesser splanchnic nerve

T12

Least splanchnic nerve

L1

Upper lumbar splanchnic nerves

L2

L3

Gray ramus communicans

L4

Testicular artery and plexus

Ductus deferens and plexus

Inferior extent of peritoneum

S1

Pelvic splanchnic nerves

S2

S3
S4

Sacral plexus

S5

Pudendal nerve

Inferior hypogastric (pelvic) plexus

Vesical plexus

Prostatic plexus

(Greater and lesser) cavernous nerves of penis

Celiac ganglia

Superior mesenteric ganglion

Left aorticorenal ganglion

Renal ganglion

Intermesenteric (aortic) plexus

Inferior mesenteric ganglion

Testicular artery and plexus

Superior hypogastric plexus

Hypogastric nerves

Ductus deferens and plexus

S1

Pelvic splanchnic nerves

S2

Sacral plexus

S3

S4

S5

Pudendal nerve

Dorsal nerves of penis

Epididymis

Testis

Sympathetic fibers	Preganglionic ————	Parasympathetic fibers	Preganglionic ————	Afferent fibers ————
	Postganglionic – – – –		Postganglionic – – – –	

Plate 416 | **Innervation**

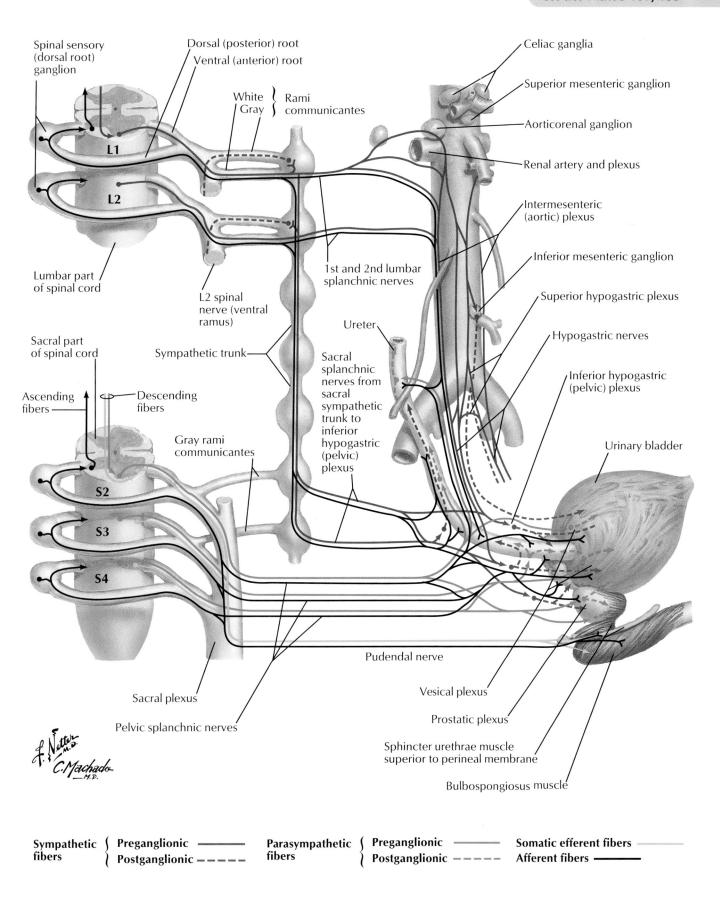

Spinal sensory (dorsal root) ganglion

Dorsal (posterior) root

Ventral (anterior) root

White } Rami
Gray } communicantes

Celiac ganglia

Superior mesenteric ganglion

Aorticorenal ganglion

Renal artery and plexus

Intermesenteric (aortic) plexus

Inferior mesenteric ganglion

Superior hypogastric plexus

Hypogastric nerves

Inferior hypogastric (pelvic) plexus

Urinary bladder

L1

L2

Lumbar part of spinal cord

L2 spinal nerve (ventral ramus)

1st and 2nd lumbar splanchnic nerves

Sympathetic trunk

Ureter

Sacral splanchnic nerves from sacral sympathetic trunk to inferior hypogastric (pelvic) plexus

Sacral part of spinal cord

Ascending fibers

Descending fibers

Gray rami communicantes

S2

S3

S4

Pudendal nerve

Sacral plexus

Vesical plexus

Pelvic splanchnic nerves

Prostatic plexus

Sphincter urethrae muscle superior to perineal membrane

Bulbospongiosus muscle

Sympathetic fibers	{	Preganglionic ———	Parasympathetic fibers	{	Preganglionic ———	Somatic efferent fibers ———
		Postganglionic - - - -			Postganglionic - - - -	Afferent fibers ———

Section 6 Upper Limb

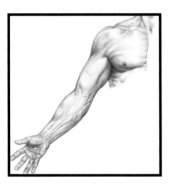
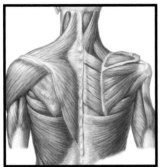
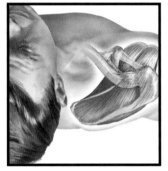
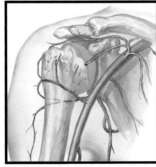

6 Upper Limb

Elbow and Forearm
Plates 436–451

Wrist and Hand
Plates 452–471

Neurovasculature
Plates 472–483

Regional Scans
Plate 484

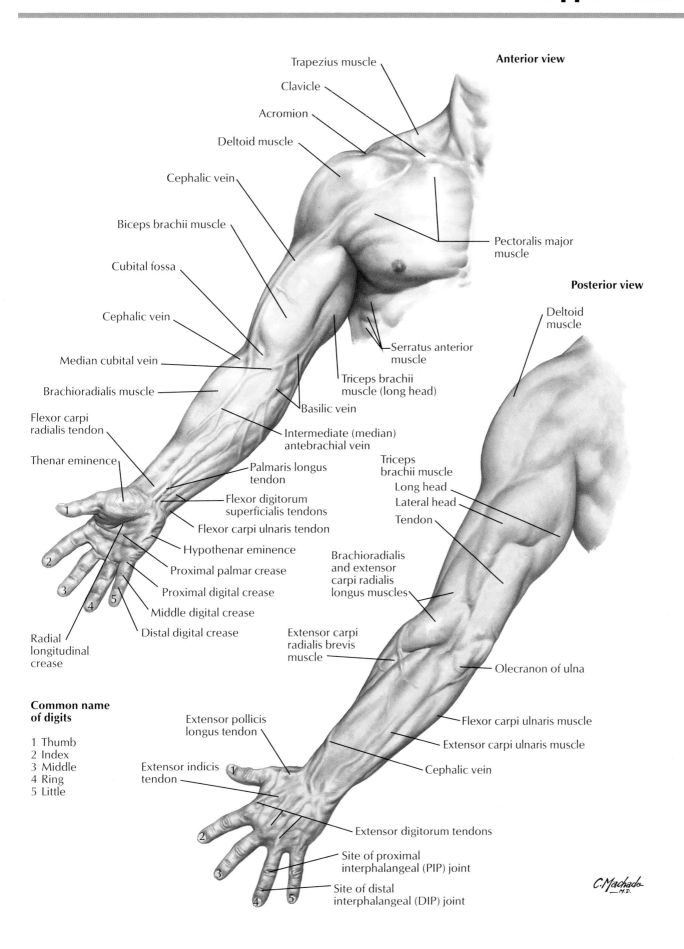

Anterior view

Trapezius muscle

Clavicle

Acromion

Deltoid muscle

Cephalic vein

Biceps brachii muscle

Cubital fossa

Cephalic vein

Median cubital vein

Brachioradialis muscle

Flexor carpi radialis tendon

Thenar eminence

Pectoralis major muscle

Posterior view

Deltoid muscle

Serratus anterior muscle

Triceps brachii muscle (long head)

Basilic vein

Intermediate (median) antebrachial vein

Palmaris longus tendon

Flexor digitorum superficialis tendons

Flexor carpi ulnaris tendon

Hypothenar eminence

Proximal palmar crease

Proximal digital crease

Middle digital crease

Distal digital crease

Radial longitudinal crease

Triceps brachii muscle

Long head

Lateral head

Tendon

Brachioradialis and extensor carpi radialis longus muscles

Extensor carpi radialis brevis muscle

Olecranon of ulna

Flexor carpi ulnaris muscle

Extensor carpi ulnaris muscle

Cephalic vein

Common name of digits

1 Thumb
2 Index
3 Middle
4 Ring
5 Little

Extensor pollicis longus tendon

Extensor indicis tendon

Extensor digitorum tendons

Site of proximal interphalangeal (PIP) joint

Site of distal interphalangeal (DIP) joint

C. Machado _M.D._

Topographic Anatomy

Plate 418

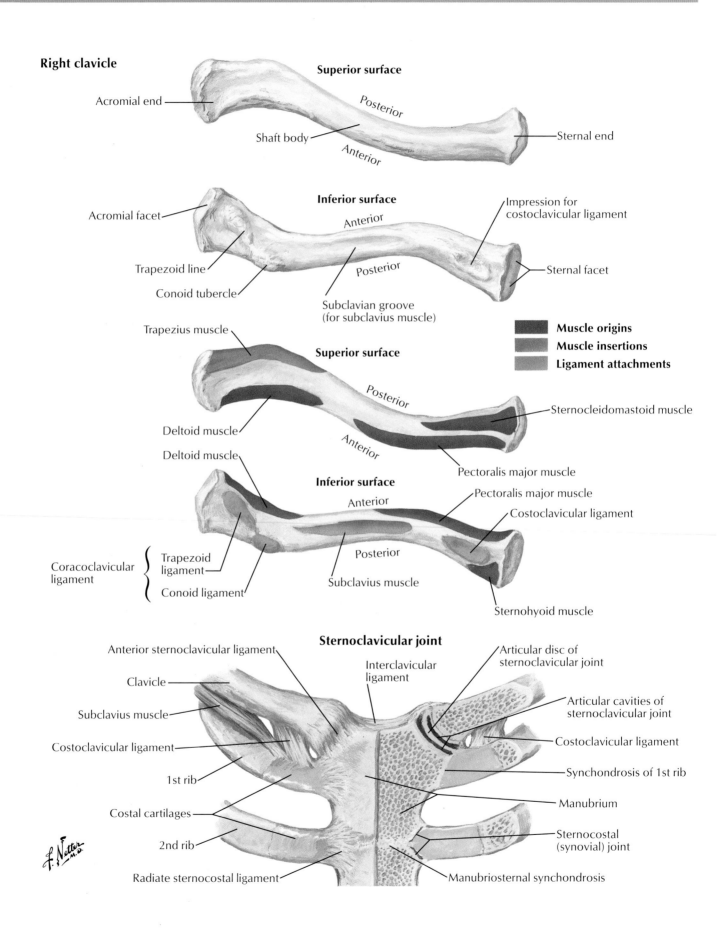

Right clavicle

Superior surface

Acromial end

Posterior

Shaft body

Anterior

Sternal end

Inferior surface

Acromial facet

Anterior

Impression for costoclavicular ligament

Trapezoid line

Posterior

Conoid tubercle

Subclavian groove (for subclavius muscle)

Sternal facet

Trapezius muscle

Superior surface

Muscle origins
Muscle insertions
Ligament attachments

Posterior

Deltoid muscle

Anterior

Sternocleidomastoid muscle

Deltoid muscle

Pectoralis major muscle

Inferior surface

Pectoralis major muscle

Anterior

Costoclavicular ligament

Coracoclavicular ligament

Trapezoid ligament

Posterior

Conoid ligament

Subclavius muscle

Sternohyoid muscle

Sternoclavicular joint

Anterior sternoclavicular ligament

Interclavicular ligament

Articular disc of sternoclavicular joint

Clavicle

Articular cavities of sternoclavicular joint

Subclavius muscle

Costoclavicular ligament

Costoclavicular ligament

Synchondrosis of 1st rib

1st rib

Manubrium

Costal cartilages

Sternocostal (synovial) joint

2nd rib

Radiate sternocostal ligament

Manubriosternal synchondrosis

Plate 419

Shoulder and Axilla

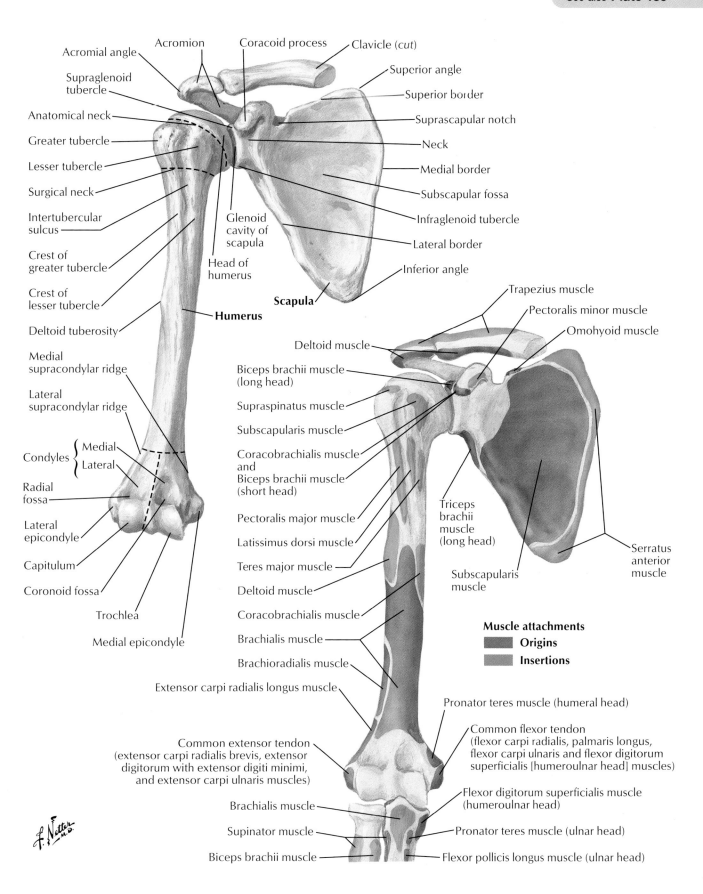

Acromial angle

Supraglenoid
tubercle

Acromion

Coracoid process

Clavicle (cut)

Superior angle

Superior border

Anatomical neck

Suprascapular notch

Greater tubercle

Neck

Lesser tubercle

Medial border

Surgical neck

Subscapular fossa

Intertubercular
sulcus

Glenoid
cavity of
scapula

Infraglenoid tubercle

Crest of
greater tubercle

Lateral border

Head of
humerus

Inferior angle

Crest of
lesser tubercle

Scapula

Deltoid tuberosity

Humerus

Trapezius muscle

Pectoralis minor muscle

Omohyoid muscle

Deltoid muscle

Medial
supracondylar ridge

Biceps brachii muscle
(long head)

Lateral
supracondylar ridge

Supraspinatus muscle

Subscapularis muscle

Condyles { Medial
Lateral

Coracobrachialis muscle
and
Biceps brachii muscle
(short head)

Radial
fossa

Triceps
brachii
muscle
(long head)

Lateral
epicondyle

Pectoralis major muscle

Capitulum

Latissimus dorsi muscle

Serratus
anterior
muscle

Coronoid fossa

Teres major muscle

Subscapularis
muscle

Trochlea

Deltoid muscle

Medial epicondyle

Coracobrachialis muscle

Muscle attachments

Brachialis muscle

Origins

Brachioradialis muscle

Insertions

Extensor carpi radialis longus muscle

Pronator teres muscle (humeral head)

Common flexor tendon
(flexor carpi radialis, palmaris longus,
flexor carpi ulnaris and flexor digitorum
superficialis [humeroulnar head] muscles)

Common extensor tendon
(extensor carpi radialis brevis, extensor
digitorum with extensor digiti minimi,
and extensor carpi ulnaris muscles)

Flexor digitorum superficialis muscle
(humeroulnar head)

Brachialis muscle

Supinator muscle

Pronator teres muscle (ulnar head)

Biceps brachii muscle

Flexor pollicis longus muscle (ulnar head)

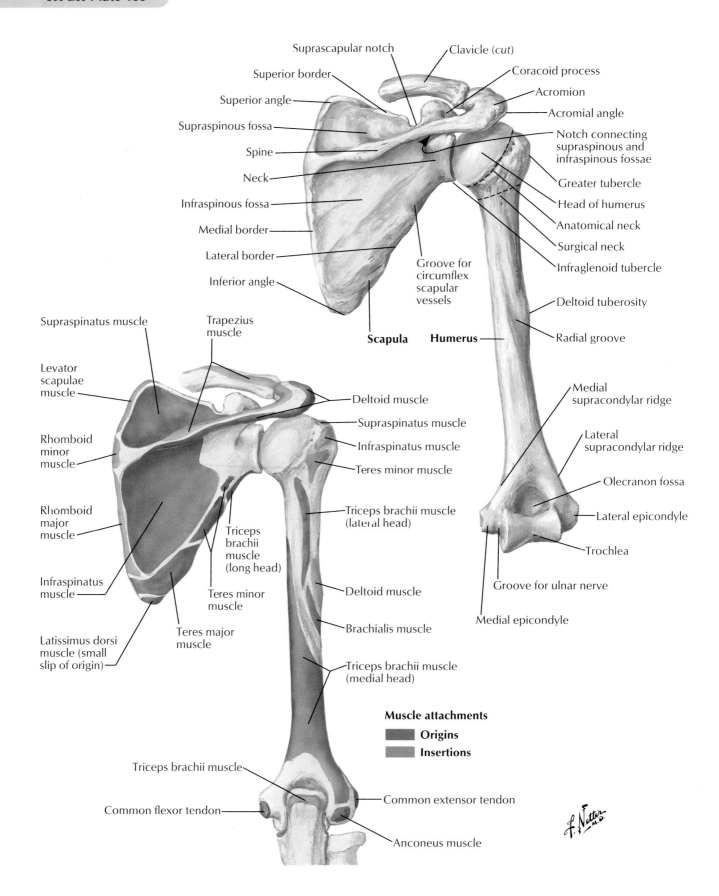

Suprascapular notch

Clavicle (cut)

Superior border

Coracoid process

Superior angle

Acromion

Supraspinous fossa

Acromial angle

Spine

Notch connecting supraspinous and infraspinous fossae

Neck

Greater tubercle

Infraspinous fossa

Head of humerus

Medial border

Anatomical neck

Lateral border

Surgical neck

Inferior angle

Infraglenoid tubercle

Groove for circumflex scapular vessels

Deltoid tuberosity

Scapula   **Humerus**

Radial groove

Supraspinatus muscle

Trapezius muscle

Levator scapulae muscle

Deltoid muscle

Medial supracondylar ridge

Rhomboid minor muscle

Supraspinatus muscle

Lateral supracondylar ridge

Infraspinatus muscle

Teres minor muscle

Olecranon fossa

Rhomboid major muscle

Triceps brachii muscle (lateral head)

Lateral epicondyle

Triceps brachii muscle (long head)

Deltoid muscle

Trochlea

Infraspinatus muscle

Teres minor muscle

Brachialis muscle

Groove for ulnar nerve

Latissimus dorsi muscle (small slip of origin)

Teres major muscle

Triceps brachii muscle (medial head)

Medial epicondyle

Muscle attachments
- **Origins**
- **Insertions**

Triceps brachii muscle

Common extensor tendon

Common flexor tendon

Anconeus muscle

Plate 421   **Shoulder and Axilla**

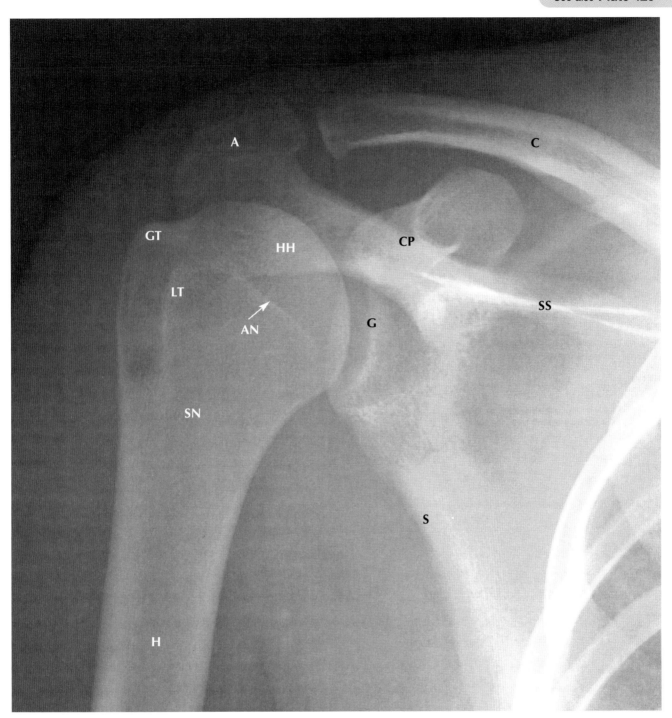

A	Acromion
AN	Anatomical neck of humerus
C	Clavicle
CP	Coracoid process
G	Glenoid cavity of scapula
GT	Greater tubercle
H	Humerus
HH	Head of humerus
LT	Lesser tubercle
S	Scapula (lateral border)
SN	Surgical neck of humerus
SS	Spine of scapula

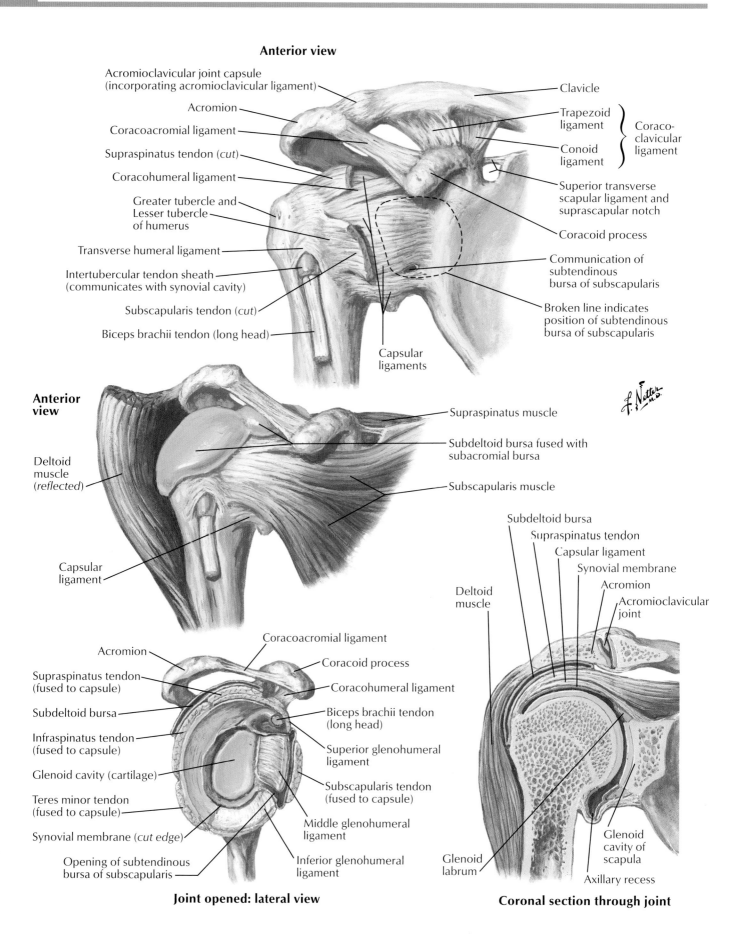

Anterior view

Acromioclavicular joint capsule
(incorporating acromioclavicular ligament)

Acromion

Coracoacromial ligament

Supraspinatus tendon (cut)

Coracohumeral ligament

Greater tubercle and
Lesser tubercle
of humerus

Transverse humeral ligament

Intertubercular tendon sheath
(communicates with synovial cavity)

Subscapularis tendon (cut)

Biceps brachii tendon (long head)

Clavicle

Trapezoid
ligament

Conoid
ligament

} Coraco-
clavicular
ligament

Superior transverse
scapular ligament and
suprascapular notch

Coracoid process

Communication of
subtendinous
bursa of subscapularis

Broken line indicates
position of subtendinous
bursa of subscapularis

Capsular
ligaments

**Anterior
view**

Deltoid
muscle
(reflected)

Capsular
ligament

Supraspinatus muscle

Subdeltoid bursa fused with
subacromial bursa

Subscapularis muscle

Subdeltoid bursa

Supraspinatus tendon

Capsular ligament

Synovial membrane

Acromion

Acromioclavicular
joint

Deltoid
muscle

Acromion

Supraspinatus tendon
(fused to capsule)

Subdeltoid bursa

Infraspinatus tendon
(fused to capsule)

Glenoid cavity (cartilage)

Teres minor tendon
(fused to capsule)

Synovial membrane (cut edge)

Opening of subtendinous
bursa of subscapularis

Coracoacromial ligament

Coracoid process

Coracohumeral ligament

Biceps brachii tendon
(long head)

Superior glenohumeral
ligament

Subscapularis tendon
(fused to capsule)

Middle glenohumeral
ligament

Inferior glenohumeral
ligament

Glenoid
labrum

Glenoid
cavity
of
scapula

Axillary recess

Joint opened: lateral view

Coronal section through joint

Plate 423

Shoulder and Axilla

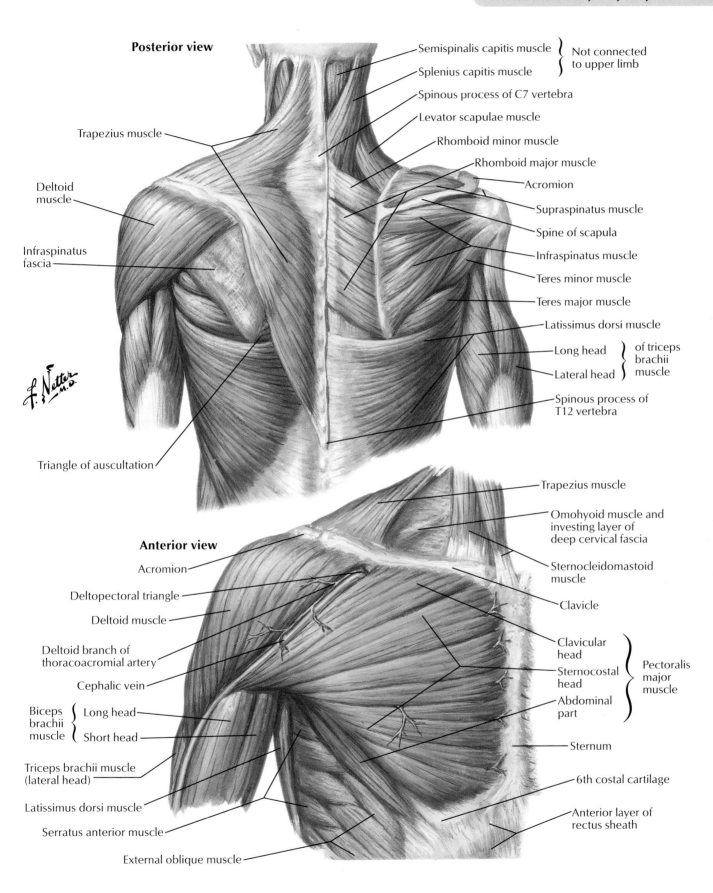

Posterior view

Semispinalis capitis muscle ⎫
Splenius capitis muscle ⎬ Not connected to upper limb

Spinous process of C7 vertebra

Levator scapulae muscle

Rhomboid minor muscle

Rhomboid major muscle

Acromion

Trapezius muscle

Deltoid muscle

Infraspinatus fascia

Supraspinatus muscle

Spine of scapula

Infraspinatus muscle

Teres minor muscle

Teres major muscle

Latissimus dorsi muscle

Long head ⎫ of triceps brachii muscle
Lateral head ⎬

Spinous process of T12 vertebra

Triangle of auscultation

Anterior view

Trapezius muscle

Omohyoid muscle and investing layer of deep cervical fascia

Sternocleidomastoid muscle

Acromion

Deltopectoral triangle

Deltoid muscle

Clavicle

Deltoid branch of thoracoacromial artery

Cephalic vein

Clavicular head ⎫
Sternocostal head ⎬ Pectoralis major muscle
Abdominal part ⎭

Biceps brachii muscle ⎰ Long head
⎱ Short head

Triceps brachii muscle (lateral head)

Sternum

Latissimus dorsi muscle

6th costal cartilage

Serratus anterior muscle

Anterior layer of rectus sheath

External oblique muscle

Shoulder and Axilla

Plate 424

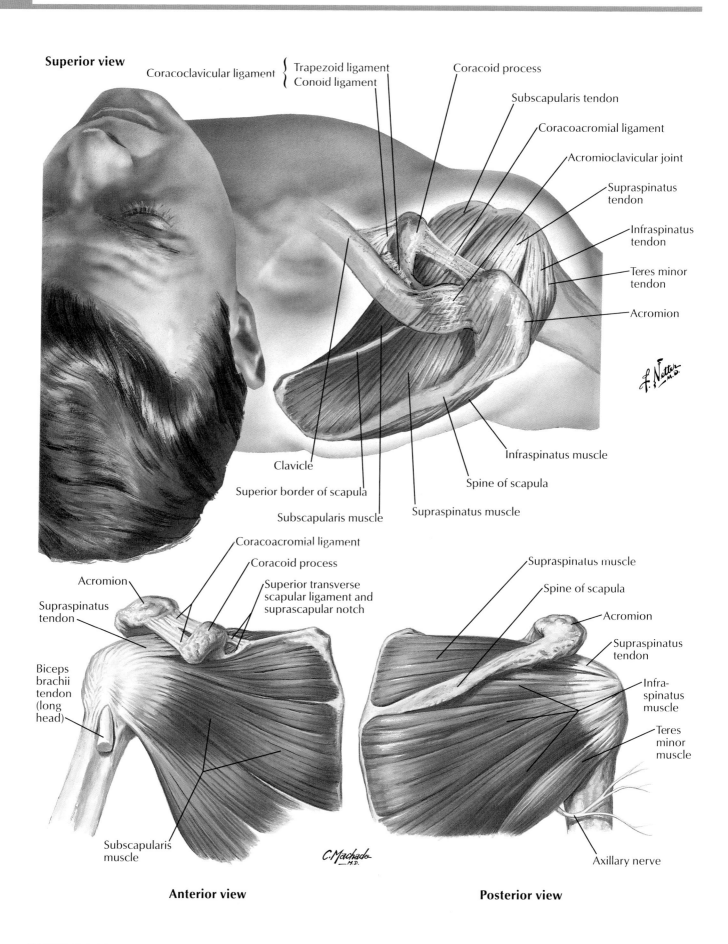

Superior view

Coracoclavicular ligament { Trapezoid ligament
Conoid ligament

Coracoid process

Subscapularis tendon

Coracoacromial ligament

Acromioclavicular joint

Supraspinatus tendon

Infraspinatus tendon

Teres minor tendon

Acromion

Clavicle

Superior border of scapula

Subscapularis muscle

Supraspinatus muscle

Spine of scapula

Infraspinatus muscle

Coracoacromial ligament

Coracoid process

Acromion

Superior transverse scapular ligament and suprascapular notch

Supraspinatus tendon

Biceps brachii tendon (long head)

Subscapularis muscle

Anterior view

Supraspinatus muscle

Spine of scapula

Acromion

Supraspinatus tendon

Infraspinatus muscle

Teres minor muscle

Axillary nerve

Posterior view

Plate 425   **Shoulder and Axilla**

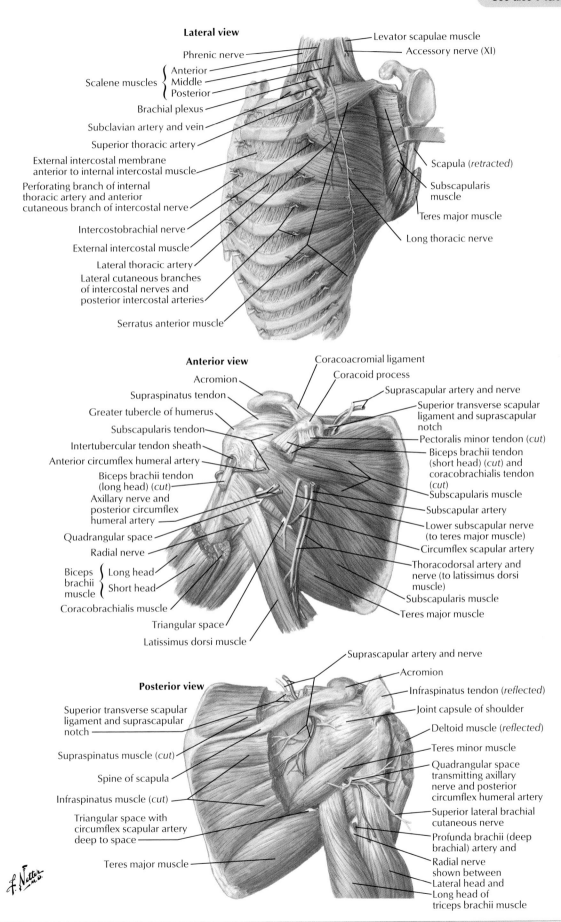

Lateral view

Levator scapulae muscle

Accessory nerve (XI)

Phrenic nerve

Anterior
Middle — Scalene muscles
Posterior

Brachial plexus

Subclavian artery and vein

Superior thoracic artery

External intercostal membrane anterior to internal intercostal muscle

Perforating branch of internal thoracic artery and anterior cutaneous branch of intercostal nerve

Intercostobrachial nerve

External intercostal muscle

Lateral thoracic artery

Lateral cutaneous branches of intercostal nerves and posterior intercostal arteries

Serratus anterior muscle

Scapula (*retracted*)

Subscapularis muscle

Teres major muscle

Long thoracic nerve

Anterior view

Coracoacromial ligament

Coracoid process

Acromion

Suprascapular artery and nerve

Supraspinatus tendon

Greater tubercle of humerus

Subscapularis tendon

Intertubercular tendon sheath

Anterior circumflex humeral artery

Biceps brachii tendon (long head) (*cut*)

Axillary nerve and posterior circumflex humeral artery

Quadrangular space

Radial nerve

Biceps brachii muscle { Long head
Short head

Coracobrachialis muscle

Triangular space

Latissimus dorsi muscle

Superior transverse scapular ligament and suprascapular notch

Pectoralis minor tendon (*cut*)

Biceps brachii tendon (short head) (*cut*) and coracobrachialis tendon (*cut*)

Subscapularis muscle

Subscapular artery

Lower subscapular nerve (to teres major muscle)

Circumflex scapular artery

Thoracodorsal artery and nerve (to latissimus dorsi muscle)

Subscapularis muscle

Teres major muscle

Posterior view

Suprascapular artery and nerve

Acromion

Infraspinatus tendon (*reflected*)

Joint capsule of shoulder

Deltoid muscle (*reflected*)

Teres minor muscle

Quadrangular space transmitting axillary nerve and posterior circumflex humeral artery

Superior lateral brachial cutaneous nerve

Profunda brachii (deep brachial) artery and

Radial nerve shown between

Lateral head and

Long head of triceps brachii muscle

Superior transverse scapular ligament and suprascapular notch

Supraspinatus muscle (*cut*)

Spine of scapula

Infraspinatus muscle (*cut*)

Triangular space with circumflex scapular artery deep to space

Teres major muscle

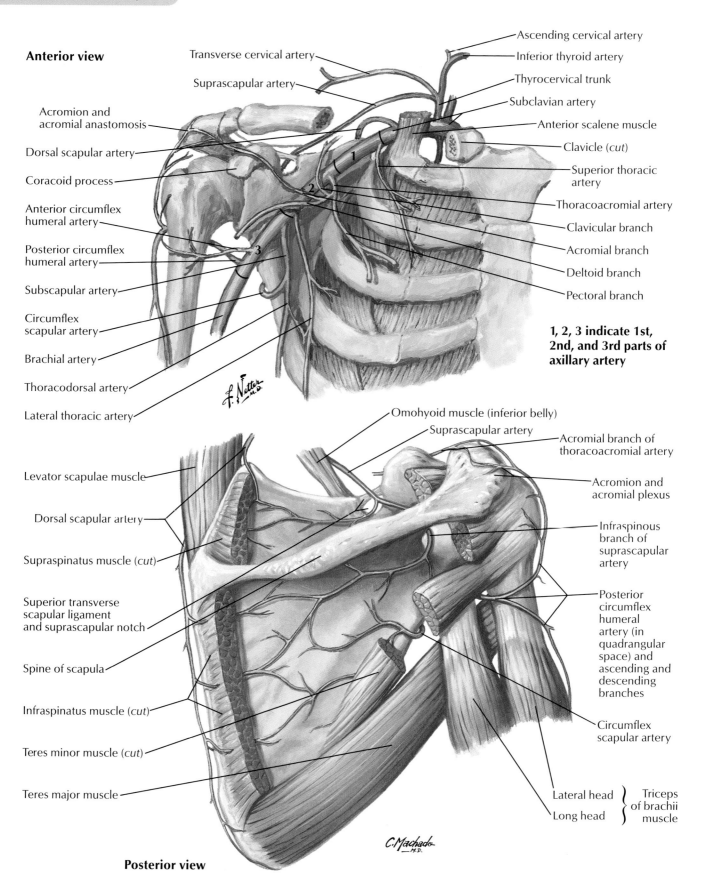

Anterior view

Transverse cervical artery

Suprascapular artery

Ascending cervical artery

Inferior thyroid artery

Thyrocervical trunk

Subclavian artery

Anterior scalene muscle

Clavicle (cut)

Superior thoracic artery

Thoracoacromial artery

Clavicular branch

Acromial branch

Deltoid branch

Pectoral branch

Acromion and acromial anastomosis

Dorsal scapular artery

Coracoid process

Anterior circumflex humeral artery

Posterior circumflex humeral artery

Subscapular artery

Circumflex scapular artery

Brachial artery

Thoracodorsal artery

Lateral thoracic artery

1, 2, 3 indicate 1st, 2nd, and 3rd parts of axillary artery

Omohyoid muscle (inferior belly)

Suprascapular artery

Acromial branch of thoracoacromial artery

Acromion and acromial plexus

Infraspinous branch of suprascapular artery

Posterior circumflex humeral artery (in quadrangular space) and ascending and descending branches

Circumflex scapular artery

Levator scapulae muscle

Dorsal scapular artery

Supraspinatus muscle (cut)

Superior transverse scapular ligament and suprascapular notch

Spine of scapula

Infraspinatus muscle (cut)

Teres minor muscle (cut)

Teres major muscle

Lateral head ⎫ Triceps
Long head ⎬ of brachii
⎭ muscle

Posterior view

Plate 427   **Shoulder and Axilla**

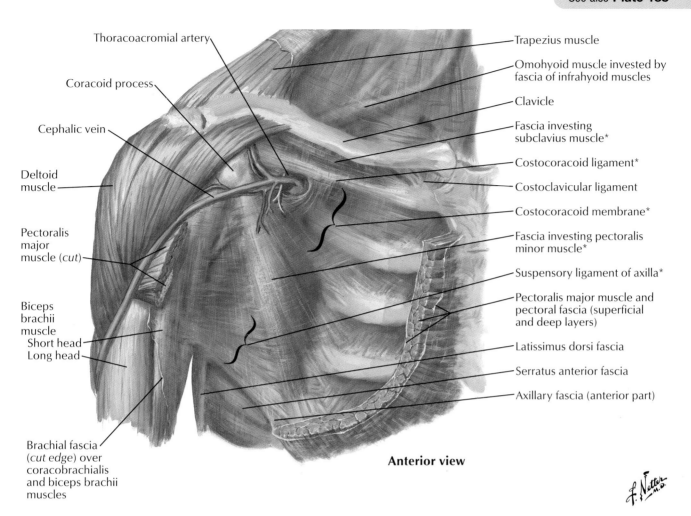

Thoracoacromial artery

Coracoid process

Cephalic vein

Deltoid muscle

Pectoralis major muscle (*cut*)

Biceps brachii muscle
Short head
Long head

Brachial fascia (*cut edge*) over coracobrachialis and biceps brachii muscles

Trapezius muscle

Omohyoid muscle invested by fascia of infrahyoid muscles

Clavicle

Fascia investing subclavius muscle*

Costocoracoid ligament*

Costoclavicular ligament

Costocoracoid membrane*

Fascia investing pectoralis minor muscle*

Suspensory ligament of axilla*

Pectoralis major muscle and pectoral fascia (superficial and deep layers)

Latissimus dorsi fascia

Serratus anterior fascia

Axillary fascia (anterior part)

Anterior view

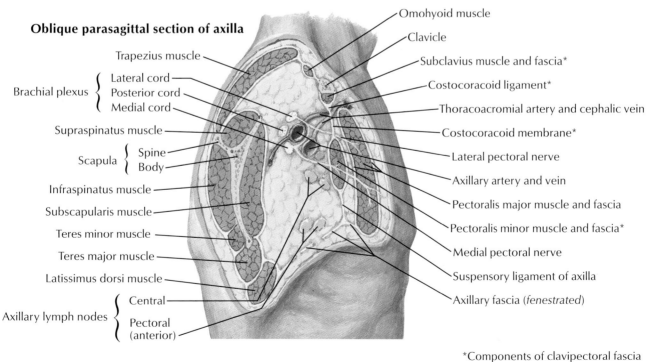

Oblique parasagittal section of axilla

Trapezius muscle

Brachial plexus {
Lateral cord
Posterior cord
Medial cord

Supraspinatus muscle

Scapula {
Spine
Body

Infraspinatus muscle

Subscapularis muscle

Teres minor muscle

Teres major muscle

Latissimus dorsi muscle

Axillary lymph nodes {
Central
Pectoral (anterior)

Omohyoid muscle

Clavicle

Subclavius muscle and fascia*

Costocoracoid ligament*

Thoracoacromial artery and cephalic vein

Costocoracoid membrane*

Lateral pectoral nerve

Axillary artery and vein

Pectoralis major muscle and fascia

Pectoralis minor muscle and fascia*

Medial pectoral nerve

Suspensory ligament of axilla

Axillary fascia (*fenestrated*)

*Components of clavipectoral fascia

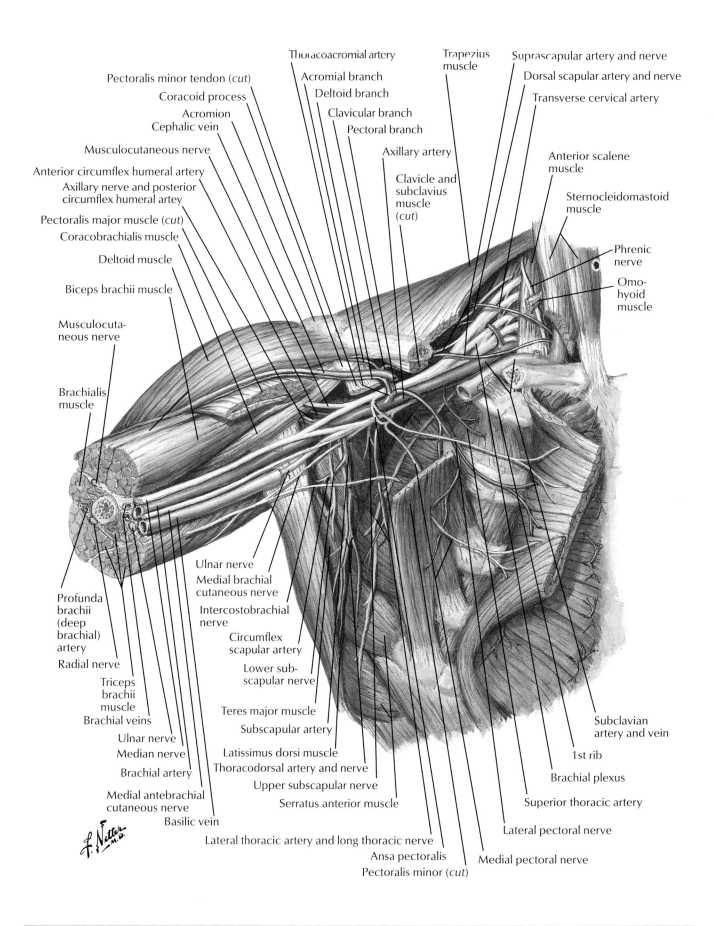

Thoracoacromial artery

Acromial branch

Deltoid branch

Clavicular branch

Pectoral branch

Axillary artery

Trapezius muscle

Suprascapular artery and nerve

Dorsal scapular artery and nerve

Transverse cervical artery

Pectoralis minor tendon (cut)

Coracoid process

Acromion

Cephalic vein

Musculocutaneous nerve

Anterior circumflex humeral artery

Axillary nerve and posterior circumflex humeral artery

Pectoralis major muscle (cut)

Coracobrachialis muscle

Deltoid muscle

Biceps brachii muscle

Musculocuta-neous nerve

Brachialis muscle

Clavicle and subclavius muscle (cut)

Anterior scalene muscle

Sternocleidomastoid muscle

Phrenic nerve

Omo-hyoid muscle

Profunda brachii (deep brachial) artery

Radial nerve

Triceps brachii muscle

Brachial veins

Ulnar nerve

Median nerve

Brachial artery

Medial antebrachial cutaneous nerve

Basilic vein

Ulnar nerve

Medial brachial cutaneous nerve

Intercostobrachial nerve

Circumflex scapular artery

Lower sub-scapular nerve

Teres major muscle

Subscapular artery

Latissimus dorsi muscle

Thoracodorsal artery and nerve

Upper subscapular nerve

Serratus anterior muscle

Lateral thoracic artery and long thoracic nerve

Ansa pectoralis

Pectoralis minor (cut)

Subclavian artery and vein

1st rib

Brachial plexus

Superior thoracic artery

Lateral pectoral nerve

Medial pectoral nerve

f. Netter M.D.

Plate 429 **Shoulder and Axilla**

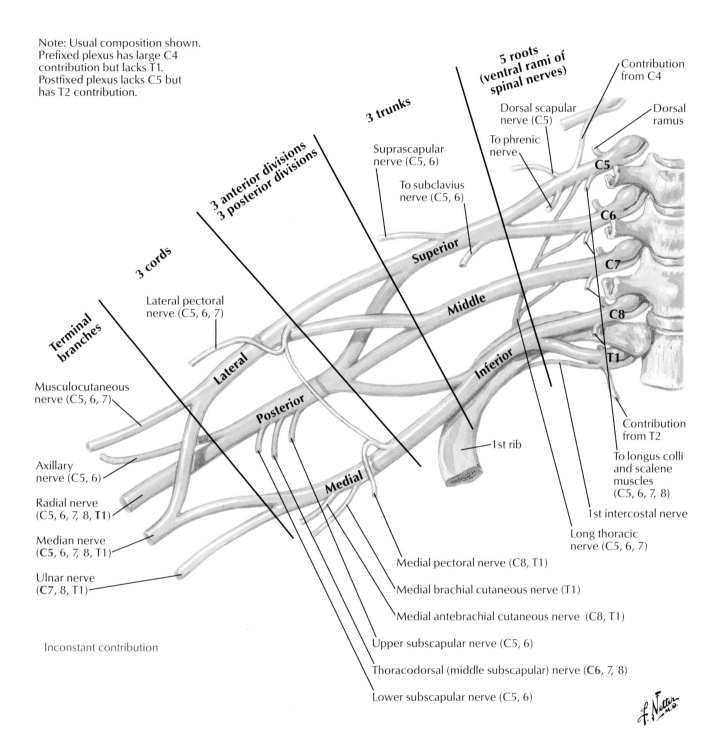

Note: Usual composition shown.
Prefixed plexus has large C4
contribution but lacks T1.
Postfixed plexus lacks C5 but
has T2 contribution.

5 roots
(ventral rami of
spinal nerves)

Contribution
from C4

Dorsal scapular
nerve (C5)

3 trunks

Dorsal
ramus

Suprascapular
nerve (C5, 6)

To phrenic
nerve

3 anterior divisions
3 posterior divisions

To subclavius
nerve (C5, 6)

C5

C6

Superior

C7

3 cords

Lateral pectoral
nerve (C5, 6, 7)

Middle

C8

Lateral

T1

Terminal
branches

Posterior

Inferior

Musculocutaneous
nerve (C5, 6, 7)

Contribution
from T2

Axillary
nerve (C5, 6)

1st rib

To longus colli
and scalene
muscles
(C5, 6, 7, 8)

Radial nerve
(C5, 6, 7, 8, **T1**)

Medial

1st intercostal nerve

Median nerve
(**C5**, 6, 7, 8, T1)

Long thoracic
nerve (C5, 6, 7)

Ulnar nerve
(**C7**, 8, T1)

Medial pectoral nerve (C8, T1)

Medial brachial cutaneous nerve (T1)

Medial antebrachial cutaneous nerve (C8, T1)

Inconstant contribution

Upper subscapular nerve (C5, 6)

Thoracodorsal (middle subscapular) nerve (**C6**, 7, 8)

Lower subscapular nerve (C5, 6)

f. Netter

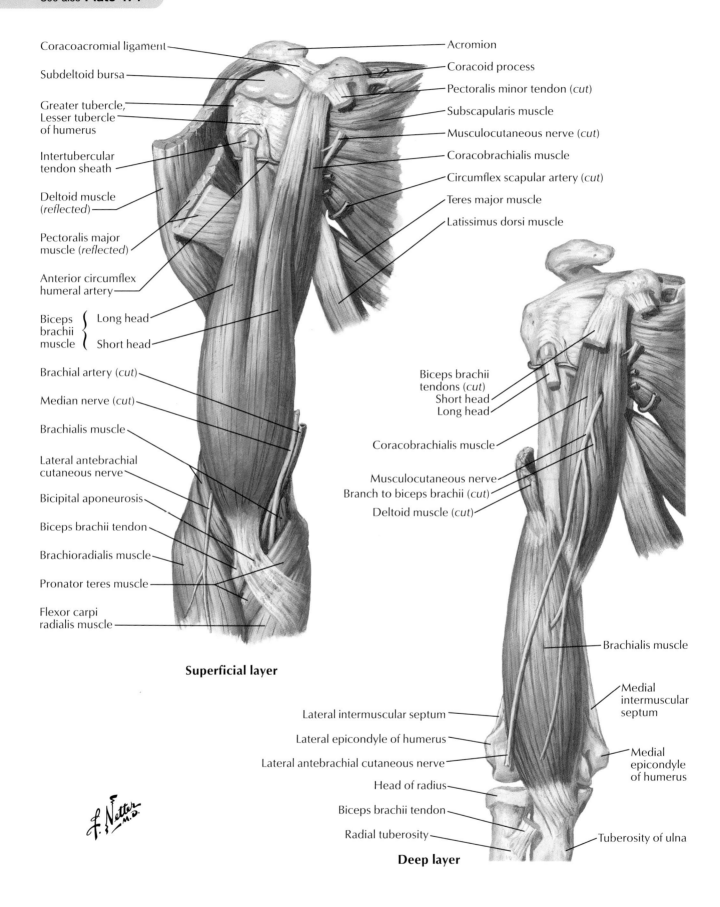

Coracoacromial ligament

Subdeltoid bursa

Greater tubercle, Lesser tubercle of humerus

Intertubercular tendon sheath

Deltoid muscle (reflected)

Pectoralis major muscle (reflected)

Anterior circumflex humeral artery

Biceps brachii muscle { Long head / Short head }

Brachial artery (cut)

Median nerve (cut)

Brachialis muscle

Lateral antebrachial cutaneous nerve

Bicipital aponeurosis

Biceps brachii tendon

Brachioradialis muscle

Pronator teres muscle

Flexor carpi radialis muscle

Acromion

Coracoid process

Pectoralis minor tendon (cut)

Subscapularis muscle

Musculocutaneous nerve (cut)

Coracobrachialis muscle

Circumflex scapular artery (cut)

Teres major muscle

Latissimus dorsi muscle

Superficial layer

Biceps brachii tendons (cut)
Short head
Long head

Coracobrachialis muscle

Musculocutaneous nerve
Branch to biceps brachii (cut)
Deltoid muscle (cut)

Brachialis muscle

Medial intermuscular septum

Lateral intermuscular septum

Lateral epicondyle of humerus

Lateral antebrachial cutaneous nerve

Medial epicondyle of humerus

Head of radius

Biceps brachii tendon

Radial tuberosity

Tuberosity of ulna

Deep layer

Plate 431

Arm

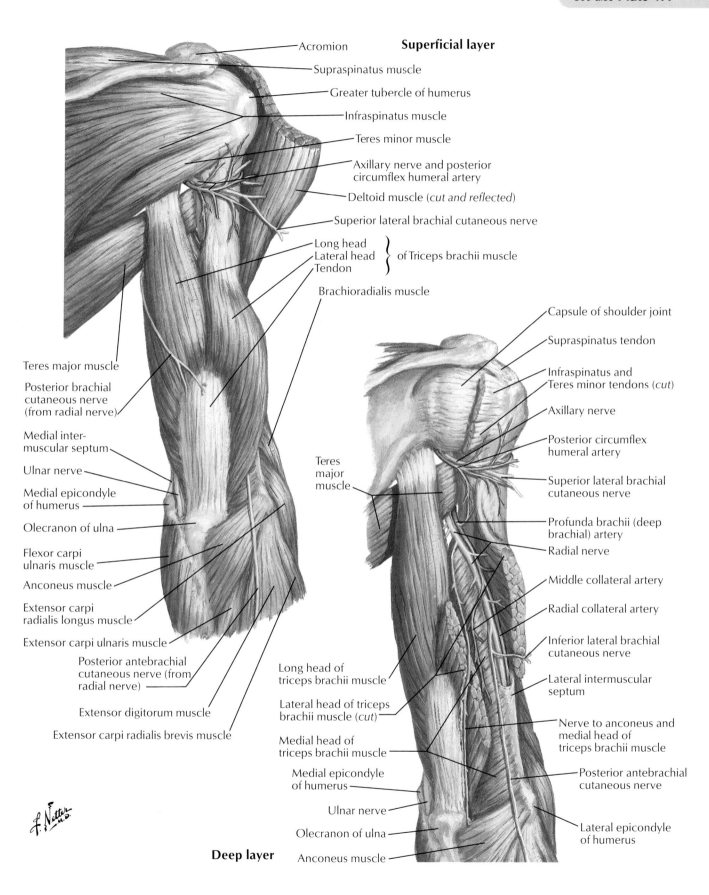

Superficial layer

Acromion

Supraspinatus muscle

Greater tubercle of humerus

Infraspinatus muscle

Teres minor muscle

Axillary nerve and posterior circumflex humeral artery

Deltoid muscle (*cut and reflected*)

Superior lateral brachial cutaneous nerve

Long head
Lateral head } of Triceps brachii muscle
Tendon

Brachioradialis muscle

Capsule of shoulder joint

Supraspinatus tendon

Infraspinatus and Teres minor tendons (*cut*)

Axillary nerve

Posterior circumflex humeral artery

Superior lateral brachial cutaneous nerve

Profunda brachii (deep brachial) artery

Radial nerve

Middle collateral artery

Radial collateral artery

Inferior lateral brachial cutaneous nerve

Lateral intermuscular septum

Nerve to anconeus and medial head of triceps brachii muscle

Posterior antebrachial cutaneous nerve

Lateral epicondyle of humerus

Teres major muscle

Posterior brachial cutaneous nerve (from radial nerve)

Medial intermuscular septum

Ulnar nerve

Medial epicondyle of humerus

Olecranon of ulna

Flexor carpi ulnaris muscle

Anconeus muscle

Extensor carpi radialis longus muscle

Extensor carpi ulnaris muscle

Posterior antebrachial cutaneous nerve (from radial nerve)

Extensor digitorum muscle

Extensor carpi radialis brevis muscle

Teres major muscle

Long head of triceps brachii muscle

Lateral head of triceps brachii muscle (*cut*)

Medial head of triceps brachii muscle

Medial epicondyle of humerus

Ulnar nerve

Olecranon of ulna

Deep layer Anconeus muscle

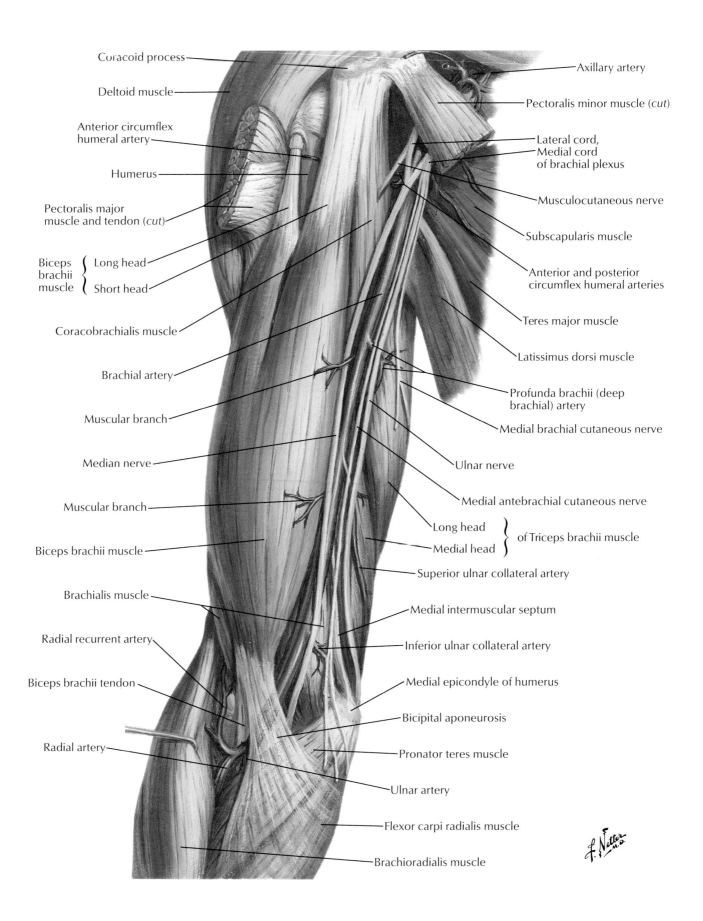

Coracoid process

Deltoid muscle

Anterior circumflex humeral artery

Humerus

Pectoralis major muscle and tendon (cut)

Biceps brachii muscle { Long head / Short head

Coracobrachialis muscle

Brachial artery

Muscular branch

Median nerve

Muscular branch

Biceps brachii muscle

Brachialis muscle

Radial recurrent artery

Biceps brachii tendon

Radial artery

Axillary artery

Pectoralis minor muscle (cut)

Lateral cord, Medial cord of brachial plexus

Musculocutaneous nerve

Subscapularis muscle

Anterior and posterior circumflex humeral arteries

Teres major muscle

Latissimus dorsi muscle

Profunda brachii (deep brachial) artery

Medial brachial cutaneous nerve

Ulnar nerve

Medial antebrachial cutaneous nerve

Long head / Medial head } of Triceps brachii muscle

Superior ulnar collateral artery

Medial intermuscular septum

Inferior ulnar collateral artery

Medial epicondyle of humerus

Bicipital aponeurosis

Pronator teres muscle

Ulnar artery

Flexor carpi radialis muscle

Brachioradialis muscle

Plate 433   **Arm**

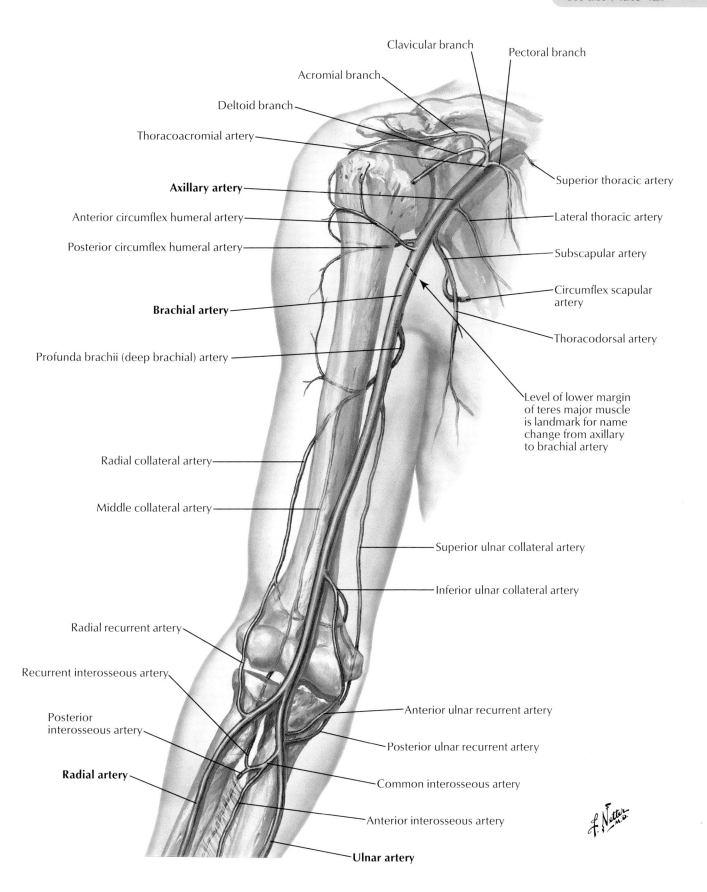

Clavicular branch

Pectoral branch

Acromial branch

Deltoid branch

Thoracoacromial artery

Axillary artery

Anterior circumflex humeral artery

Posterior circumflex humeral artery

Brachial artery

Profunda brachii (deep brachial) artery

Radial collateral artery

Middle collateral artery

Radial recurrent artery

Recurrent interosseous artery

Posterior interosseous artery

Radial artery

Superior thoracic artery

Lateral thoracic artery

Subscapular artery

Circumflex scapular artery

Thoracodorsal artery

Level of lower margin of teres major muscle is landmark for name change from axillary to brachial artery

Superior ulnar collateral artery

Inferior ulnar collateral artery

Anterior ulnar recurrent artery

Posterior ulnar recurrent artery

Common interosseous artery

Anterior interosseous artery

Ulnar artery

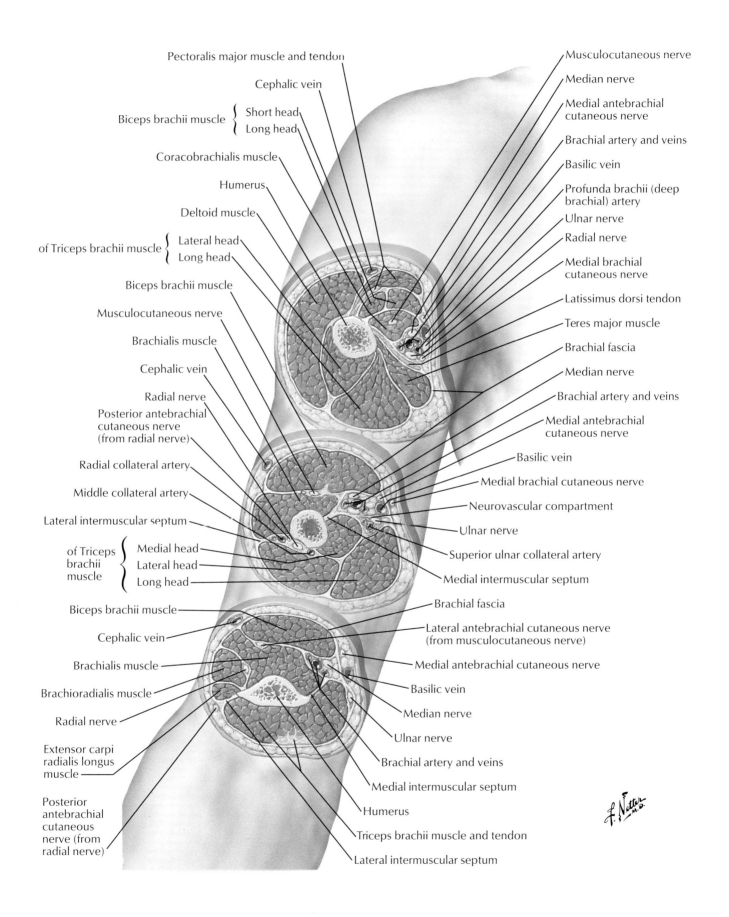

Pectoralis major muscle and tendon

Cephalic vein

Biceps brachii muscle { Short head / Long head

Coracobrachialis muscle

Humerus

Deltoid muscle

of Triceps brachii muscle { Lateral head / Long head

Biceps brachii muscle

Musculocutaneous nerve

Brachialis muscle

Cephalic vein

Radial nerve

Posterior antebrachial cutaneous nerve (from radial nerve)

Radial collateral artery

Middle collateral artery

Lateral intermuscular septum

of Triceps brachii muscle { Medial head / Lateral head / Long head

Biceps brachii muscle

Cephalic vein

Brachialis muscle

Brachioradialis muscle

Radial nerve

Extensor carpi radialis longus muscle

Posterior antebrachial cutaneous nerve (from radial nerve)

Musculocutaneous nerve

Median nerve

Medial antebrachial cutaneous nerve

Brachial artery and veins

Basilic vein

Profunda brachii (deep brachial) artery

Ulnar nerve

Radial nerve

Medial brachial cutaneous nerve

Latissimus dorsi tendon

Teres major muscle

Brachial fascia

Median nerve

Brachial artery and veins

Medial antebrachial cutaneous nerve

Basilic vein

Medial brachial cutaneous nerve

Neurovascular compartment

Ulnar nerve

Superior ulnar collateral artery

Medial intermuscular septum

Brachial fascia

Lateral antebrachial cutaneous nerve (from musculocutaneous nerve)

Medial antebrachial cutaneous nerve

Basilic vein

Median nerve

Ulnar nerve

Brachial artery and veins

Medial intermuscular septum

Humerus

Triceps brachii muscle and tendon

Lateral intermuscular septum

Plate 435

Arm

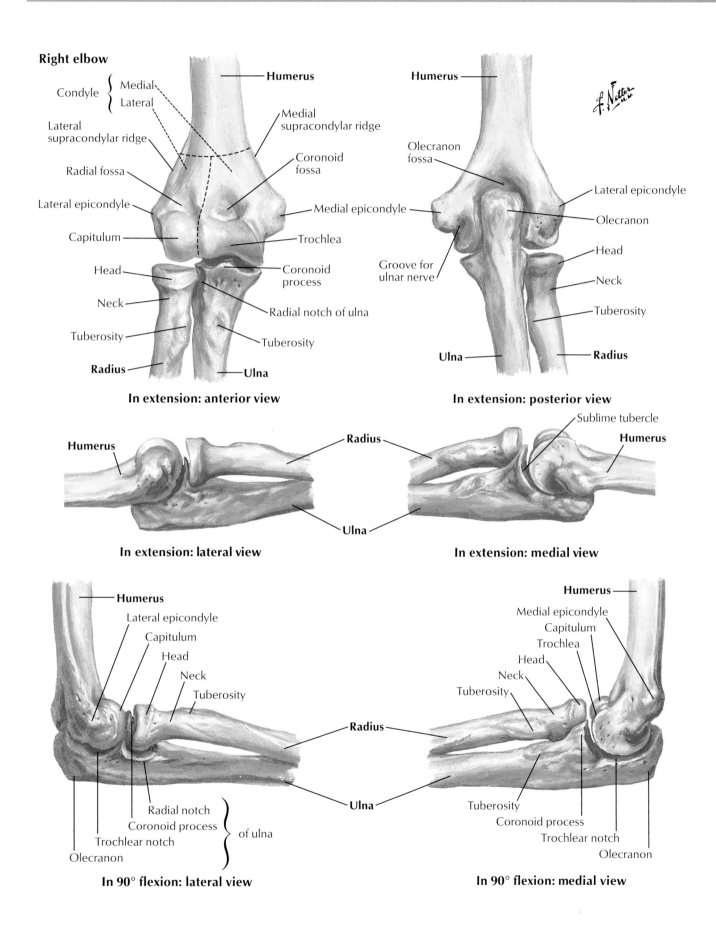

Right elbow

Condyle { Medial
         { Lateral

Lateral supracondylar ridge

Radial fossa

Lateral epicondyle

Capitulum

Head

Neck

Tuberosity

Radius

Humerus

Medial supracondylar ridge

Coronoid fossa

Medial epicondyle

Trochlea

Coronoid process

Radial notch of ulna

Tuberosity

Ulna

In extension: anterior view

Humerus

Olecranon fossa

Groove for ulnar nerve

Lateral epicondyle

Olecranon

Head

Neck

Tuberosity

Ulna   **Radius**

In extension: posterior view

Humerus

Radius

Ulna

In extension: lateral view

Sublime tubercle

Humerus

Radius

Ulna

In extension: medial view

Humerus

Lateral epicondyle

Capitulum

Head

Neck

Tuberosity

Radius

Radial notch
Coronoid process } of ulna
Trochlear notch

Olecranon

Ulna

In 90° flexion: lateral view

Humerus

Medial epicondyle

Capitulum

Trochlea

Head

Neck

Tuberosity

Radius

Tuberosity

Coronoid process

Trochlear notch

Olecranon

Ulna

In 90° flexion: medial view

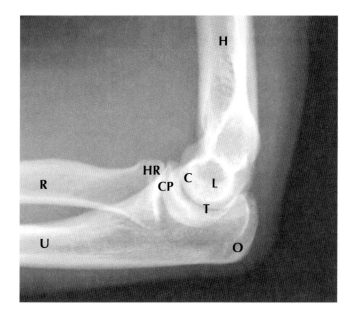

Lateral radiograph

C	Capitulum
CP	Coronoid process of ulna
H	Humerus
HR	Head of radius
L	Lateral epicondyle
O	Olecranon
R	Radius
T	Trochlear notch
U	Ulna

Anteroposterior radiograph

C	Capitulum
CP	Coronoid process of ulna
H	Humerus
HR	Head of radius
L	Lateral epicondyle
M	Medial of epicondyle
NR	Neck of radius
O	Olecranon
OF	Olecranon fossa
R	Radius
T	Trochlea of humerus
RT	Radial tuberosity
U	Ulna

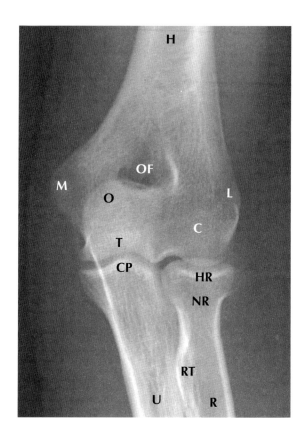

Plate 437   **Elbow and Forearm**

Right elbow

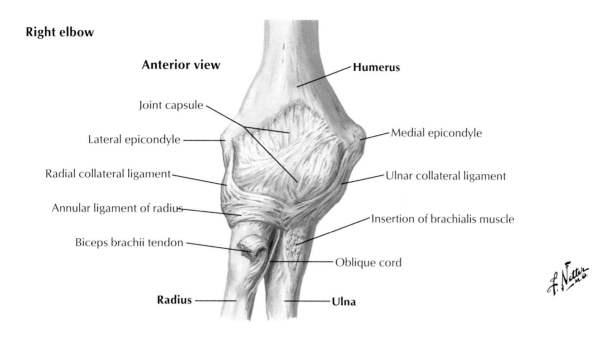

Anterior view

Joint capsule

Lateral epicondyle

Radial collateral ligament

Annular ligament of radius

Biceps brachii tendon

Humerus

Medial epicondyle

Ulnar collateral ligament

Insertion of brachialis muscle

Oblique cord

Radius

Ulna

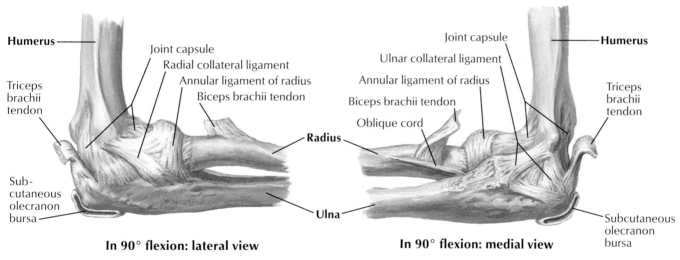

Humerus

Triceps brachii tendon

Sub-cutaneous olecranon bursa

Joint capsule
Radial collateral ligament
Annular ligament of radius
Biceps brachii tendon

In 90° flexion: lateral view

Joint capsule
Ulnar collateral ligament
Annular ligament of radius
Biceps brachii tendon
Oblique cord

Radius

Ulna

Humerus

Triceps brachii tendon

Subcutaneous olecranon bursa

In 90° flexion: medial view

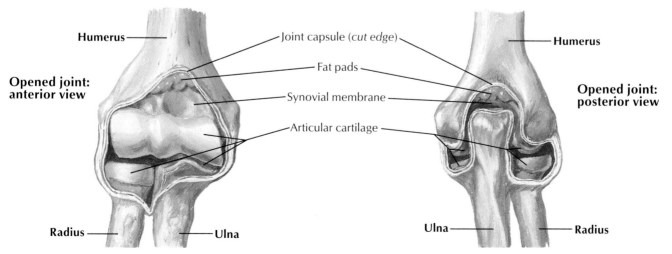

Humerus

Opened joint: anterior view

Radius

Ulna

Joint capsule (*cut edge*)

Fat pads

Synovial membrane

Articular cartilage

Humerus

Opened joint: posterior view

Ulna

Radius

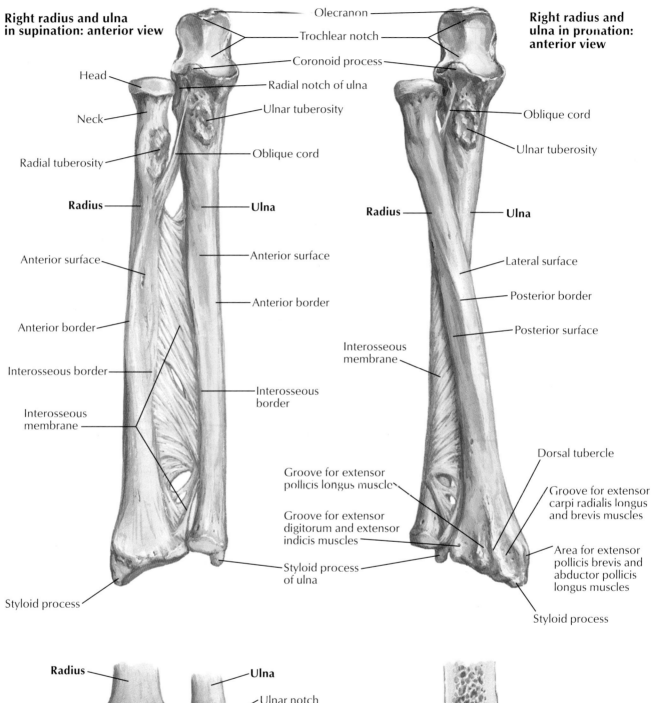

Right radius and ulna in supination: anterior view

Olecranon

Trochlear notch

Coronoid process

Head

Radial notch of ulna

Neck

Ulnar tuberosity

Radial tuberosity

Oblique cord

Radius

Ulna

Anterior surface

Anterior surface

Anterior border

Anterior border

Interosseous border

Interosseous border

Interosseous membrane

Interosseous membrane

Groove for extensor pollicis longus muscle

Groove for extensor digitorum and extensor indicis muscles

Styloid process of ulna

Styloid process

Right radius and ulna in pronation: anterior view

Oblique cord

Ulnar tuberosity

Radius

Ulna

Lateral surface

Posterior border

Posterior surface

Dorsal tubercle

Groove for extensor carpi radialis longus and brevis muscles

Area for extensor pollicis brevis and abductor pollicis longus muscles

Styloid process

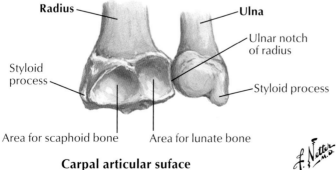

Radius

Ulna

Ulnar notch of radius

Styloid process

Styloid process

Area for scaphoid bone

Area for lunate bone

Carpal articular suface

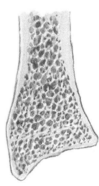

Coronal section of radius demonstrates how thickness of cortical bone of shaft diminishes to thin layer over cancellous bone at distal end

Plate 439 **Elbow and Forearm**

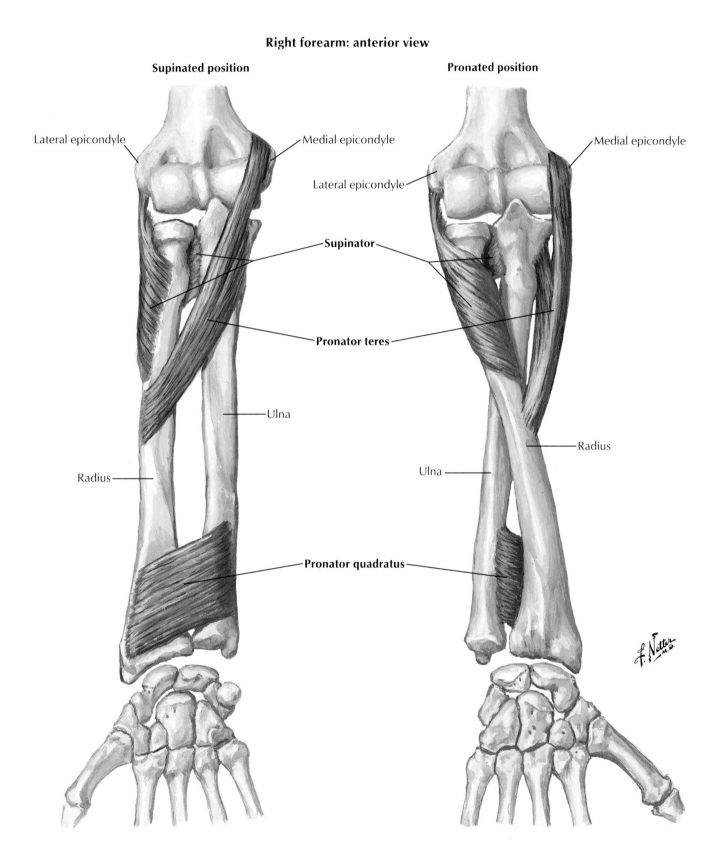

Right forearm: anterior view

Supinated position

Pronated position

Lateral epicondyle

Medial epicondyle

Medial epicondyle

Lateral epicondyle

Supinator

Pronator teres

Ulna

Radius

Radius

Ulna

Pronator quadratus

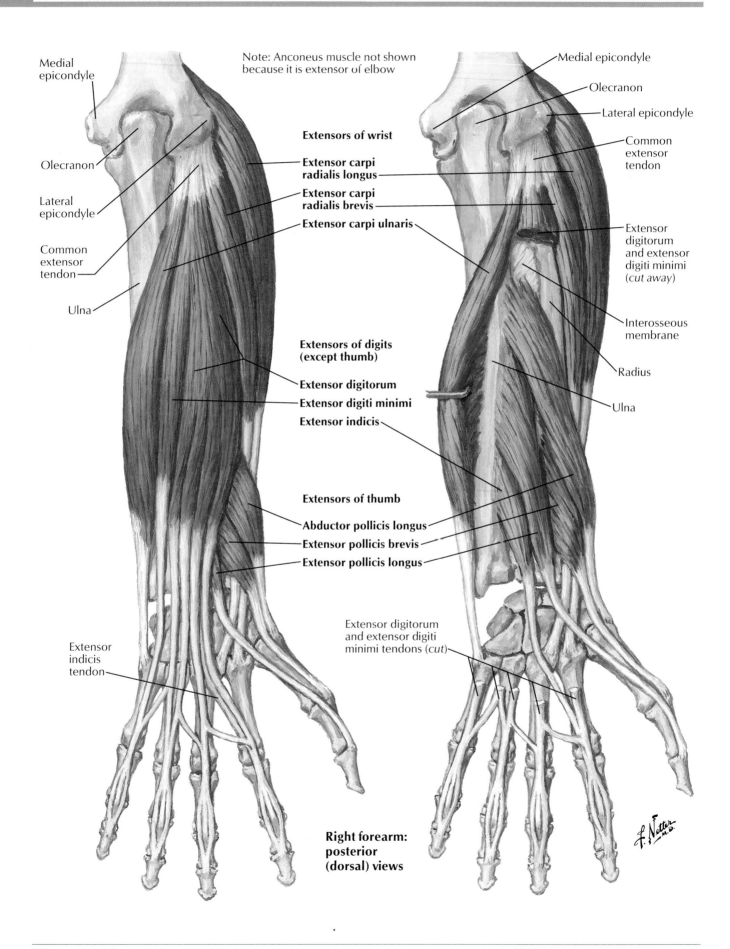

Medial epicondyle

Olecranon

Lateral epicondyle

Common extensor tendon

Ulna

Note: Anconeus muscle not shown because it is extensor of elbow

Extensors of wrist

Extensor carpi radialis longus

Extensor carpi radialis brevis

Extensor carpi ulnaris

Extensors of digits (except thumb)

Extensor digitorum

Extensor digiti minimi

Extensor indicis

Extensors of thumb

Abductor pollicis longus

Extensor pollicis brevis

Extensor pollicis longus

Extensor indicis tendon

Medial epicondyle

Olecranon

Lateral epicondyle

Common extensor tendon

Extensor digitorum and extensor digiti minimi (*cut away*)

Interosseous membrane

Radius

Ulna

Extensor digitorum and extensor digiti minimi tendons (*cut*)

Right forearm: posterior (dorsal) views

Plate 441   **Elbow and Forearm**

Note: Brachioradialis muscle not shown because it is flexor of elbow

Lateral epicondyle

Medial epicondyle

Common flexor tendon

Flexor carpi radialis

Palmaris longus

Flexor carpi ulnaris

Radius

Ulna

Pisiform

Hook of hamate

Palmar aponeurosis (*cut*)

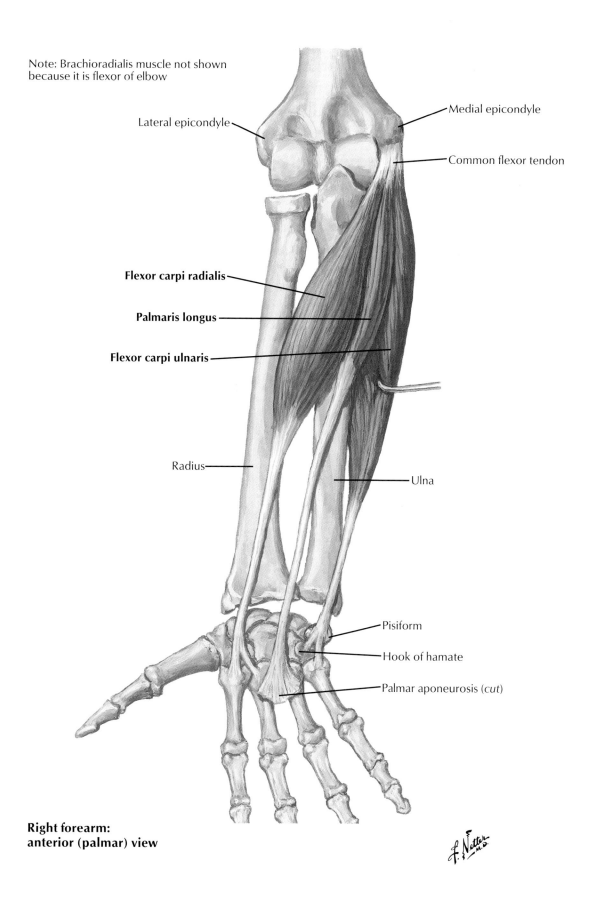

Right forearm:
anterior (palmar) view

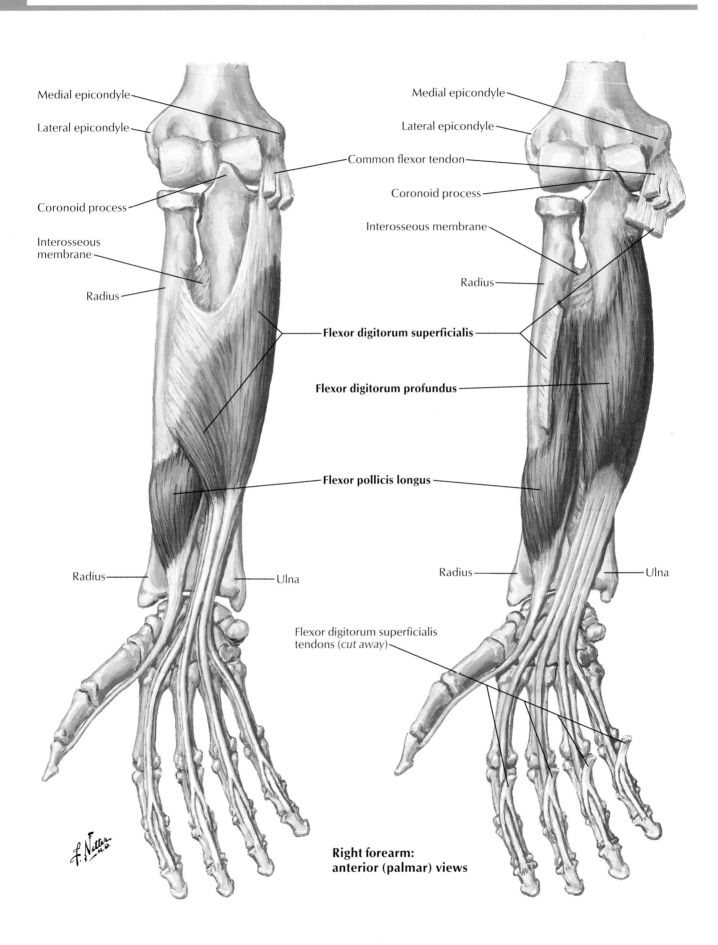

Medial epicondyle

Lateral epicondyle

Common flexor tendon

Coronoid process

Interosseous membrane

Radius

Flexor digitorum superficialis

Flexor digitorum profundus

Flexor pollicis longus

Radius

Ulna

Medial epicondyle

Lateral epicondyle

Coronoid process

Interosseous membrane

Radius

Radius

Ulna

Flexor digitorum superficialis tendons (*cut away*)

Right forearm: anterior (palmar) views

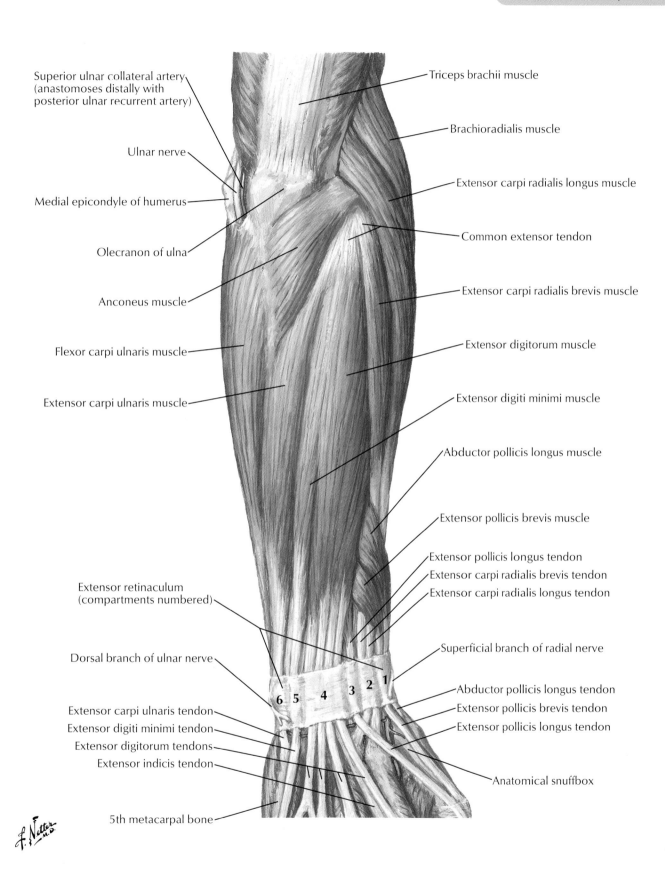

Superior ulnar collateral artery (anastomoses distally with posterior ulnar recurrent artery)

Ulnar nerve

Medial epicondyle of humerus

Olecranon of ulna

Anconeus muscle

Flexor carpi ulnaris muscle

Extensor carpi ulnaris muscle

Extensor retinaculum (compartments numbered)

Dorsal branch of ulnar nerve

Extensor carpi ulnaris tendon
Extensor digiti minimi tendon
Extensor digitorum tendons
Extensor indicis tendon

5th metacarpal bone

Triceps brachii muscle

Brachioradialis muscle

Extensor carpi radialis longus muscle

Common extensor tendon

Extensor carpi radialis brevis muscle

Extensor digitorum muscle

Extensor digiti minimi muscle

Abductor pollicis longus muscle

Extensor pollicis brevis muscle

Extensor pollicis longus tendon
Extensor carpi radialis brevis tendon
Extensor carpi radialis longus tendon

Superficial branch of radial nerve

Abductor pollicis longus tendon
Extensor pollicis brevis tendon
Extensor pollicis longus tendon

Anatomical snuffbox

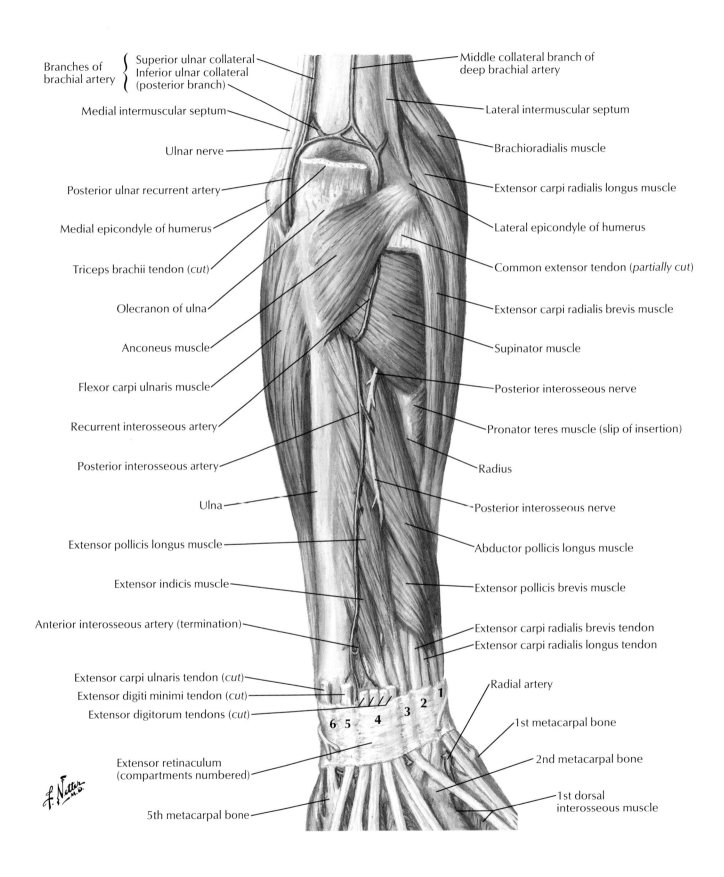

Branches of brachial artery {
Superior ulnar collateral
Inferior ulnar collateral (posterior branch)

Medial intermuscular septum

Ulnar nerve

Posterior ulnar recurrent artery

Medial epicondyle of humerus

Triceps brachii tendon (cut)

Olecranon of ulna

Anconeus muscle

Flexor carpi ulnaris muscle

Recurrent interosseous artery

Posterior interosseous artery

Ulna

Extensor pollicis longus muscle

Extensor indicis muscle

Anterior interosseous artery (termination)

Extensor carpi ulnaris tendon (cut)

Extensor digiti minimi tendon (cut)

Extensor digitorum tendons (cut)

Extensor retinaculum (compartments numbered)

5th metacarpal bone

Middle collateral branch of deep brachial artery

Lateral intermuscular septum

Brachioradialis muscle

Extensor carpi radialis longus muscle

Lateral epicondyle of humerus

Common extensor tendon (partially cut)

Extensor carpi radialis brevis muscle

Supinator muscle

Posterior interosseous nerve

Pronator teres muscle (slip of insertion)

Radius

Posterior interosseous nerve

Abductor pollicis longus muscle

Extensor pollicis brevis muscle

Extensor carpi radialis brevis tendon

Extensor carpi radialis longus tendon

Radial artery

1st metacarpal bone

2nd metacarpal bone

1st dorsal interosseous muscle

Plate 445

Elbow and Forearm

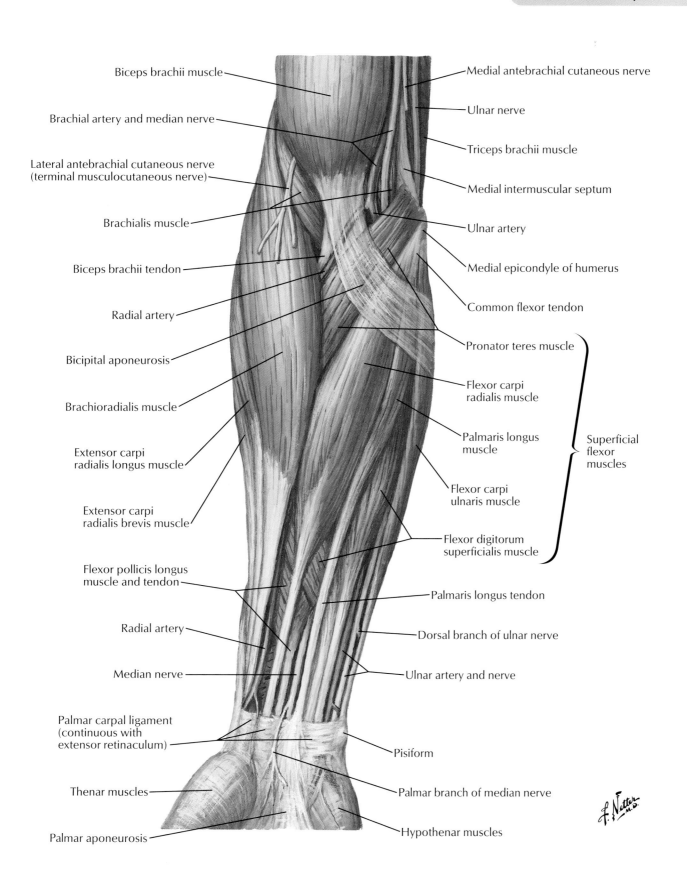

Biceps brachii muscle

Brachial artery and median nerve

Lateral antebrachial cutaneous nerve (terminal musculocutaneous nerve)

Brachialis muscle

Biceps brachii tendon

Radial artery

Bicipital aponeurosis

Brachioradialis muscle

Extensor carpi radialis longus muscle

Extensor carpi radialis brevis muscle

Flexor pollicis longus muscle and tendon

Radial artery

Median nerve

Palmar carpal ligament (continuous with extensor retinaculum)

Thenar muscles

Palmar aponeurosis

Medial antebrachial cutaneous nerve

Ulnar nerve

Triceps brachii muscle

Medial intermuscular septum

Ulnar artery

Medial epicondyle of humerus

Common flexor tendon

Pronator teres muscle

Flexor carpi radialis muscle

Palmaris longus muscle

Flexor carpi ulnaris muscle

Flexor digitorum superficialis muscle

Superficial flexor muscles

Palmaris longus tendon

Dorsal branch of ulnar nerve

Ulnar artery and nerve

Pisiform

Palmar branch of median nerve

Hypothenar muscles

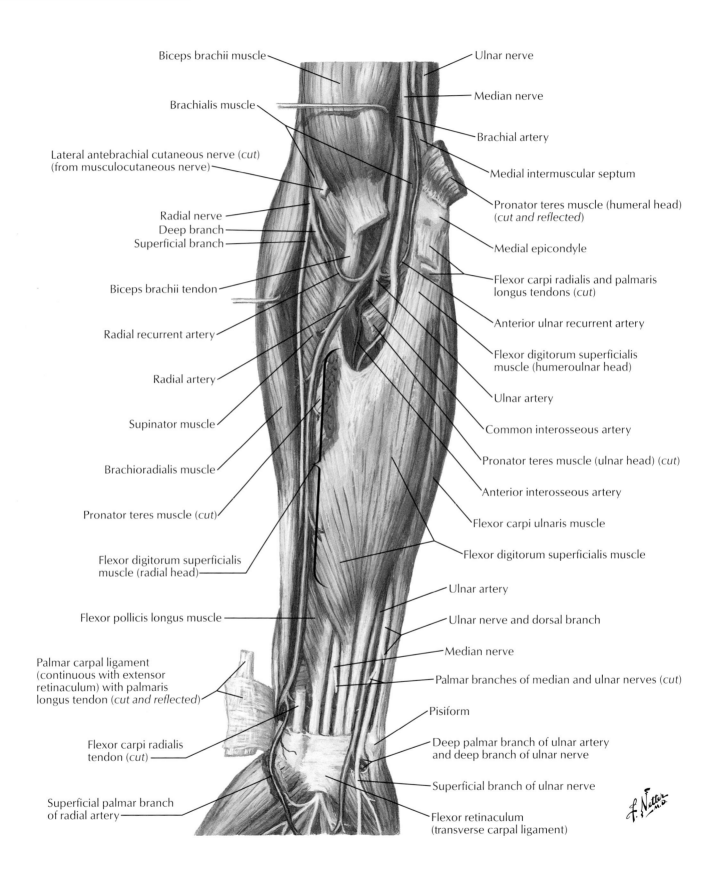

Biceps brachii muscle

Brachialis muscle

Lateral antebrachial cutaneous nerve (*cut*)
(from musculocutaneous nerve)

Radial nerve
Deep branch
Superficial branch

Biceps brachii tendon

Radial recurrent artery

Radial artery

Supinator muscle

Brachioradialis muscle

Pronator teres muscle (*cut*)

Flexor digitorum superficialis
muscle (radial head)

Flexor pollicis longus muscle

Palmar carpal ligament
(continuous with extensor
retinaculum) with palmaris
longus tendon (*cut and reflected*)

Flexor carpi radialis
tendon (*cut*)

Superficial palmar branch
of radial artery

Ulnar nerve

Median nerve

Brachial artery

Medial intermuscular septum

Pronator teres muscle (humeral head)
(*cut and reflected*)

Medial epicondyle

Flexor carpi radialis and palmaris
longus tendons (*cut*)

Anterior ulnar recurrent artery

Flexor digitorum superficialis
muscle (humeroulnar head)

Ulnar artery

Common interosseous artery

Pronator teres muscle (ulnar head) (*cut*)

Anterior interosseous artery

Flexor carpi ulnaris muscle

Flexor digitorum superficialis muscle

Ulnar artery

Ulnar nerve and dorsal branch

Median nerve

Palmar branches of median and ulnar nerves (*cut*)

Pisiform

Deep palmar branch of ulnar artery
and deep branch of ulnar nerve

Superficial branch of ulnar nerve

Flexor retinaculum
(transverse carpal ligament)

Plate 447   **Elbow and Forearm**

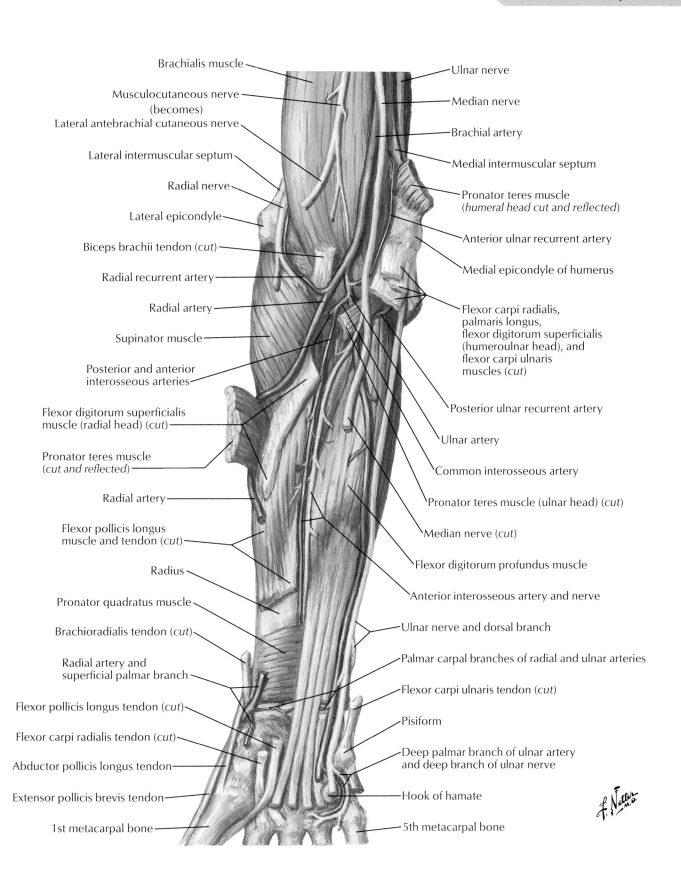

Brachialis muscle

Musculocutaneous nerve (becomes)

Lateral antebrachial cutaneous nerve

Lateral intermuscular septum

Radial nerve

Lateral epicondyle

Biceps brachii tendon (cut)

Radial recurrent artery

Radial artery

Supinator muscle

Posterior and anterior interosseous arteries

Flexor digitorum superficialis muscle (radial head) (cut)

Pronator teres muscle (cut and reflected)

Radial artery

Flexor pollicis longus muscle and tendon (cut)

Radius

Pronator quadratus muscle

Brachioradialis tendon (cut)

Radial artery and superficial palmar branch

Flexor pollicis longus tendon (cut)

Flexor carpi radialis tendon (cut)

Abductor pollicis longus tendon

Extensor pollicis brevis tendon

1st metacarpal bone

Ulnar nerve

Median nerve

Brachial artery

Medial intermuscular septum

Pronator teres muscle (humeral head cut and reflected)

Anterior ulnar recurrent artery

Medial epicondyle of humerus

Flexor carpi radialis, palmaris longus, flexor digitorum superficialis (humeroulnar head), and flexor carpi ulnaris muscles (cut)

Posterior ulnar recurrent artery

Ulnar artery

Common interosseous artery

Pronator teres muscle (ulnar head) (cut)

Median nerve (cut)

Flexor digitorum profundus muscle

Anterior interosseous artery and nerve

Ulnar nerve and dorsal branch

Palmar carpal branches of radial and ulnar arteries

Flexor carpi ulnaris tendon (cut)

Pisiform

Deep palmar branch of ulnar artery and deep branch of ulnar nerve

Hook of hamate

5th metacarpal bone

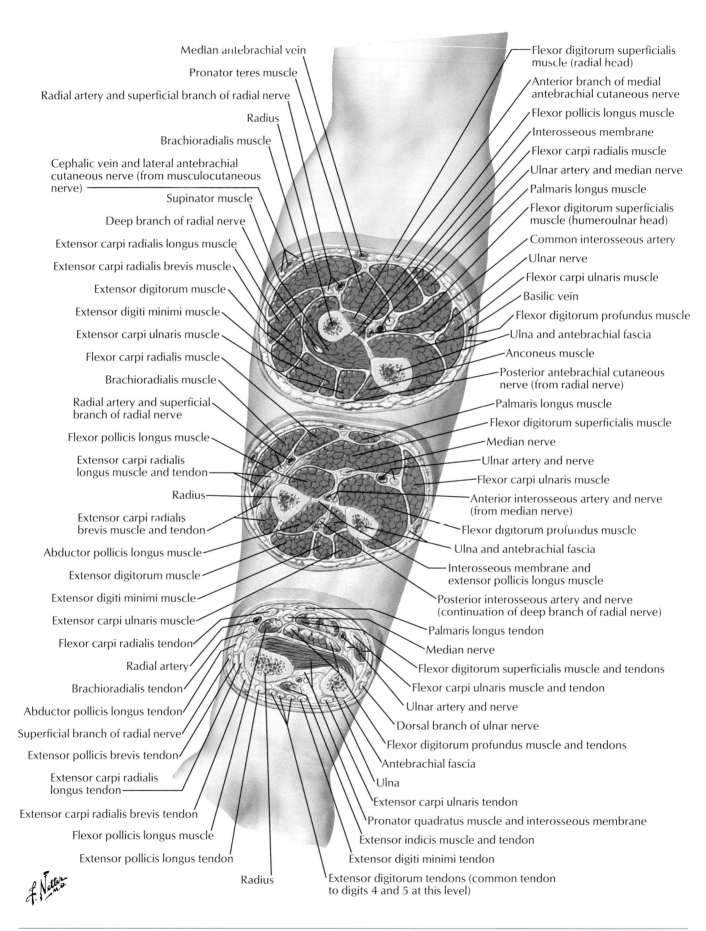

Median antebrachial vein

Pronator teres muscle

Radial artery and superficial branch of radial nerve

Radius

Brachioradialis muscle

Cephalic vein and lateral antebrachial cutaneous nerve (from musculocutaneous nerve)

Supinator muscle

Deep branch of radial nerve

Extensor carpi radialis longus muscle

Extensor carpi radialis brevis muscle

Extensor digitorum muscle

Extensor digiti minimi muscle

Extensor carpi ulnaris muscle

Flexor carpi radialis muscle

Brachioradialis muscle

Radial artery and superficial branch of radial nerve

Flexor pollicis longus muscle

Extensor carpi radialis longus muscle and tendon

Radius

Extensor carpi radialis brevis muscle and tendon

Abductor pollicis longus muscle

Extensor digitorum muscle

Extensor digiti minimi muscle

Extensor carpi ulnaris muscle

Flexor carpi radialis tendon

Radial artery

Brachioradialis tendon

Abductor pollicis longus tendon

Superficial branch of radial nerve

Extensor pollicis brevis tendon

Extensor carpi radialis longus tendon

Extensor carpi radialis brevis tendon

Flexor pollicis longus muscle

Extensor pollicis longus tendon

Radius

Flexor digitorum superficialis muscle (radial head)

Anterior branch of medial antebrachial cutaneous nerve

Flexor pollicis longus muscle

Interosseous membrane

Flexor carpi radialis muscle

Ulnar artery and median nerve

Palmaris longus muscle

Flexor digitorum superficialis muscle (humeroulnar head)

Common interosseous artery

Ulnar nerve

Flexor carpi ulnaris muscle

Basilic vein

Flexor digitorum profundus muscle

Ulna and antebrachial fascia

Anconeus muscle

Posterior antebrachial cutaneous nerve (from radial nerve)

Palmaris longus muscle

Flexor digitorum superficialis muscle

Median nerve

Ulnar artery and nerve

Flexor carpi ulnaris muscle

Anterior interosseous artery and nerve (from median nerve)

Flexor digitorum profundus muscle

Ulna and antebrachial fascia

Interosseous membrane and extensor pollicis longus muscle

Posterior interosseous artery and nerve (continuation of deep branch of radial nerve)

Palmaris longus tendon

Median nerve

Flexor digitorum superficialis muscle and tendons

Flexor carpi ulnaris muscle and tendon

Ulnar artery and nerve

Dorsal branch of ulnar nerve

Flexor digitorum profundus muscle and tendons

Antebrachial fascia

Ulna

Extensor carpi ulnaris tendon

Pronator quadratus muscle and interosseous membrane

Extensor indicis muscle and tendon

Extensor digiti minimi tendon

Extensor digitorum tendons (common tendon to digits 4 and 5 at this level)

Plate 449   **Elbow and Forearm**

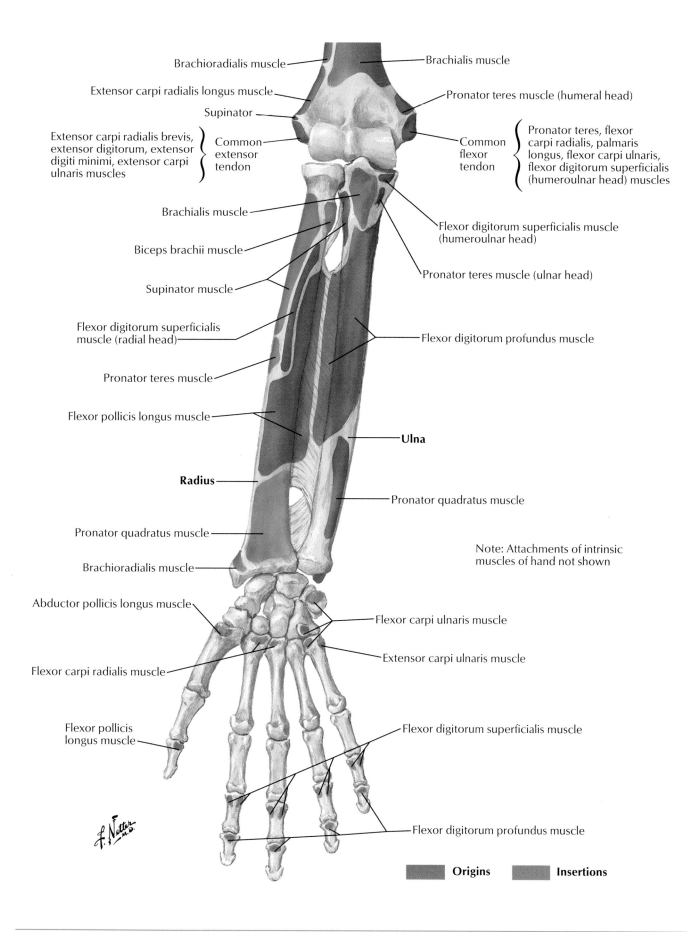

Brachioradialis muscle

Brachialis muscle

Extensor carpi radialis longus muscle

Pronator teres muscle (humeral head)

Supinator

Extensor carpi radialis brevis, extensor digitorum, extensor digiti minimi, extensor carpi ulnaris muscles

Common extensor tendon

Common flexor tendon

Pronator teres, flexor carpi radialis, palmaris longus, flexor carpi ulnaris, flexor digitorum superficialis (humeroulnar head) muscles

Brachialis muscle

Flexor digitorum superficialis muscle (humeroulnar head)

Biceps brachii muscle

Pronator teres muscle (ulnar head)

Supinator muscle

Flexor digitorum superficialis muscle (radial head)

Flexor digitorum profundus muscle

Pronator teres muscle

Flexor pollicis longus muscle

Ulna

Radius

Pronator quadratus muscle

Pronator quadratus muscle

Note: Attachments of intrinsic muscles of hand not shown

Brachioradialis muscle

Abductor pollicis longus muscle

Flexor carpi ulnaris muscle

Extensor carpi ulnaris muscle

Flexor carpi radialis muscle

Flexor pollicis longus muscle

Flexor digitorum superficialis muscle

Flexor digitorum profundus muscle

Origins

Insertions

Attachments of Muscles of Forearm: Posterior View

Note: Attachments of intrinsic
muscles of hand not shown

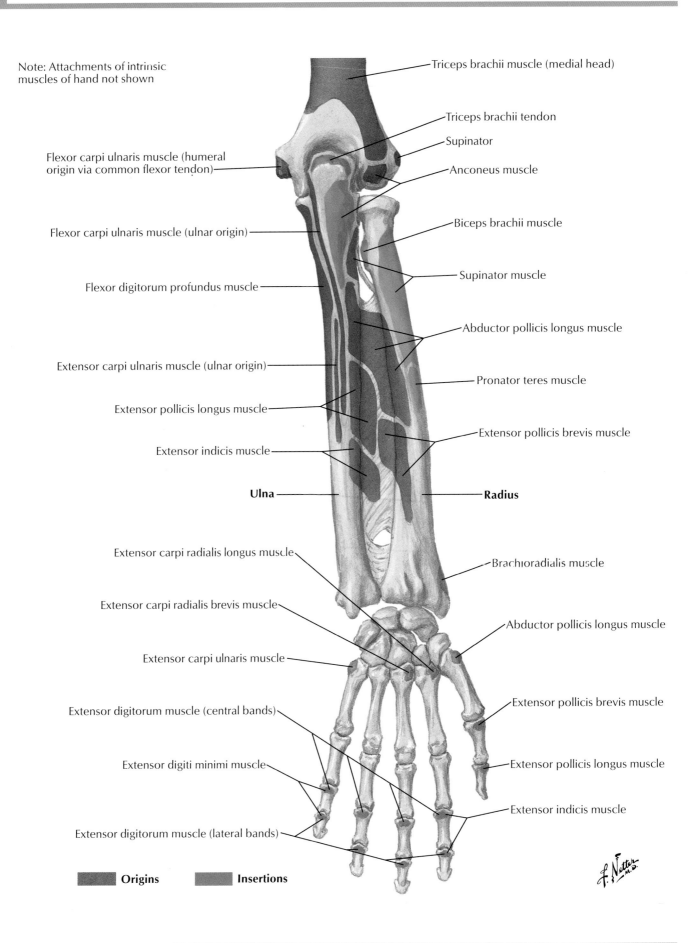

Triceps brachii muscle (medial head)

Triceps brachii tendon

Supinator

Anconeus muscle

Biceps brachii muscle

Supinator muscle

Abductor pollicis longus muscle

Pronator teres muscle

Extensor pollicis brevis muscle

Radius

Brachioradialis muscle

Abductor pollicis longus muscle

Extensor pollicis brevis muscle

Extensor pollicis longus muscle

Extensor indicis muscle

Flexor carpi ulnaris muscle (humeral
origin via common flexor tendon)

Flexor carpi ulnaris muscle (ulnar origin)

Flexor digitorum profundus muscle

Extensor carpi ulnaris muscle (ulnar origin)

Extensor pollicis longus muscle

Extensor indicis muscle

Ulna

Extensor carpi radialis longus muscle

Extensor carpi radialis brevis muscle

Extensor carpi ulnaris muscle

Extensor digitorum muscle (central bands)

Extensor digiti minimi muscle

Extensor digitorum muscle (lateral bands)

Origins   Insertions

Plate 451   **Elbow and Forearm**

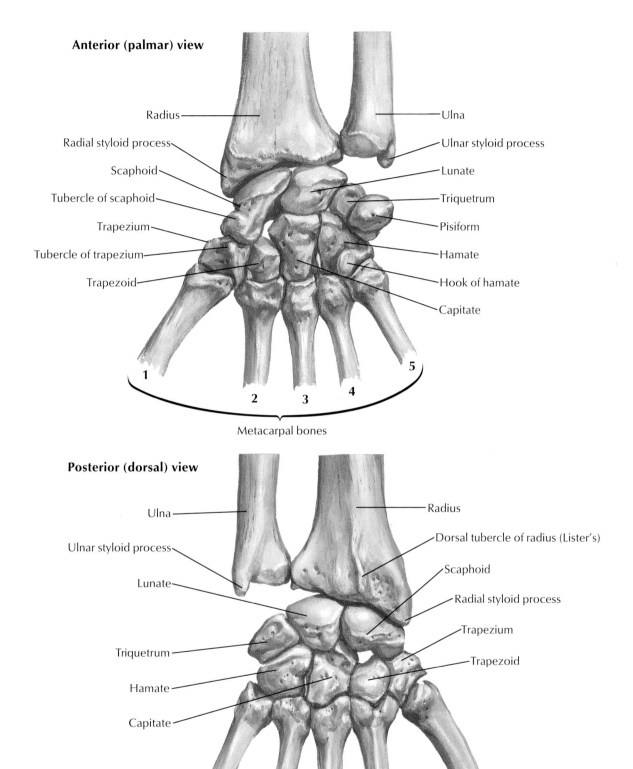

Anterior (palmar) view

Radius
Radial styloid process
Scaphoid
Tubercle of scaphoid
Trapezium
Tubercle of trapezium
Trapezoid

Ulna
Ulnar styloid process
Lunate
Triquetrum
Pisiform
Hamate
Hook of hamate
Capitate

1   2   3   4   5

Metacarpal bones

Posterior (dorsal) view

Ulna
Ulnar styloid process
Lunate
Triquetrum
Hamate
Capitate

Radius
Dorsal tubercle of radius (Lister's)
Scaphoid
Radial styloid process
Trapezium
Trapezoid

5   4   3   2   1

Metacarpal bones

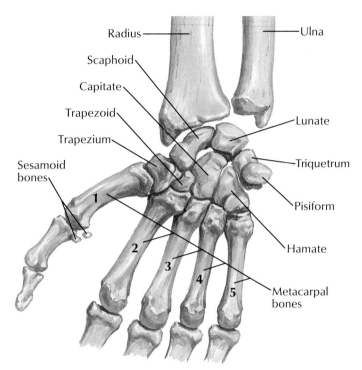

Position of carpal bones with hand in abduction: anterior (palmar) view

Position of carpal bones with hand in adduction: anterior (palmar) view

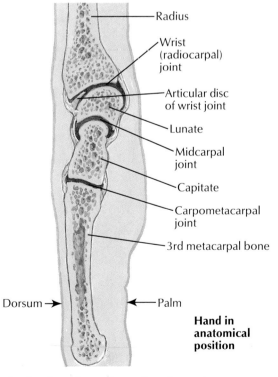

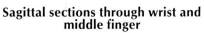

Sagittal sections through wrist and middle finger

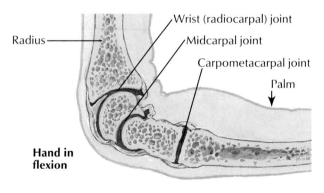

Hand in flexion

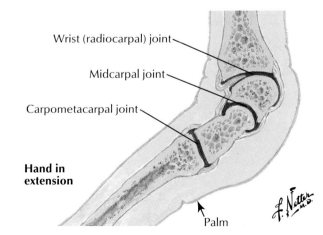

Hand in extension

Carpal tunnel: palmar view

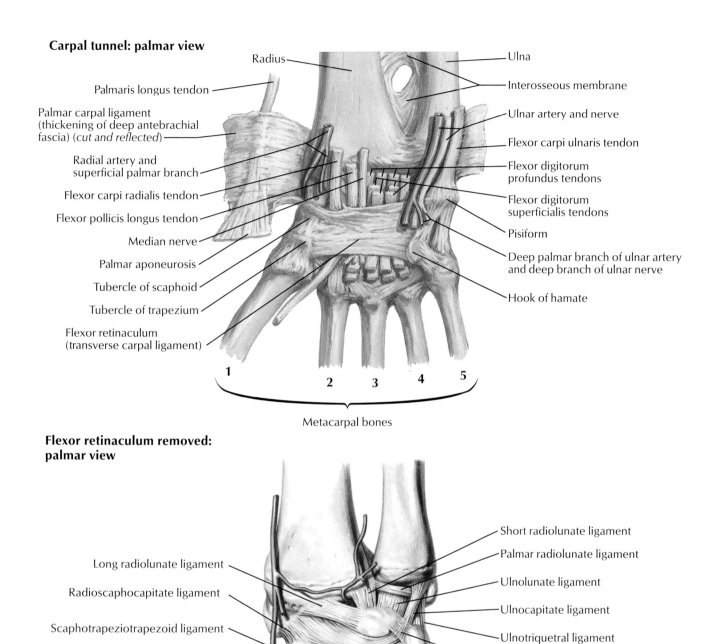

Radius

Ulna

Palmaris longus tendon

Interosseous membrane

Palmar carpal ligament (thickening of deep antebrachial fascia) (cut and reflected)

Ulnar artery and nerve

Flexor carpi ulnaris tendon

Radial artery and superficial palmar branch

Flexor digitorum profundus tendons

Flexor carpi radialis tendon

Flexor digitorum superficialis tendons

Flexor pollicis longus tendon

Median nerve

Pisiform

Palmar aponeurosis

Deep palmar branch of ulnar artery and deep branch of ulnar nerve

Tubercle of scaphoid

Tubercle of trapezium

Hook of hamate

Flexor retinaculum (transverse carpal ligament)

1   2   3   4   5

Metacarpal bones

Flexor retinaculum removed: palmar view

Short radiolunate ligament

Palmar radiolunate ligament

Long radiolunate ligament

Radioscaphocapitate ligament

Ulnolunate ligament

Scaphotrapeziotrapezoid ligament

Ulnocapitate ligament

Scaphocapitate ligment

Ulnotriquetral ligament

Trapeziotrapezoid ligament

Lunotriquetral ligament

Triquetrohamate ligament

Triquetrocapitate ligament

Capitohamate ligament

Trapeziocapitate ligament

1   2   3   4   5

Metacarpal bones

Posterior (dorsal) view

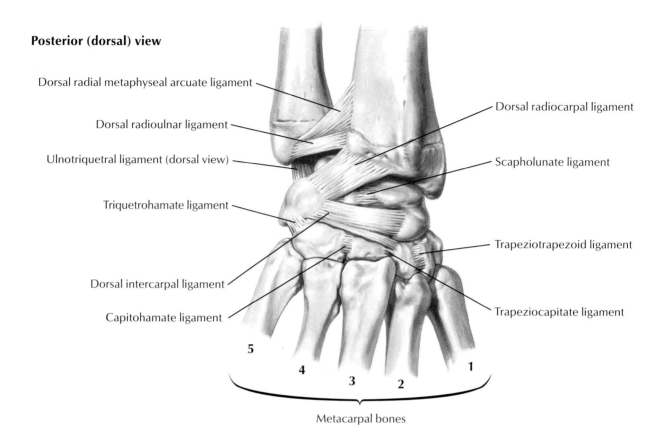

Dorsal radial metaphyseal arcuate ligament

Dorsal radioulnar ligament

Ulnotriquetral ligament (dorsal view)

Triquetrohamate ligament

Dorsal intercarpal ligament

Capitohamate ligament

Dorsal radiocarpal ligament

Scapholunate ligament

Trapeziotrapezoid ligament

Trapeziocapitate ligament

5 4 3 2 1

Metacarpal bones

Coronal section: dorsal view

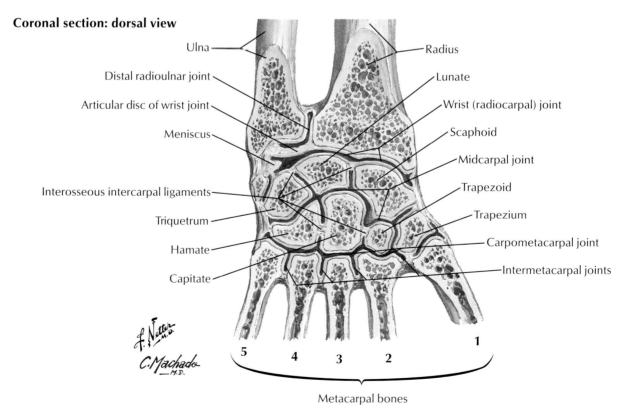

Ulna

Distal radioulnar joint

Articular disc of wrist joint

Meniscus

Interosseous intercarpal ligaments

Triquetrum

Hamate

Capitate

Radius

Lunate

Wrist (radiocarpal) joint

Scaphoid

Midcarpal joint

Trapezoid

Trapezium

Carpometacarpal joint

Intermetacarpal joints

5 4 3 2 1

Metacarpal bones

Plate 455   **Wrist and Hand**

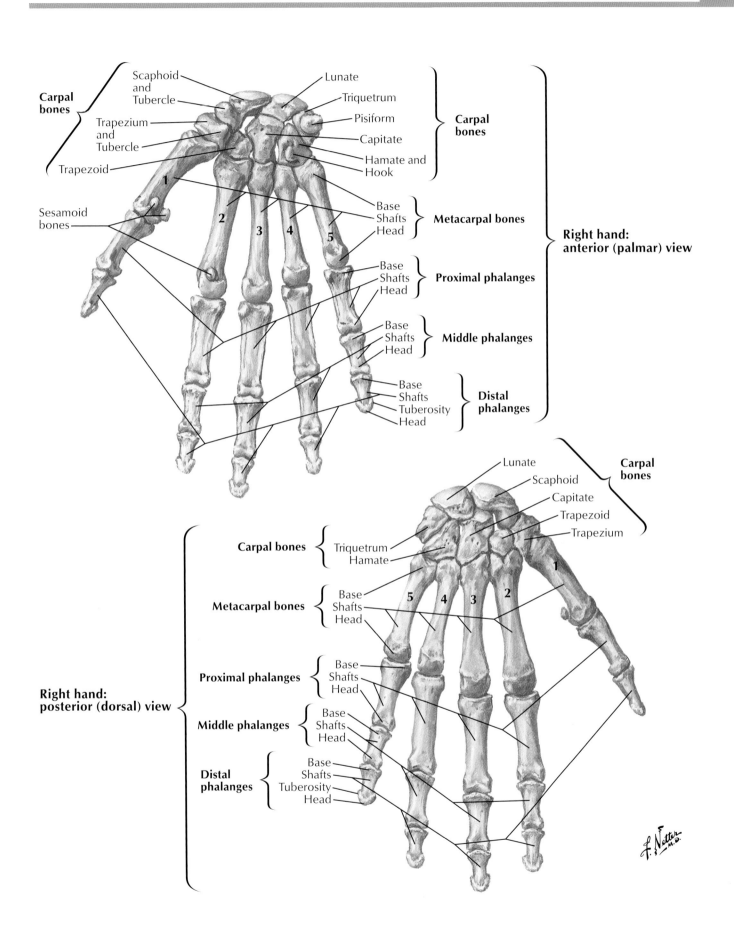

Carpal bones
Scaphoid and Tubercle
Trapezium and Tubercle
Trapezoid

Lunate
Triquetrum
Pisiform
Capitate
Hamate and Hook
Carpal bones

Sesamoid bones

1
2
3 4 5

Base
Shafts
Head
Metacarpal bones

Base
Shafts
Head
Proximal phalanges

Base
Shafts
Head
Middle phalanges

Base
Shafts
Tuberosity
Head
Distal phalanges

Right hand: anterior (palmar) view

Lunate
Scaphoid
Capitate
Trapezoid
Trapezium
Carpal bones

Carpal bones
Triquetrum
Hamate

Metacarpal bones
Base
Shafts
Head

5 4 3 2 1

Proximal phalanges
Base
Shafts
Head

Middle phalanges
Base
Shafts
Head

Distal phalanges
Base
Shafts
Tuberosity
Head

Right hand: posterior (dorsal) view

f. Netter M.D.

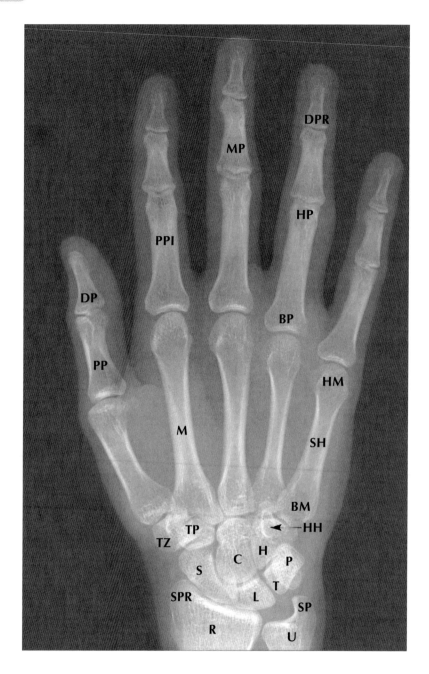

BM	Base of 5th metacarpal	**P**	Pisiform
BP	Base of 4th proximal phalanx	**PP**	Proximal phalanx of thumb
C	Capitate	**PPI**	Proximal phalanx of index finger
DP	Distal phalanx of thumb	**R**	Radius
DPR	Distal phalanx of ring finger	**S**	Scaphoid
H	Hamate	**SH**	Shaft of 5th metacarpal
HH	Hook of hamate	**SP**	Styloid process of ulna
HM	Head of 5th metacarpal	**SPR**	Styloid process of radius
HP	Head of proximal phalanx	**T**	Triquetrum
L	Lunate	**TP**	Trapezoid
M	Metacarpal of index finger	**TZ**	Trapezium
MP	Middle phalanx of middle finger	**U**	Ulna

Plate 457　　　　　　　　　　　　　　　　　　　　　　　　　　　　**Wrist and Hand**

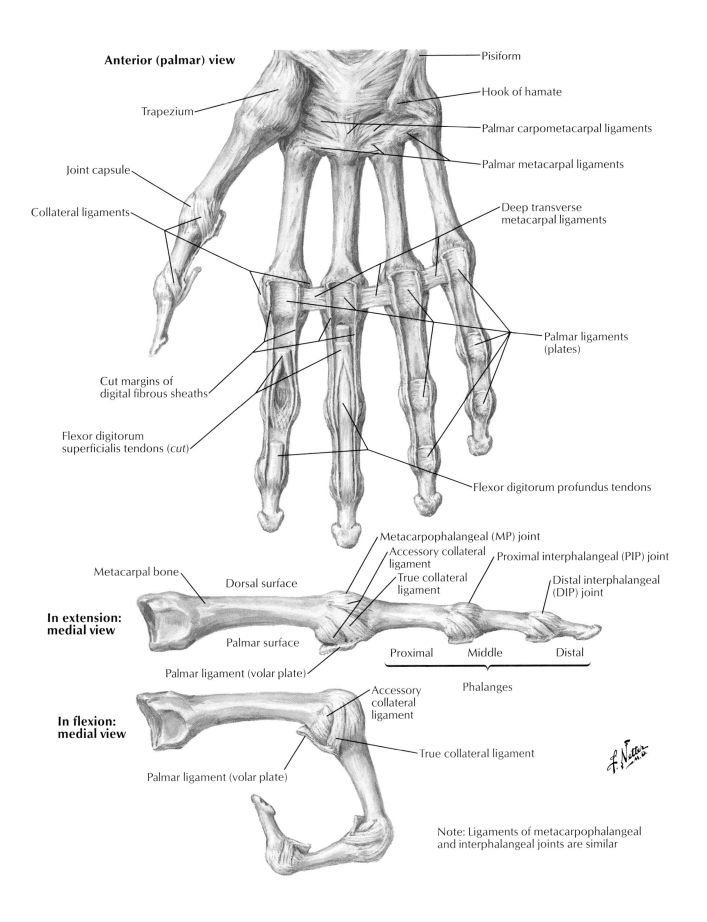

Anterior (palmar) view

Pisiform

Hook of hamate

Trapezium

Palmar carpometacarpal ligaments

Palmar metacarpal ligaments

Joint capsule

Collateral ligaments

Deep transverse metacarpal ligaments

Palmar ligaments (plates)

Cut margins of digital fibrous sheaths

Flexor digitorum superficialis tendons (*cut*)

Flexor digitorum profundus tendons

Metacarpophalangeal (MP) joint

Accessory collateral ligament

Proximal interphalangeal (PIP) joint

Metacarpal bone

Dorsal surface

True collateral ligament

Distal interphalangeal (DIP) joint

In extension: medial view

Palmar surface

Proximal   Middle   Distal

Palmar ligament (volar plate)

Phalanges

Accessory collateral ligament

In flexion: medial view

True collateral ligament

Palmar ligament (volar plate)

Note: Ligaments of metacarpophalangeal and interphalangeal joints are similar

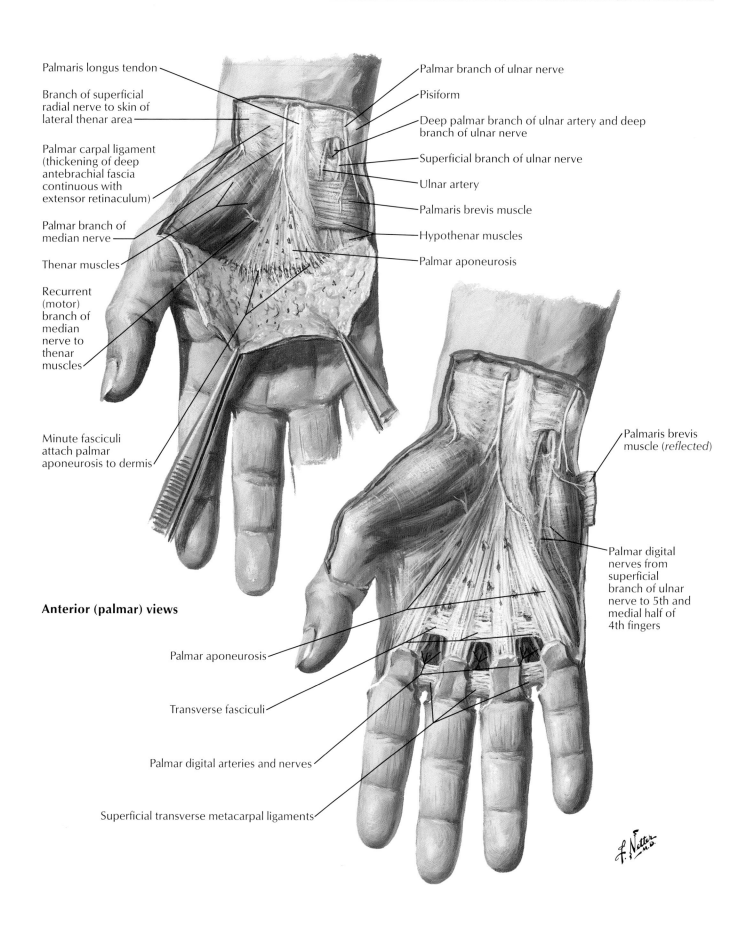

Palmaris longus tendon

Branch of superficial radial nerve to skin of lateral thenar area

Palmar carpal ligament (thickening of deep antebrachial fascia continuous with extensor retinaculum)

Palmar branch of median nerve

Thenar muscles

Recurrent (motor) branch of median nerve to thenar muscles

Minute fasciculi attach palmar aponeurosis to dermis

Palmar branch of ulnar nerve

Pisiform

Deep palmar branch of ulnar artery and deep branch of ulnar nerve

Superficial branch of ulnar nerve

Ulnar artery

Palmaris brevis muscle

Hypothenar muscles

Palmar aponeurosis

Palmaris brevis muscle (reflected)

Palmar digital nerves from superficial branch of ulnar nerve to 5th and medial half of 4th fingers

Anterior (palmar) views

Palmar aponeurosis

Transverse fasciculi

Palmar digital arteries and nerves

Superficial transverse metacarpal ligaments

Plate 459   **Wrist and Hand**

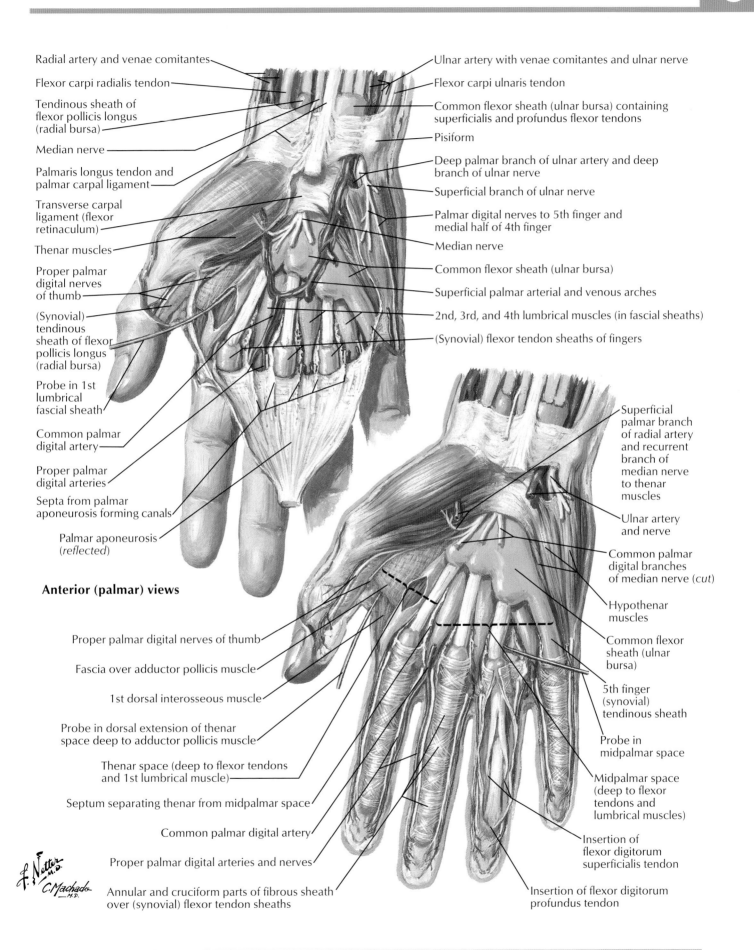

Radial artery and venae comitantes

Flexor carpi radialis tendon

Tendinous sheath of flexor pollicis longus (radial bursa)

Median nerve

Palmaris longus tendon and palmar carpal ligament

Transverse carpal ligament (flexor retinaculum)

Thenar muscles

Proper palmar digital nerves of thumb

(Synovial) tendinous sheath of flexor pollicis longus (radial bursa)

Probe in 1st lumbrical fascial sheath

Common palmar digital artery

Proper palmar digital arteries

Septa from palmar aponeurosis forming canals

Palmar aponeurosis (reflected)

Ulnar artery with venae comitantes and ulnar nerve

Flexor carpi ulnaris tendon

Common flexor sheath (ulnar bursa) containing superficialis and profundus flexor tendons

Pisiform

Deep palmar branch of ulnar artery and deep branch of ulnar nerve

Superficial branch of ulnar nerve

Palmar digital nerves to 5th finger and medial half of 4th finger

Median nerve

Common flexor sheath (ulnar bursa)

Superficial palmar arterial and venous arches

2nd, 3rd, and 4th lumbrical muscles (in fascial sheaths)

(Synovial) flexor tendon sheaths of fingers

Anterior (palmar) views

Proper palmar digital nerves of thumb

Fascia over adductor pollicis muscle

1st dorsal interosseous muscle

Probe in dorsal extension of thenar space deep to adductor pollicis muscle

Thenar space (deep to flexor tendons and 1st lumbrical muscle)

Septum separating thenar from midpalmar space

Common palmar digital artery

Proper palmar digital arteries and nerves

Annular and cruciform parts of fibrous sheath over (synovial) flexor tendon sheaths

Superficial palmar branch of radial artery and recurrent branch of median nerve to thenar muscles

Ulnar artery and nerve

Common palmar digital branches of median nerve (cut)

Hypothenar muscles

Common flexor sheath (ulnar bursa)

5th finger (synovial) tendinous sheath

Probe in midpalmar space

Midpalmar space (deep to flexor tendons and lumbrical muscles)

Insertion of flexor digitorum superficialis tendon

Insertion of flexor digitorum profundus tendon

Palmar view

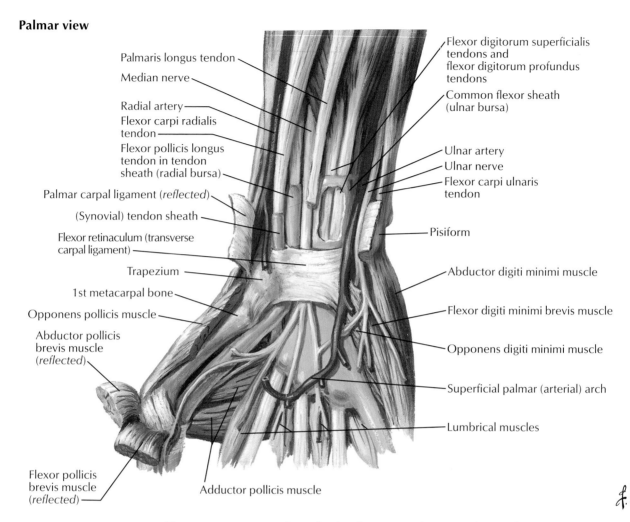

Palmaris longus tendon

Median nerve

Radial artery

Flexor carpi radialis tendon

Flexor pollicis longus tendon in tendon sheath (radial bursa)

Palmar carpal ligament (*reflected*)

(Synovial) tendon sheath

Flexor retinaculum (transverse carpal ligament)

Trapezium

1st metacarpal bone

Opponens pollicis muscle

Abductor pollicis brevis muscle (*reflected*)

Flexor pollicis brevis muscle (*reflected*)

Adductor pollicis muscle

Flexor digitorum superficialis tendons and flexor digitorum profundus tendons

Common flexor sheath (ulnar bursa)

Ulnar artery

Ulnar nerve

Flexor carpi ulnaris tendon

Pisiform

Abductor digiti minimi muscle

Flexor digiti minimi brevis muscle

Opponens digiti minimi muscle

Superficial palmar (arterial) arch

Lumbrical muscles

Transverse cross section of wrist demonstrating carpal tunnel

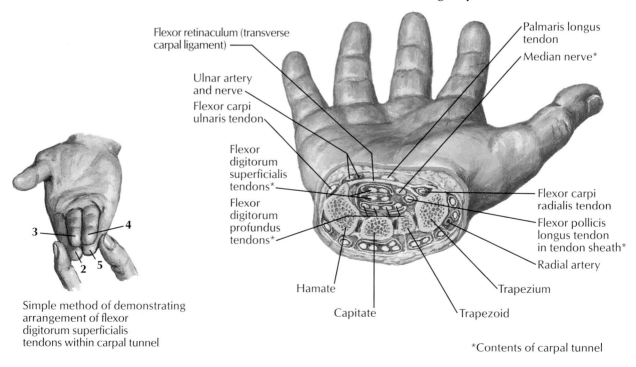

Flexor retinaculum (transverse carpal ligament)

Ulnar artery and nerve

Flexor carpi ulnaris tendon

Flexor digitorum superficialis tendons*

Flexor digitorum profundus tendons*

Palmaris longus tendon

Median nerve*

Flexor carpi radialis tendon

Flexor pollicis longus tendon in tendon sheath*

Radial artery

Trapezium

Trapezoid

Capitate

Hamate

Simple method of demonstrating arrangement of flexor digitorum superficialis tendons within carpal tunnel

3   4

2   5

*Contents of carpal tunnel

Plate 461   **Wrist and Hand**

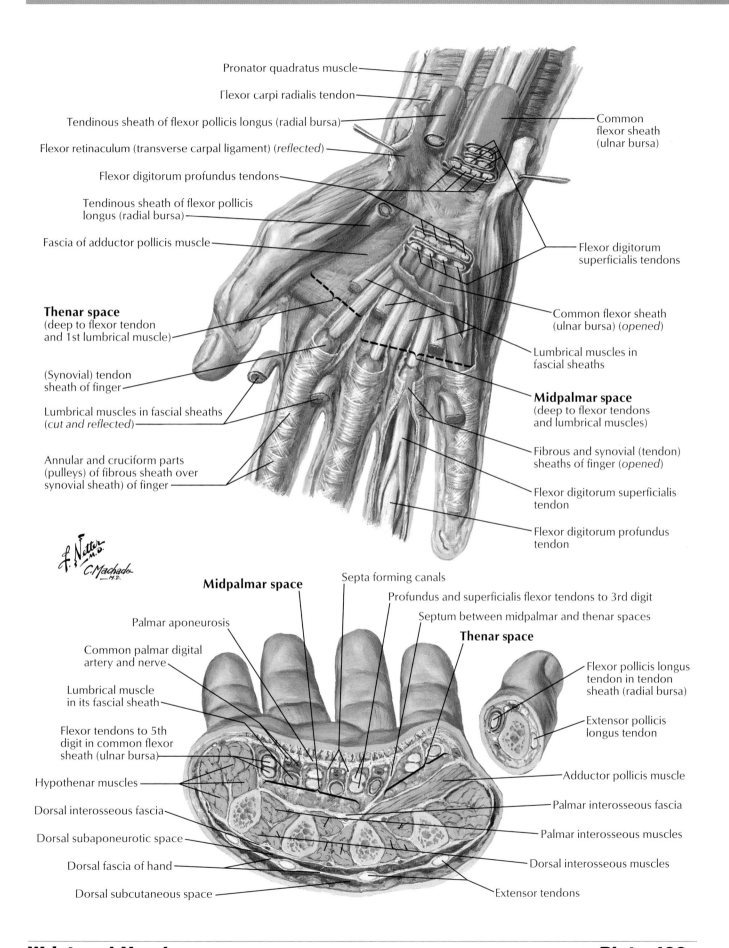

Pronator quadratus muscle

Flexor carpi radialis tendon

Tendinous sheath of flexor pollicis longus (radial bursa)

Flexor retinaculum (transverse carpal ligament) (*reflected*)

Flexor digitorum profundus tendons

Tendinous sheath of flexor pollicis longus (radial bursa)

Fascia of adductor pollicis muscle

Thenar space
(deep to flexor tendon and 1st lumbrical muscle)

(Synovial) tendon sheath of finger

Lumbrical muscles in fascial sheaths (*cut and reflected*)

Annular and cruciform parts (pulleys) of fibrous sheath over synovial sheath) of finger

Common flexor sheath (ulnar bursa)

Flexor digitorum superficialis tendons

Common flexor sheath (ulnar bursa) (*opened*)

Lumbrical muscles in fascial sheaths

Midpalmar space
(deep to flexor tendons and lumbrical muscles)

Fibrous and synovial (tendon) sheaths of finger (*opened*)

Flexor digitorum superficialis tendon

Flexor digitorum profundus tendon

Midpalmar space

Palmar aponeurosis

Common palmar digital artery and nerve

Lumbrical muscle in its fascial sheath

Flexor tendons to 5th digit in common flexor sheath (ulnar bursa)

Hypothenar muscles

Dorsal interosseous fascia

Dorsal subaponeurotic space

Dorsal fascia of hand

Dorsal subcutaneous space

Septa forming canals

Profundus and superficialis flexor tendons to 3rd digit

Septum between midpalmar and thenar spaces

Thenar space

Flexor pollicis longus tendon in tendon sheath (radial bursa)

Extensor pollicis longus tendon

Adductor pollicis muscle

Palmar interosseous fascia

Palmar interosseous muscles

Dorsal interosseous muscles

Extensor tendons

Lumbrical Muscles and Bursae, Spaces, and Sheaths: Schema

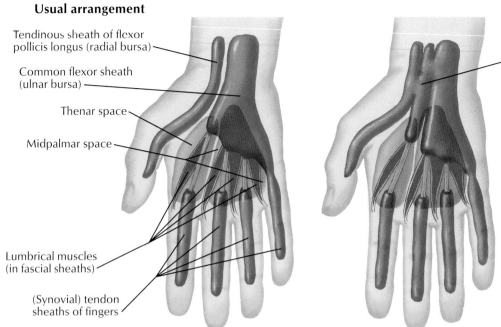

Usual arrangement

Common variation

Tendinous sheath of flexor pollicis longus (radial bursa)

Common flexor sheath (ulnar bursa)

Thenar space

Midpalmar space

Lumbrical muscles (in fascial sheaths)

(Synovial) tendon sheaths of fingers

Intermediate bursa (communication between common flexor sheath [ulnar bursa] and tendinous sheath of flexor pollicis longus [radial bursa])

Lumbrical muscles: schema

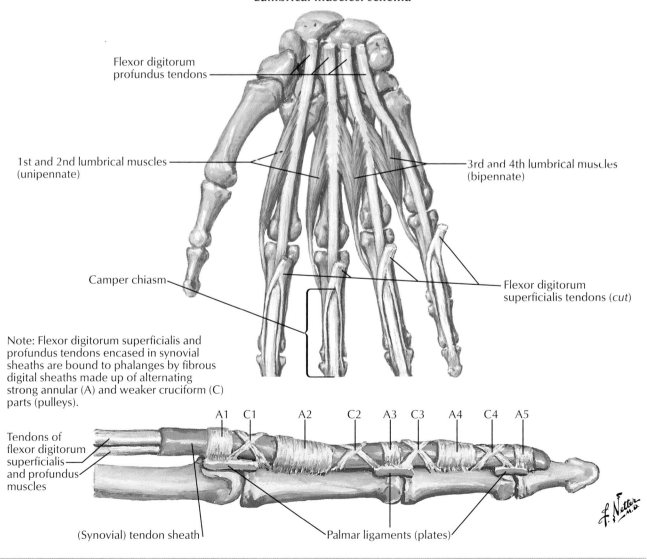

Flexor digitorum profundus tendons

1st and 2nd lumbrical muscles (unipennate)

3rd and 4th lumbrical muscles (bipennate)

Camper chiasm

Flexor digitorum superficialis tendons (*cut*)

Note: Flexor digitorum superficialis and profundus tendons encased in synovial sheaths are bound to phalanges by fibrous digital sheaths made up of alternating strong annular (A) and weaker cruciform (C) parts (pulleys).

A1 C1 A2 C2 A3 C3 A4 C4 A5

Tendons of flexor digitorum superficialis and profundus muscles

(Synovial) tendon sheath

Palmar ligaments (plates)

Plate 463   **Wrist and Hand**

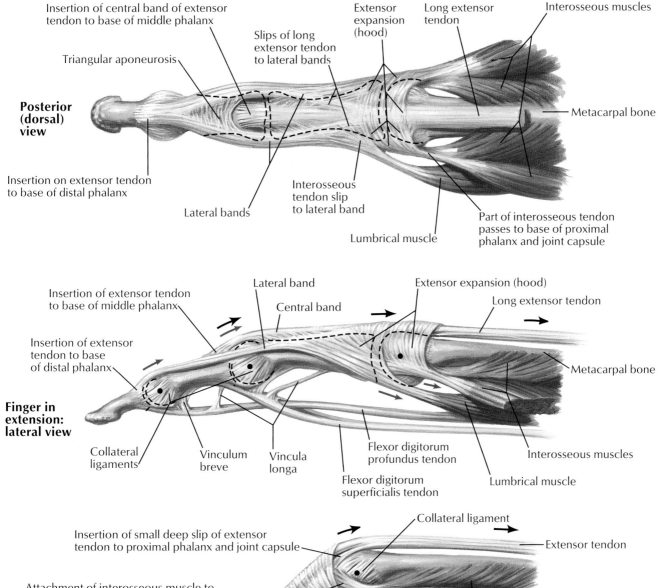

Insertion of central band of extensor tendon to base of middle phalanx

Triangular aponeurosis

Slips of long extensor tendon to lateral bands

Extensor expansion (hood)

Long extensor tendon

Interosseous muscles

Posterior (dorsal) view

Metacarpal bone

Insertion on extensor tendon to base of distal phalanx

Lateral bands

Interosseous tendon slip to lateral band

Lumbrical muscle

Part of interosseous tendon passes to base of proximal phalanx and joint capsule

Insertion of extensor tendon to base of middle phalanx

Lateral band

Central band

Extensor expansion (hood)

Long extensor tendon

Insertion of extensor tendon to base of distal phalanx

Metacarpal bone

Finger in extension: lateral view

Collateral ligaments

Vinculum breve

Vincula longa

Flexor digitorum profundus tendon

Flexor digitorum superficialis tendon

Interosseous muscles

Lumbrical muscle

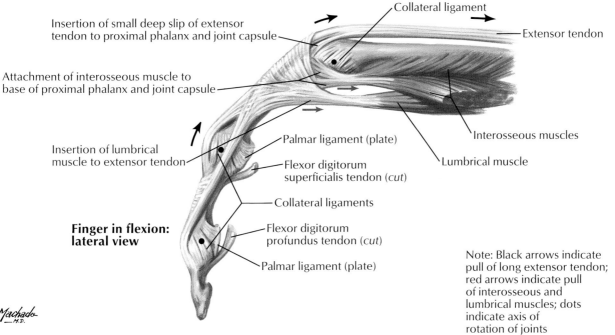

Insertion of small deep slip of extensor tendon to proximal phalanx and joint capsule

Collateral ligament

Extensor tendon

Attachment of interosseous muscle to base of proximal phalanx and joint capsule

Insertion of lumbrical muscle to extensor tendon

Palmar ligament (plate)

Flexor digitorum superficialis tendon (cut)

Collateral ligaments

Flexor digitorum profundus tendon (cut)

Palmar ligament (plate)

Interosseous muscles

Lumbrical muscle

Finger in flexion: lateral view

Note: Black arrows indicate pull of long extensor tendon; red arrows indicate pull of interosseous and lumbrical muscles; dots indicate axis of rotation of joints

C. Machado _M.D._

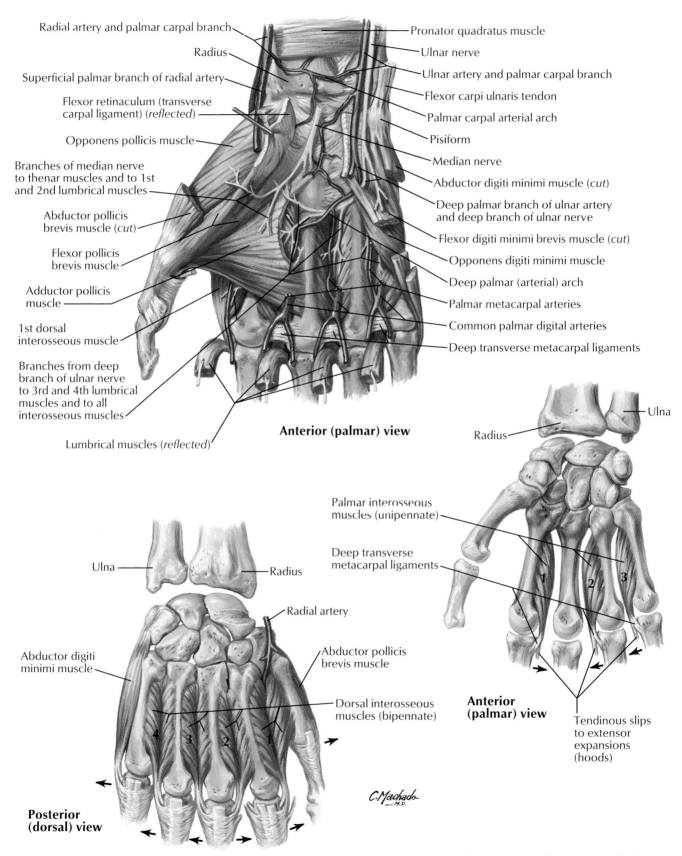

Radial artery and palmar carpal branch

Radius

Superficial palmar branch of radial artery

Flexor retinaculum (transverse carpal ligament) (*reflected*)

Opponens pollicis muscle

Branches of median nerve to thenar muscles and to 1st and 2nd lumbrical muscles

Abductor pollicis brevis muscle (*cut*)

Flexor pollicis brevis muscle

Adductor pollicis muscle

1st dorsal interosseous muscle

Branches from deep branch of ulnar nerve to 3rd and 4th lumbrical muscles and to all interosseous muscles

Lumbrical muscles (*reflected*)

Pronator quadratus muscle

Ulnar nerve

Ulnar artery and palmar carpal branch

Flexor carpi ulnaris tendon

Palmar carpal arterial arch

Pisiform

Median nerve

Abductor digiti minimi muscle (*cut*)

Deep palmar branch of ulnar artery and deep branch of ulnar nerve

Flexor digiti minimi brevis muscle (*cut*)

Opponens digiti minimi muscle

Deep palmar (arterial) arch

Palmar metacarpal arteries

Common palmar digital arteries

Deep transverse metacarpal ligaments

Anterior (palmar) view

Ulna

Radius

Radial artery

Abductor pollicis brevis muscle

Abductor digiti minimi muscle

Dorsal interosseous muscles (bipennate)

Posterior (dorsal) view

Ulna

Radius

Palmar interosseous muscles (unipennate)

Deep transverse metacarpal ligaments

Anterior (palmar) view

Tendinous slips to extensor expansions (hoods)

C.Machado M.D.

Note: Arrows indicate action of muscles.

Plate 465

Wrist and Hand

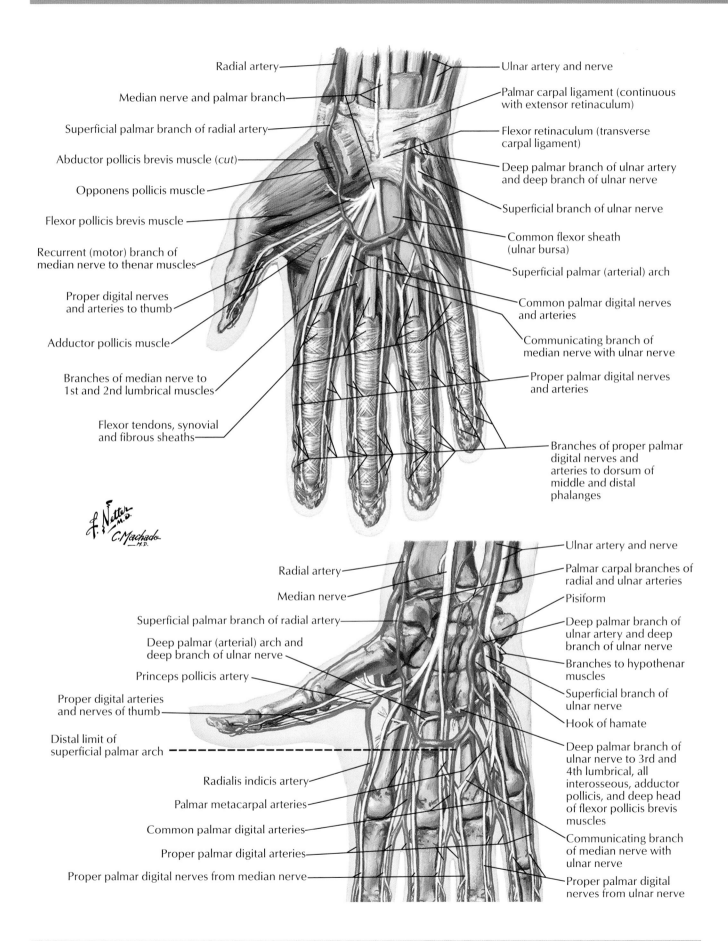

Radial artery

Median nerve and palmar branch

Superficial palmar branch of radial artery

Abductor pollicis brevis muscle (cut)

Opponens pollicis muscle

Flexor pollicis brevis muscle

Recurrent (motor) branch of
median nerve to thenar muscles

Proper digital nerves
and arteries to thumb

Adductor pollicis muscle

Branches of median nerve to
1st and 2nd lumbrical muscles

Flexor tendons, synovial
and fibrous sheaths

Ulnar artery and nerve

Palmar carpal ligament (continuous
with extensor retinaculum)

Flexor retinaculum (transverse
carpal ligament)

Deep palmar branch of ulnar artery
and deep branch of ulnar nerve

Superficial branch of ulnar nerve

Common flexor sheath
(ulnar bursa)

Superficial palmar (arterial) arch

Common palmar digital nerves
and arteries

Communicating branch of
median nerve with ulnar nerve

Proper palmar digital nerves
and arteries

Branches of proper palmar
digital nerves and
arteries to dorsum of
middle and distal
phalanges

Radial artery

Median nerve

Superficial palmar branch of radial artery

Deep palmar (arterial) arch and
deep branch of ulnar nerve

Princeps pollicis artery

Proper digital arteries
and nerves of thumb

Distal limit of
superficial palmar arch

Radialis indicis artery

Palmar metacarpal arteries

Common palmar digital arteries

Proper palmar digital arteries

Proper palmar digital nerves from median nerve

Ulnar artery and nerve

Palmar carpal branches of
radial and ulnar arteries

Pisiform

Deep palmar branch of
ulnar artery and deep
branch of ulnar nerve

Branches to hypothenar
muscles

Superficial branch of
ulnar nerve

Hook of hamate

Deep palmar branch of
ulnar nerve to 3rd and
4th lumbrical, all
interosseous, adductor
pollicis, and deep head
of flexor pollicis brevis
muscles

Communicating branch
of median nerve with
ulnar nerve

Proper palmar digital
nerves from ulnar nerve

Lateral (radial) view

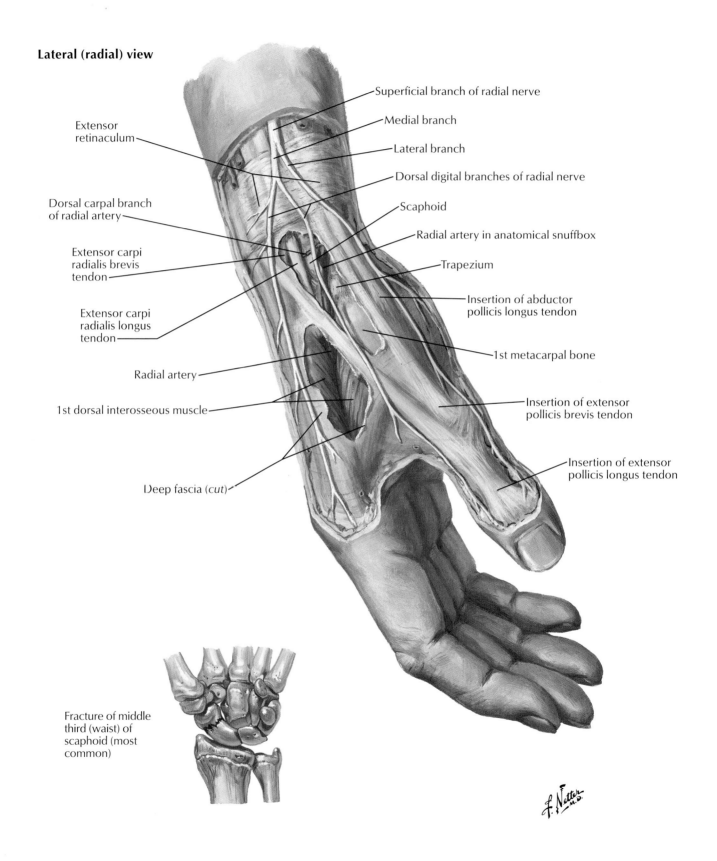

Extensor retinaculum

Dorsal carpal branch of radial artery

Extensor carpi radialis brevis tendon

Extensor carpi radialis longus tendon

Radial artery

1st dorsal interosseous muscle

Deep fascia (cut)

Superficial branch of radial nerve

Medial branch

Lateral branch

Dorsal digital branches of radial nerve

Scaphoid

Radial artery in anatomical snuffbox

Trapezium

Insertion of abductor pollicis longus tendon

1st metacarpal bone

Insertion of extensor pollicis brevis tendon

Insertion of extensor pollicis longus tendon

Fracture of middle third (waist) of scaphoid (most common)

Plate 467

Wrist and Hand

Posterior (dorsal) view

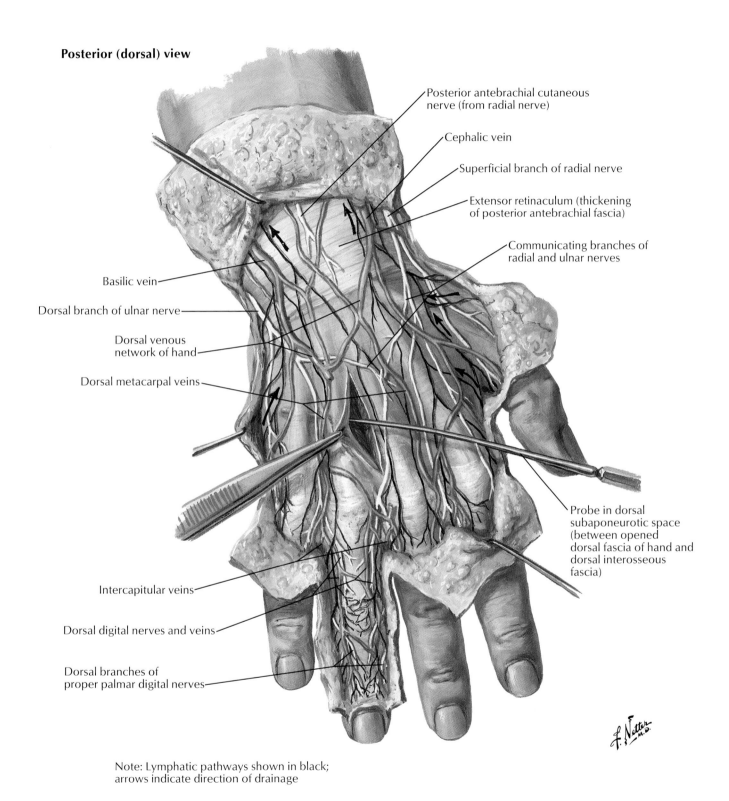

Posterior antebrachial cutaneous nerve (from radial nerve)

Cephalic vein

Superficial branch of radial nerve

Extensor retinaculum (thickening of posterior antebrachial fascia)

Communicating branches of radial and ulnar nerves

Basilic vein

Dorsal branch of ulnar nerve

Dorsal venous network of hand

Dorsal metacarpal veins

Probe in dorsal subaponeurotic space (between opened dorsal fascia of hand and dorsal interosseous fascia)

Intercapitular veins

Dorsal digital nerves and veins

Dorsal branches of proper palmar digital nerves

Note: Lymphatic pathways shown in black; arrows indicate direction of drainage

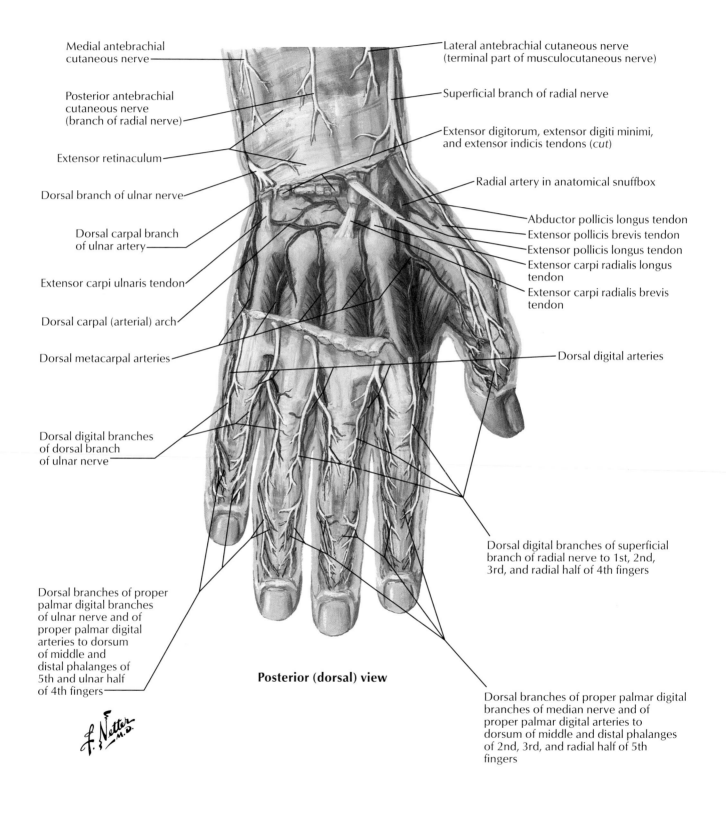

Medial antebrachial cutaneous nerve

Posterior antebrachial cutaneous nerve (branch of radial nerve)

Extensor retinaculum

Dorsal branch of ulnar nerve

Dorsal carpal branch of ulnar artery

Extensor carpi ulnaris tendon

Dorsal carpal (arterial) arch

Dorsal metacarpal arteries

Dorsal digital branches of dorsal branch of ulnar nerve

Dorsal branches of proper palmar digital branches of ulnar nerve and of proper palmar digital arteries to dorsum of middle and distal phalanges of 5th and ulnar half of 4th fingers

Lateral antebrachial cutaneous nerve (terminal part of musculocutaneous nerve)

Superficial branch of radial nerve

Extensor digitorum, extensor digiti minimi, and extensor indicis tendons (*cut*)

Radial artery in anatomical snuffbox

Abductor pollicis longus tendon
Extensor pollicis brevis tendon
Extensor pollicis longus tendon
Extensor carpi radialis longus tendon
Extensor carpi radialis brevis tendon

Dorsal digital arteries

Dorsal digital branches of superficial branch of radial nerve to 1st, 2nd, 3rd, and radial half of 4th fingers

Posterior (dorsal) view

Dorsal branches of proper palmar digital branches of median nerve and of proper palmar digital arteries to dorsum of middle and distal phalanges of 2nd, 3rd, and radial half of 5th fingers

f. Netter M.D.

Plate 469   **Wrist and Hand**

Posterior (dorsal) view

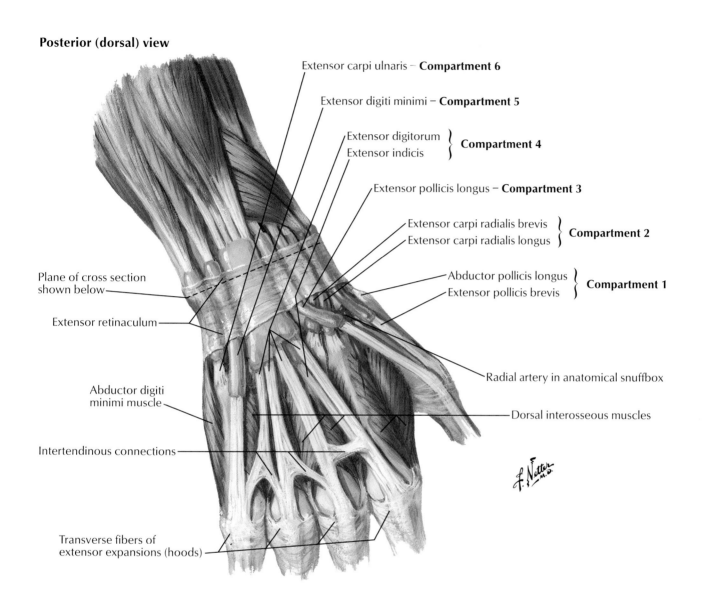

Extensor carpi ulnaris – **Compartment 6**

Extensor digiti minimi – **Compartment 5**

Extensor digitorum
Extensor indicis } **Compartment 4**

Extensor pollicis longus – **Compartment 3**

Extensor carpi radialis brevis
Extensor carpi radialis longus } **Compartment 2**

Abductor pollicis longus
Extensor pollicis brevis } **Compartment 1**

Plane of cross section shown below

Extensor retinaculum

Radial artery in anatomical snuffbox

Abductor digiti minimi muscle

Dorsal interosseous muscles

Intertendinous connections

Transverse fibers of extensor expansions (hoods)

Cross section of most distal portion of forearm

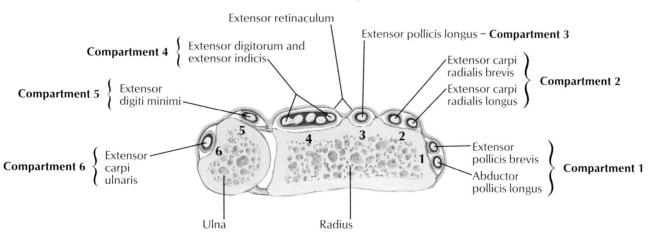

Extensor retinaculum

Extensor pollicis longus – **Compartment 3**

Compartment 4 { Extensor digitorum and extensor indicis

Extensor carpi radialis brevis
Extensor carpi radialis longus } **Compartment 2**

Compartment 5 { Extensor digiti minimi

Compartment 6 { Extensor carpi ulnaris

Extensor pollicis brevis
Abductor pollicis longus } **Compartment 1**

Ulna

Radius

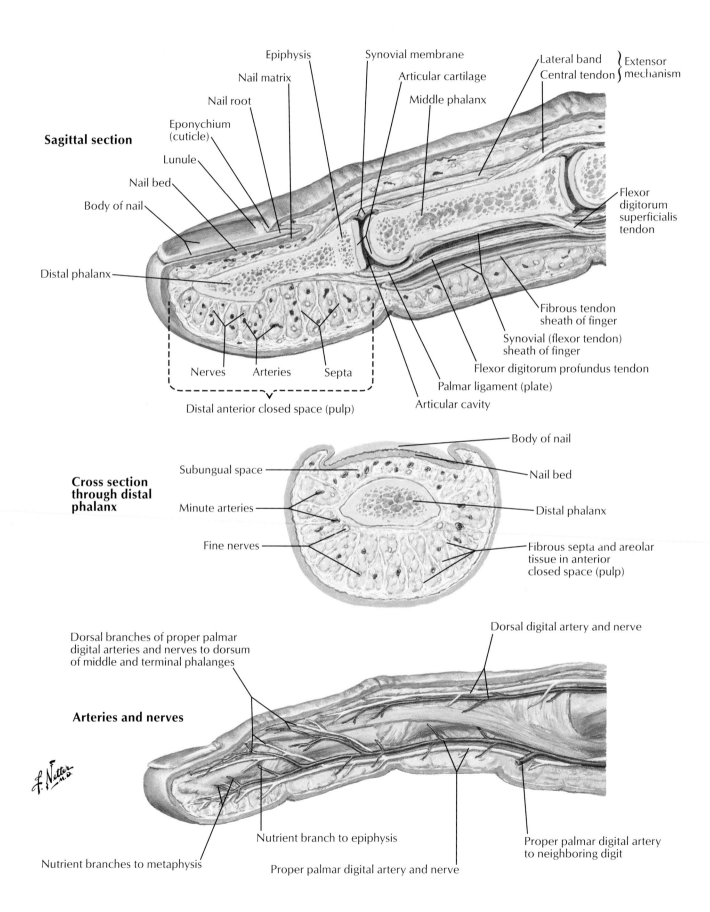

Sagittal section

Epiphysis
Nail matrix
Nail root
Eponychium (cuticle)
Lunule
Nail bed
Body of nail
Distal phalanx

Synovial membrane
Articular cartilage
Middle phalanx

Lateral band ⎫ Extensor
Central tendon ⎬ mechanism

Flexor digitorum superficialis tendon

Fibrous tendon sheath of finger
Synovial (flexor tendon) sheath of finger
Flexor digitorum profundus tendon
Palmar ligament (plate)
Articular cavity

Nerves   Arteries   Septa

Distal anterior closed space (pulp)

Cross section through distal phalanx

Subungual space
Minute arteries
Fine nerves

Body of nail
Nail bed
Distal phalanx
Fibrous septa and areolar tissue in anterior closed space (pulp)

Arteries and nerves

Dorsal branches of proper palmar digital arteries and nerves to dorsum of middle and terminal phalanges

Dorsal digital artery and nerve

Nutrient branches to metaphysis
Nutrient branch to epiphysis
Proper palmar digital artery and nerve
Proper palmar digital artery to neighboring digit

Plate 471   **Wrist and Hand**

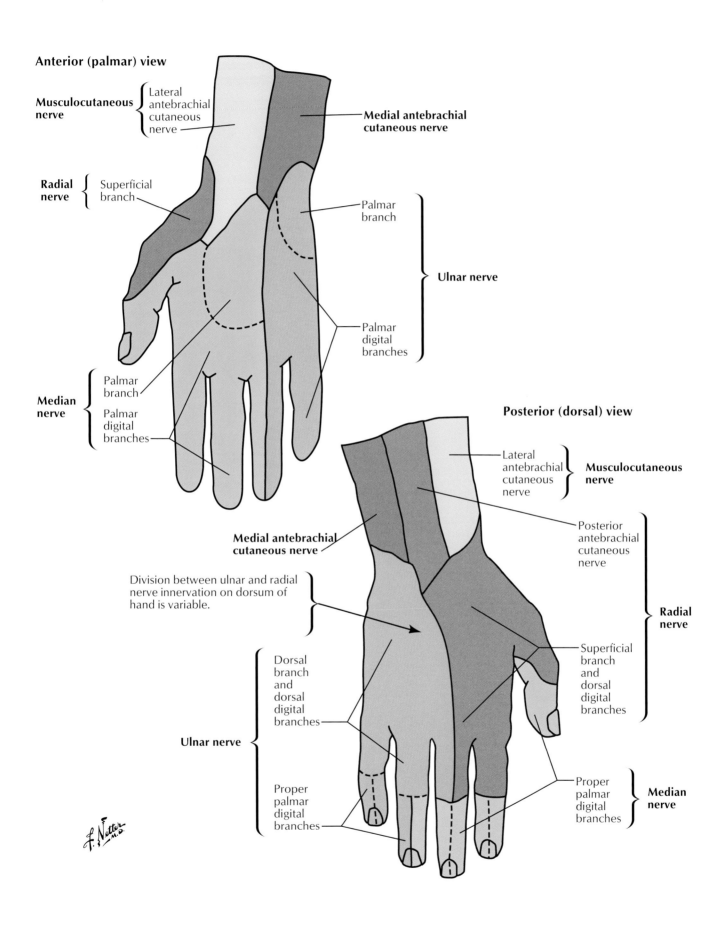

Anterior (palmar) view

Musculocutaneous nerve { Lateral antebrachial cutaneous nerve

Medial antebrachial cutaneous nerve

Radial nerve { Superficial branch

Palmar branch

Ulnar nerve

Palmar digital branches

Median nerve { Palmar branch / Palmar digital branches

Posterior (dorsal) view

Lateral antebrachial cutaneous nerve } **Musculocutaneous nerve**

Posterior antebrachial cutaneous nerve

Medial antebrachial cutaneous nerve

Division between ulnar and radial nerve innervation on dorsum of hand is variable.

Radial nerve

Superficial branch and dorsal digital branches

Ulnar nerve { Dorsal branch and dorsal digital branches / Proper palmar digital branches

Proper palmar digital branches } **Median nerve**

Anterior view

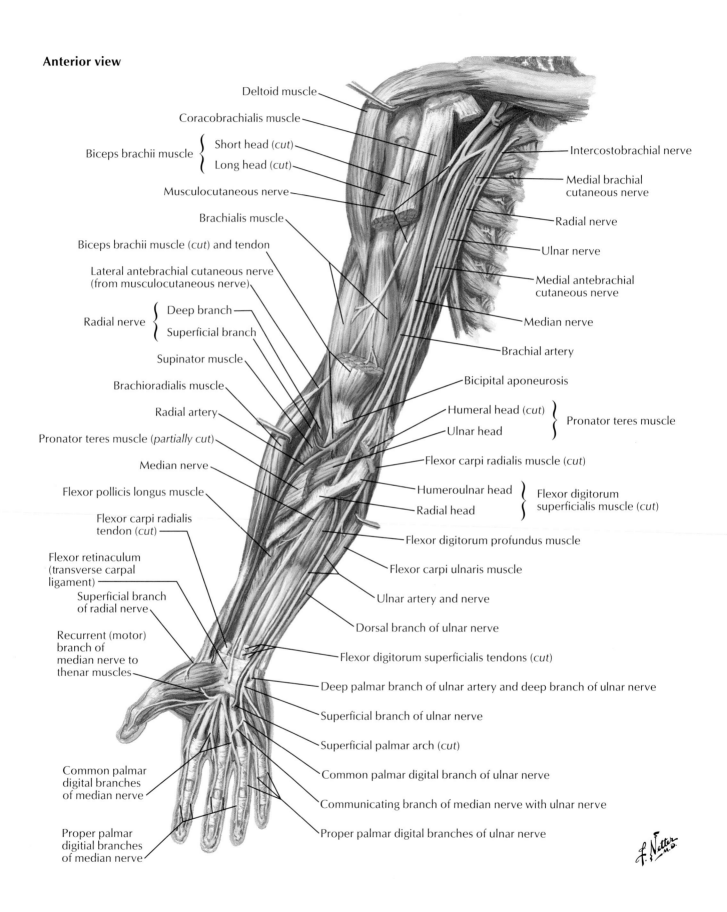

Deltoid muscle

Coracobrachialis muscle

Biceps brachii muscle { Short head (*cut*)
Long head (*cut*)

Musculocutaneous nerve

Brachialis muscle

Biceps brachii muscle (*cut*) and tendon

Lateral antebrachial cutaneous nerve (from musculocutaneous nerve)

Radial nerve { Deep branch
Superficial branch

Supinator muscle

Brachioradialis muscle

Radial artery

Pronator teres muscle (*partially cut*)

Median nerve

Flexor pollicis longus muscle

Flexor carpi radialis tendon (*cut*)

Flexor retinaculum (transverse carpal ligament)

Superficial branch of radial nerve

Recurrent (motor) branch of median nerve to thenar muscles

Common palmar digital branches of median nerve

Proper palmar digitial branches of median nerve

Intercostobrachial nerve

Medial brachial cutaneous nerve

Radial nerve

Ulnar nerve

Medial antebrachial cutaneous nerve

Median nerve

Brachial artery

Bicipital aponeurosis

Humeral head (*cut*)
Ulnar head } Pronator teres muscle

Flexor carpi radialis muscle (*cut*)

Humeroulnar head
Radial head } Flexor digitorum superficialis muscle (*cut*)

Flexor digitorum profundus muscle

Flexor carpi ulnaris muscle

Ulnar artery and nerve

Dorsal branch of ulnar nerve

Flexor digitorum superficialis tendons (*cut*)

Deep palmar branch of ulnar artery and deep branch of ulnar nerve

Superficial branch of ulnar nerve

Superficial palmar arch (*cut*)

Common palmar digital branch of ulnar nerve

Communicating branch of median nerve with ulnar nerve

Proper palmar digital branches of ulnar nerve

f. Netter M.D.

Plate 473 **Neurovasculature**

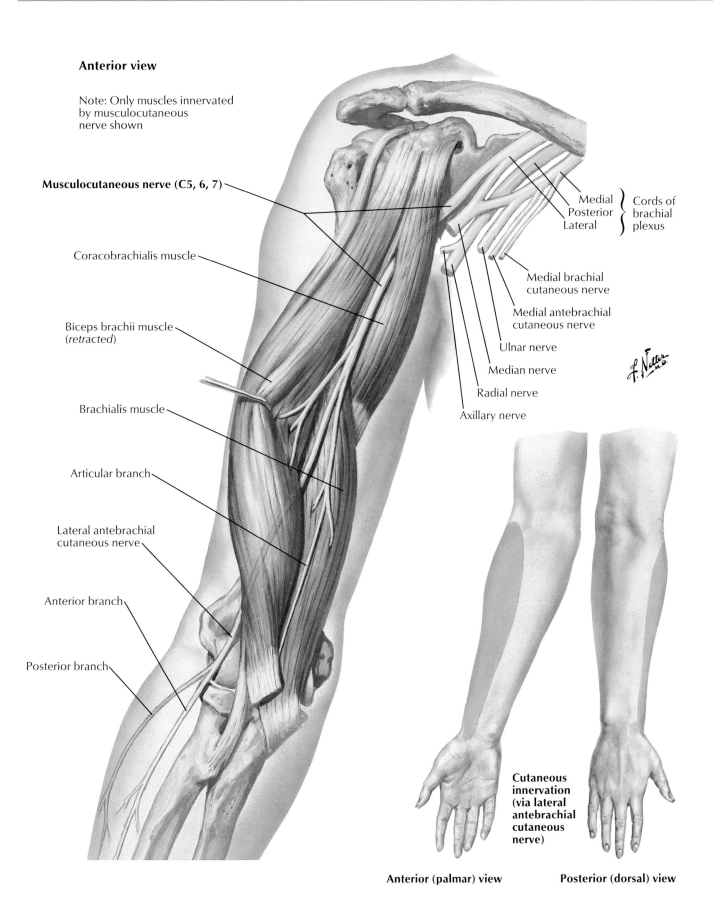

Anterior view

Note: Only muscles innervated by musculocutaneous nerve shown

Musculocutaneous nerve (C5, 6, 7)

Coracobrachialis muscle

Biceps brachii muscle (*retracted*)

Brachialis muscle

Articular branch

Lateral antebrachial cutaneous nerve

Anterior branch

Posterior branch

Medial
Posterior } Cords of brachial plexus
Lateral

Medial brachial cutaneous nerve

Medial antebrachial cutaneous nerve

Ulnar nerve

Median nerve

Radial nerve

Axillary nerve

Cutaneous innervation (via lateral antebrachial cutaneous nerve)

Anterior (palmar) view

Posterior (dorsal) view

Anterior view

Note: Only muscles innervated by median nerve shown

Musculocutaneous nerve

Median nerve (C5, 6, 7, 8, T1)
Inconstant contribution

Pronator teres muscle (humeral head)

Articular branch

Flexor carpi radialis muscle

Palmaris longus muscle

Pronator teres muscle (ulnar head)

Flexor digitorum superficialis muscle (*turned up*)

Flexor digitorum profundus muscle (lateral part supplied by median [anterior interosseous] nerve; medial part supplied by ulnar nerve)

Anterior interosseous nerve

Flexor pollicis longus muscle

Pronator quadratus muscle

Palmar branch of median nerve

Thenar muscles
{ Abductor pollicis brevis
Opponens pollicis
Superficial head of flexor pollicis brevis (deep head supplied by ulnar nerve)

1st and 2nd lumbrical muscles

Dorsal branches to dorsum of middle and distal phalanges

Medial
Posterior
Lateral
} Cords of brachial plexus

Medial brachial cutaneous nerve

Medial antebrachial cutaneous nerve

Axillary nerve

Radial nerve

Ulnar nerve

Communicating branch of median nerve with ulnar nerve

Common palmar digital nerves

Proper palmar digital nerves

Cutaneous innervation

Palmar view

Posterior (dorsal) view

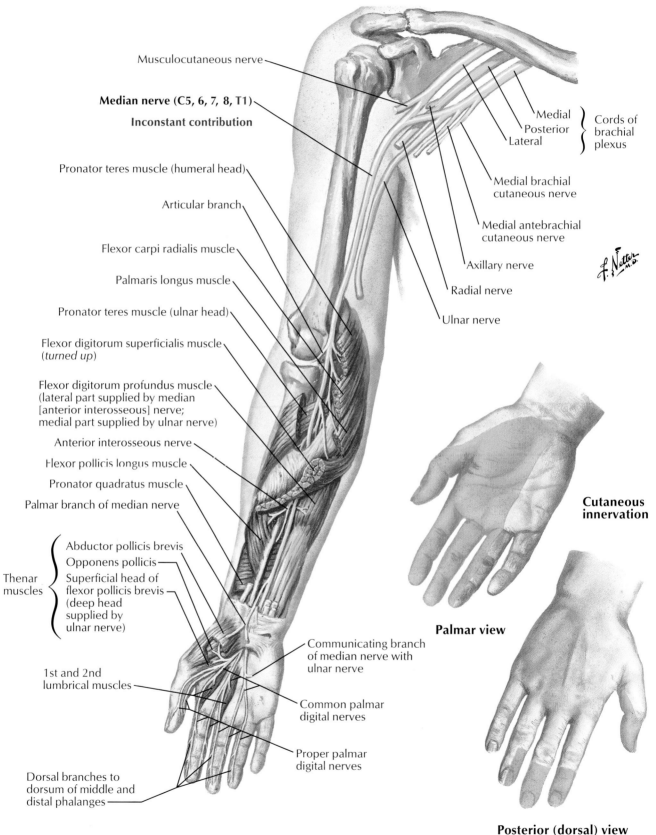

Plate 475   **Neurovasculature**

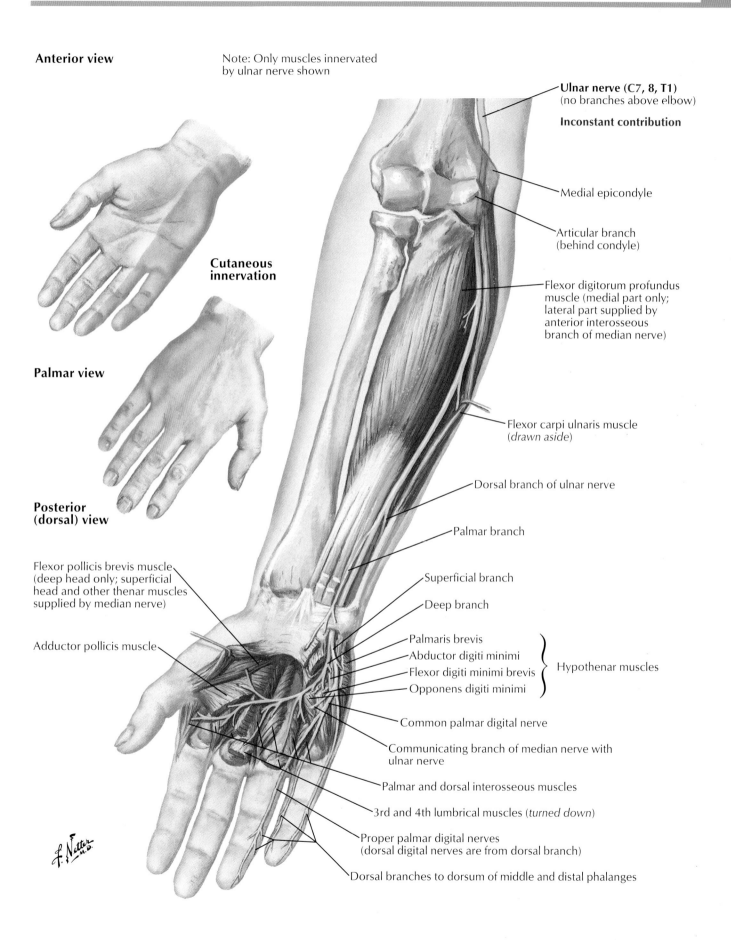

Anterior view

Note: Only muscles innervated
by ulnar nerve shown

Ulnar nerve (C7, 8, T1)
(no branches above elbow)

Inconstant contribution

Medial epicondyle

Articular branch
(behind condyle)

Flexor digitorum profundus
muscle (medial part only;
lateral part supplied by
anterior interosseous
branch of median nerve)

Flexor carpi ulnaris muscle
(*drawn aside*)

Dorsal branch of ulnar nerve

Palmar branch

Superficial branch

Deep branch

Palmaris brevis
Abductor digiti minimi   } Hypothenar muscles
Flexor digiti minimi brevis
Opponens digiti minimi

Common palmar digital nerve

Communicating branch of median nerve with
ulnar nerve

Palmar and dorsal interosseous muscles

3rd and 4th lumbrical muscles (*turned down*)

Proper palmar digital nerves
(dorsal digital nerves are from dorsal branch)

Dorsal branches to dorsum of middle and distal phalanges

**Cutaneous
innervation**

Palmar view

Posterior
(dorsal) view

Flexor pollicis brevis muscle
(deep head only; superficial
head and other thenar muscles
supplied by median nerve)

Adductor pollicis muscle

Radial Nerve in Arm and Nerves of Posterior Shoulder

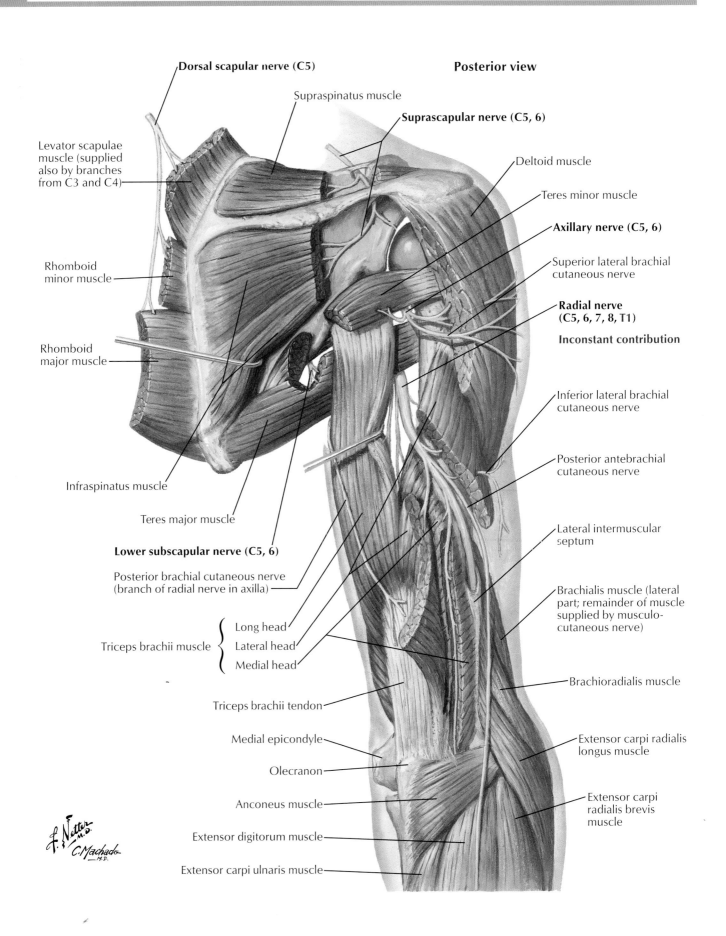

Dorsal scapular nerve (C5)

Posterior view

Supraspinatus muscle

Suprascapular nerve (C5, 6)

Levator scapulae muscle (supplied also by branches from C3 and C4)

Deltoid muscle

Teres minor muscle

Axillary nerve (C5, 6)

Superior lateral brachial cutaneous nerve

Rhomboid minor muscle

Radial nerve (C5, 6, 7, 8, T1)

Inconstant contribution

Rhomboid major muscle

Inferior lateral brachial cutaneous nerve

Posterior antebrachial cutaneous nerve

Infraspinatus muscle

Teres major muscle

Lateral intermuscular septum

Lower subscapular nerve (C5, 6)

Posterior brachial cutaneous nerve (branch of radial nerve in axilla)

Brachialis muscle (lateral part; remainder of muscle supplied by musculo-cutaneous nerve)

Triceps brachii muscle { Long head / Lateral head / Medial head

Triceps brachii tendon

Brachioradialis muscle

Medial epicondyle

Extensor carpi radialis longus muscle

Olecranon

Anconeus muscle

Extensor carpi radialis brevis muscle

Extensor digitorum muscle

Extensor carpi ulnaris muscle

Plate 477

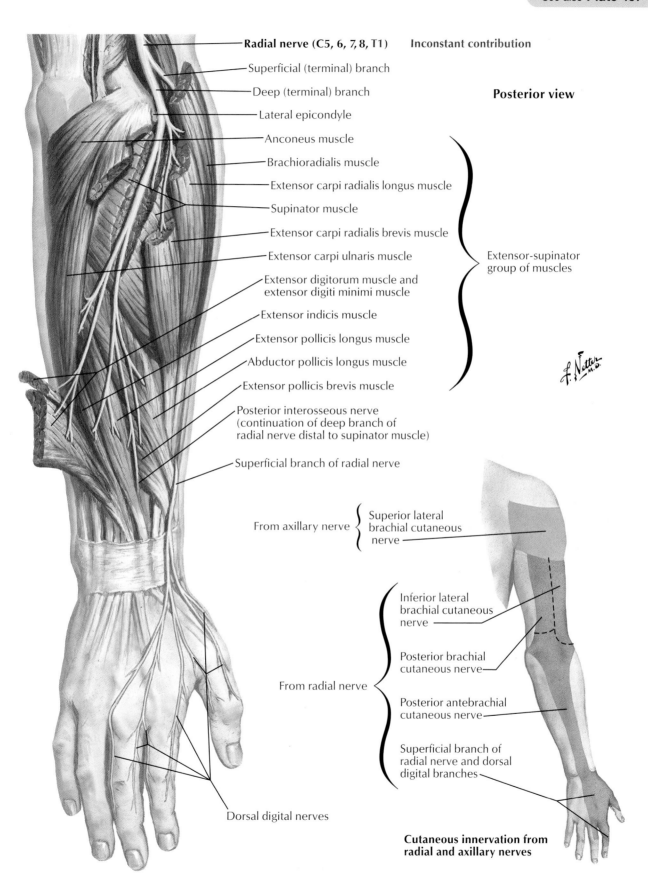

Radial nerve (C5, 6, 7, 8, T1)   Inconstant contribution

Superficial (terminal) branch

Deep (terminal) branch   **Posterior view**

Lateral epicondyle

Anconeus muscle

Brachioradialis muscle

Extensor carpi radialis longus muscle

Supinator muscle

Extensor carpi radialis brevis muscle   Extensor-supinator group of muscles

Extensor carpi ulnaris muscle

Extensor digitorum muscle and extensor digiti minimi muscle

Extensor indicis muscle

Extensor pollicis longus muscle

Abductor pollicis longus muscle

Extensor pollicis brevis muscle

Posterior interosseous nerve (continuation of deep branch of radial nerve distal to supinator muscle)

Superficial branch of radial nerve

From axillary nerve { Superior lateral brachial cutaneous nerve

Inferior lateral brachial cutaneous nerve

Posterior brachial cutaneous nerve

From radial nerve

Posterior antebrachial cutaneous nerve

Superficial branch of radial nerve and dorsal digital branches

Dorsal digital nerves

Cutaneous innervation from radial and axillary nerves

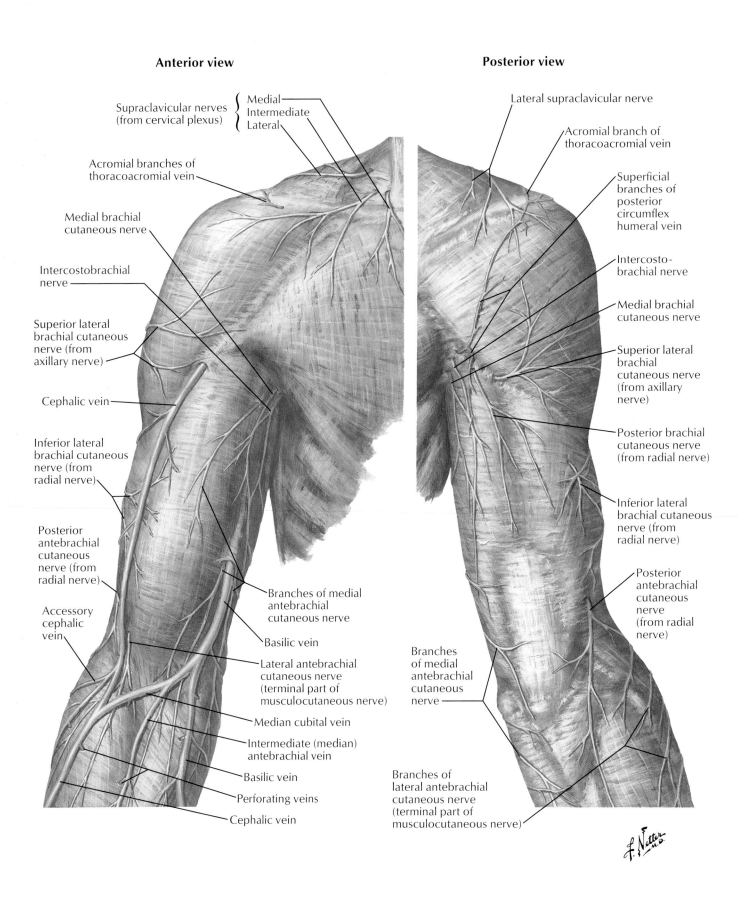

Anterior view

Supraclavicular nerves (from cervical plexus) { Medial / Intermediate / Lateral

Acromial branches of thoracoacromial vein

Medial brachial cutaneous nerve

Intercostobrachial nerve

Superior lateral brachial cutaneous nerve (from axillary nerve)

Cephalic vein

Inferior lateral brachial cutaneous nerve (from radial nerve)

Posterior antebrachial cutaneous nerve (from radial nerve)

Accessory cephalic vein

Branches of medial antebrachial cutaneous nerve

Basilic vein

Lateral antebrachial cutaneous nerve (terminal part of musculocutaneous nerve)

Median cubital vein

Intermediate (median) antebrachial vein

Basilic vein

Perforating veins

Cephalic vein

Posterior view

Lateral supraclavicular nerve

Acromial branch of thoracoacromial vein

Superficial branches of posterior circumflex humeral vein

Intercosto-brachial nerve

Medial brachial cutaneous nerve

Superior lateral brachial cutaneous nerve (from axillary nerve)

Posterior brachial cutaneous nerve (from radial nerve)

Inferior lateral brachial cutaneous nerve (from radial nerve)

Posterior antebrachial cutaneous nerve (from radial nerve)

Branches of medial antebrachial cutaneous nerve

Branches of lateral antebrachial cutaneous nerve (terminal part of musculocutaneous nerve)

Plate 479   **Neurovasculature**

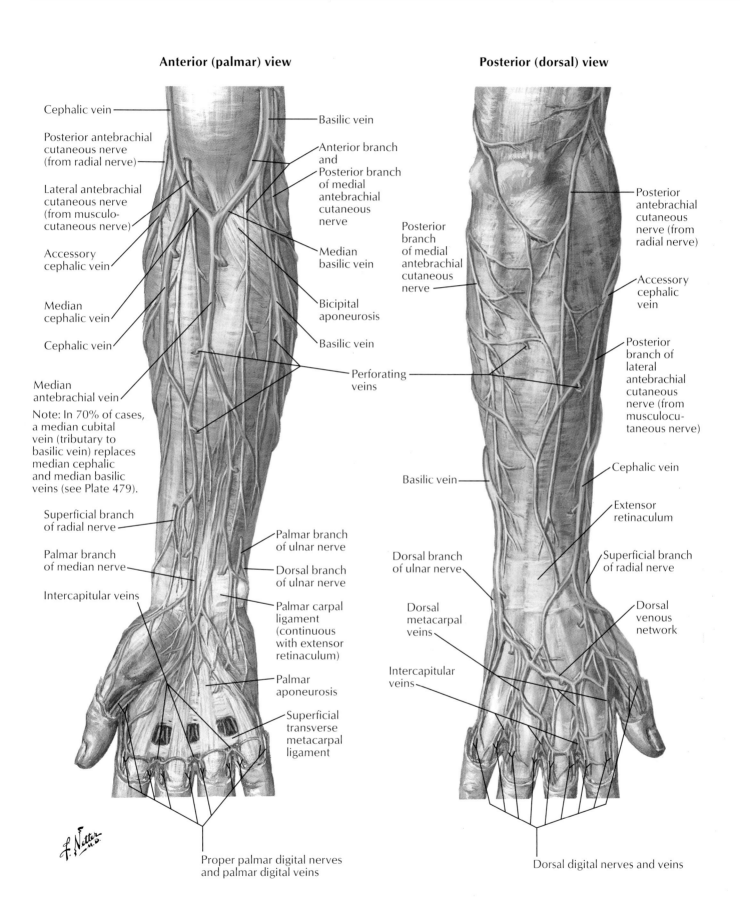

Anterior (palmar) view

Cephalic vein

Posterior antebrachial cutaneous nerve (from radial nerve)

Lateral antebrachial cutaneous nerve (from musculo-cutaneous nerve)

Accessory cephalic vein

Median cephalic vein

Cephalic vein

Median antebrachial vein

Note: In 70% of cases, a median cubital vein (tributary to basilic vein) replaces median cephalic and median basilic veins (see Plate 479).

Superficial branch of radial nerve

Palmar branch of median nerve

Intercapitular veins

Basilic vein

Anterior branch and Posterior branch of medial antebrachial cutaneous nerve

Median basilic vein

Bicipital aponeurosis

Basilic vein

Perforating veins

Palmar branch of ulnar nerve

Dorsal branch of ulnar nerve

Palmar carpal ligament (continuous with extensor retinaculum)

Palmar aponeurosis

Superficial transverse metacarpal ligament

Proper palmar digital nerves and palmar digital veins

Posterior (dorsal) view

Posterior branch of medial antebrachial cutaneous nerve

Basilic vein

Dorsal branch of ulnar nerve

Dorsal metacarpal veins

Intercapitular veins

Posterior antebrachial cutaneous nerve (from radial nerve)

Accessory cephalic vein

Posterior branch of lateral antebrachial cutaneous nerve (from musculocutaneous nerve)

Cephalic vein

Extensor retinaculum

Superficial branch of radial nerve

Dorsal venous network

Dorsal digital nerves and veins

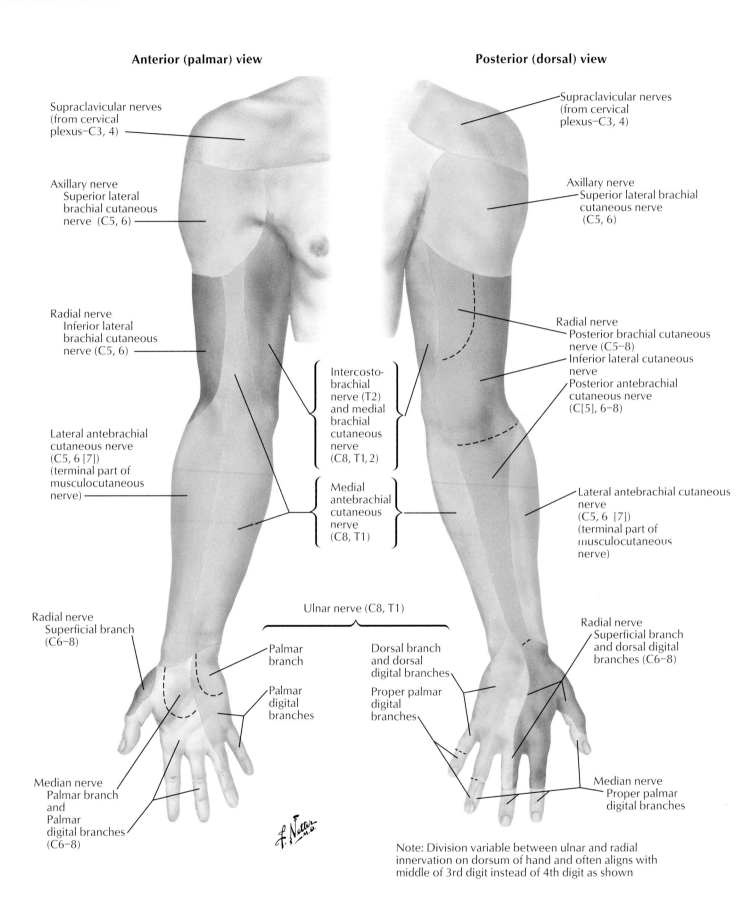

Anterior (palmar) view

Posterior (dorsal) view

Supraclavicular nerves
(from cervical
plexus–C3, 4)

Supraclavicular nerves
(from cervical
plexus–C3, 4)

Axillary nerve
Superior lateral
brachial cutaneous
nerve (C5, 6)

Axillary nerve
Superior lateral brachial
cutaneous nerve
(C5, 6)

Radial nerve
Inferior lateral
brachial cutaneous
nerve (C5, 6)

Radial nerve
Posterior brachial cutaneous
nerve (C5–8)
Inferior lateral cutaneous
nerve
Posterior antebrachial
cutaneous nerve
(C[5], 6–8)

Intercosto-
brachial
nerve (T2)
and medial
brachial
cutaneous
nerve
(C8, T1, 2)

Lateral antebrachial
cutaneous nerve
(C5, 6 [7])
(terminal part of
musculocutaneous
nerve)

Medial
antebrachial
cutaneous
nerve
(C8, T1)

Lateral antebrachial cutaneous
nerve
(C5, 6 [7])
(terminal part of
musculocutaneous
nerve)

Ulnar nerve (C8, T1)

Radial nerve
Superficial branch
(C6–8)

Palmar
branch

Dorsal branch
and dorsal
digital branches

Radial nerve
Superficial branch
and dorsal digital
branches (C6–8)

Palmar
digital
branches

Proper palmar
digital
branches

Median nerve
Palmar branch
and
Palmar
digital branches
(C6–8)

Median nerve
Proper palmar
digital branches

Note: Division variable between ulnar and radial
innervation on dorsum of hand and often aligns with
middle of 3rd digit instead of 4th digit as shown

Plate 481   **Neurovasculature**

Note: Schematic demarcation of dermatomes (according to Keegan and Garrett) shown as distinct segments. There is actually considerable overlap between adjacent dermatomes. An alternative dermatome map is provided by Foerster (see references).

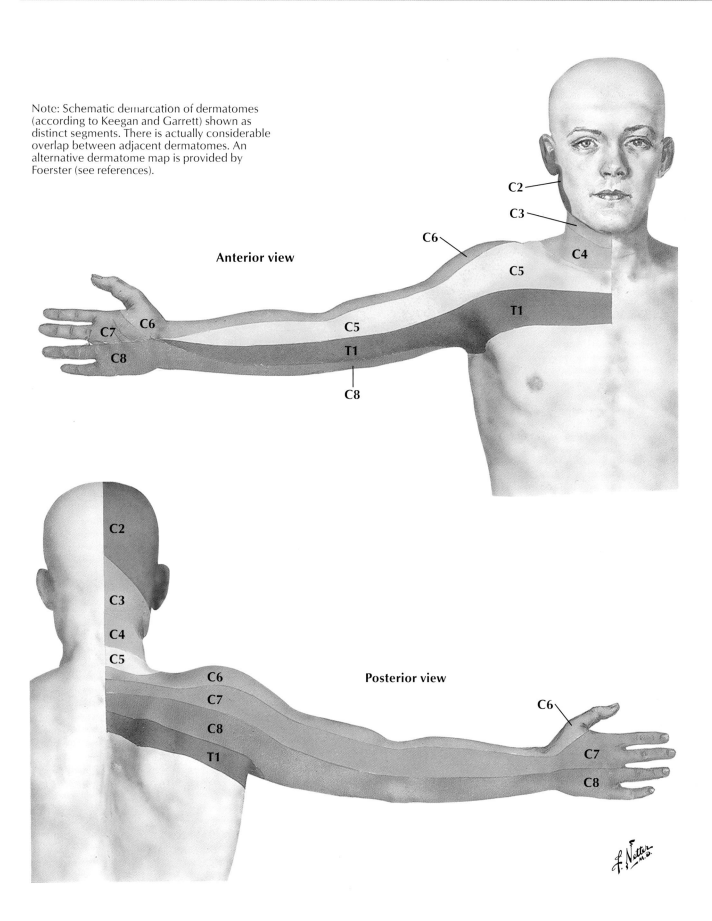

Anterior view

Posterior view

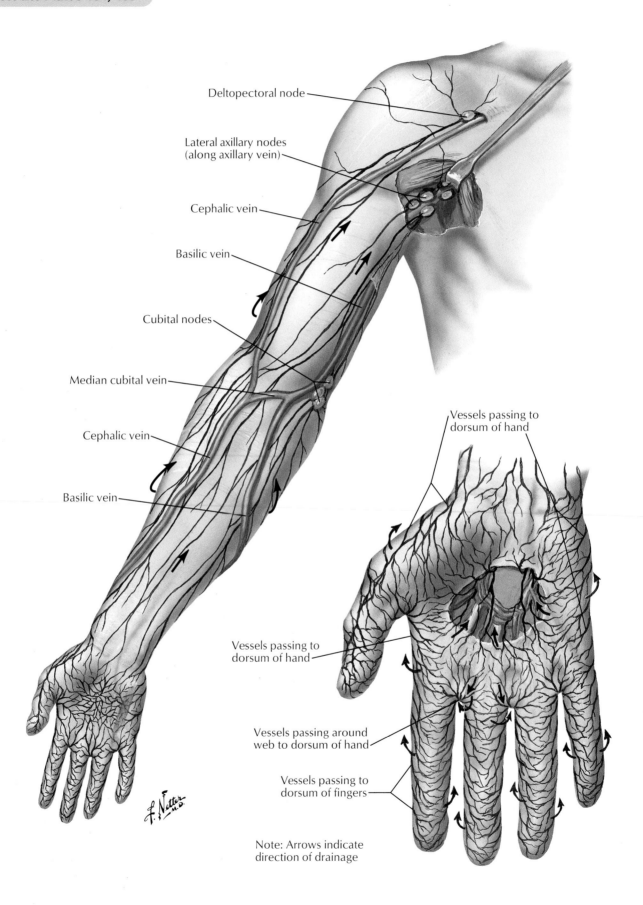

Deltopectoral node

Lateral axillary nodes (along axillary vein)

Cephalic vein

Basilic vein

Cubital nodes

Median cubital vein

Cephalic vein

Basilic vein

Vessels passing to dorsum of hand

Vessels passing to dorsum of hand

Vessels passing around web to dorsum of hand

Vessels passing to dorsum of fingers

Note: Arrows indicate direction of drainage

Plate 483

Neurovasculature

Regional Scans

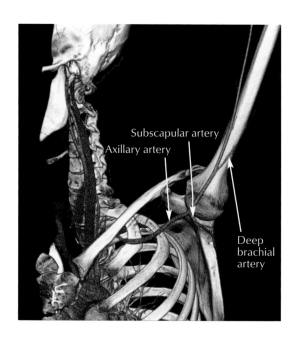

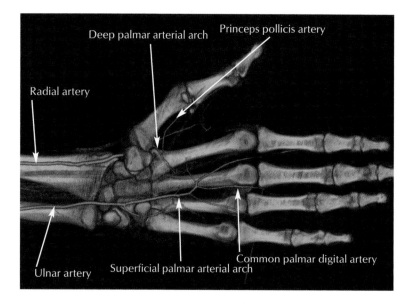

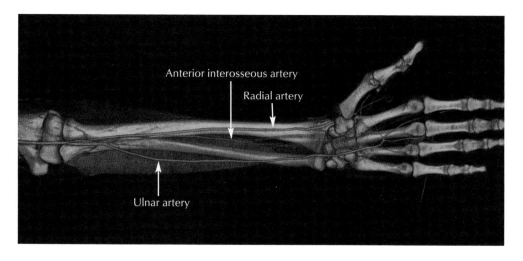

Section 7 **Lower Limb**

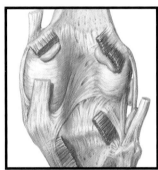
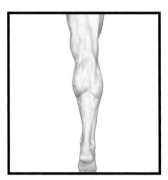
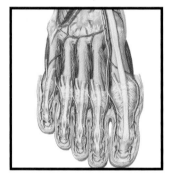
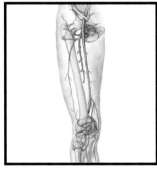

Topographic Anatomy
Plate 485

Hip and Thigh
Plates 486–505

7 Lower Limb

Knee
Plates 506–512

Leg
Plates 513–522

Ankle and Foot
Plates 523–537

Neurovasculature
Plates 538–546

Regional Scans
Plate 547

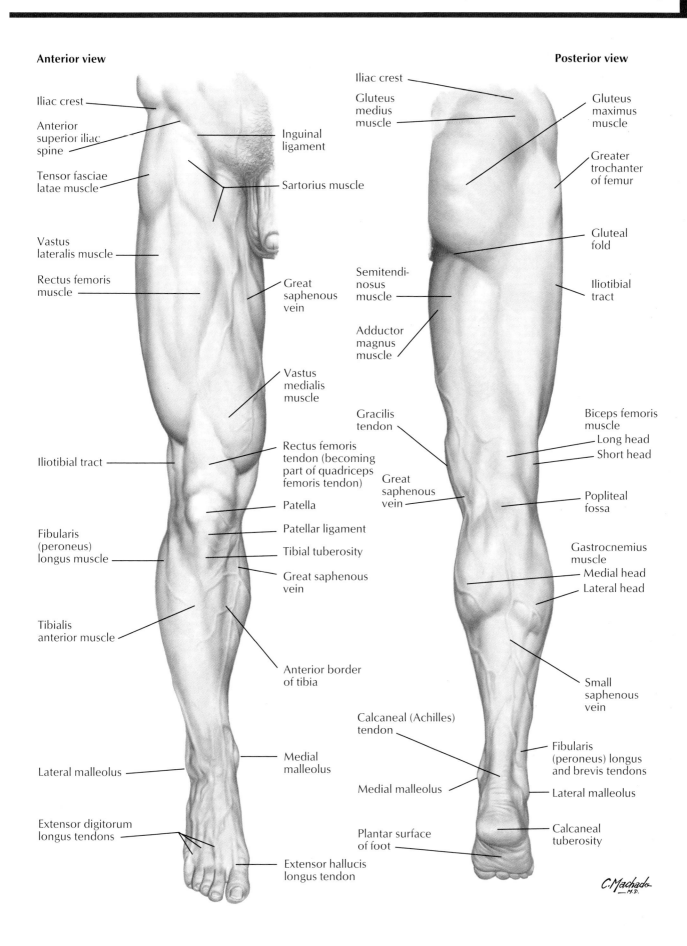

Anterior view

Posterior view

Iliac crest

Anterior superior iliac spine

Tensor fasciae latae muscle

Vastus lateralis muscle

Rectus femoris muscle

Iliotibial tract

Fibularis (peroneus) longus muscle

Tibialis anterior muscle

Lateral malleolus

Extensor digitorum longus tendons

Inguinal ligament

Sartorius muscle

Great saphenous vein

Vastus medialis muscle

Rectus femoris tendon (becoming part of quadriceps femoris tendon)

Patella

Patellar ligament

Tibial tuberosity

Great saphenous vein

Anterior border of tibia

Medial malleolus

Extensor hallucis longus tendon

Iliac crest

Gluteus medius muscle

Semitendinosus muscle

Adductor magnus muscle

Gracilis tendon

Great saphenous vein

Calcaneal (Achilles) tendon

Medial malleolus

Plantar surface of foot

Gluteus maximus muscle

Greater trochanter of femur

Gluteal fold

Iliotibial tract

Biceps femoris muscle
Long head
Short head

Popliteal fossa

Gastrocnemius muscle
Medial head
Lateral head

Small saphenous vein

Fibularis (peroneus) longus and brevis tendons

Lateral malleolus

Calcaneal tuberosity

C. Machado —M.D.

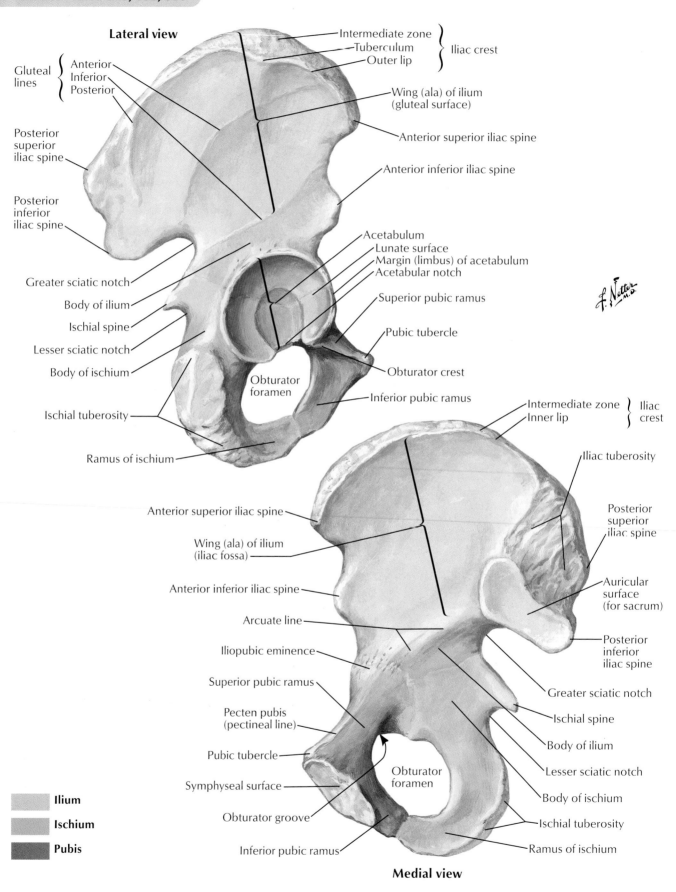

Lateral view

Gluteal lines {
- Anterior
- Inferior
- Posterior

Intermediate zone
Tuberculum } Iliac crest
Outer lip

Posterior superior iliac spine

Wing (ala) of ilium (gluteal surface)

Anterior superior iliac spine

Anterior inferior iliac spine

Posterior inferior iliac spine

Acetabulum
Lunate surface
Margin (limbus) of acetabulum
Acetabular notch

Greater sciatic notch

Superior pubic ramus

Body of ilium

Pubic tubercle

Ischial spine

Lesser sciatic notch

Obturator crest

Body of ischium

Obturator foramen

Inferior pubic ramus

Ischial tuberosity

Ramus of ischium

Intermediate zone
Inner lip } Iliac crest

Iliac tuberosity

Anterior superior iliac spine

Posterior superior iliac spine

Wing (ala) of ilium (iliac fossa)

Anterior inferior iliac spine

Auricular surface (for sacrum)

Arcuate line

Iliopubic eminence

Posterior inferior iliac spine

Superior pubic ramus

Greater sciatic notch

Pecten pubis (pectineal line)

Ischial spine

Body of ilium

Pubic tubercle

Lesser sciatic notch

Symphyseal surface

Obturator foramen

Body of ischium

Obturator groove

Ischial tuberosity

Inferior pubic ramus

Ramus of ischium

Medial view

- Ilium
- Ischium
- Pubis

Plate 486

Hip and Thigh

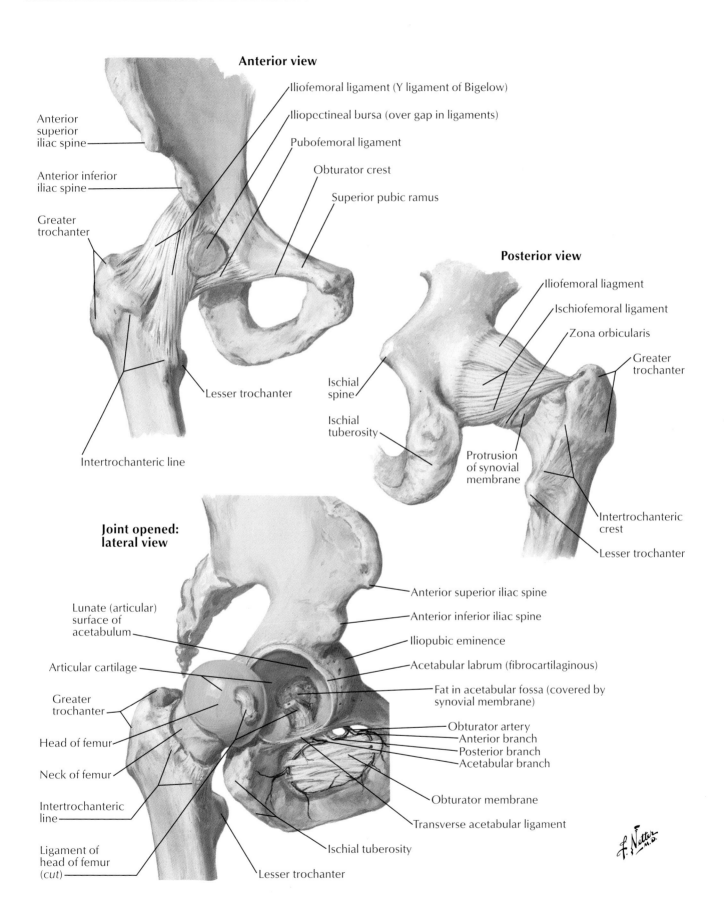

Anterior view

Anterior superior iliac spine

Anterior inferior iliac spine

Greater trochanter

Iliofemoral ligament (Y ligament of Bigelow)

Iliopectineal bursa (over gap in ligaments)

Pubofemoral ligament

Obturator crest

Superior pubic ramus

Lesser trochanter

Intertrochanteric line

Posterior view

Iliofemoral liagment

Ischiofemoral ligament

Zona orbicularis

Greater trochanter

Ischial spine

Ischial tuberosity

Protrusion of synovial membrane

Intertrochanteric crest

Lesser trochanter

Joint opened: lateral view

Lunate (articular) surface of acetabulum

Articular cartilage

Greater trochanter

Head of femur

Neck of femur

Intertrochanteric line

Ligament of head of femur (*cut*)

Lesser trochanter

Ischial tuberosity

Anterior superior iliac spine

Anterior inferior iliac spine

Iliopubic eminence

Acetabular labrum (fibrocartilaginous)

Fat in acetabular fossa (covered by synovial membrane)

Obturator artery
Anterior branch
Posterior branch
Acetabular branch

Obturator membrane

Transverse acetabular ligament

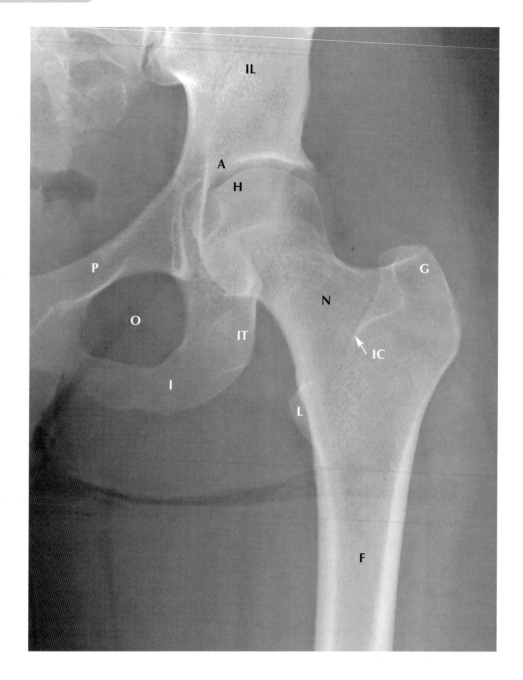

A	Acetabulum
F	Femur
G	Greater trochanter
H	Head of femur
I	Ischium
IC	Intertrochanteric crest
IL	Ilium
IT	Ischial tuberosity
L	Lesser trochanter
N	Neck
O	Obturator foramen
P	Pubis (superior ramus)

Plate 488   **Hip and Thigh**

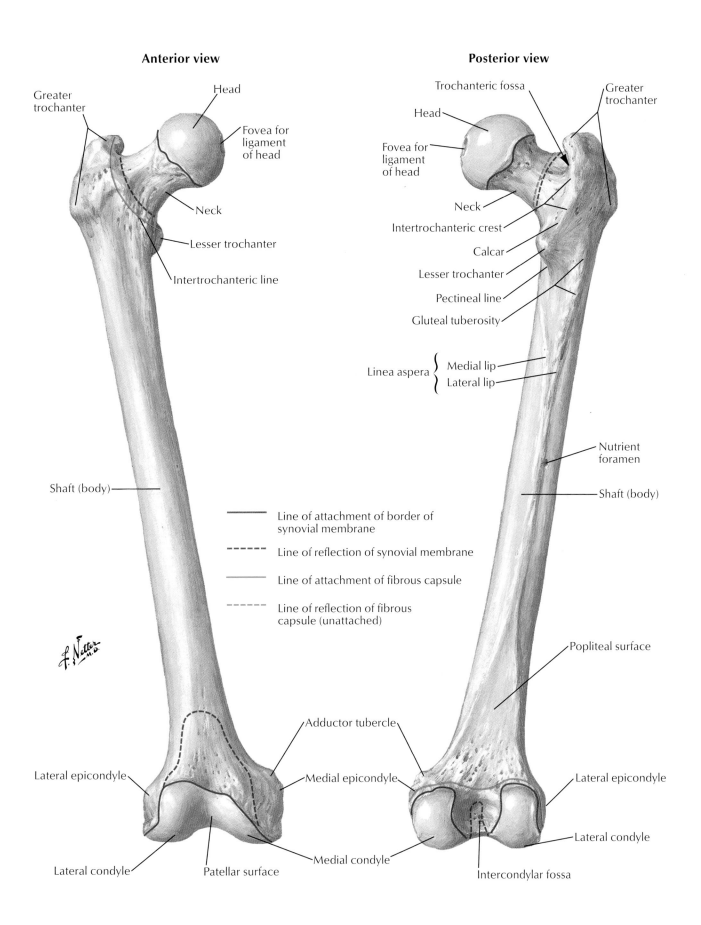

Anterior view

Greater trochanter

Head

Fovea for ligament of head

Neck

Lesser trochanter

Intertrochanteric line

Shaft (body)

——— Line of attachment of border of synovial membrane

- - - - Line of reflection of synovial membrane

——— Line of attachment of fibrous capsule

- - - - Line of reflection of fibrous capsule (unattached)

Lateral epicondyle

Adductor tubercle

Medial epicondyle

Lateral condyle

Patellar surface

Medial condyle

Posterior view

Trochanteric fossa

Greater trochanter

Head

Fovea for ligament of head

Neck

Intertrochanteric crest

Calcar

Lesser trochanter

Pectineal line

Gluteal tuberosity

Linea aspera { Medial lip / Lateral lip

Nutrient foramen

Shaft (body)

Popliteal surface

Medial epicondyle

Lateral epicondyle

Lateral condyle

Intercondylar fossa

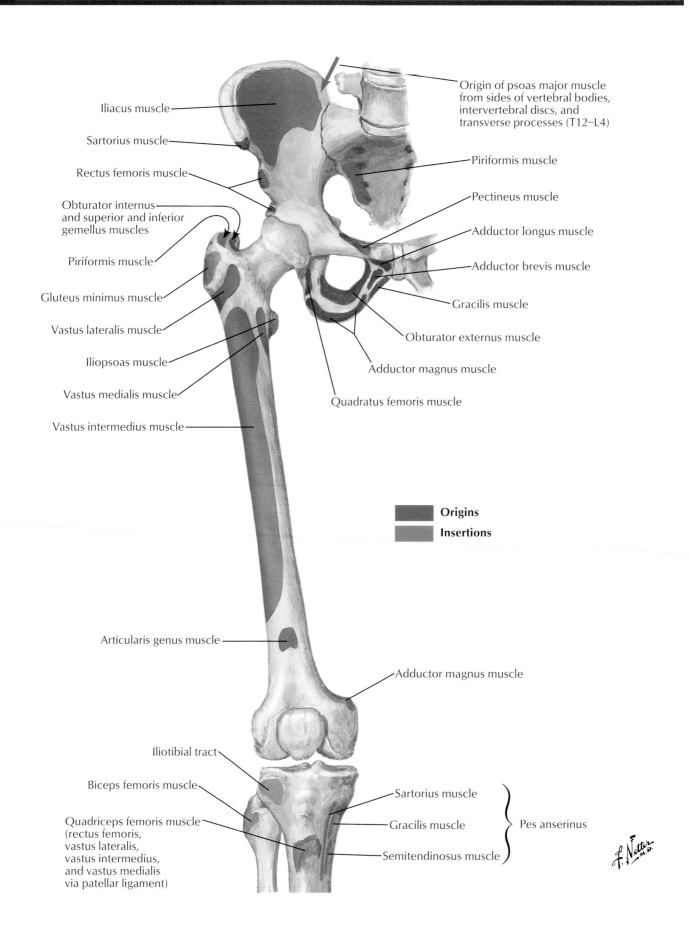

Iliacus muscle

Sartorius muscle

Rectus femoris muscle

Obturator internus
and superior and inferior
gemellus muscles

Piriformis muscle

Gluteus minimus muscle

Vastus lateralis muscle

Iliopsoas muscle

Vastus medialis muscle

Vastus intermedius muscle

Origin of psoas major muscle
from sides of vertebral bodies,
intervertebral discs, and
transverse processes (T12–L4)

Piriformis muscle

Pectineus muscle

Adductor longus muscle

Adductor brevis muscle

Gracilis muscle

Obturator externus muscle

Adductor magnus muscle

Quadratus femoris muscle

■ Origins
■ Insertions

Articularis genus muscle

Adductor magnus muscle

Iliotibial tract

Biceps femoris muscle

Quadriceps femoris muscle
(rectus femoris,
vastus lateralis,
vastus intermedius,
and vastus medialis
via patellar ligament)

Sartorius muscle

Gracilis muscle

Semitendinosus muscle

⎫
⎬ Pes anserinus
⎭

F. Netter
M.D.

Plate 490

Hip and Thigh

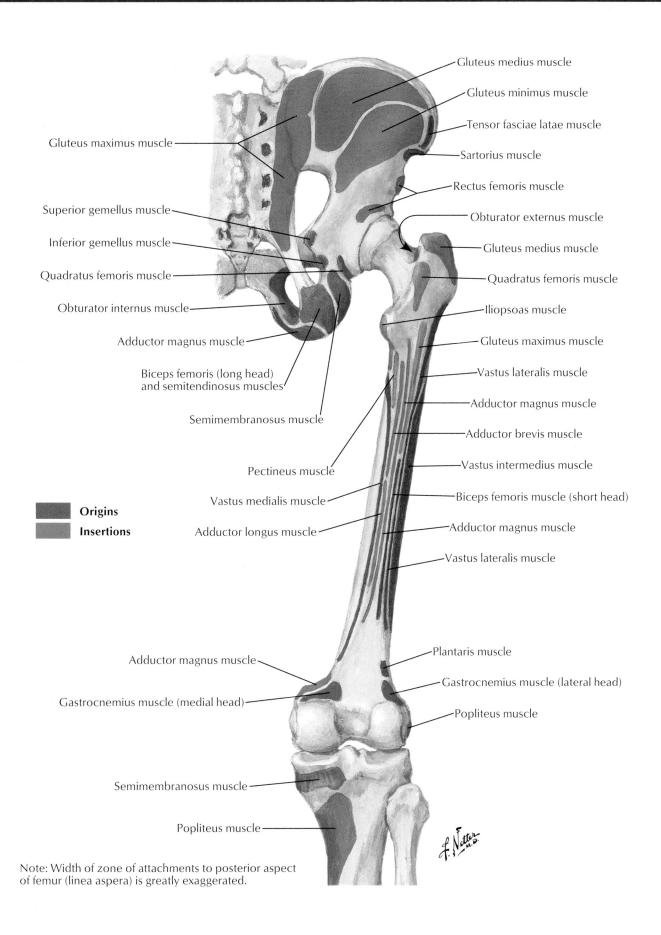

Gluteus medius muscle

Gluteus minimus muscle

Tensor fasciae latae muscle

Sartorius muscle

Gluteus maximus muscle

Rectus femoris muscle

Obturator externus muscle

Gluteus medius muscle

Superior gemellus muscle

Inferior gemellus muscle

Quadratus femoris muscle

Quadratus femoris muscle

Obturator internus muscle

Iliopsoas muscle

Gluteus maximus muscle

Adductor magnus muscle

Vastus lateralis muscle

Biceps femoris (long head)
and semitendinosus muscles

Adductor magnus muscle

Adductor brevis muscle

Semimembranosus muscle

Vastus intermedius muscle

Origins

Insertions

Pectineus muscle

Biceps femoris muscle (short head)

Vastus medialis muscle

Adductor magnus muscle

Adductor longus muscle

Vastus lateralis muscle

Adductor magnus muscle

Plantaris muscle

Gastrocnemius muscle (lateral head)

Gastrocnemius muscle (medial head)

Popliteus muscle

Semimembranosus muscle

Popliteus muscle

Note: Width of zone of attachments to posterior aspect
of femur (linea aspera) is greatly exaggerated.

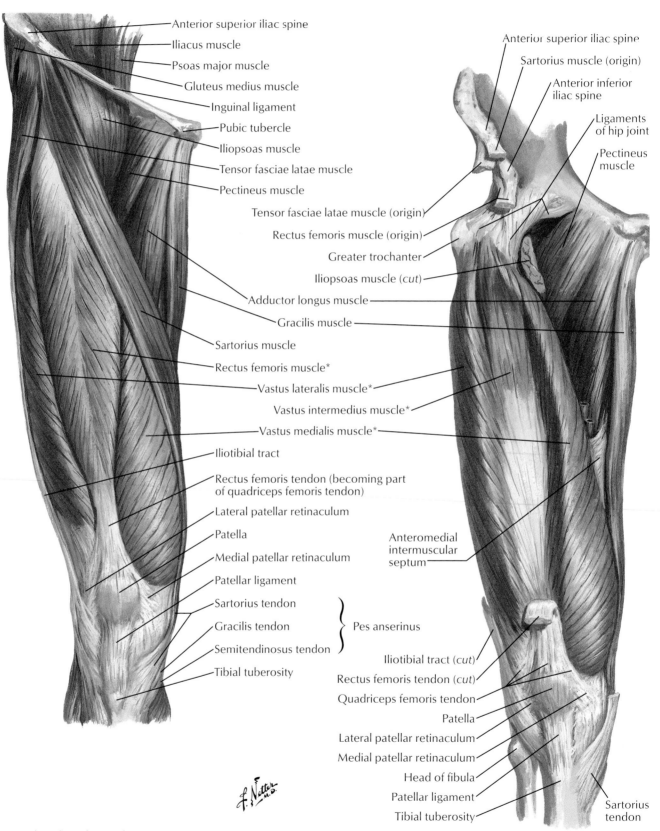

Anterior superior iliac spine

Iliacus muscle

Psoas major muscle

Gluteus medius muscle

Inguinal ligament

Pubic tubercle

Iliopsoas muscle

Tensor fasciae latae muscle

Pectineus muscle

Tensor fasciae latae muscle (origin)

Rectus femoris muscle (origin)

Greater trochanter

Iliopsoas muscle (*cut*)

Adductor longus muscle

Gracilis muscle

Sartorius muscle

Rectus femoris muscle*

Vastus lateralis muscle*

Vastus intermedius muscle*

Vastus medialis muscle*

Iliotibial tract

Rectus femoris tendon (becoming part of quadriceps femoris tendon)

Lateral patellar retinaculum

Patella

Medial patellar retinaculum

Patellar ligament

Sartorius tendon

Gracilis tendon

Semitendinosus tendon

Tibial tuberosity

Pes anserinus

Anterior superior iliac spine

Sartorius muscle (origin)

Anterior inferior iliac spine

Ligaments of hip joint

Pectineus muscle

Anteromedial intermuscular septum

Iliotibial tract (*cut*)

Rectus femoris tendon (*cut*)

Quadriceps femoris tendon

Patella

Lateral patellar retinaculum

Medial patellar retinaculum

Head of fibula

Patellar ligament

Tibial tuberosity

Sartorius tendon

*Muscles of quadriceps femoris

Plate 492

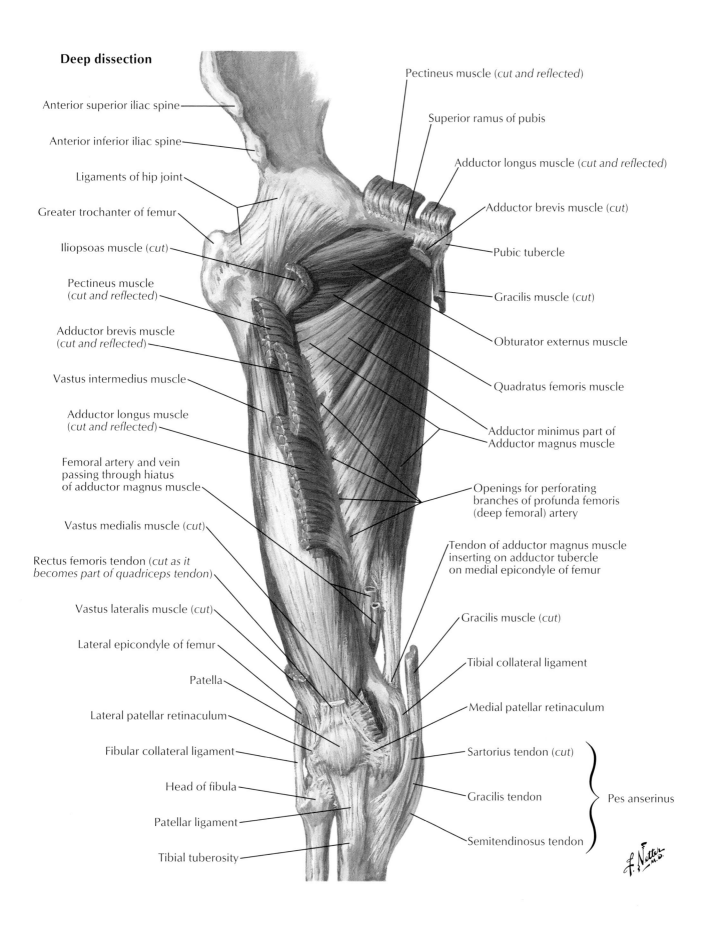

Deep dissection

Anterior superior iliac spine

Anterior inferior iliac spine

Ligaments of hip joint

Greater trochanter of femur

Iliopsoas muscle (*cut*)

Pectineus muscle
(*cut and reflected*)

Adductor brevis muscle
(*cut and reflected*)

Vastus intermedius muscle

Adductor longus muscle
(*cut and reflected*)

Femoral artery and vein
passing through hiatus
of adductor magnus muscle

Vastus medialis muscle (*cut*)

Rectus femoris tendon (*cut as it
becomes part of quadriceps tendon*)

Vastus lateralis muscle (*cut*)

Lateral epicondyle of femur

Patella

Lateral patellar retinaculum

Fibular collateral ligament

Head of fibula

Patellar ligament

Tibial tuberosity

Pectineus muscle (*cut and reflected*)

Superior ramus of pubis

Adductor longus muscle (*cut and reflected*)

Adductor brevis muscle (*cut*)

Pubic tubercle

Gracilis muscle (*cut*)

Obturator externus muscle

Quadratus femoris muscle

Adductor minimus part of
Adductor magnus muscle

Openings for perforating
branches of profunda femoris
(deep femoral) artery

Tendon of adductor magnus muscle
inserting on adductor tubercle
on medial epicondyle of femur

Gracilis muscle (*cut*)

Tibial collateral ligament

Medial patellar retinaculum

Sartorius tendon (*cut*)

Gracilis tendon

Semitendinosus tendon

Pes anserinus

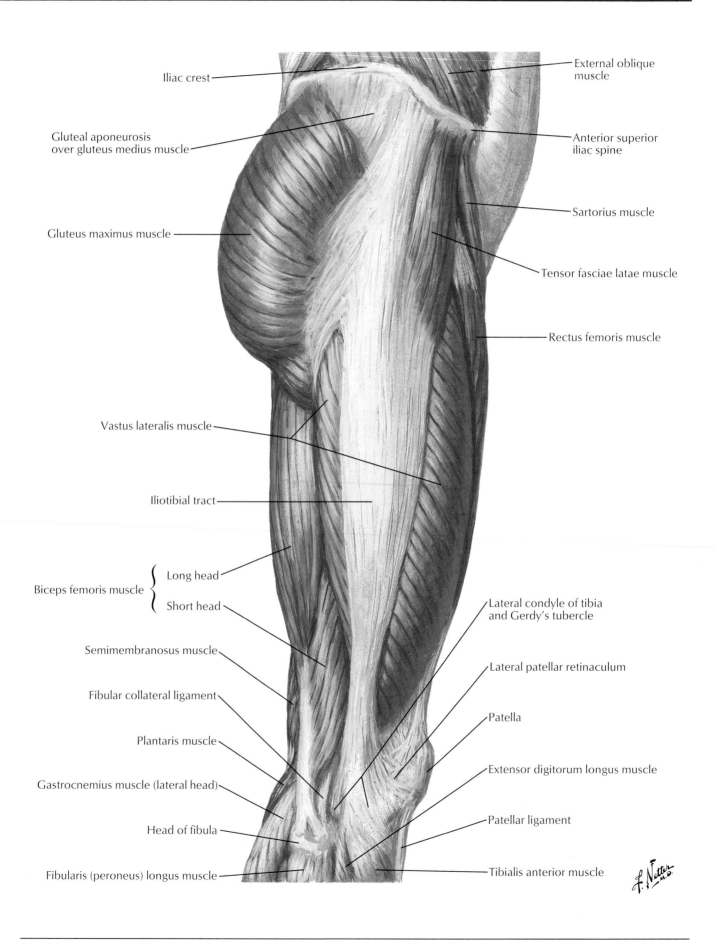

Iliac crest

Gluteal aponeurosis over gluteus medius muscle

Gluteus maximus muscle

Vastus lateralis muscle

Iliotibial tract

Biceps femoris muscle { Long head

Short head

Semimembranosus muscle

Fibular collateral ligament

Plantaris muscle

Gastrocnemius muscle (lateral head)

Head of fibula

Fibularis (peroneus) longus muscle

External oblique muscle

Anterior superior iliac spine

Sartorius muscle

Tensor fasciae latae muscle

Rectus femoris muscle

Lateral condyle of tibia and Gerdy's tubercle

Lateral patellar retinaculum

Patella

Extensor digitorum longus muscle

Patellar ligament

Tibialis anterior muscle

Plate 494

Hip and Thigh

For piriformis and obturator internus see also **Plates 356, 357**; For obturator externus see **Plate 501**

Superficial dissection

Deeper dissection

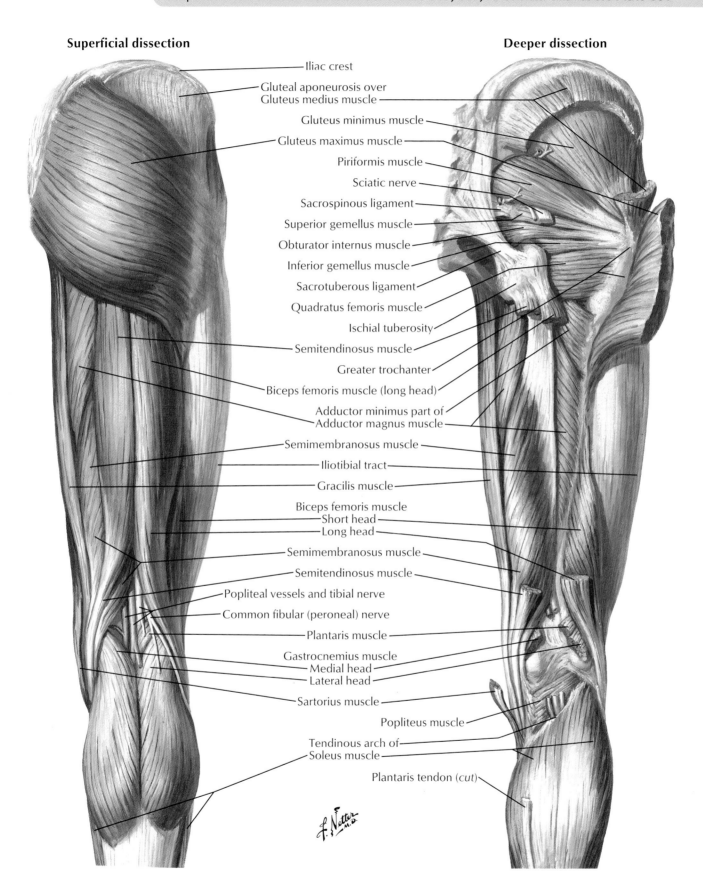

Iliac crest

Gluteal aponeurosis over
Gluteus medius muscle

Gluteus minimus muscle

Gluteus maximus muscle

Piriformis muscle

Sciatic nerve

Sacrospinous ligament

Superior gemellus muscle

Obturator internus muscle

Inferior gemellus muscle

Sacrotuberous ligament

Quadratus femoris muscle

Ischial tuberosity

Semitendinosus muscle

Greater trochanter

Biceps femoris muscle (long head)

Adductor minimus part of
Adductor magnus muscle

Semimembranosus muscle

Iliotibial tract

Gracilis muscle

Biceps femoris muscle
Short head
Long head

Semimembranosus muscle

Semitendinosus muscle

Popliteal vessels and tibial nerve

Common fibular (peroneal) nerve

Plantaris muscle

Gastrocnemius muscle
Medial head
Lateral head

Sartorius muscle

Popliteus muscle

Tendinous arch of
Soleus muscle

Plantaris tendon (*cut*)

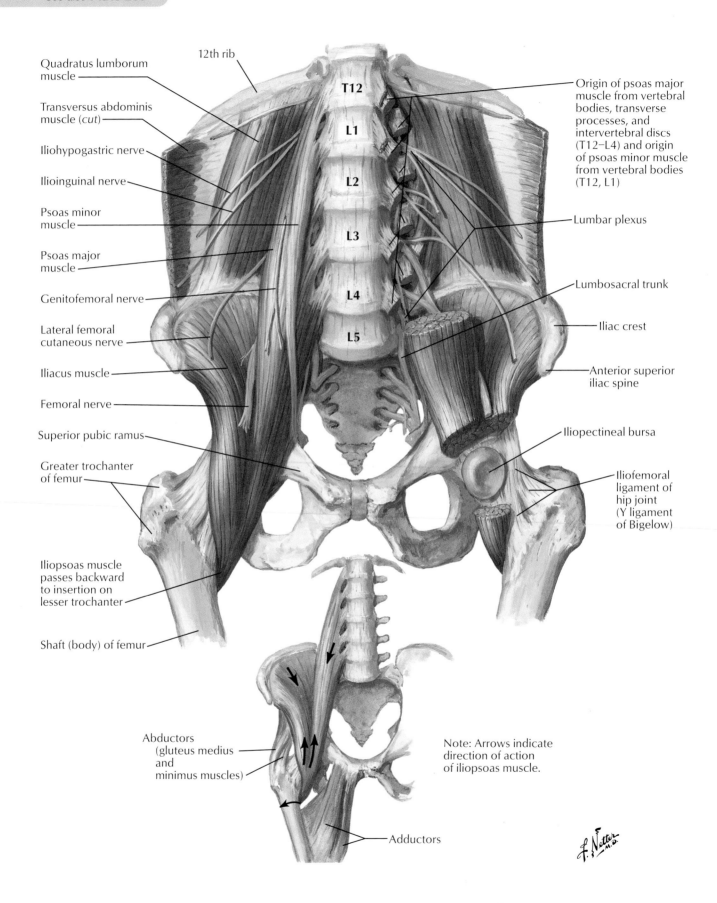

Quadratus lumborum muscle

Transversus abdominis muscle (*cut*)

Iliohypogastric nerve

Ilioinguinal nerve

Psoas minor muscle

Psoas major muscle

Genitofemoral nerve

Lateral femoral cutaneous nerve

Iliacus muscle

Femoral nerve

Superior pubic ramus

Greater trochanter of femur

Iliopsoas muscle passes backward to insertion on lesser trochanter

Shaft (body) of femur

12th rib

T12

L1

L2

L3

L4

L5

Origin of psoas major muscle from vertebral bodies, transverse processes, and intervertebral discs (T12–L4) and origin of psoas minor muscle from vertebral bodies (T12, L1)

Lumbar plexus

Lumbosacral trunk

Iliac crest

Anterior superior iliac spine

Iliopectineal bursa

Iliofemoral ligament of hip joint (Y ligament of Bigelow)

Abductors (gluteus medius and minimus muscles)

Adductors

Note: Arrows indicate direction of action of iliopsoas muscle.

f. Netter m.d.

Plate 496   **Hip and Thigh**

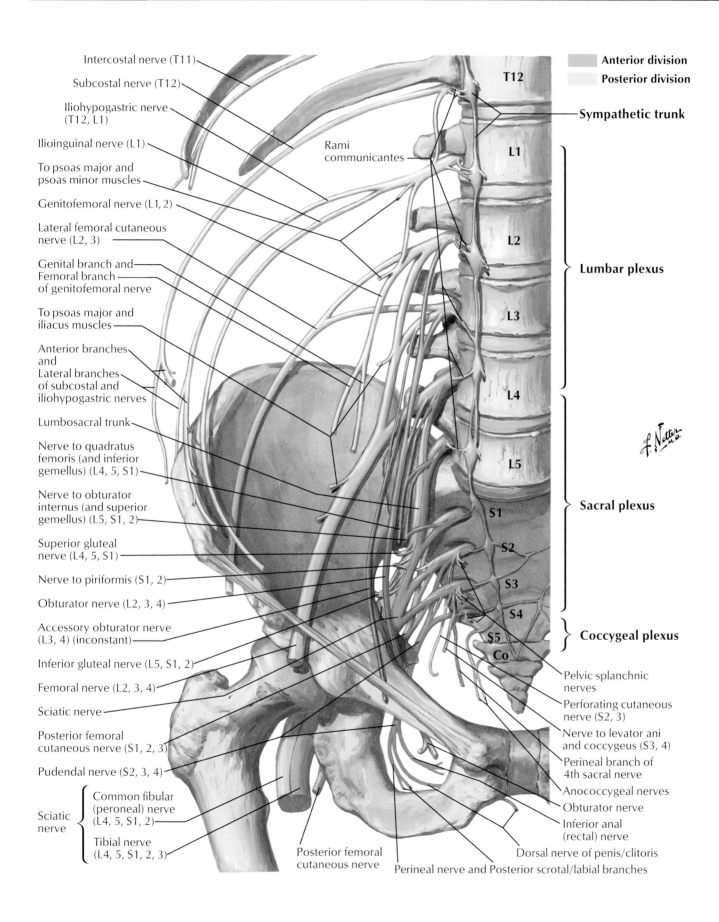

Intercostal nerve (T11)

Subcostal nerve (T12)

Iliohypogastric nerve (T12, L1)

Ilioinguinal nerve (L1)

To psoas major and psoas minor muscles

Genitofemoral nerve (L1, 2)

Lateral femoral cutaneous nerve (L2, 3)

Genital branch and Femoral branch of genitofemoral nerve

To psoas major and iliacus muscles

Anterior branches and Lateral branches of subcostal and iliohypogastric nerves

Lumbosacral trunk

Nerve to quadratus femoris (and inferior gemellus) (L4, 5, S1)

Nerve to obturator internus (and superior gemellus) (L5, S1, 2)

Superior gluteal nerve (L4, 5, S1)

Nerve to piriformis (S1, 2)

Obturator nerve (L2, 3, 4)

Accessory obturator nerve (L3, 4) (inconstant)

Inferior gluteal nerve (L5, S1, 2)

Femoral nerve (L2, 3, 4)

Sciatic nerve

Posterior femoral cutaneous nerve (S1, 2, 3)

Pudendal nerve (S2, 3, 4)

Sciatic nerve {
Common fibular (peroneal) nerve (L4, 5, S1, 2)

Tibial nerve (L4, 5, S1, 2, 3)
}

Rami communicantes

T12

L1

L2

L3

L4

L5

S1

S2

S3

S4

S5

Co

Anterior division

Posterior division

Sympathetic trunk

Lumbar plexus

Sacral plexus

Coccygeal plexus

Pelvic splanchnic nerves

Perforating cutaneous nerve (S2, 3)

Nerve to levator ani and coccygeus (S3, 4)

Perineal branch of 4th sacral nerve

Anococcygeal nerves

Obturator nerve

Inferior anal (rectal) nerve

Dorsal nerve of penis/clitoris

Posterior femoral cutaneous nerve

Perineal nerve and Posterior scrotal/labial branches

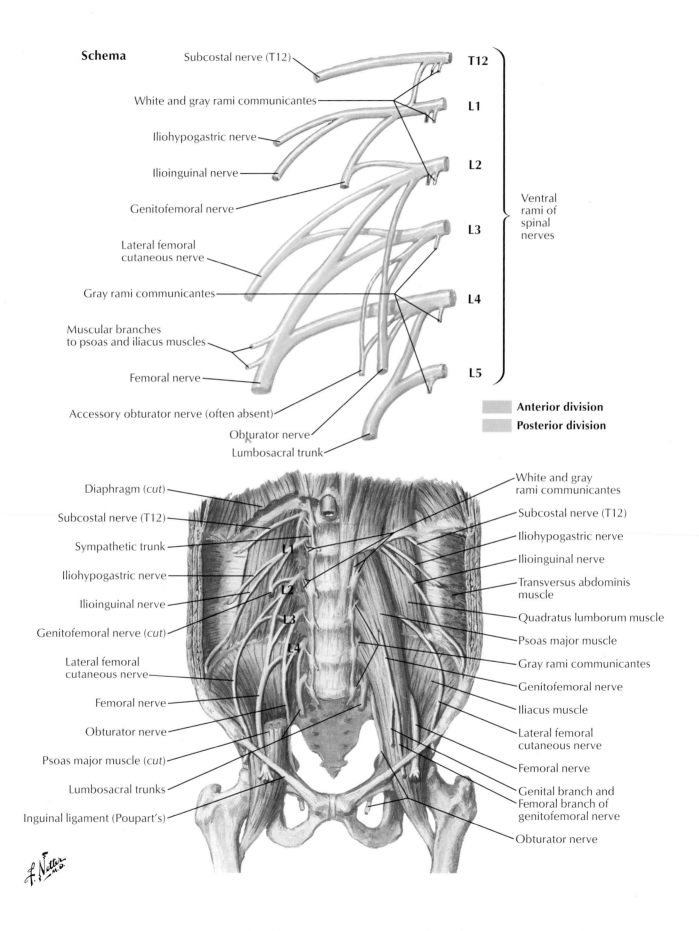

Schema

Subcostal nerve (T12)

White and gray rami communicantes

Iliohypogastric nerve

Ilioinguinal nerve

Genitofemoral nerve

Lateral femoral cutaneous nerve

Gray rami communicantes

Muscular branches to psoas and iliacus muscles

Femoral nerve

Accessory obturator nerve (often absent)

Obturator nerve

Lumbosacral trunk

T12

L1

L2

L3

L4

L5

Ventral rami of spinal nerves

Anterior division

Posterior division

Diaphragm (cut)

Subcostal nerve (T12)

Sympathetic trunk

Iliohypogastric nerve

Ilioinguinal nerve

Genitofemoral nerve (cut)

Lateral femoral cutaneous nerve

Femoral nerve

Obturator nerve

Psoas major muscle (cut)

Lumbosacral trunks

Inguinal ligament (Poupart's)

White and gray rami communicantes

Subcostal nerve (T12)

Iliohypogastric nerve

Ilioinguinal nerve

Transversus abdominis muscle

Quadratus lumborum muscle

Psoas major muscle

Gray rami communicantes

Genitofemoral nerve

Iliacus muscle

Lateral femoral cutaneous nerve

Femoral nerve

Genital branch and Femoral branch of genitofemoral nerve

Obturator nerve

Plate 498

Hip and Thigh

Schema

Anterior division
Posterior division

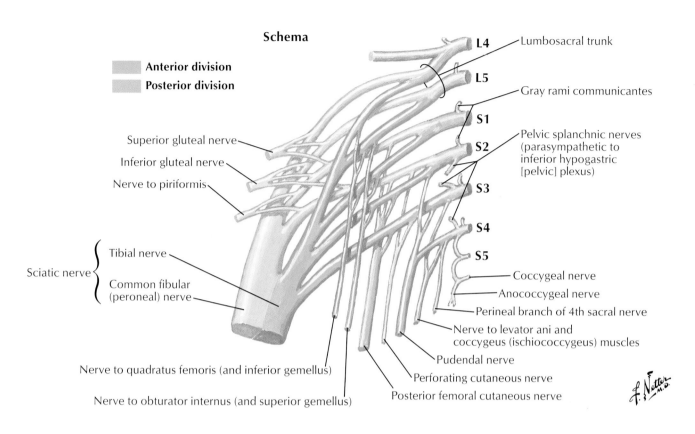

L4 — Lumbosacral trunk

L5

Gray rami communicantes

S1

S2 — Pelvic splanchnic nerves (parasympathetic to inferior hypogastric [pelvic] plexus)

Superior gluteal nerve

Inferior gluteal nerve

Nerve to piriformis

S3

S4

S5

Coccygeal nerve

Anococcygeal nerve

Sciatic nerve { Tibial nerve

Common fibular (peroneal) nerve

Perineal branch of 4th sacral nerve

Nerve to levator ani and coccygeus (ischiococcygeus) muscles

Nerve to quadratus femoris (and inferior gemellus)

Pudendal nerve

Perforating cutaneous nerve

Nerve to obturator internus (and superior gemellus)

Posterior femoral cutaneous nerve

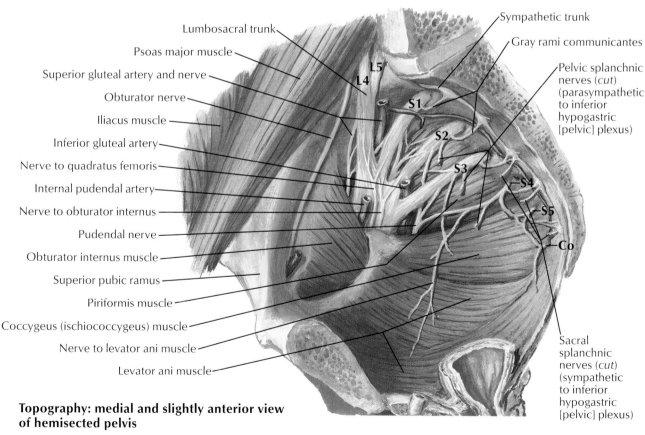

Lumbosacral trunk

Psoas major muscle

Superior gluteal artery and nerve

Obturator nerve

Iliacus muscle

Inferior gluteal artery

Nerve to quadratus femoris

Internal pudendal artery

Nerve to obturator internus

Pudendal nerve

Obturator internus muscle

Superior pubic ramus

Piriformis muscle

Coccygeus (ischiococcygeus) muscle

Nerve to levator ani muscle

Levator ani muscle

Sympathetic trunk

Gray rami communicantes

Pelvic splanchnic nerves (cut) (parasympathetic to inferior hypogastric [pelvic] plexus)

L5
L4

S1

S2

S3

S4

S5

Co

Sacral splanchnic nerves (cut) (sympathetic to inferior hypogastric [pelvic] plexus)

Topography: medial and slightly anterior view of hemisected pelvis

Superficial dissections

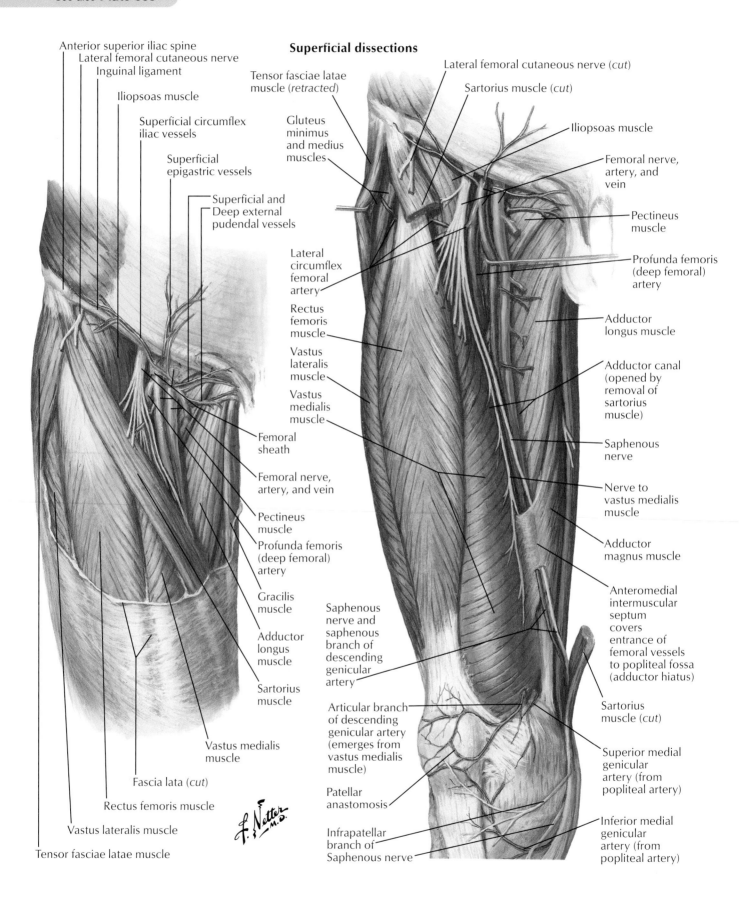

Anterior superior iliac spine

Lateral femoral cutaneous nerve

Inguinal ligament

Iliopsoas muscle

Superficial circumflex iliac vessels

Superficial epigastric vessels

Superficial and Deep external pudendal vessels

Tensor fasciae latae muscle (retracted)

Gluteus minimus and medius muscles

Lateral circumflex femoral artery

Rectus femoris muscle

Vastus lateralis muscle

Vastus medialis muscle

Femoral sheath

Femoral nerve, artery, and vein

Pectineus muscle

Profunda femoris (deep femoral) artery

Gracilis muscle

Adductor longus muscle

Sartorius muscle

Saphenous nerve and saphenous branch of descending genicular artery

Vastus medialis muscle

Articular branch of descending genicular artery (emerges from vastus medialis muscle)

Fascia lata (cut)

Patellar anastomosis

Rectus femoris muscle

Infrapatellar branch of Saphenous nerve

Vastus lateralis muscle

Tensor fasciae latae muscle

Lateral femoral cutaneous nerve (cut)

Sartorius muscle (cut)

Iliopsoas muscle

Femoral nerve, artery, and vein

Pectineus muscle

Profunda femoris (deep femoral) artery

Adductor longus muscle

Adductor canal (opened by removal of sartorius muscle)

Saphenous nerve

Nerve to vastus medialis muscle

Adductor magnus muscle

Anteromedial intermuscular septum covers entrance of femoral vessels to popliteal fossa (adductor hiatus)

Sartorius muscle (cut)

Superior medial genicular artery (from popliteal artery)

Inferior medial genicular artery (from popliteal artery)

Plate 500

Hip and Thigh

Deep dissection

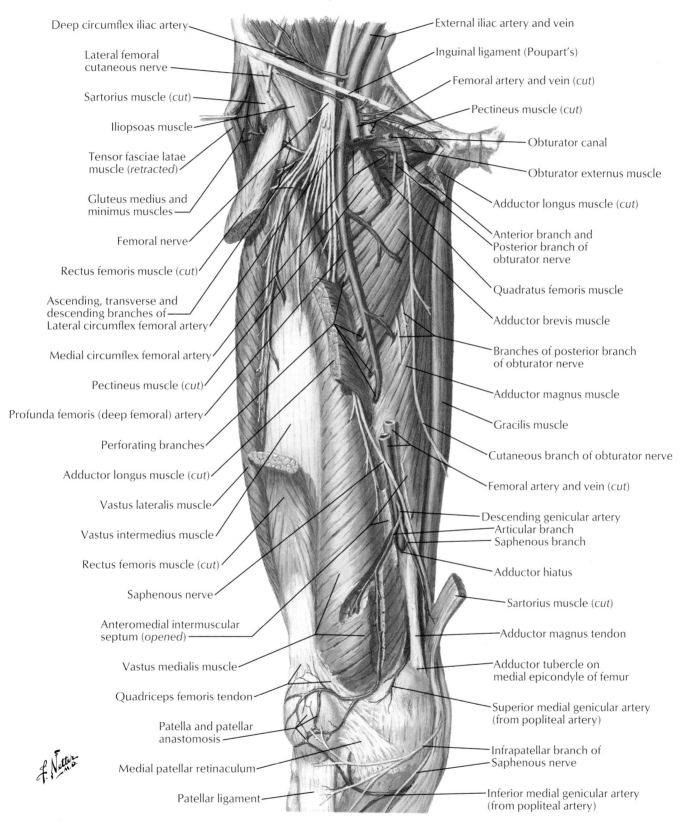

Deep circumflex iliac artery

Lateral femoral cutaneous nerve

Sartorius muscle (*cut*)

Iliopsoas muscle

Tensor fasciae latae muscle (*retracted*)

Gluteus medius and minimus muscles

Femoral nerve

Rectus femoris muscle (*cut*)

Ascending, transverse and descending branches of Lateral circumflex femoral artery

Medial circumflex femoral artery

Pectineus muscle (*cut*)

Profunda femoris (deep femoral) artery

Perforating branches

Adductor longus muscle (*cut*)

Vastus lateralis muscle

Vastus intermedius muscle

Rectus femoris muscle (*cut*)

Saphenous nerve

Anteromedial intermuscular septum (*opened*)

Vastus medialis muscle

Quadriceps femoris tendon

Patella and patellar anastomosis

Medial patellar retinaculum

Patellar ligament

External iliac artery and vein

Inguinal ligament (Poupart's)

Femoral artery and vein (*cut*)

Pectineus muscle (*cut*)

Obturator canal

Obturator externus muscle

Adductor longus muscle (*cut*)

Anterior branch and Posterior branch of obturator nerve

Quadratus femoris muscle

Adductor brevis muscle

Branches of posterior branch of obturator nerve

Adductor magnus muscle

Gracilis muscle

Cutaneous branch of obturator nerve

Femoral artery and vein (*cut*)

Descending genicular artery

Articular branch

Saphenous branch

Adductor hiatus

Sartorius muscle (*cut*)

Adductor magnus tendon

Adductor tubercle on medial epicondyle of femur

Superior medial genicular artery (from popliteal artery)

Infrapatellar branch of Saphenous nerve

Inferior medial genicular artery (from popliteal artery)

Deep dissection

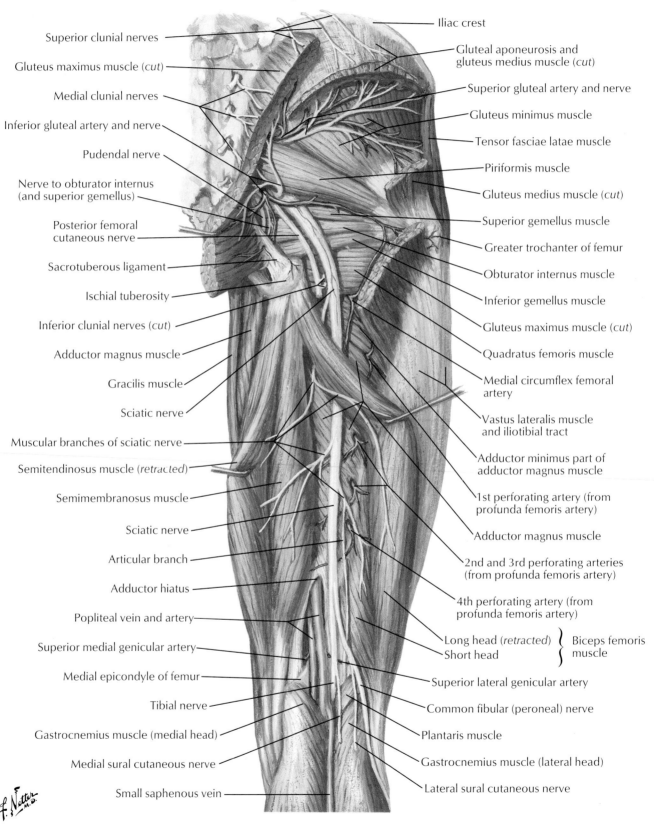

Superior clunial nerves

Gluteus maximus muscle (*cut*)

Medial clunial nerves

Inferior gluteal artery and nerve

Pudendal nerve

Nerve to obturator internus
(and superior gemellus)

Posterior femoral
cutaneous nerve

Sacrotuberous ligament

Ischial tuberosity

Inferior clunial nerves (*cut*)

Adductor magnus muscle

Gracilis muscle

Sciatic nerve

Muscular branches of sciatic nerve

Semitendinosus muscle (*retracted*)

Semimembranosus muscle

Sciatic nerve

Articular branch

Adductor hiatus

Popliteal vein and artery

Superior medial genicular artery

Medial epicondyle of femur

Tibial nerve

Gastrocnemius muscle (medial head)

Medial sural cutaneous nerve

Small saphenous vein

Iliac crest

Gluteal aponeurosis and
gluteus medius muscle (*cut*)

Superior gluteal artery and nerve

Gluteus minimus muscle

Tensor fasciae latae muscle

Piriformis muscle

Gluteus medius muscle (*cut*)

Superior gemellus muscle

Greater trochanter of femur

Obturator internus muscle

Inferior gemellus muscle

Gluteus maximus muscle (*cut*)

Quadratus femoris muscle

Medial circumflex femoral
artery

Vastus lateralis muscle
and iliotibial tract

Adductor minimus part of
adductor magnus muscle

1st perforating artery (from
profunda femoris artery)

Adductor magnus muscle

2nd and 3rd perforating arteries
(from profunda femoris artery)

4th perforating artery (from
profunda femoris artery)

Long head (*retracted*) ⎫ Biceps femoris
Short head   ⎭ muscle

Superior lateral genicular artery

Common fibular (peroneal) nerve

Plantaris muscle

Gastrocnemius muscle (lateral head)

Lateral sural cutaneous nerve

Plate 502

Hip and Thigh

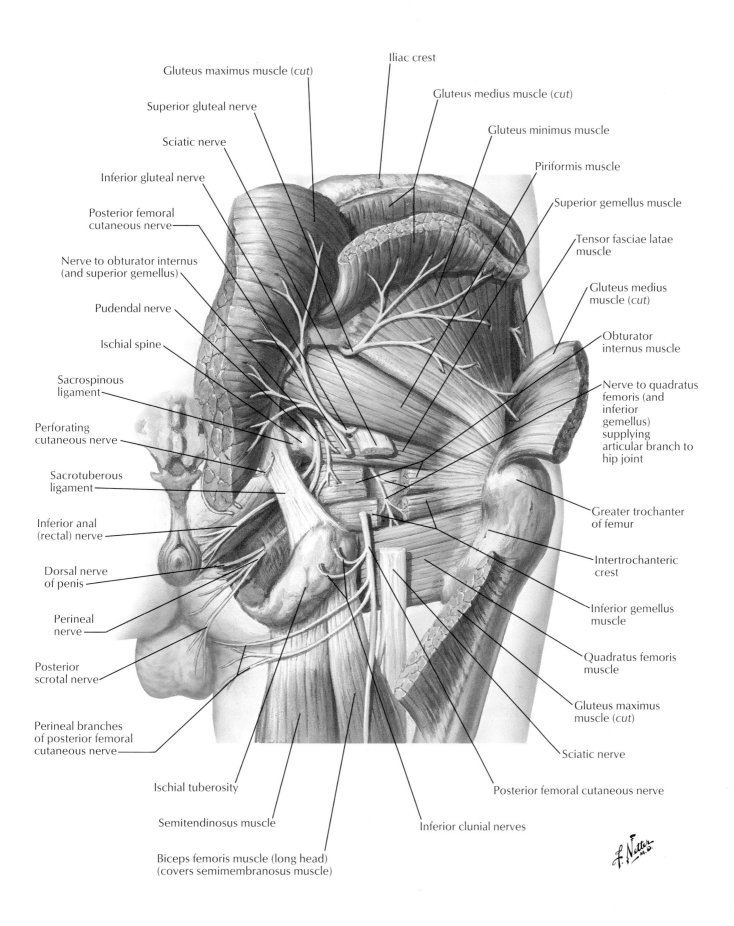

Gluteus maximus muscle (*cut*)

Iliac crest

Superior gluteal nerve

Gluteus medius muscle (*cut*)

Sciatic nerve

Gluteus minimus muscle

Inferior gluteal nerve

Piriformis muscle

Posterior femoral cutaneous nerve

Superior gemellus muscle

Tensor fasciae latae muscle

Nerve to obturator internus (and superior gemellus)

Gluteus medius muscle (*cut*)

Pudendal nerve

Obturator internus muscle

Ischial spine

Nerve to quadratus femoris (and inferior gemellus) supplying articular branch to hip joint

Sacrospinous ligament

Perforating cutaneous nerve

Greater trochanter of femur

Sacrotuberous ligament

Intertrochanteric crest

Inferior anal (rectal) nerve

Dorsal nerve of penis

Inferior gemellus muscle

Perineal nerve

Quadratus femoris muscle

Posterior scrotal nerve

Gluteus maximus muscle (*cut*)

Perineal branches of posterior femoral cutaneous nerve

Sciatic nerve

Ischial tuberosity

Posterior femoral cutaneous nerve

Semitendinosus muscle

Inferior clunial nerves

Biceps femoris muscle (long head) (covers semimembranosus muscle)

Anterior view

Retinacular arteries (subsynovial) { Superior, Anterior, Inferior

Anastomosis between medial and lateral circumflex femoral arteries

Iliofemoral (Y) ligament and joint capsule

Ascending, Transverse, Descending branches of Lateral circumflex femoral artery

Acetabular branch of obturator artery (often minute)

Iliopsoas tendon

Medial circumflex femoral artery

Profunda femoris (deep femoral) artery

Nutrient artery of femur

Posterior view

Retinacular arteries (subsynovial) { Superior, Posterior, Inferior

Anastomosis

Ischiofemoral ligament and joint capsule

Medial circumflex femoral artery

Lateral circumflex femoral artery

Nutrient artery of femur

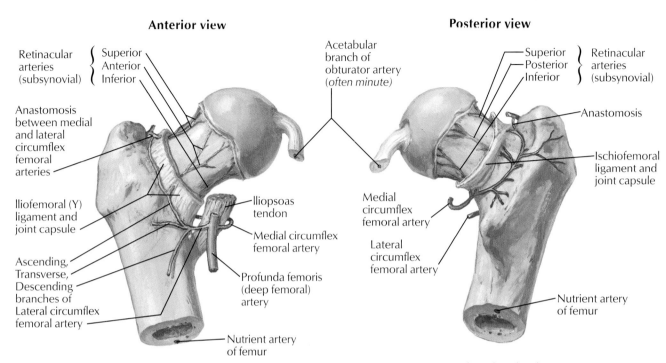

Coronal section

Acetabular labrum

Ligaments and joint capsule

Synovial membrane

Retinacular arteries

Acetabular branch

Obturator artery

Epiphyseal plate

Medial circumflex femoral artery

Anterior view in situ

Medial circumflex femoral artery

Anastomosis

Lateral circumflex femoral artery
Ascending, Transverse, Descending branches

Iliopsoas muscle

Femoral artery

Pectineus muscle

Medial circumflex femoral artery

Profunda femoris (deep femoral) artery

Medial circumflex femoral artery

Iliopsoas tendon

Lateral circumflex femoral artery

Femur of child: anterior view

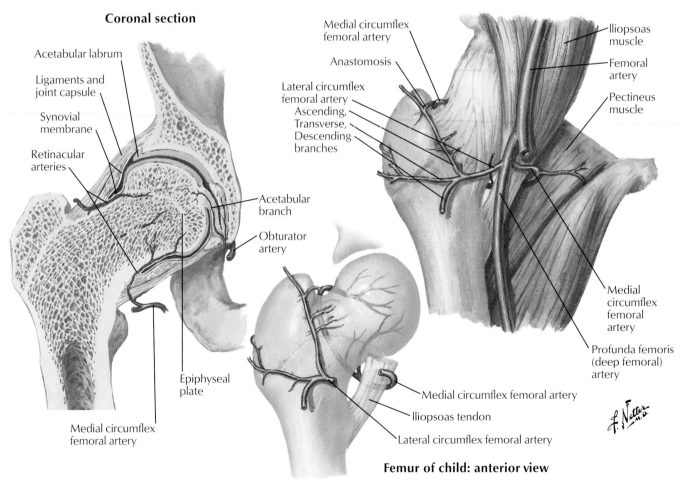

Plate 504   **Hip and Thigh**

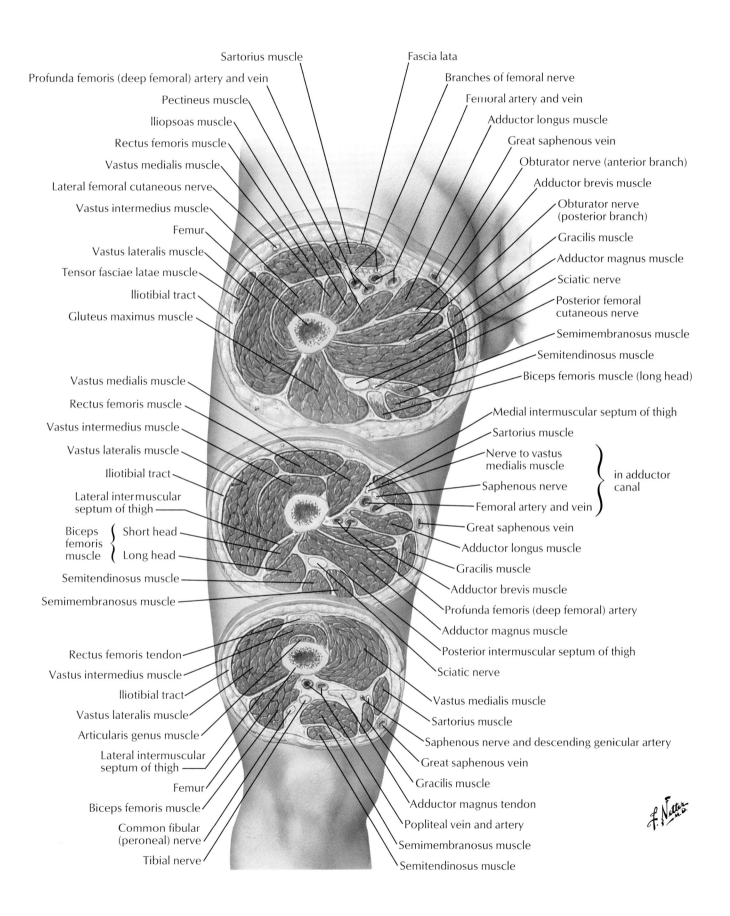

Sartorius muscle

Profunda femoris (deep femoral) artery and vein

Pectineus muscle

Iliopsoas muscle

Rectus femoris muscle

Vastus medialis muscle

Lateral femoral cutaneous nerve

Vastus intermedius muscle

Femur

Vastus lateralis muscle

Tensor fasciae latae muscle

Iliotibial tract

Gluteus maximus muscle

Fascia lata

Branches of femoral nerve

Femoral artery and vein

Adductor longus muscle

Great saphenous vein

Obturator nerve (anterior branch)

Adductor brevis muscle

Obturator nerve (posterior branch)

Gracilis muscle

Adductor magnus muscle

Sciatic nerve

Posterior femoral cutaneous nerve

Semimembranosus muscle

Semitendinosus muscle

Biceps femoris muscle (long head)

Vastus medialis muscle

Rectus femoris muscle

Vastus intermedius muscle

Vastus lateralis muscle

Iliotibial tract

Lateral intermuscular septum of thigh

Biceps femoris muscle { Short head / Long head }

Semitendinosus muscle

Semimembranosus muscle

Medial intermuscular septum of thigh

Sartorius muscle

Nerve to vastus medialis muscle

Saphenous nerve

Femoral artery and vein

} in adductor canal

Great saphenous vein

Adductor longus muscle

Gracilis muscle

Adductor brevis muscle

Profunda femoris (deep femoral) artery

Adductor magnus muscle

Posterior intermuscular septum of thigh

Sciatic nerve

Rectus femoris tendon

Vastus intermedius muscle

Iliotibial tract

Vastus lateralis muscle

Articularis genus muscle

Lateral intermuscular septum of thigh

Femur

Biceps femoris muscle

Common fibular (peroneal) nerve

Tibial nerve

Vastus medialis muscle

Sartorius muscle

Saphenous nerve and descending genicular artery

Great saphenous vein

Gracilis muscle

Adductor magnus tendon

Popliteal vein and artery

Semimembranosus muscle

Semitendinosus muscle

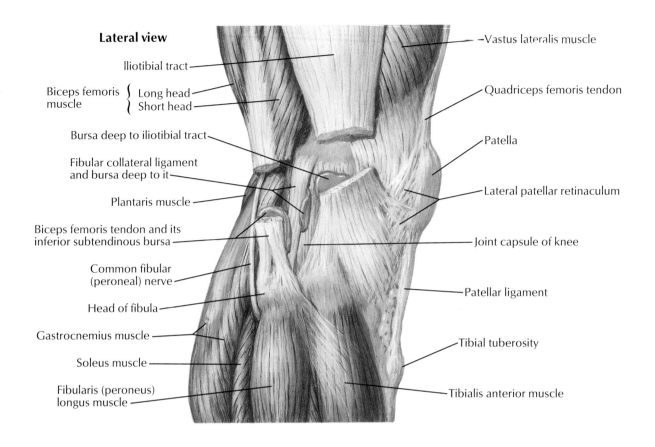

Lateral view

Iliotibial tract

Biceps femoris muscle { Long head / Short head

Bursa deep to iliotibial tract

Fibular collateral ligament and bursa deep to it

Plantaris muscle

Biceps femoris tendon and its inferior subtendinous bursa

Common fibular (peroneal) nerve

Head of fibula

Gastrocnemius muscle

Soleus muscle

Fibularis (peroneus) longus muscle

Vastus lateralis muscle

Quadriceps femoris tendon

Patella

Lateral patellar retinaculum

Joint capsule of knee

Patellar ligament

Tibial tuberosity

Tibialis anterior muscle

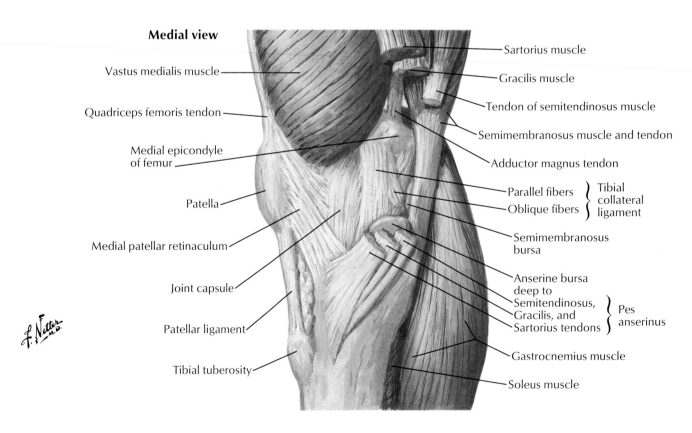

Medial view

Vastus medialis muscle

Quadriceps femoris tendon

Medial epicondyle of femur

Patella

Medial patellar retinaculum

Joint capsule

Patellar ligament

Tibial tuberosity

Sartorius muscle

Gracilis muscle

Tendon of semitendinosus muscle

Semimembranosus muscle and tendon

Adductor magnus tendon

Parallel fibers } Tibial collateral ligament
Oblique fibers }

Semimembranosus bursa

Anserine bursa deep to Semitendinosus, Gracilis, and Sartorius tendons } Pes anserinus

Gastrocnemius muscle

Soleus muscle

Plate 506

Knee

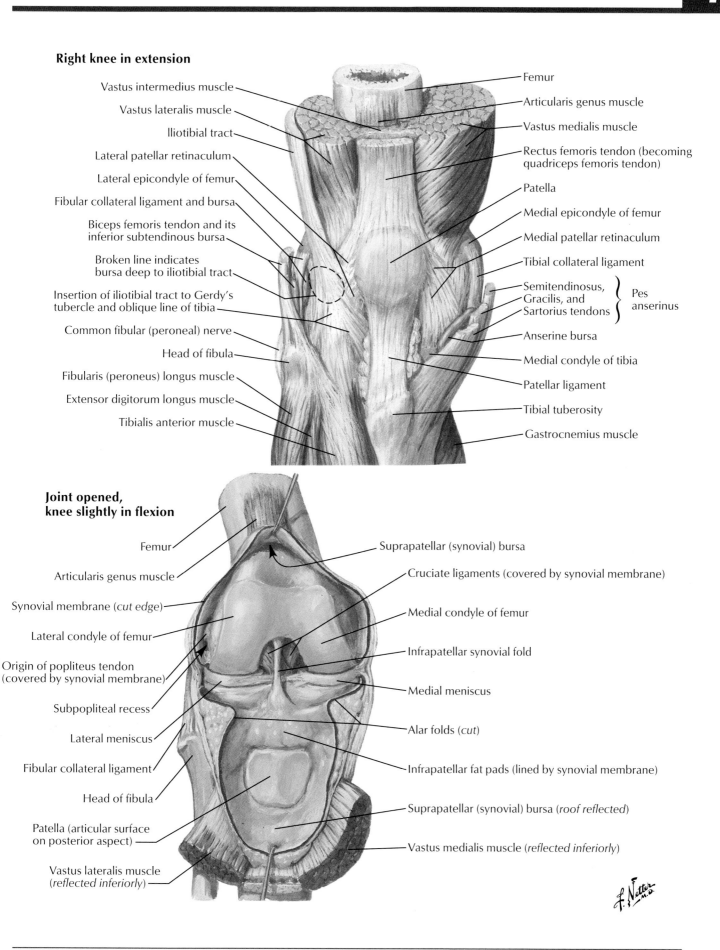

Right knee in extension

Vastus intermedius muscle

Vastus lateralis muscle

Iliotibial tract

Lateral patellar retinaculum

Lateral epicondyle of femur

Fibular collateral ligament and bursa

Biceps femoris tendon and its inferior subtendinous bursa

Broken line indicates bursa deep to iliotibial tract

Insertion of iliotibial tract to Gerdy's tubercle and oblique line of tibia

Common fibular (peroneal) nerve

Head of fibula

Fibularis (peroneus) longus muscle

Extensor digitorum longus muscle

Tibialis anterior muscle

Femur

Articularis genus muscle

Vastus medialis muscle

Rectus femoris tendon (becoming quadriceps femoris tendon)

Patella

Medial epicondyle of femur

Medial patellar retinaculum

Tibial collateral ligament

Semitendinosus, Gracilis, and Sartorius tendons } Pes anserinus

Anserine bursa

Medial condyle of tibia

Patellar ligament

Tibial tuberosity

Gastrocnemius muscle

Joint opened, knee slightly in flexion

Femur

Articularis genus muscle

Synovial membrane (*cut edge*)

Lateral condyle of femur

Origin of popliteus tendon (covered by synovial membrane)

Subpopliteal recess

Lateral meniscus

Fibular collateral ligament

Head of fibula

Patella (articular surface on posterior aspect)

Vastus lateralis muscle (*reflected inferiorly*)

Suprapatellar (synovial) bursa

Cruciate ligaments (covered by synovial membrane)

Medial condyle of femur

Infrapatellar synovial fold

Medial meniscus

Alar folds (*cut*)

Infrapatellar fat pads (lined by synovial membrane)

Suprapatellar (synovial) bursa (*roof reflected*)

Vastus medialis muscle (*reflected inferiorly*)

Inferior view

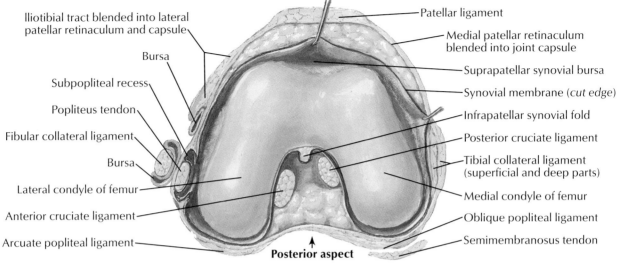

Iliotibial tract blended into lateral patellar retinaculum and capsule

Bursa

Subpopliteal recess

Popliteus tendon

Fibular collateral ligament

Bursa

Lateral condyle of femur

Anterior cruciate ligament

Arcuate popliteal ligament

Patellar ligament

Medial patellar retinaculum blended into joint capsule

Suprapatellar synovial bursa

Synovial membrane (*cut edge*)

Infrapatellar synovial fold

Posterior cruciate ligament

Tibial collateral ligament (superficial and deep parts)

Medial condyle of femur

Oblique popliteal ligament

Semimembranosus tendon

Posterior aspect

Superior view

Posterior meniscofemoral ligament

Arcuate popliteal ligament

Fibular collateral ligament

Bursa

Popliteus tendon

Subpopliteal recess

Lateral meniscus

Superior articular surface of tibia (lateral facet)

Iliotibial tract blended into capsule

Infrapatellar fat pad

Semimembranosus tendon

Oblique popliteal ligament

Posterior cruciate ligament

Tibial collateral ligament (deep part bound to medial meniscus)

Medial meniscus

Synovial membrane

Superior articular surface of tibia (medial facet)

Joint capsule

Anterior cruciate ligament

Patellar ligament

Anterior aspect

Superior view: ligaments and cartilage removed

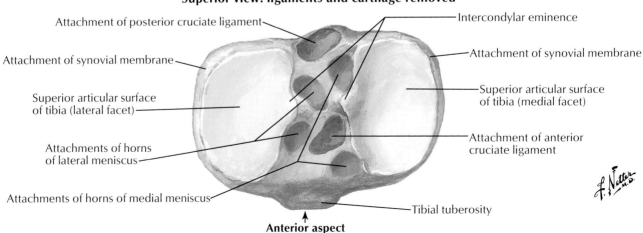

Attachment of posterior cruciate ligament

Attachment of synovial membrane

Superior articular surface of tibia (lateral facet)

Attachments of horns of lateral meniscus

Attachments of horns of medial meniscus

Intercondylar eminence

Attachment of synovial membrane

Superior articular surface of tibia (medial facet)

Attachment of anterior cruciate ligament

Tibial tuberosity

Anterior aspect

Plate 508

Knee

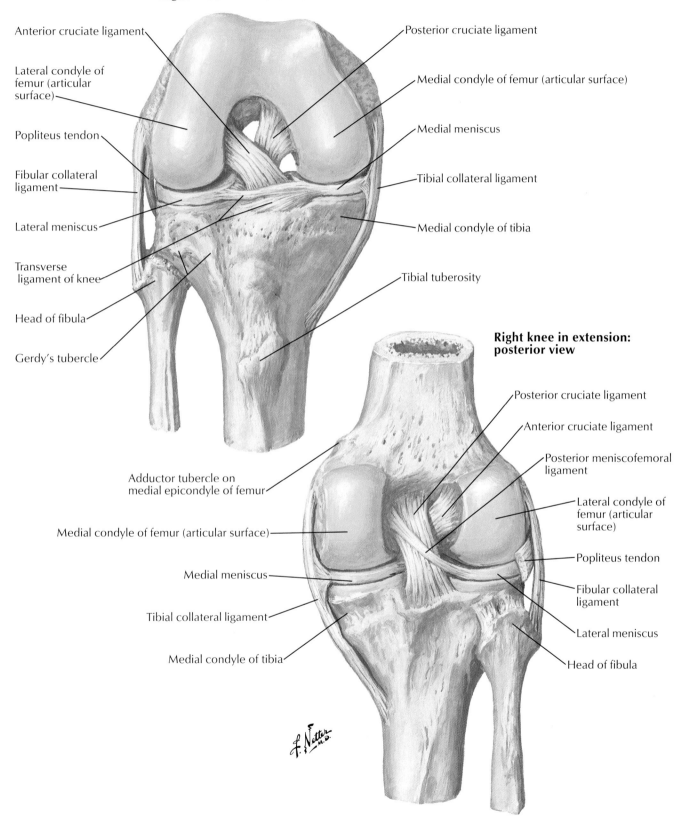

Right knee in flexion: anterior view

Anterior cruciate ligament

Lateral condyle of femur (articular surface)

Popliteus tendon

Fibular collateral ligament

Lateral meniscus

Transverse ligament of knee

Head of fibula

Gerdy's tubercle

Posterior cruciate ligament

Medial condyle of femur (articular surface)

Medial meniscus

Tibial collateral ligament

Medial condyle of tibia

Tibial tuberosity

Right knee in extension: posterior view

Posterior cruciate ligament

Anterior cruciate ligament

Posterior meniscofemoral ligament

Lateral condyle of femur (articular surface)

Popliteus tendon

Fibular collateral ligament

Lateral meniscus

Head of fibula

Adductor tubercle on medial epicondyle of femur

Medial condyle of femur (articular surface)

Medial meniscus

Tibial collateral ligament

Medial condyle of tibia

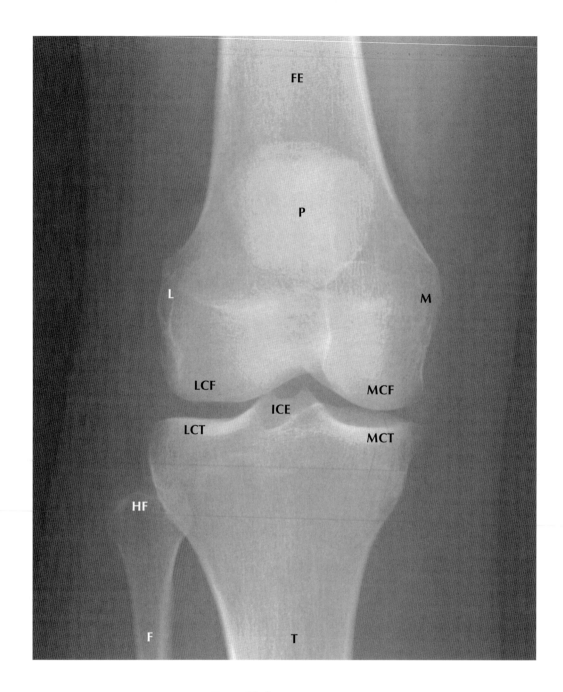

F	Fibula
FE	Femur
HF	Head of fibula
ICE	Intercondylar eminence
L	Lateral epicondyle
LCF	Lateral condyle of femur
LCT	Lateral condyle of tibia
M	Medial epicondyle
MCF	Medial condyle of femur
MCT	Medial condyle of tibia
P	Patella
T	Tibia

Plate 510   **Knee**

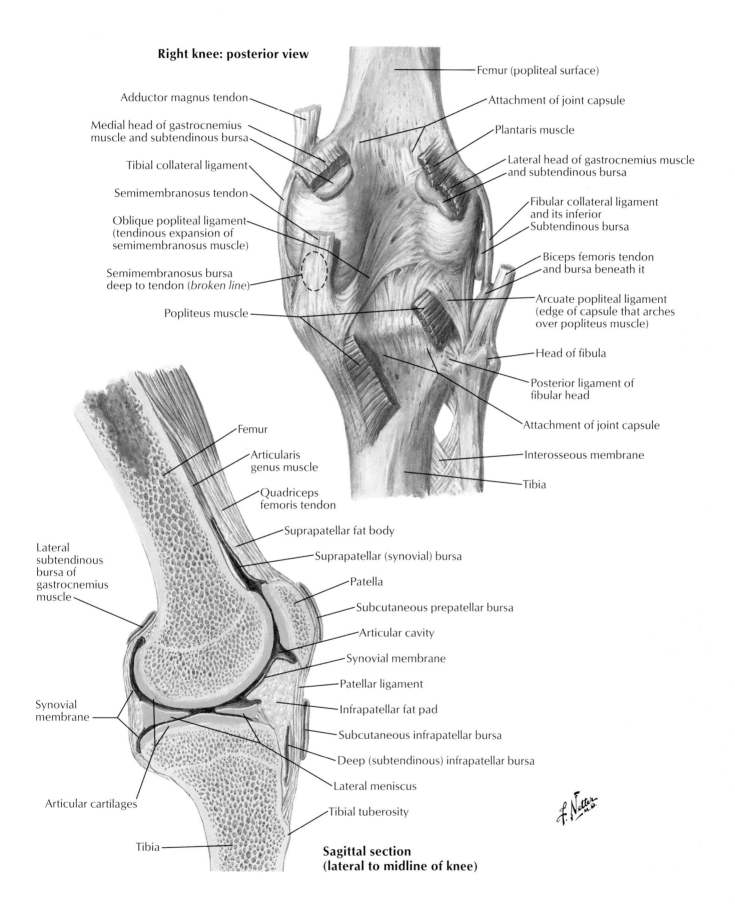

Right knee: posterior view

Adductor magnus tendon

Medial head of gastrocnemius muscle and subtendinous bursa

Tibial collateral ligament

Semimembranosus tendon

Oblique popliteal ligament (tendinous expansion of semimembranosus muscle)

Semimembranosus bursa deep to tendon (*broken line*)

Popliteus muscle

Femur (popliteal surface)

Attachment of joint capsule

Plantaris muscle

Lateral head of gastrocnemius muscle and subtendinous bursa

Fibular collateral ligament and its inferior Subtendinous bursa

Biceps femoris tendon and bursa beneath it

Arcuate popliteal ligament (edge of capsule that arches over popliteus muscle)

Head of fibula

Posterior ligament of fibular head

Attachment of joint capsule

Interosseous membrane

Tibia

Femur

Articularis genus muscle

Quadriceps femoris tendon

Suprapatellar fat body

Suprapatellar (synovial) bursa

Patella

Subcutaneous prepatellar bursa

Articular cavity

Synovial membrane

Patellar ligament

Infrapatellar fat pad

Subcutaneous infrapatellar bursa

Deep (subtendinous) infrapatellar bursa

Lateral meniscus

Tibial tuberosity

Lateral subtendinous bursa of gastrocnemius muscle

Synovial membrane

Articular cartilages

Tibia

Sagittal section (lateral to midline of knee)

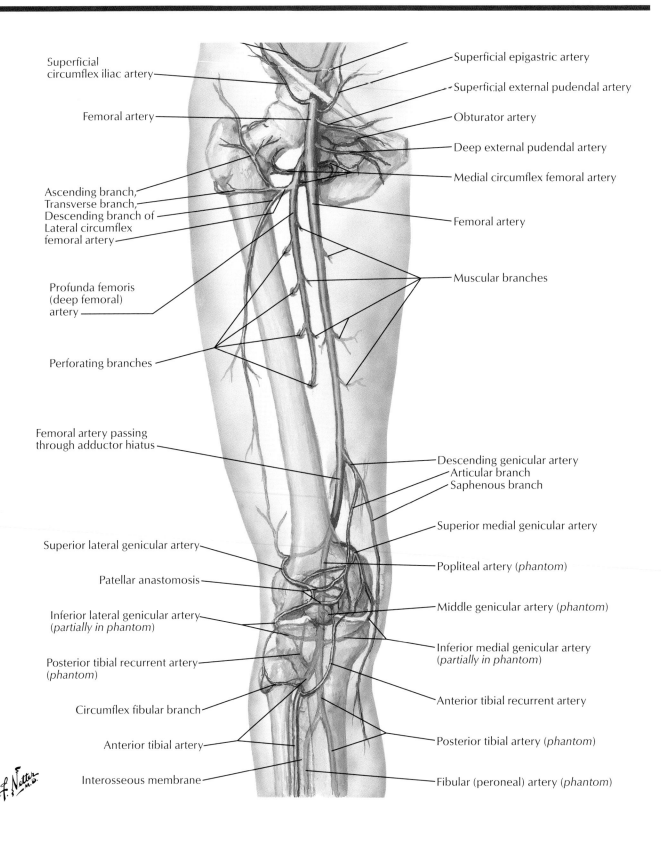

Superficial circumflex iliac artery

Femoral artery

Ascending branch, Transverse branch, Descending branch of Lateral circumflex femoral artery

Profunda femoris (deep femoral) artery

Perforating branches

Femoral artery passing through adductor hiatus

Superior lateral genicular artery

Patellar anastomosis

Inferior lateral genicular artery (partially in phantom)

Posterior tibial recurrent artery (phantom)

Circumflex fibular branch

Anterior tibial artery

Interosseous membrane

Superficial epigastric artery

Superficial external pudendal artery

Obturator artery

Deep external pudendal artery

Medial circumflex femoral artery

Femoral artery

Muscular branches

Descending genicular artery
Articular branch
Saphenous branch

Superior medial genicular artery

Popliteal artery (phantom)

Middle genicular artery (phantom)

Inferior medial genicular artery (partially in phantom)

Anterior tibial recurrent artery

Posterior tibial artery (phantom)

Fibular (peroneal) artery (phantom)

Plate 512   **Knee**

**Bones of
right leg**

Anterior view

Posterior view

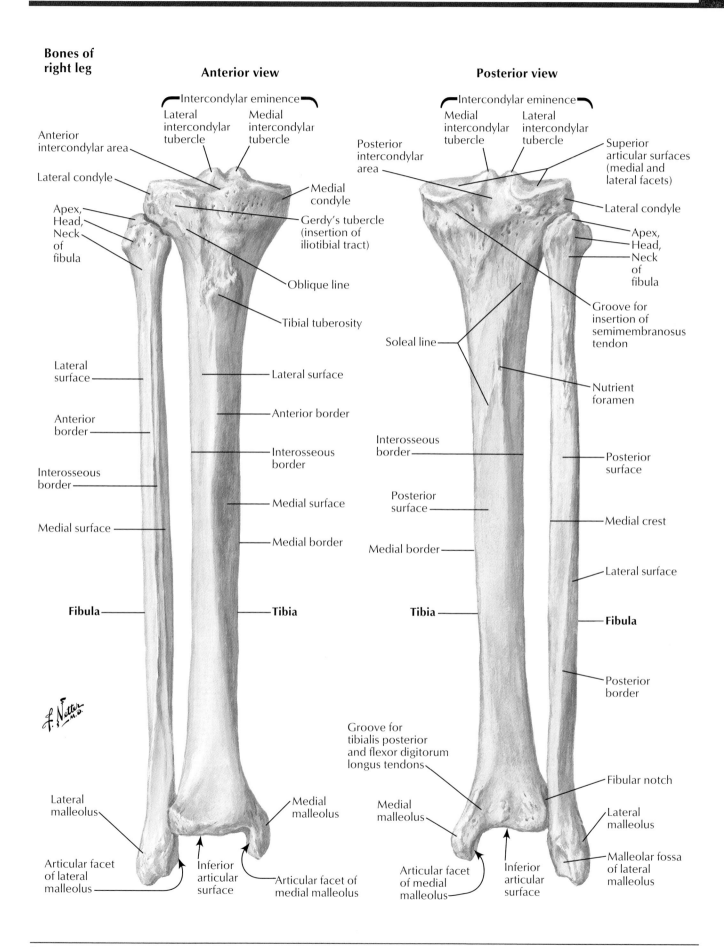

Intercondylar eminence
Lateral
intercondylar
tubercle
Medial
intercondylar
tubercle
Anterior
intercondylar area
Lateral condyle
Medial
condyle
Apex,
Head,
Neck
of
fibula
Gerdy's tubercle
(insertion of
iliotibial tract)
Oblique line
Tibial tuberosity
Lateral
surface
Lateral surface
Anterior
border
Anterior border
Interosseous
border
Interosseous
border
Medial surface
Medial surface
Medial border
Fibula
Tibia
Lateral
malleolus
Medial
malleolus
Articular facet
of lateral
malleolus
Inferior
articular
surface
Articular facet of
medial malleolus

Intercondylar eminence
Medial
intercondylar
tubercle
Lateral
intercondylar
tubercle
Posterior
intercondylar
area
Superior
articular surfaces
(medial and
lateral facets)
Lateral condyle
Apex,
Head,
Neck
of
fibula
Groove for
insertion of
semimembranosus
tendon
Soleal line
Nutrient
foramen
Interosseous
border
Posterior
surface
Posterior
surface
Medial crest
Medial border
Lateral surface
Tibia
Fibula
Posterior
border
Groove for
tibialis posterior
and flexor digitorum
longus tendons
Fibular notch
Medial
malleolus
Lateral
malleolus
Articular facet
of medial
malleolus
Inferior
articular
surface
Malleolar fossa
of lateral
malleolus

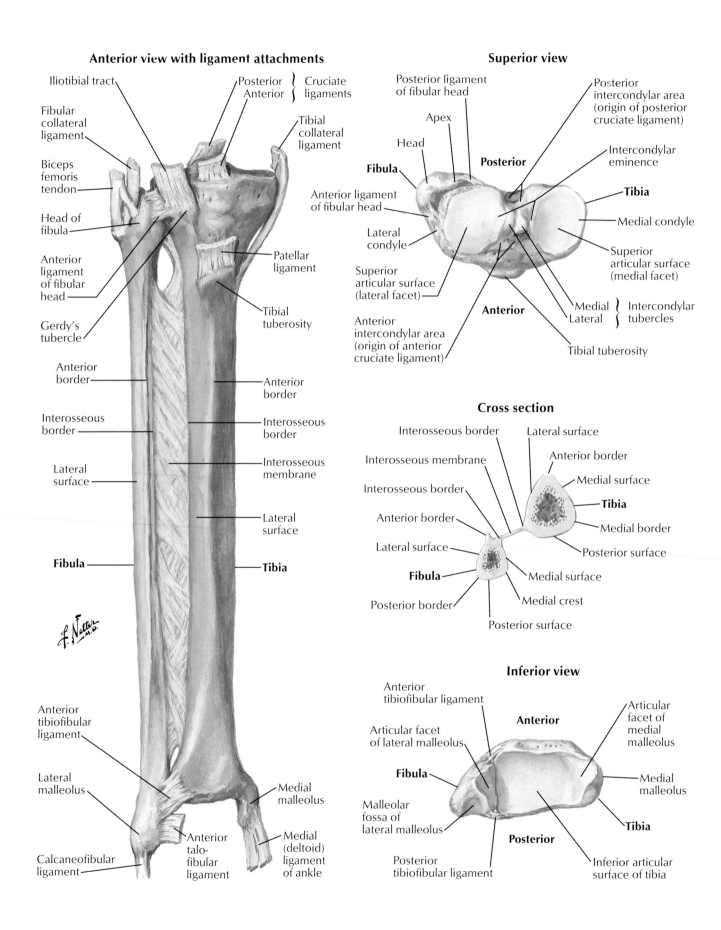

Anterior view with ligament attachments

Iliotibial tract

Fibular collateral ligament

Biceps femoris tendon

Head of fibula

Anterior ligament of fibular head

Gerdy's tubercle

Anterior border

Interosseous border

Lateral surface

Fibula

Anterior tibiofibular ligament

Lateral malleolus

Calcaneofibular ligament

Posterior Anterior } Cruciate ligaments

Tibial collateral ligament

Patellar ligament

Tibial tuberosity

Anterior border

Interosseous border

Interosseous membrane

Lateral surface

Tibia

Anterior talo-fibular ligament

Medial malleolus

Medial (deltoid) ligament of ankle

Superior view

Posterior ligament of fibular head

Apex

Head

Fibula

Anterior ligament of fibular head

Lateral condyle

Superior articular surface (lateral facet)

Anterior intercondylar area (origin of anterior cruciate ligament)

Posterior

Posterior intercondylar area (origin of posterior cruciate ligament)

Intercondylar eminence

Tibia

Medial condyle

Superior articular surface (medial facet)

Medial } Intercondylar
Lateral } tubercles

Anterior

Tibial tuberosity

Cross section

Interosseous border

Interosseous membrane

Interosseous border

Anterior border

Lateral surface

Fibula

Posterior border

Lateral surface

Anterior border

Medial surface

Tibia

Medial border

Posterior surface

Medial surface

Medial crest

Posterior surface

Inferior view

Anterior tibiofibular ligament

Articular facet of lateral malleolus

Fibula

Malleolar fossa of lateral malleolus

Posterior tibiofibular ligament

Anterior

Articular facet of medial malleolus

Medial malleolus

Tibia

Posterior

Inferior articular surface of tibia

f. Netter m.d.

Plate 514   **Leg**

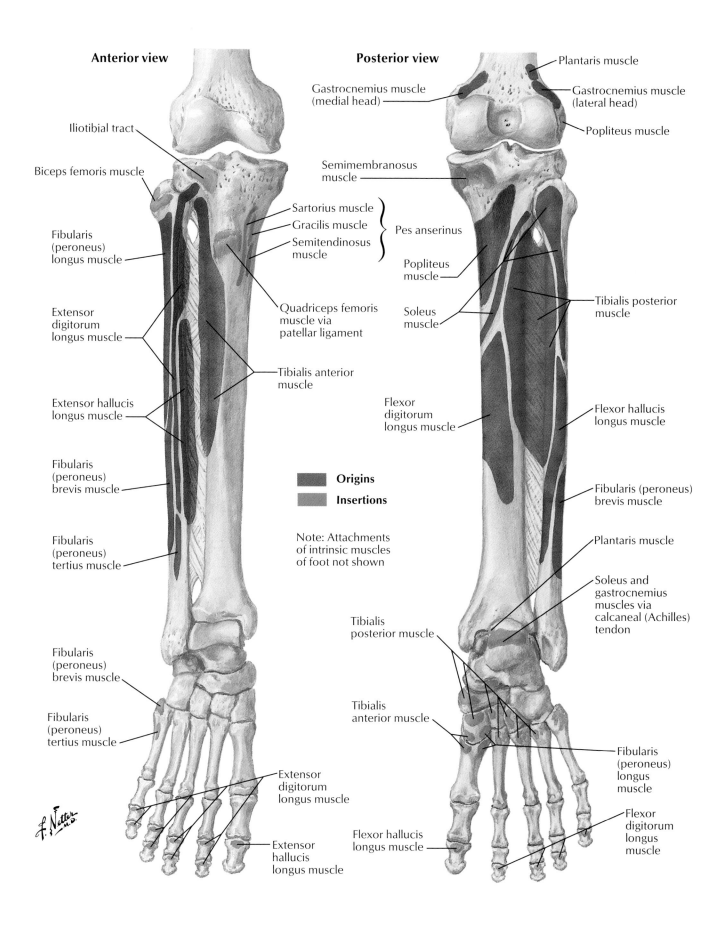

Anterior view

Iliotibial tract

Biceps femoris muscle

Fibularis (peroneus) longus muscle

Extensor digitorum longus muscle

Extensor hallucis longus muscle

Fibularis (peroneus) brevis muscle

Fibularis (peroneus) tertius muscle

Fibularis (peroneus) brevis muscle

Fibularis (peroneus) tertius muscle

Sartorius muscle
Gracilis muscle
Semitendinosus muscle
} Pes anserinus

Quadriceps femoris muscle via patellar ligament

Tibialis anterior muscle

Extensor digitorum longus muscle

Extensor hallucis longus muscle

Posterior view

Plantaris muscle

Gastrocnemius muscle (medial head)

Gastrocnemius muscle (lateral head)

Popliteus muscle

Semimembranosus muscle

Popliteus muscle

Soleus muscle

Tibialis posterior muscle

Flexor digitorum longus muscle

Flexor hallucis longus muscle

Fibularis (peroneus) brevis muscle

Plantaris muscle

Soleus and gastrocnemius muscles via calcaneal (Achilles) tendon

Tibialis posterior muscle

Tibialis anterior muscle

Fibularis (peroneus) longus muscle

Flexor hallucis longus muscle

Flexor digitorum longus muscle

Origins
Insertions

Note: Attachments of intrinsic muscles of foot not shown

Muscles of Leg (Superficial Dissection): Posterior View

See also Plate 540

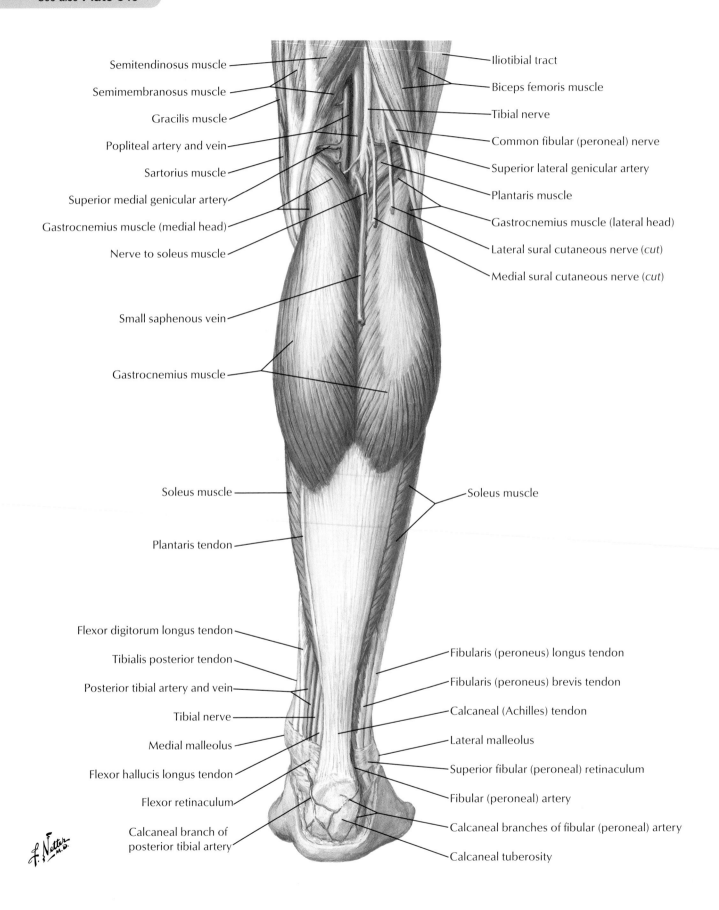

Semitendinosus muscle

Semimembranosus muscle

Gracilis muscle

Popliteal artery and vein

Sartorius muscle

Superior medial genicular artery

Gastrocnemius muscle (medial head)

Nerve to soleus muscle

Small saphenous vein

Gastrocnemius muscle

Soleus muscle

Plantaris tendon

Flexor digitorum longus tendon

Tibialis posterior tendon

Posterior tibial artery and vein

Tibial nerve

Medial malleolus

Flexor hallucis longus tendon

Flexor retinaculum

Calcaneal branch of posterior tibial artery

Iliotibial tract

Biceps femoris muscle

Tibial nerve

Common fibular (peroneal) nerve

Superior lateral genicular artery

Plantaris muscle

Gastrocnemius muscle (lateral head)

Lateral sural cutaneous nerve (cut)

Medial sural cutaneous nerve (cut)

Soleus muscle

Fibularis (peroneus) longus tendon

Fibularis (peroneus) brevis tendon

Calcaneal (Achilles) tendon

Lateral malleolus

Superior fibular (peroneal) retinaculum

Fibular (peroneal) artery

Calcaneal branches of fibular (peroneal) artery

Calcaneal tuberosity

Plate 516

Leg

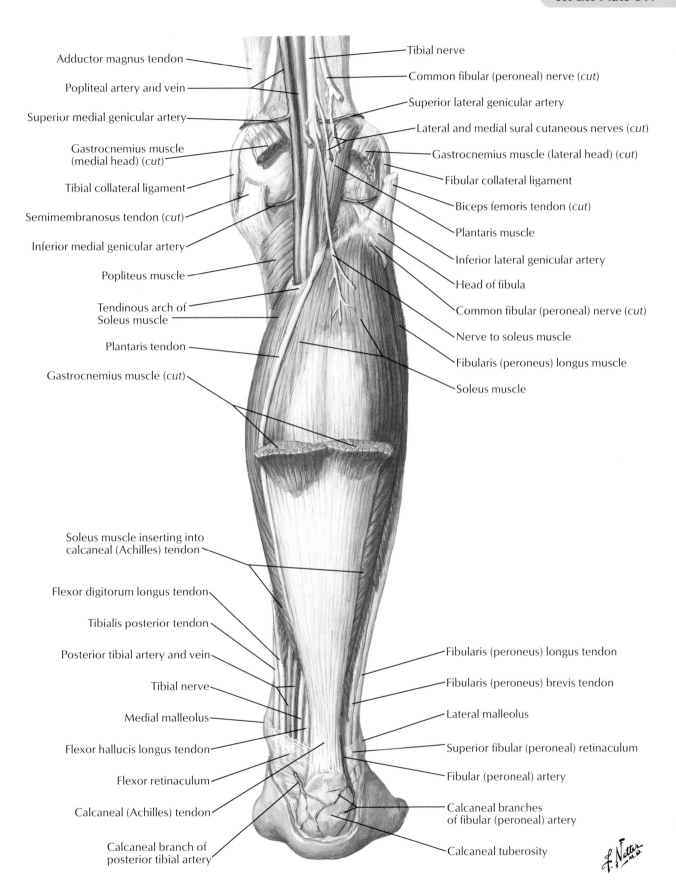

Adductor magnus tendon

Popliteal artery and vein

Superior medial genicular artery

Gastrocnemius muscle (medial head) (*cut*)

Tibial collateral ligament

Semimembranosus tendon (*cut*)

Inferior medial genicular artery

Popliteus muscle

Tendinous arch of Soleus muscle

Plantaris tendon

Gastrocnemius muscle (*cut*)

Soleus muscle inserting into calcaneal (Achilles) tendon

Flexor digitorum longus tendon

Tibialis posterior tendon

Posterior tibial artery and vein

Tibial nerve

Medial malleolus

Flexor hallucis longus tendon

Flexor retinaculum

Calcaneal (Achilles) tendon

Calcaneal branch of posterior tibial artery

Tibial nerve

Common fibular (peroneal) nerve (*cut*)

Superior lateral genicular artery

Lateral and medial sural cutaneous nerves (*cut*)

Gastrocnemius muscle (lateral head) (*cut*)

Fibular collateral ligament

Biceps femoris tendon (*cut*)

Plantaris muscle

Inferior lateral genicular artery

Head of fibula

Common fibular (peroneal) nerve (*cut*)

Nerve to soleus muscle

Fibularis (peroneus) longus muscle

Soleus muscle

Fibularis (peroneus) longus tendon

Fibularis (peroneus) brevis tendon

Lateral malleolus

Superior fibular (peroneal) retinaculum

Fibular (peroneal) artery

Calcaneal branches of fibular (peroneal) artery

Calcaneal tuberosity

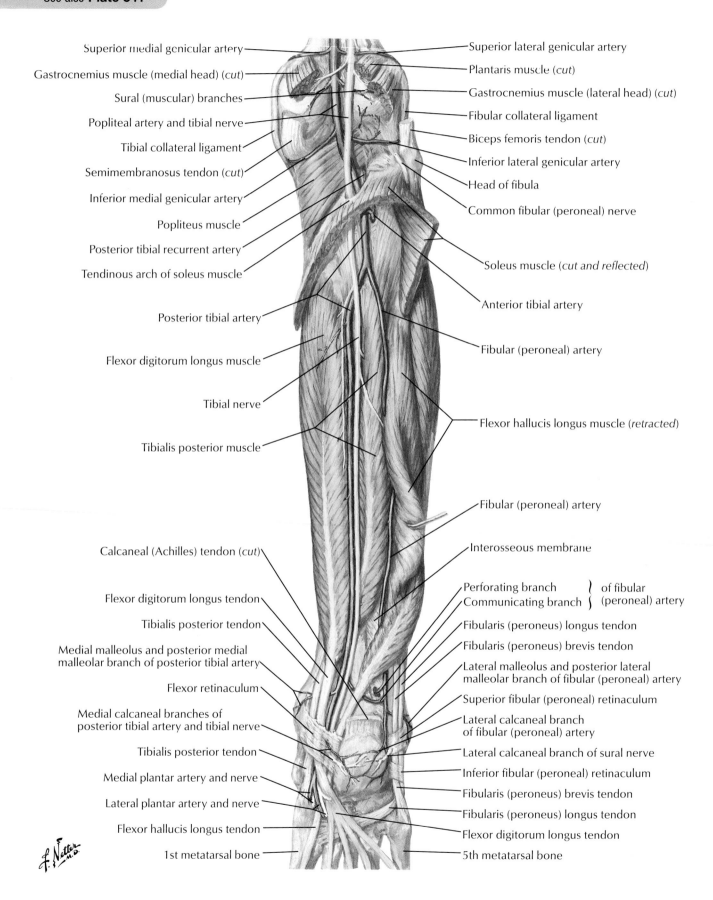

Superior medial genicular artery

Gastrocnemius muscle (medial head) (*cut*)

Sural (muscular) branches

Popliteal artery and tibial nerve

Tibial collateral ligament

Semimembranosus tendon (*cut*)

Inferior medial genicular artery

Popliteus muscle

Posterior tibial recurrent artery

Tendinous arch of soleus muscle

Posterior tibial artery

Flexor digitorum longus muscle

Tibial nerve

Tibialis posterior muscle

Calcaneal (Achilles) tendon (*cut*)

Flexor digitorum longus tendon

Tibialis posterior tendon

Medial malleolus and posterior medial malleolar branch of posterior tibial artery

Flexor retinaculum

Medial calcaneal branches of posterior tibial artery and tibial nerve

Tibialis posterior tendon

Medial plantar artery and nerve

Lateral plantar artery and nerve

Flexor hallucis longus tendon

1st metatarsal bone

Superior lateral genicular artery

Plantaris muscle (*cut*)

Gastrocnemius muscle (lateral head) (*cut*)

Fibular collateral ligament

Biceps femoris tendon (*cut*)

Inferior lateral genicular artery

Head of fibula

Common fibular (peroneal) nerve

Soleus muscle (*cut and reflected*)

Anterior tibial artery

Fibular (peroneal) artery

Flexor hallucis longus muscle (*retracted*)

Fibular (peroneal) artery

Interosseous membrane

Perforating branch   } of fibular
Communicating branch } (peroneal) artery

Fibularis (peroneus) longus tendon

Fibularis (peroneus) brevis tendon

Lateral malleolus and posterior lateral malleolar branch of fibular (peroneal) artery

Superior fibular (peroneal) retinaculum

Lateral calcaneal branch of fibular (peroneal) artery

Lateral calcaneal branch of sural nerve

Inferior fibular (peroneal) retinaculum

Fibularis (peroneus) brevis tendon

Fibularis (peroneus) longus tendon

Flexor digitorum longus tendon

5th metatarsal bone

Plate 518

Leg

See also **Plate 542**

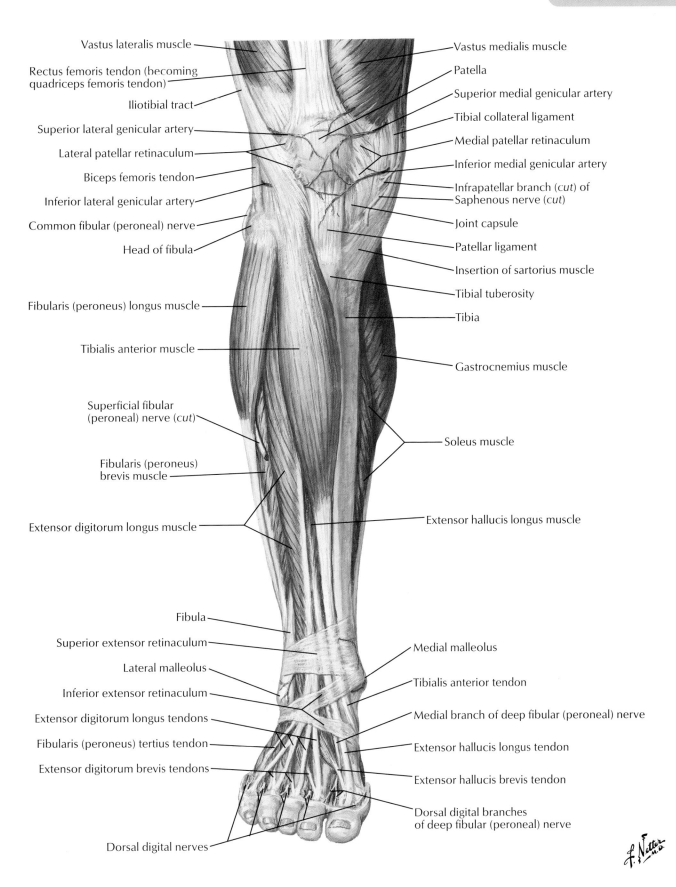

Vastus lateralis muscle

Rectus femoris tendon (becoming quadriceps femoris tendon)

Iliotibial tract

Superior lateral genicular artery

Lateral patellar retinaculum

Biceps femoris tendon

Inferior lateral genicular artery

Common fibular (peroneal) nerve

Head of fibula

Fibularis (peroneus) longus muscle

Tibialis anterior muscle

Superficial fibular (peroneal) nerve (cut)

Fibularis (peroneus) brevis muscle

Extensor digitorum longus muscle

Fibula

Superior extensor retinaculum

Lateral malleolus

Inferior extensor retinaculum

Extensor digitorum longus tendons

Fibularis (peroneus) tertius tendon

Extensor digitorum brevis tendons

Dorsal digital nerves

Vastus medialis muscle

Patella

Superior medial genicular artery

Tibial collateral ligament

Medial patellar retinaculum

Inferior medial genicular artery

Infrapatellar branch (cut) of Saphenous nerve (cut)

Joint capsule

Patellar ligament

Insertion of sartorius muscle

Tibial tuberosity

Tibia

Gastrocnemius muscle

Soleus muscle

Extensor hallucis longus muscle

Medial malleolus

Tibialis anterior tendon

Medial branch of deep fibular (peroneal) nerve

Extensor hallucis longus tendon

Extensor hallucis brevis tendon

Dorsal digital branches of deep fibular (peroneal) nerve

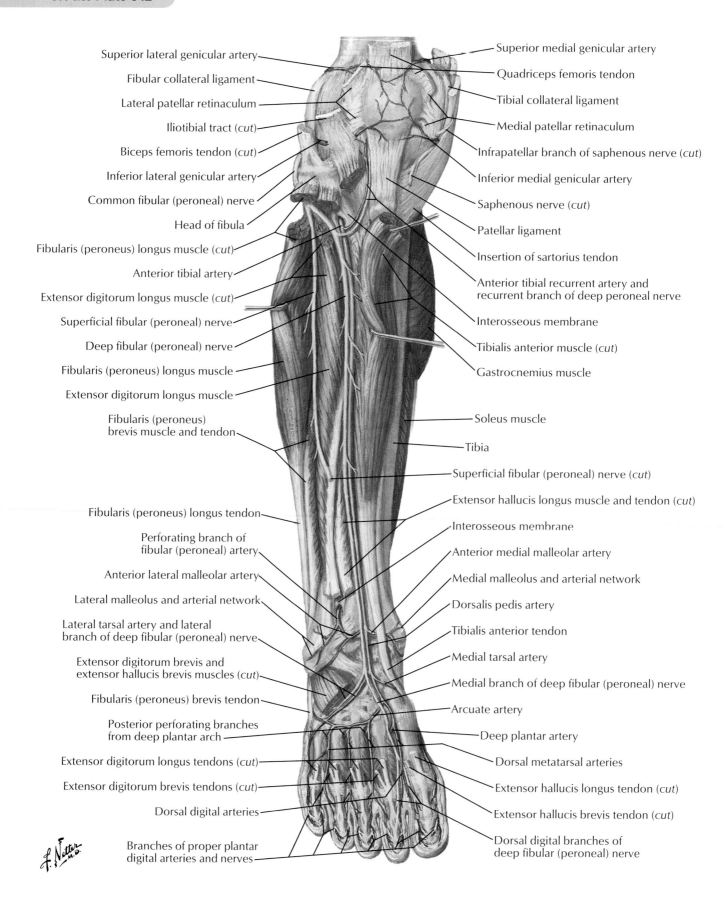

Superior lateral genicular artery

Fibular collateral ligament

Lateral patellar retinaculum

Iliotibial tract (*cut*)

Biceps femoris tendon (*cut*)

Inferior lateral genicular artery

Common fibular (peroneal) nerve

Head of fibula

Fibularis (peroneus) longus muscle (*cut*)

Anterior tibial artery

Extensor digitorum longus muscle (*cut*)

Superficial fibular (peroneal) nerve

Deep fibular (peroneal) nerve

Fibularis (peroneus) longus muscle

Extensor digitorum longus muscle

Fibularis (peroneus) brevis muscle and tendon

Fibularis (peroneus) longus tendon

Perforating branch of fibular (peroneal) artery

Anterior lateral malleolar artery

Lateral malleolus and arterial network

Lateral tarsal artery and lateral branch of deep fibular (peroneal) nerve

Extensor digitorum brevis and extensor hallucis brevis muscles (*cut*)

Fibularis (peroneus) brevis tendon

Posterior perforating branches from deep plantar arch

Extensor digitorum longus tendons (*cut*)

Extensor digitorum brevis tendons (*cut*)

Dorsal digital arteries

Branches of proper plantar digital arteries and nerves

Superior medial genicular artery

Quadriceps femoris tendon

Tibial collateral ligament

Medial patellar retinaculum

Infrapatellar branch of saphenous nerve (*cut*)

Inferior medial genicular artery

Saphenous nerve (*cut*)

Patellar ligament

Insertion of sartorius tendon

Anterior tibial recurrent artery and recurrent branch of deep peroneal nerve

Interosseous membrane

Tibialis anterior muscle (*cut*)

Gastrocnemius muscle

Soleus muscle

Tibia

Superficial fibular (peroneal) nerve (*cut*)

Extensor hallucis longus muscle and tendon (*cut*)

Interosseous membrane

Anterior medial malleolar artery

Medial malleolus and arterial network

Dorsalis pedis artery

Tibialis anterior tendon

Medial tarsal artery

Medial branch of deep fibular (peroneal) nerve

Arcuate artery

Deep plantar artery

Dorsal metatarsal arteries

Extensor hallucis longus tendon (*cut*)

Extensor hallucis brevis tendon (*cut*)

Dorsal digital branches of deep fibular (peroneal) nerve

Plate 520

Leg

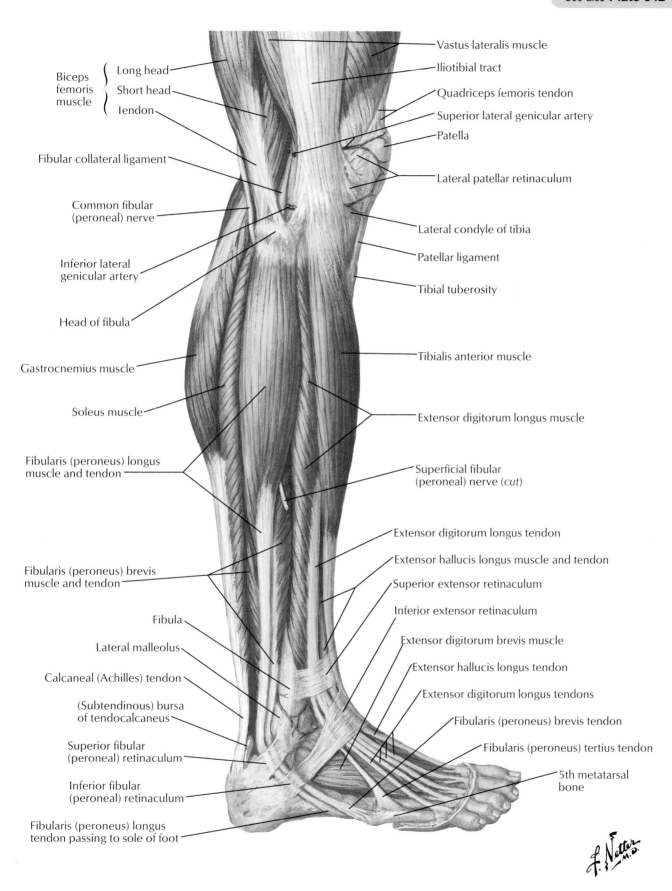

Vastus lateralis muscle

Iliotibial tract

Biceps femoris muscle
- Long head
- Short head
- Tendon

Quadriceps femoris tendon

Superior lateral genicular artery

Patella

Fibular collateral ligament

Lateral patellar retinaculum

Common fibular (peroneal) nerve

Lateral condyle of tibia

Inferior lateral genicular artery

Patellar ligament

Tibial tuberosity

Head of fibula

Tibialis anterior muscle

Gastrocnemius muscle

Soleus muscle

Extensor digitorum longus muscle

Fibularis (peroneus) longus muscle and tendon

Superficial fibular (peroneal) nerve (*cut*)

Extensor digitorum longus tendon

Extensor hallucis longus muscle and tendon

Superior extensor retinaculum

Fibularis (peroneus) brevis muscle and tendon

Inferior extensor retinaculum

Extensor digitorum brevis muscle

Fibula

Extensor hallucis longus tendon

Lateral malleolus

Extensor digitorum longus tendons

Calcaneal (Achilles) tendon

Fibularis (peroneus) brevis tendon

(Subtendinous) bursa of tendocalcaneus

Fibularis (peroneus) tertius tendon

Superior fibular (peroneal) retinaculum

5th metatarsal bone

Inferior fibular (peroneal) retinaculum

Fibularis (peroneus) longus tendon passing to sole of foot

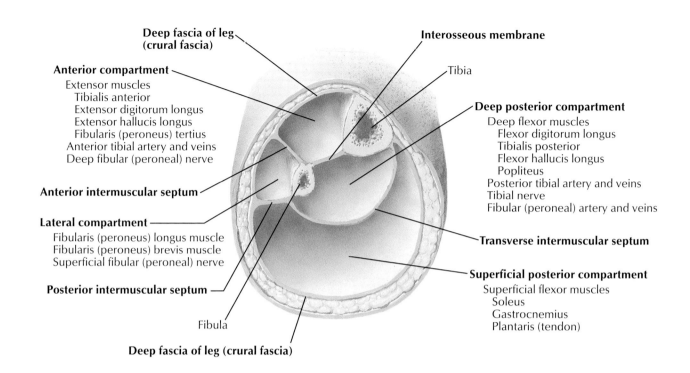

Deep fascia of leg (crural fascia)

Interosseous membrane

Anterior compartment
Extensor muscles
Tibialis anterior
Extensor digitorum longus
Extensor hallucis longus
Fibularis (peroneus) tertius
Anterior tibial artery and veins
Deep fibular (peroneal) nerve

Tibia

Deep posterior compartment
Deep flexor muscles
Flexor digitorum longus
Tibialis posterior
Flexor hallucis longus
Popliteus
Posterior tibial artery and veins
Tibial nerve
Fibular (peroneal) artery and veins

Anterior intermuscular septum

Lateral compartment
Fibularis (peroneus) longus muscle
Fibularis (peroneus) brevis muscle
Superficial fibular (peroneal) nerve

Transverse intermuscular septum

Posterior intermuscular septum

Superficial posterior compartment
Superficial flexor muscles
Soleus
Gastrocnemius
Plantaris (tendon)

Fibula

Deep fascia of leg (crural fascia)

Cross section just above middle of leg

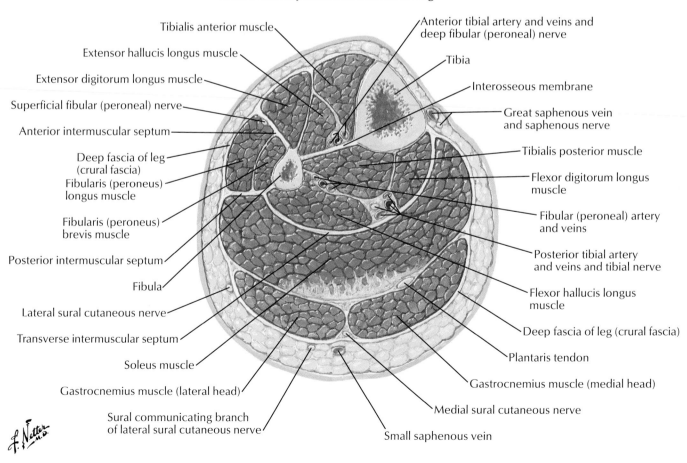

Tibialis anterior muscle

Anterior tibial artery and veins and deep fibular (peroneal) nerve

Extensor hallucis longus muscle

Tibia

Extensor digitorum longus muscle

Interosseous membrane

Superficial fibular (peroneal) nerve

Great saphenous vein and saphenous nerve

Anterior intermuscular septum

Tibialis posterior muscle

Deep fascia of leg (crural fascia)

Flexor digitorum longus muscle

Fibularis (peroneus) longus muscle

Fibular (peroneal) artery and veins

Fibularis (peroneus) brevis muscle

Posterior intermuscular septum

Posterior tibial artery and veins and tibial nerve

Fibula

Flexor hallucis longus muscle

Lateral sural cutaneous nerve

Deep fascia of leg (crural fascia)

Transverse intermuscular septum

Plantaris tendon

Soleus muscle

Gastrocnemius muscle (medial head)

Gastrocnemius muscle (lateral head)

Medial sural cutaneous nerve

Sural communicating branch of lateral sural cutaneous nerve

Small saphenous vein

Plate 522

Leg

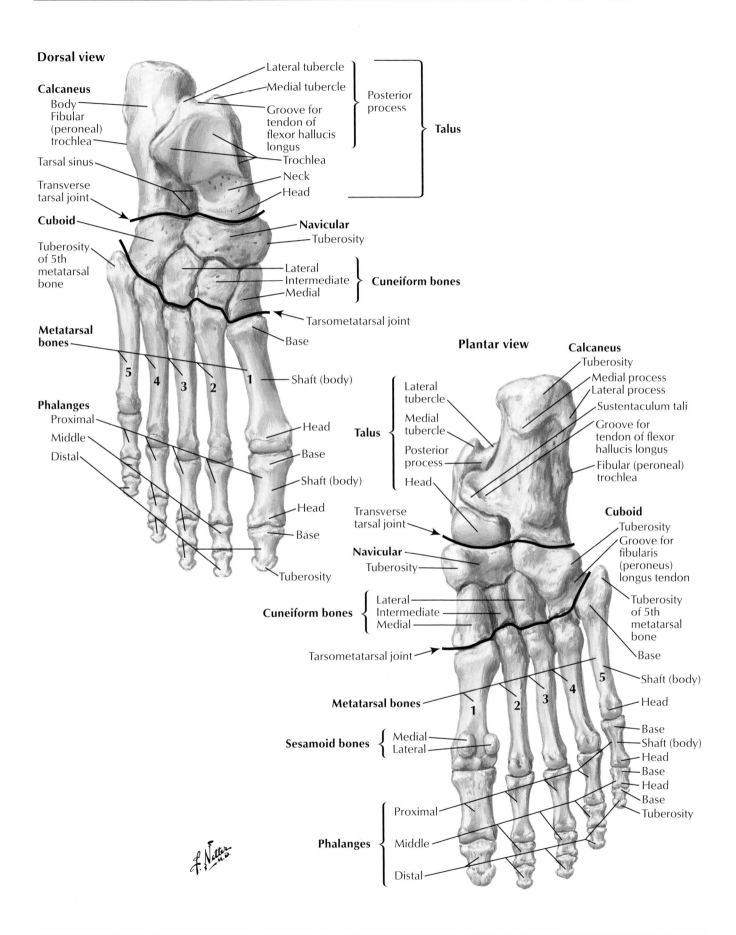

Dorsal view

Calcaneus
Body
Fibular (peroneal) trochlea
Tarsal sinus
Transverse tarsal joint
Cuboid
Tuberosity of 5th metatarsal bone

Lateral tubercle
Medial tubercle
Groove for tendon of flexor hallucis longus
Trochlea
Neck
Head

Posterior process

Talus

Navicular
Tuberosity

Lateral
Intermediate
Medial

Cuneiform bones

Tarsometatarsal joint
Base

Metatarsal bones

5 4 3 2 1

Shaft (body)

Phalanges
Proximal
Middle
Distal

Head
Base
Shaft (body)
Head
Base

Tuberosity

Plantar view

Lateral tubercle
Medial tubercle
Posterior process
Head

Talus

Transverse tarsal joint

Navicular
Tuberosity

Lateral
Intermediate
Medial

Cuneiform bones

Tarsometatarsal joint

Metatarsal bones

1 2 3 4 5

Sesamoid bones
Medial
Lateral

Phalanges
Proximal
Middle
Distal

Calcaneus
Tuberosity
Medial process
Lateral process
Sustentaculum tali
Groove for tendon of flexor hallucis longus
Fibular (peroneal) trochlea

Cuboid
Tuberosity
Groove for fibularis (peroneus) longus tendon
Tuberosity of 5th metatarsal bone
Base

Shaft (body)
Head
Base
Shaft (body)
Head
Base
Head
Base
Tuberosity

Lateral view

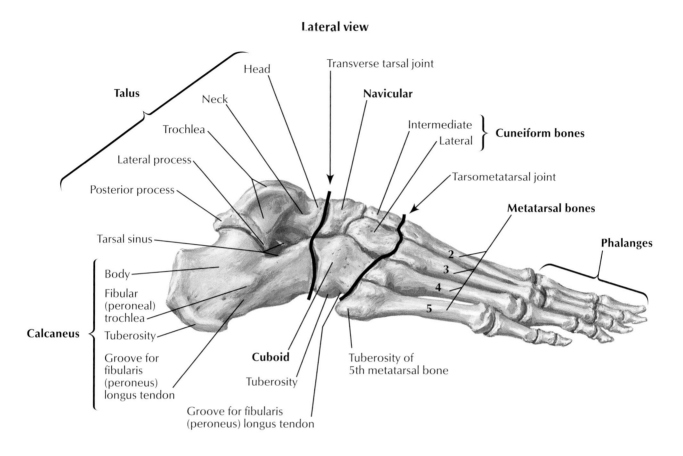

Talus
Head
Neck
Trochlea
Lateral process
Posterior process
Tarsal sinus
Calcaneus
Body
Fibular (peroneal) trochlea
Tuberosity
Groove for fibularis (peroneus) longus tendon
Groove for fibularis (peroneus) longus tendon
Cuboid
Tuberosity
Transverse tarsal joint
Navicular
Intermediate
Lateral
Cuneiform bones
Tarsometatarsal joint
Metatarsal bones
2
3
4
5
Phalanges
Tuberosity of 5th metatarsal bone

Medial view

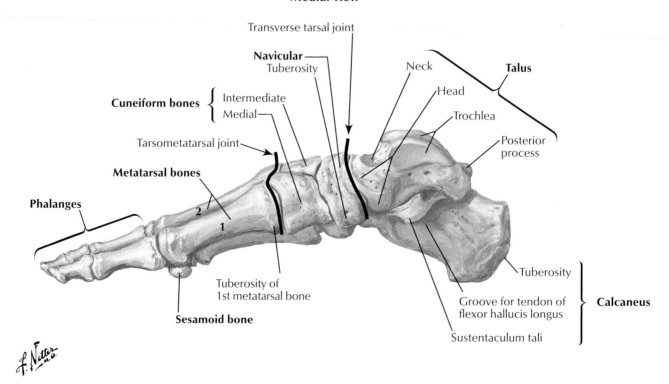

Transverse tarsal joint
Navicular
Tuberosity
Cuneiform bones
Intermediate
Medial
Tarsometatarsal joint
Metatarsal bones
2
1
Phalanges
Tuberosity of 1st metatarsal bone
Sesamoid bone
Neck
Head
Talus
Trochlea
Posterior process
Tuberosity
Groove for tendon of flexor hallucis longus
Calcaneus
Sustentaculum tali

Plate 524

Ankle and Foot

Right foot

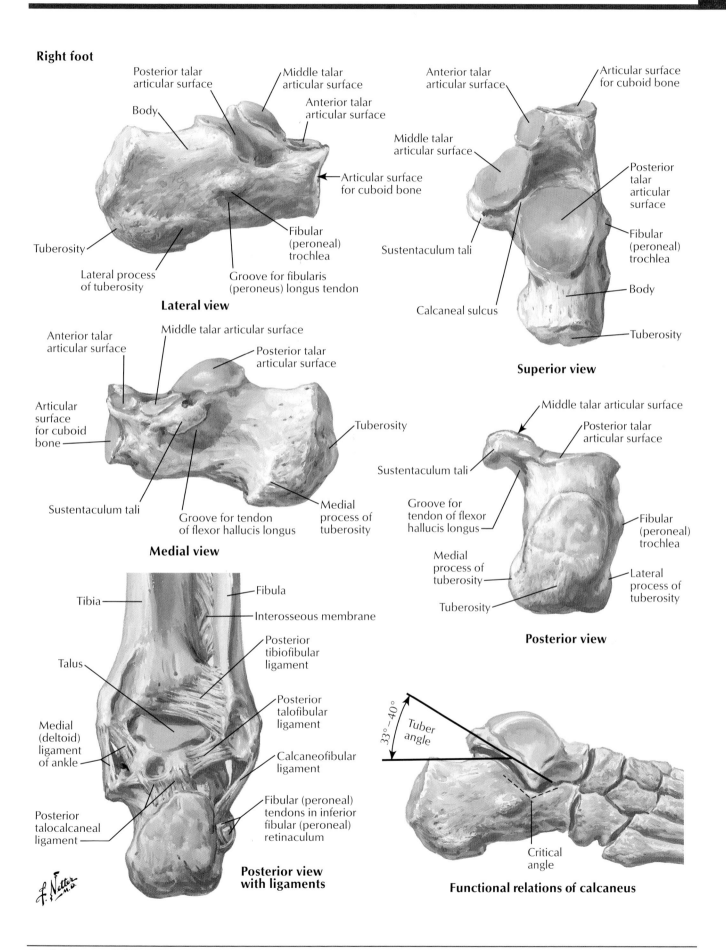

Posterior talar articular surface

Middle talar articular surface

Anterior talar articular surface

Body

Article surface for cuboid bone

Tuberosity

Fibular (peroneal) trochlea

Lateral process of tuberosity

Groove for fibularis (peroneus) longus tendon

Lateral view

Anterior talar articular surface

Articular surface for cuboid bone

Middle talar articular surface

Posterior talar articular surface

Middle talar articular surface

Posterior talar articular surface

Articular surface for cuboid bone

Sustentaculum tali

Calcaneal sulcus

Fibular (peroneal) trochlea

Body

Tuberosity

Superior view

Anterior talar articular surface

Article surface for cuboid bone

Sustentaculum tali

Groove for tendon of flexor hallucis longus

Tuberosity

Medial process of tuberosity

Medial view

Middle talar articular surface

Posterior talar articular surface

Sustentaculum tali

Groove for tendon of flexor hallucis longus

Medial process of tuberosity

Tuberosity

Fibular (peroneal) trochlea

Lateral process of tuberosity

Posterior view

Tibia

Fibula

Interosseous membrane

Talus

Posterior tibiofibular ligament

Posterior talofibular ligament

Medial (deltoid) ligament of ankle

Calcaneofibular ligament

Fibular (peroneal) tendons in inferior fibular (peroneal) retinaculum

Posterior talocalcaneal ligament

Posterior view with ligaments

33°–40°

Tuber angle

Critical angle

Functional relations of calcaneus

f. Netter

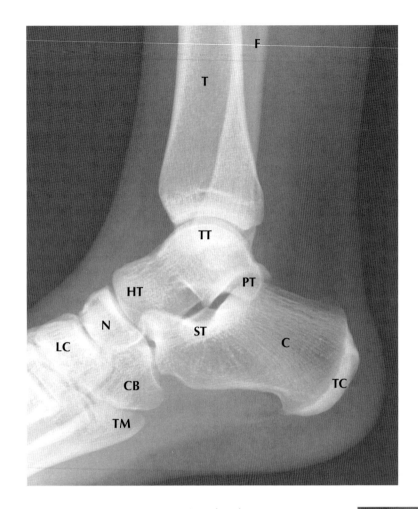

Lateral view

C	Calcaneus
CB	Cuboid
F	Fibula
HT	Head of talus
LC	Lateral cuneiform
N	Navicular
PT	Posterior process of talus
ST	Sustentaculum tali of calcaneus
T	Tibia
TC	Tuberosity of calcaneus
TM	Tuberosity of 5th metatarsal
TT	Trochlea of talus

Anterior view

F	Fibula
LM	Lateral malleolus
MM	Medial malleolus
T	Tibia
TA	Talus

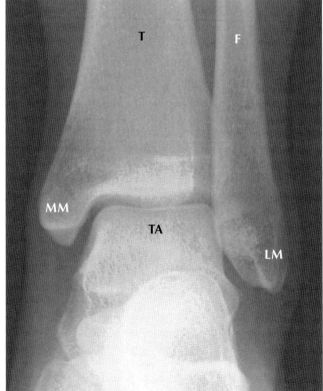

Plate 526

Ankle and Foot

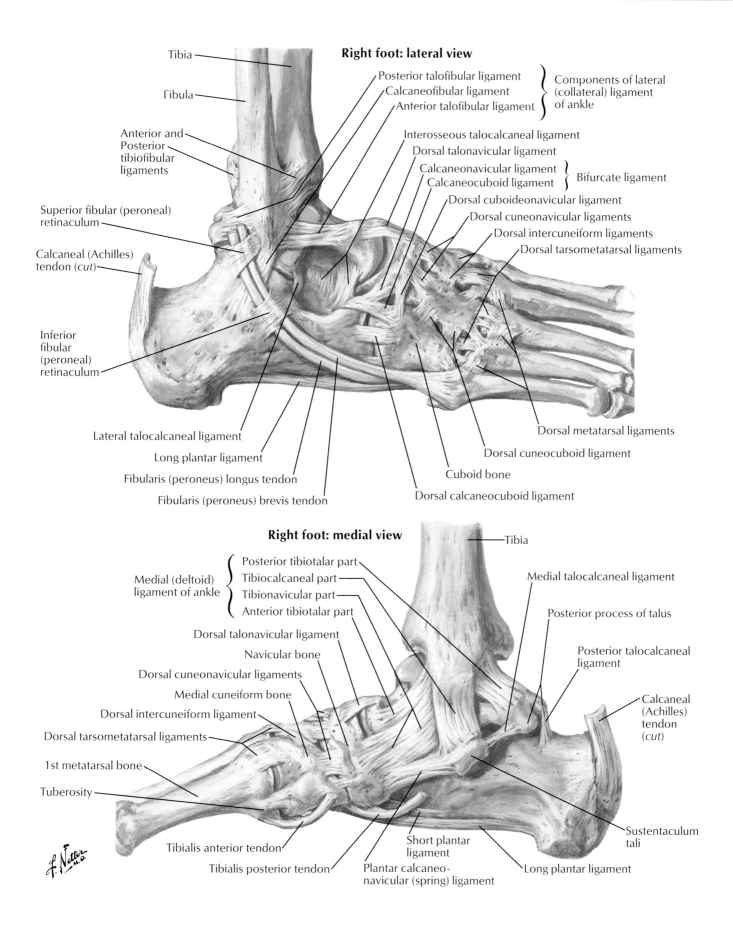

Right foot: lateral view

Tibia

Fibula

Anterior and Posterior tibiofibular ligaments

Superior fibular (peroneal) retinaculum

Calcaneal (Achilles) tendon (*cut*)

Inferior fibular (peroneal) retinaculum

Posterior talofibular ligament
Calcaneofibular ligament
Anterior talofibular ligament
} Components of lateral (collateral) ligament of ankle

Interosseous talocalcaneal ligament
Dorsal talonavicular ligament
Calcaneonavicular ligament
Calcaneocuboid ligament
} Bifurcate ligament

Dorsal cuboideonavicular ligament
Dorsal cuneonavicular ligaments
Dorsal intercuneiform ligaments
Dorsal tarsometatarsal ligaments

Lateral talocalcaneal ligament
Long plantar ligament
Fibularis (peroneus) longus tendon
Fibularis (peroneus) brevis tendon

Dorsal metatarsal ligaments
Dorsal cuneocuboid ligament
Cuboid bone
Dorsal calcaneocuboid ligament

Right foot: medial view

Tibia

Medial (deltoid) ligament of ankle {
Posterior tibiotalar part
Tibiocalcaneal part
Tibionavicular part
Anterior tibiotalar part

Dorsal talonavicular ligament
Navicular bone
Dorsal cuneonavicular ligaments
Medial cuneiform bone
Dorsal intercuneiform ligament
Dorsal tarsometatarsal ligaments
1st metatarsal bone
Tuberosity

Medial talocalcaneal ligament
Posterior process of talus
Posterior talocalcaneal ligament
Calcaneal (Achilles) tendon (*cut*)
Sustentaculum tali

Tibialis anterior tendon
Tibialis posterior tendon
Short plantar ligament
Plantar calcaneo-navicular (spring) ligament
Long plantar ligament

f. Netter m.d.

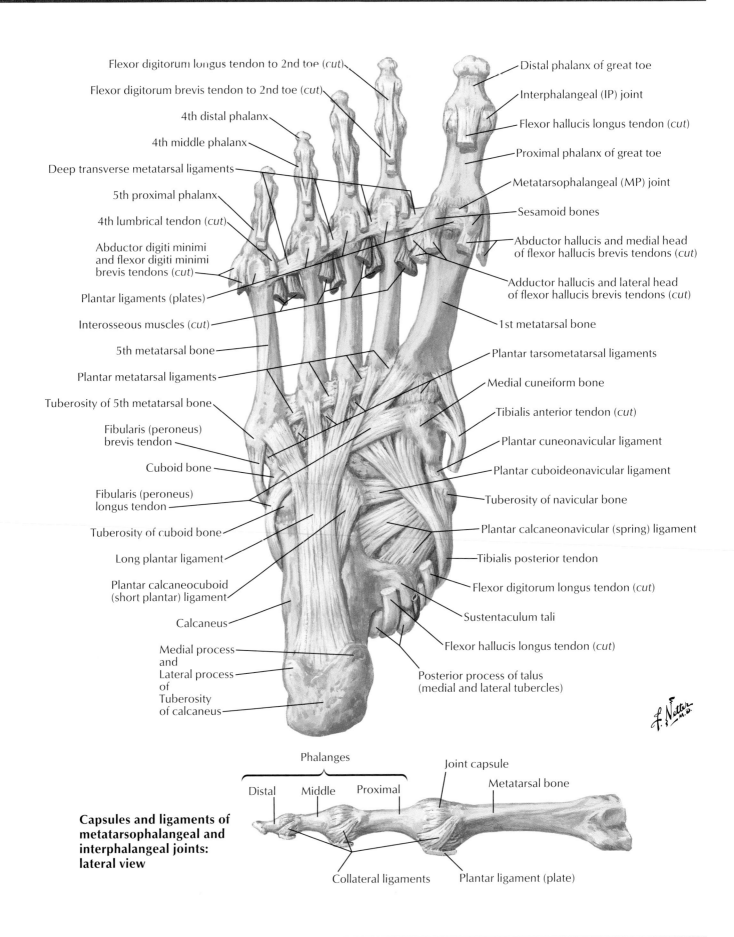

Flexor digitorum longus tendon to 2nd toe (*cut*)

Flexor digitorum brevis tendon to 2nd toe (*cut*)

4th distal phalanx

4th middle phalanx

Deep transverse metatarsal ligaments

5th proximal phalanx

4th lumbrical tendon (*cut*)

Abductor digiti minimi and flexor digiti minimi brevis tendons (*cut*)

Plantar ligaments (plates)

Interosseous muscles (*cut*)

5th metatarsal bone

Plantar metatarsal ligaments

Tuberosity of 5th metatarsal bone

Fibularis (peroneus) brevis tendon

Cuboid bone

Fibularis (peroneus) longus tendon

Tuberosity of cuboid bone

Long plantar ligament

Plantar calcaneocuboid (short plantar) ligament

Calcaneus

Medial process and Lateral process of Tuberosity of calcaneus

Distal phalanx of great toe

Interphalangeal (IP) joint

Flexor hallucis longus tendon (*cut*)

Proximal phalanx of great toe

Metatarsophalangeal (MP) joint

Sesamoid bones

Abductor hallucis and medial head of flexor hallucis brevis tendons (*cut*)

Adductor hallucis and lateral head of flexor hallucis brevis tendons (*cut*)

1st metatarsal bone

Plantar tarsometatarsal ligaments

Medial cuneiform bone

Tibialis anterior tendon (*cut*)

Plantar cuneonavicular ligament

Plantar cuboideonavicular ligament

Tuberosity of navicular bone

Plantar calcaneonavicular (spring) ligament

Tibialis posterior tendon

Flexor digitorum longus tendon (*cut*)

Sustentaculum tali

Flexor hallucis longus tendon (*cut*)

Posterior process of talus (medial and lateral tubercles)

Phalanges

Distal   Middle   Proximal

Joint capsule

Metatarsal bone

Capsules and ligaments of metatarsophalangeal and interphalangeal joints: lateral view

Collateral ligaments

Plantar ligament (plate)

Plate 528

Ankle and Foot

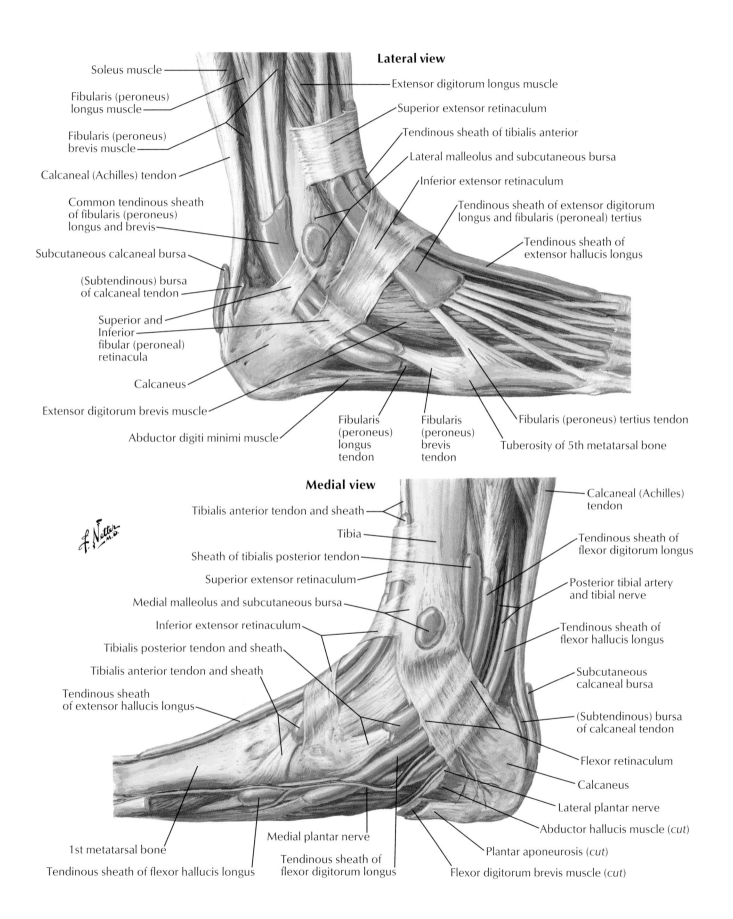

Lateral view

Soleus muscle

Fibularis (peroneus) longus muscle

Fibularis (peroneus) brevis muscle

Calcaneal (Achilles) tendon

Common tendinous sheath of fibularis (peroneus) longus and brevis

Subcutaneous calcaneal bursa

(Subtendinous) bursa of calcaneal tendon

Superior and Inferior fibular (peroneal) retinacula

Calcaneus

Extensor digitorum brevis muscle

Abductor digiti minimi muscle

Extensor digitorum longus muscle

Superior extensor retinaculum

Tendinous sheath of tibialis anterior

Lateral malleolus and subcutaneous bursa

Inferior extensor retinaculum

Tendinous sheath of extensor digitorum longus and fibularis (peroneal) tertius

Tendinous sheath of extensor hallucis longus

Fibularis (peroneus) longus tendon

Fibularis (peroneus) brevis tendon

Fibularis (peroneus) tertius tendon

Tuberosity of 5th metatarsal bone

Medial view

Tibialis anterior tendon and sheath

Tibia

Sheath of tibialis posterior tendon

Superior extensor retinaculum

Medial malleolus and subcutaneous bursa

Inferior extensor retinaculum

Tibialis posterior tendon and sheath

Tibialis anterior tendon and sheath

Tendinous sheath of extensor hallucis longus

1st metatarsal bone

Tendinous sheath of flexor hallucis longus

Medial plantar nerve

Tendinous sheath of flexor digitorum longus

Calcaneal (Achilles) tendon

Tendinous sheath of flexor digitorum longus

Posterior tibial artery and tibial nerve

Tendinous sheath of flexor hallucis longus

Subcutaneous calcaneal bursa

(Subtendinous) bursa of calcaneal tendon

Flexor retinaculum

Calcaneus

Lateral plantar nerve

Abductor hallucis muscle (*cut*)

Plantar aponeurosis (*cut*)

Flexor digitorum brevis muscle (*cut*)

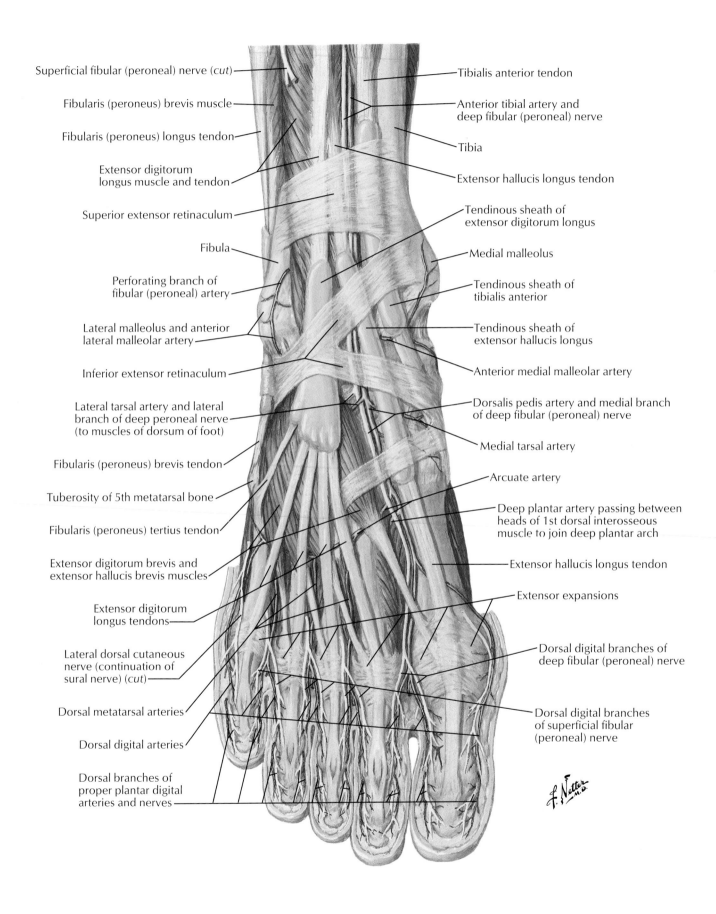

Superficial fibular (peroneal) nerve (*cut*)

Fibularis (peroneus) brevis muscle

Fibularis (peroneus) longus tendon

Extensor digitorum longus muscle and tendon

Superior extensor retinaculum

Fibula

Perforating branch of fibular (peroneal) artery

Lateral malleolus and anterior lateral malleolar artery

Inferior extensor retinaculum

Lateral tarsal artery and lateral branch of deep peroneal nerve (to muscles of dorsum of foot)

Fibularis (peroneus) brevis tendon

Tuberosity of 5th metatarsal bone

Fibularis (peroneus) tertius tendon

Extensor digitorum brevis and extensor hallucis brevis muscles

Extensor digitorum longus tendons

Lateral dorsal cutaneous nerve (continuation of sural nerve) (*cut*)

Dorsal metatarsal arteries

Dorsal digital arteries

Dorsal branches of proper plantar digital arteries and nerves

Tibialis anterior tendon

Anterior tibial artery and deep fibular (peroneal) nerve

Tibia

Extensor hallucis longus tendon

Tendinous sheath of extensor digitorum longus

Medial malleolus

Tendinous sheath of tibialis anterior

Tendinous sheath of extensor hallucis longus

Anterior medial malleolar artery

Dorsalis pedis artery and medial branch of deep fibular (peroneal) nerve

Medial tarsal artery

Arcuate artery

Deep plantar artery passing between heads of 1st dorsal interosseous muscle to join deep plantar arch

Extensor hallucis longus tendon

Extensor expansions

Dorsal digital branches of deep fibular (peroneal) nerve

Dorsal digital branches of superficial fibular (peroneal) nerve

Plate 530

Ankle and Foot

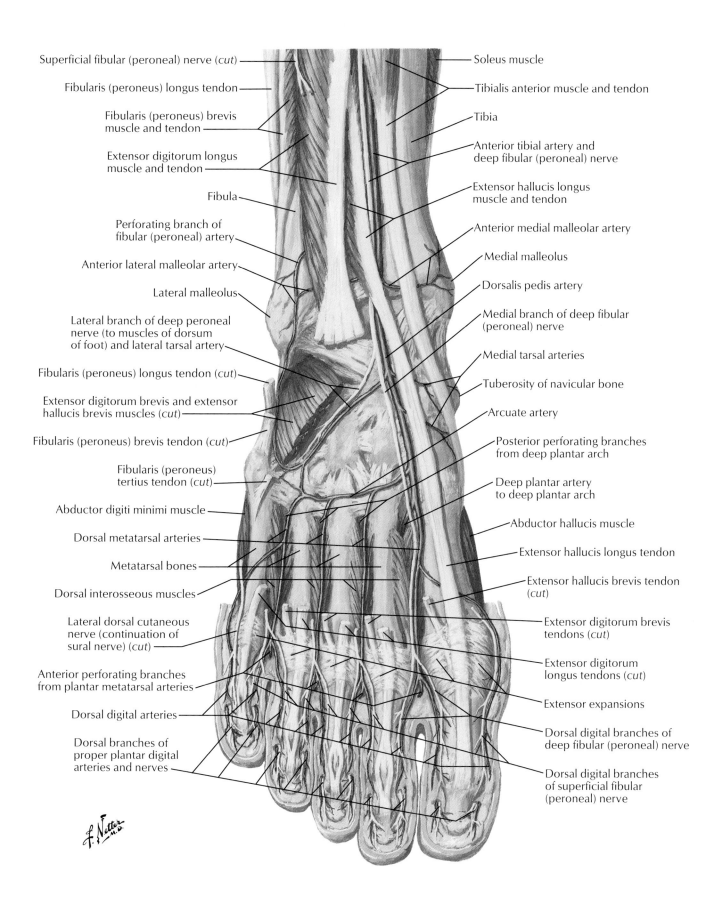

Superficial fibular (peroneal) nerve (cut)

Fibularis (peroneus) longus tendon

Fibularis (peroneus) brevis muscle and tendon

Extensor digitorum longus muscle and tendon

Fibula

Perforating branch of fibular (peroneal) artery

Anterior lateral malleolar artery

Lateral malleolus

Lateral branch of deep peroneal nerve (to muscles of dorsum of foot) and lateral tarsal artery

Fibularis (peroneus) longus tendon (cut)

Extensor digitorum brevis and extensor hallucis brevis muscles (cut)

Fibularis (peroneus) brevis tendon (cut)

Fibularis (peroneus) tertius tendon (cut)

Abductor digiti minimi muscle

Dorsal metatarsal arteries

Metatarsal bones

Dorsal interosseous muscles

Lateral dorsal cutaneous nerve (continuation of sural nerve) (cut)

Anterior perforating branches from plantar metatarsal arteries

Dorsal digital arteries

Dorsal branches of proper plantar digital arteries and nerves

Soleus muscle

Tibialis anterior muscle and tendon

Tibia

Anterior tibial artery and deep fibular (peroneal) nerve

Extensor hallucis longus muscle and tendon

Anterior medial malleolar artery

Medial malleolus

Dorsalis pedis artery

Medial branch of deep fibular (peroneal) nerve

Medial tarsal arteries

Tuberosity of navicular bone

Arcuate artery

Posterior perforating branches from deep plantar arch

Deep plantar artery to deep plantar arch

Abductor hallucis muscle

Extensor hallucis longus tendon

Extensor hallucis brevis tendon (cut)

Extensor digitorum brevis tendons (cut)

Extensor digitorum longus tendons (cut)

Extensor expansions

Dorsal digital branches of deep fibular (peroneal) nerve

Dorsal digital branches of superficial fibular (peroneal) nerve

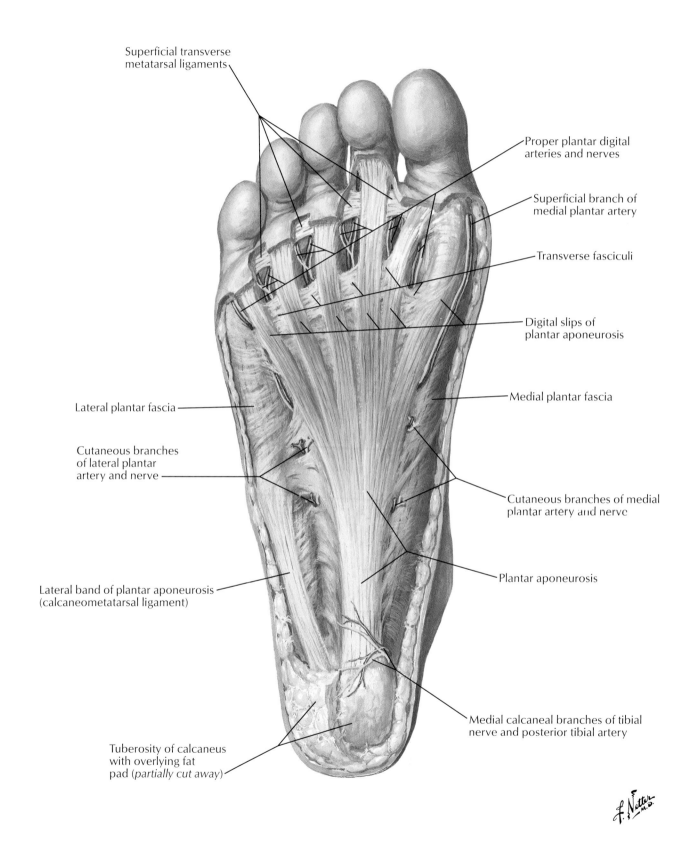

Superficial transverse
metatarsal ligaments

Proper plantar digital
arteries and nerves

Superficial branch of
medial plantar artery

Transverse fasciculi

Digital slips of
plantar aponeurosis

Medial plantar fascia

Lateral plantar fascia

Cutaneous branches
of lateral plantar
artery and nerve

Cutaneous branches of medial
plantar artery and nerve

Lateral band of plantar aponeurosis
(calcaneometatarsal ligament)

Plantar aponeurosis

Tuberosity of calcaneus
with overlying fat
pad (*partially cut away*)

Medial calcaneal branches of tibial
nerve and posterior tibial artery

Plate 532   **Ankle and Foot**

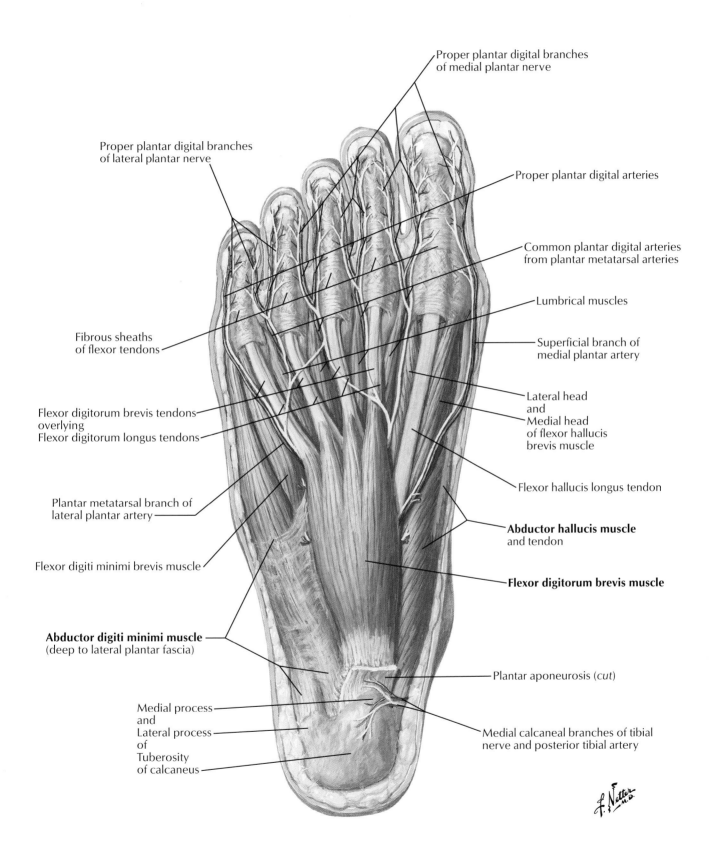

Proper plantar digital branches
of medial plantar nerve

Proper plantar digital branches
of lateral plantar nerve

Proper plantar digital arteries

Common plantar digital arteries
from plantar metatarsal arteries

Lumbrical muscles

Fibrous sheaths
of flexor tendons

Superficial branch of
medial plantar artery

Lateral head
and
Medial head
of flexor hallucis
brevis muscle

Flexor digitorum brevis tendons
overlying
Flexor digitorum longus tendons

Flexor hallucis longus tendon

Plantar metatarsal branch of
lateral plantar artery

Abductor hallucis muscle
and tendon

Flexor digiti minimi brevis muscle

Flexor digitorum brevis muscle

Abductor digiti minimi muscle
(deep to lateral plantar fascia)

Plantar aponeurosis (cut)

Medial process
and
Lateral process
of
Tuberosity
of calcaneus

Medial calcaneal branches of tibial
nerve and posterior tibial artery

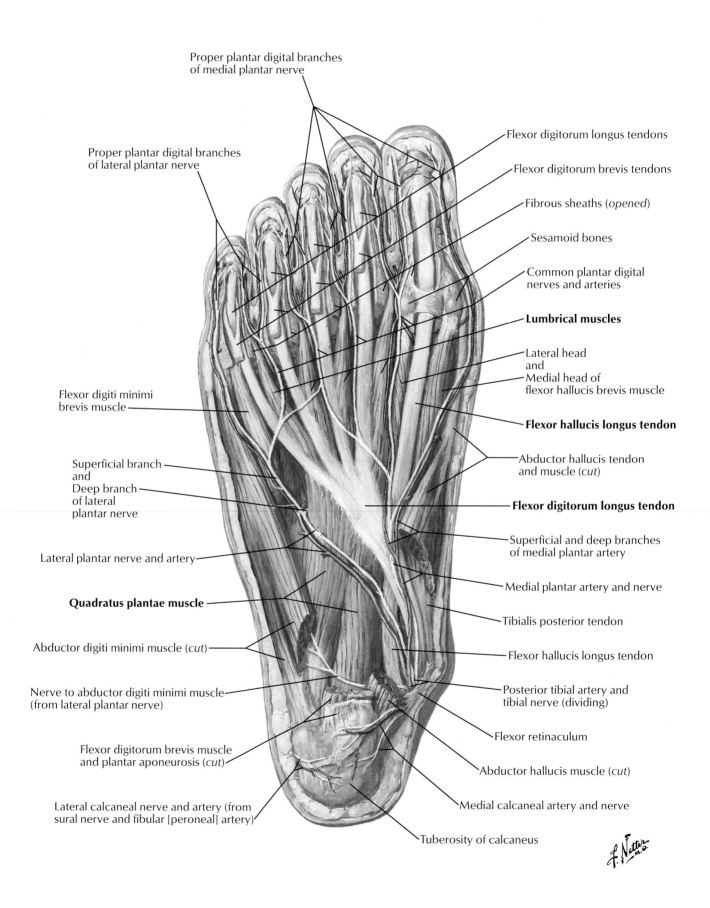

Proper plantar digital branches
of medial plantar nerve

Proper plantar digital branches
of lateral plantar nerve

Flexor digitorum longus tendons

Flexor digitorum brevis tendons

Fibrous sheaths (*opened*)

Sesamoid bones

Common plantar digital
nerves and arteries

Lumbrical muscles

Lateral head
and
Medial head of
flexor hallucis brevis muscle

Flexor hallucis longus tendon

Abductor hallucis tendon
and muscle (*cut*)

Flexor digitorum longus tendon

Superficial and deep branches
of medial plantar artery

Medial plantar artery and nerve

Tibialis posterior tendon

Flexor hallucis longus tendon

Posterior tibial artery and
tibial nerve (dividing)

Flexor retinaculum

Abductor hallucis muscle (*cut*)

Medial calcaneal artery and nerve

Flexor digiti minimi
brevis muscle

Superficial branch
and
Deep branch
of lateral
plantar nerve

Lateral plantar nerve and artery

Quadratus plantae muscle

Abductor digiti minimi muscle (*cut*)

Nerve to abductor digiti minimi muscle
(from lateral plantar nerve)

Flexor digitorum brevis muscle
and plantar aponeurosis (*cut*)

Lateral calcaneal nerve and artery (from
sural nerve and fibular [peroneal] artery)

Tuberosity of calcaneus

Plate 534   **Ankle and Foot**

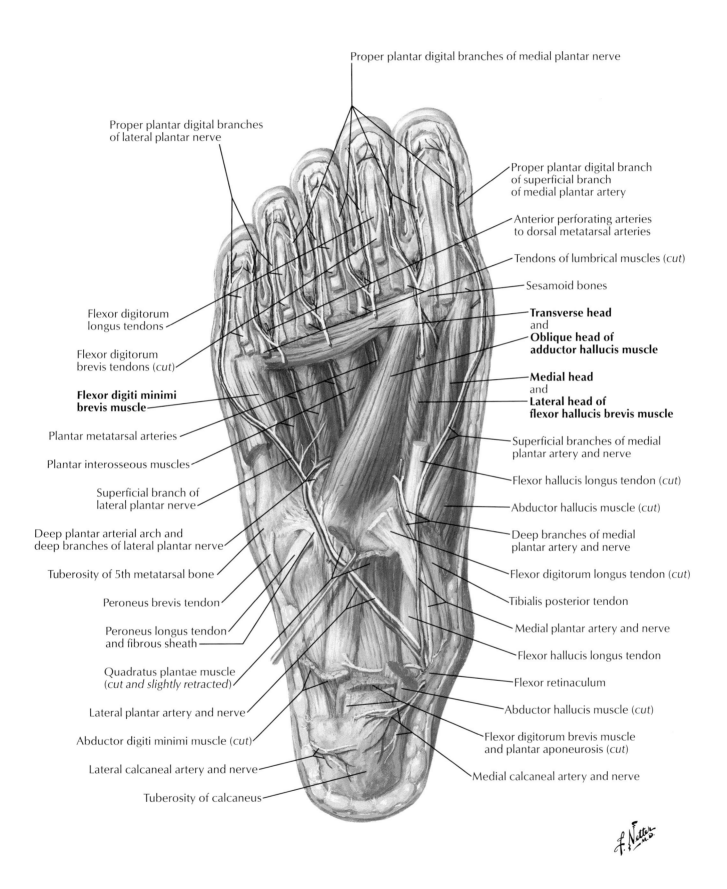

Proper plantar digital branches of medial plantar nerve

Proper plantar digital branches of lateral plantar nerve

Proper plantar digital branch of superficial branch of medial plantar artery

Anterior perforating arteries to dorsal metatarsal arteries

Tendons of lumbrical muscles (*cut*)

Sesamoid bones

Flexor digitorum longus tendons

Flexor digitorum brevis tendons (*cut*)

Transverse head and **Oblique head of adductor hallucis muscle**

Flexor digiti minimi brevis muscle

Medial head and **Lateral head of flexor hallucis brevis muscle**

Plantar metatarsal arteries

Plantar interosseous muscles

Superficial branches of medial plantar artery and nerve

Flexor hallucis longus tendon (*cut*)

Superficial branch of lateral plantar nerve

Abductor hallucis muscle (*cut*)

Deep plantar arterial arch and deep branches of lateral plantar nerve

Deep branches of medial plantar artery and nerve

Tuberosity of 5th metatarsal bone

Flexor digitorum longus tendon (*cut*)

Peroneus brevis tendon

Tibialis posterior tendon

Peroneus longus tendon and fibrous sheath

Medial plantar artery and nerve

Flexor hallucis longus tendon

Quadratus plantae muscle (*cut and slightly retracted*)

Flexor retinaculum

Lateral plantar artery and nerve

Abductor hallucis muscle (*cut*)

Abductor digiti minimi muscle (*cut*)

Flexor digitorum brevis muscle and plantar aponeurosis (*cut*)

Lateral calcaneal artery and nerve

Medial calcaneal artery and nerve

Tuberosity of calcaneus

Dorsal view

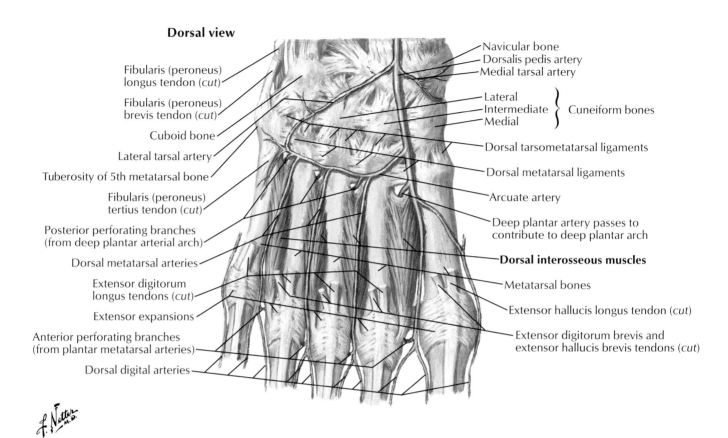

Fibularis (peroneus) longus tendon (*cut*)

Fibularis (peroneus) brevis tendon (*cut*)

Cuboid bone

Lateral tarsal artery

Tuberosity of 5th metatarsal bone

Fibularis (peroneus) tertius tendon (*cut*)

Posterior perforating branches (from deep plantar arterial arch)

Dorsal metatarsal arteries

Extensor digitorum longus tendons (*cut*)

Extensor expansions

Anterior perforating branches (from plantar metatarsal arteries)

Dorsal digital arteries

Navicular bone

Dorsalis pedis artery

Medial tarsal artery

Lateral
Intermediate } Cuneiform bones
Medial

Dorsal tarsometatarsal ligaments

Dorsal metatarsal ligaments

Arcuate artery

Deep plantar artery passes to contribute to deep plantar arch

Dorsal interosseous muscles

Metatarsal bones

Extensor hallucis longus tendon (*cut*)

Extensor digitorum brevis and extensor hallucis brevis tendons (*cut*)

Plantar view

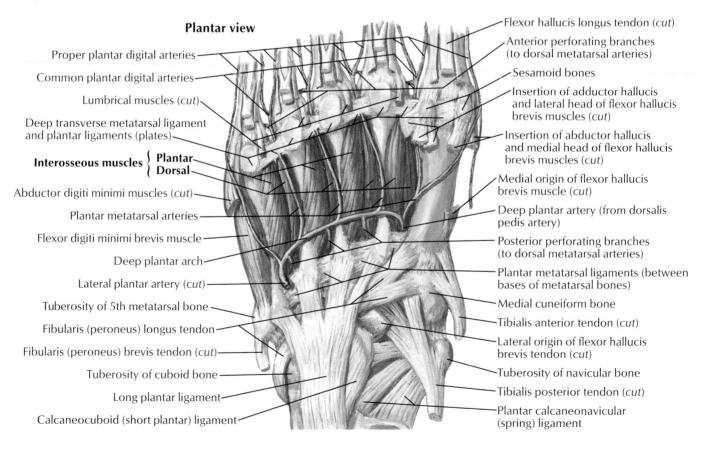

Proper plantar digital arteries

Common plantar digital arteries

Lumbrical muscles (*cut*)

Deep transverse metatarsal ligament and plantar ligaments (plates)

Interosseous muscles { **Plantar** **Dorsal**

Abductor digiti minimi muscles (*cut*)

Plantar metatarsal arteries

Flexor digiti minimi brevis muscle

Deep plantar arch

Lateral plantar artery (*cut*)

Tuberosity of 5th metatarsal bone

Fibularis (peroneus) longus tendon

Fibularis (peroneus) brevis tendon (*cut*)

Tuberosity of cuboid bone

Long plantar ligament

Calcaneocuboid (short plantar) ligament

Flexor hallucis longus tendon (*cut*)

Anterior perforating branches (to dorsal metatarsal arteries)

Sesamoid bones

Insertion of adductor hallucis and lateral head of flexor hallucis brevis muscles (*cut*)

Insertion of abductor hallucis and medial head of flexor hallucis brevis muscles (*cut*)

Medial origin of flexor hallucis brevis muscle (*cut*)

Deep plantar artery (from dorsalis pedis artery)

Posterior perforating branches (to dorsal metatarsal arteries)

Plantar metatarsal ligaments (between bases of metatarsal bones)

Medial cuneiform bone

Tibialis anterior tendon (*cut*)

Lateral origin of flexor hallucis brevis tendon (*cut*)

Tuberosity of navicular bone

Tibialis posterior tendon (*cut*)

Plantar calcaneonavicular (spring) ligament

Plate 536

Ankle and Foot

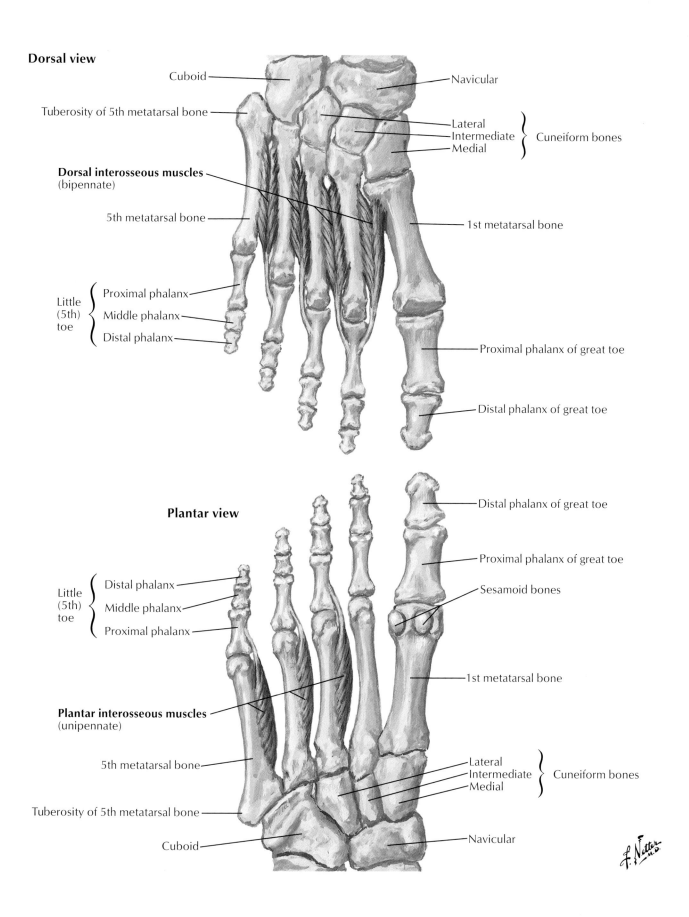

Dorsal view

Cuboid

Tuberosity of 5th metatarsal bone

Navicular

Lateral
Intermediate } Cuneiform bones
Medial

Dorsal interosseous muscles
(bipennate)

5th metatarsal bone

1st metatarsal bone

Little
(5th)
toe { Proximal phalanx
Middle phalanx
Distal phalanx

Proximal phalanx of great toe

Distal phalanx of great toe

Plantar view

Distal phalanx of great toe

Little
(5th)
toe { Distal phalanx
Middle phalanx
Proximal phalanx

Proximal phalanx of great toe

Sesamoid bones

Plantar interosseous muscles
(unipennate)

1st metatarsal bone

5th metatarsal bone

Lateral
Intermediate } Cuneiform bones
Medial

Tuberosity of 5th metatarsal bone

Cuboid

Navicular

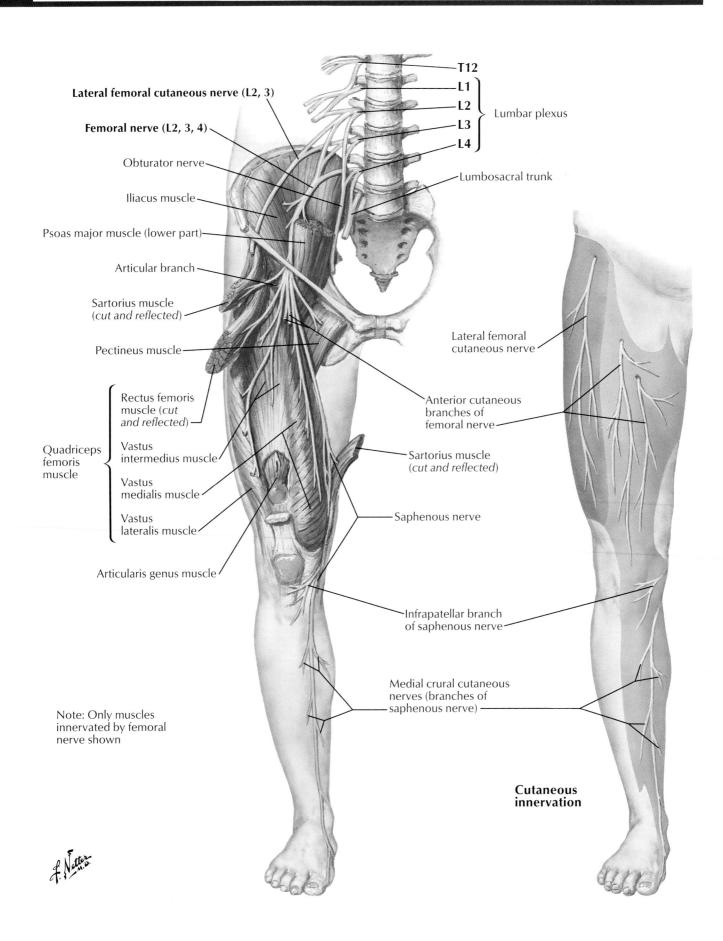

Lateral femoral cutaneous nerve (L2, 3)

Femoral nerve (L2, 3, 4)

Obturator nerve

Iliacus muscle

Psoas major muscle (lower part)

Articular branch

Sartorius muscle (cut and reflected)

Pectineus muscle

Rectus femoris muscle (cut and reflected)

Vastus intermedius muscle

Vastus medialis muscle

Vastus lateralis muscle

Quadriceps femoris muscle

Articularis genus muscle

Note: Only muscles innervated by femoral nerve shown

T12
L1
L2
L3
L4

Lumbar plexus

Lumbosacral trunk

Lateral femoral cutaneous nerve

Anterior cutaneous branches of femoral nerve

Sartorius muscle (cut and reflected)

Saphenous nerve

Infrapatellar branch of saphenous nerve

Medial crural cutaneous nerves (branches of saphenous nerve)

Cutaneous innervation

Plate 538   **Neurovasculature**

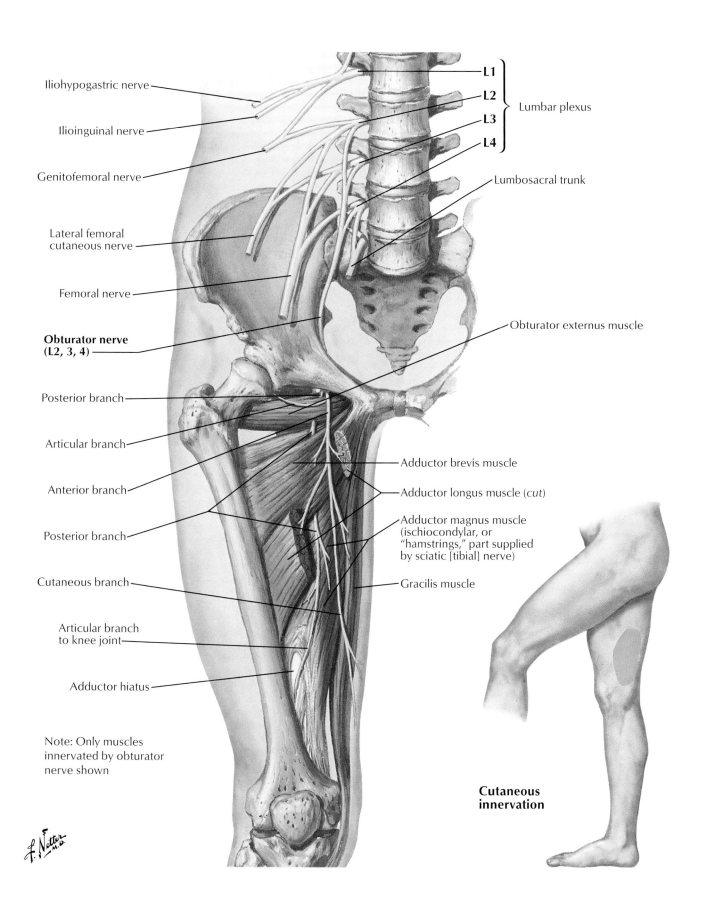

Iliohypogastric nerve

Ilioinguinal nerve

Genitofemoral nerve

Lateral femoral
cutaneous nerve

Femoral nerve

**Obturator nerve
(L2, 3, 4)**

Posterior branch

Articular branch

Anterior branch

Posterior branch

Cutaneous branch

Articular branch
to knee joint

Adductor hiatus

Note: Only muscles
innervated by obturator
nerve shown

L1
L2
L3
L4

Lumbar plexus

Lumbosacral trunk

Obturator externus muscle

Adductor brevis muscle

Adductor longus muscle (*cut*)

Adductor magnus muscle
(ischiocondylar, or
"hamstrings," part supplied
by sciatic [tibial] nerve)

Gracilis muscle

**Cutaneous
innervation**

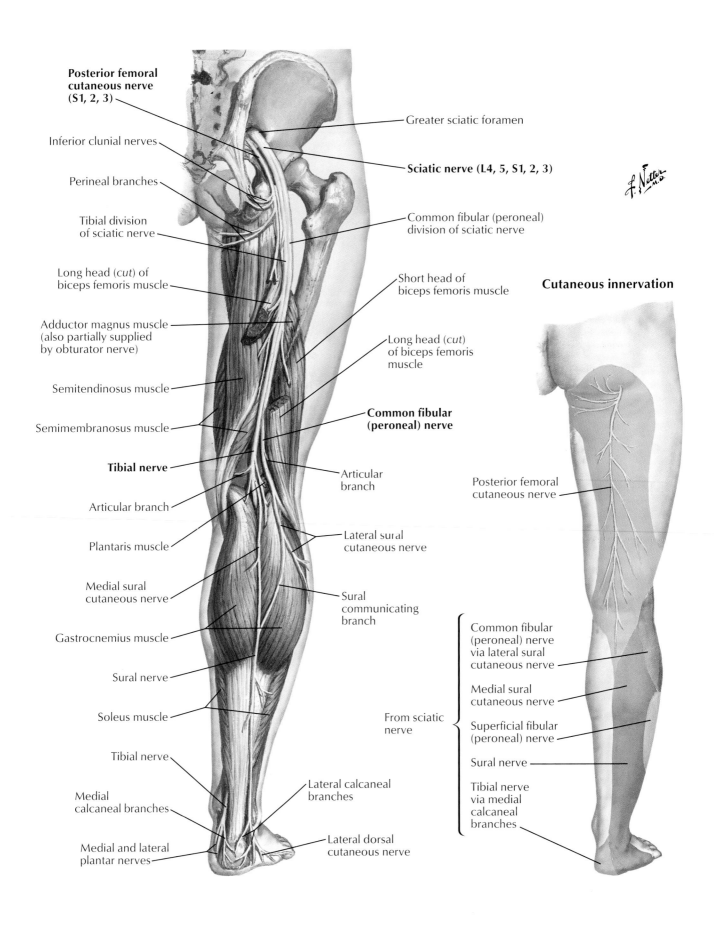

Posterior femoral cutaneous nerve (S1, 2, 3)

Inferior clunial nerves

Perineal branches

Tibial division of sciatic nerve

Long head (*cut*) of biceps femoris muscle

Adductor magnus muscle (also partially supplied by obturator nerve)

Semitendinosus muscle

Semimembranosus muscle

Tibial nerve

Articular branch

Plantaris muscle

Medial sural cutaneous nerve

Gastrocnemius muscle

Sural nerve

Soleus muscle

Tibial nerve

Medial calcaneal branches

Medial and lateral plantar nerves

Greater sciatic foramen

Sciatic nerve (L4, 5, S1, 2, 3)

Common fibular (peroneal) division of sciatic nerve

Short head of biceps femoris muscle

Long head (*cut*) of biceps femoris muscle

Common fibular (peroneal) nerve

Articular branch

Lateral sural cutaneous nerve

Sural communicating branch

Lateral calcaneal branches

Lateral dorsal cutaneous nerve

Cutaneous innervation

Posterior femoral cutaneous nerve

Common fibular (peroneal) nerve via lateral sural cutaneous nerve

Medial sural cutaneous nerve

Superficial fibular (peroneal) nerve

Sural nerve

Tibial nerve via medial calcaneal branches

From sciatic nerve

Plate 540   **Neurovasculature**

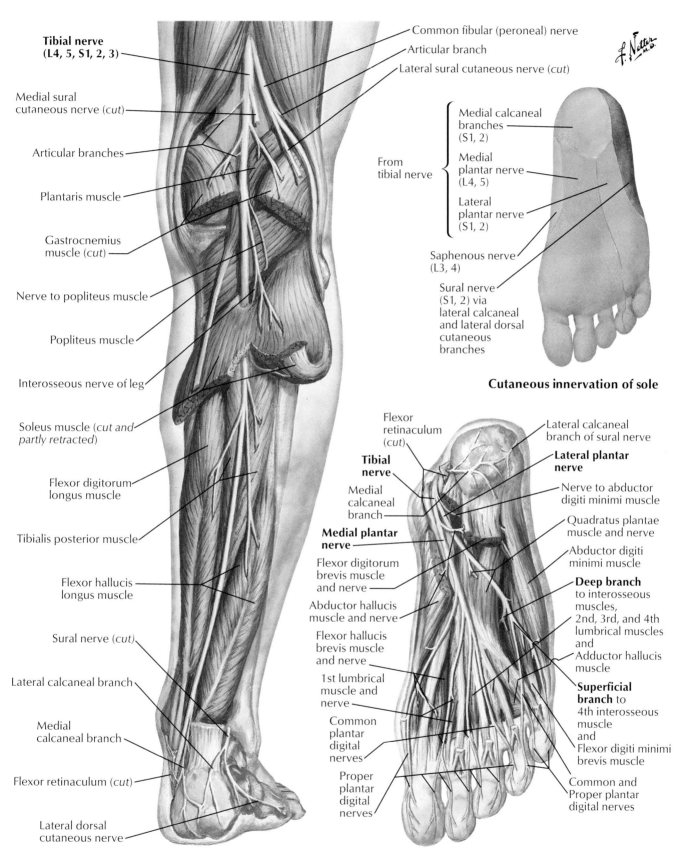

Tibial nerve
(L4, 5, S1, 2, 3)

Medial sural
cutaneous nerve (*cut*)

Articular branches

Plantaris muscle

Gastrocnemius
muscle (*cut*)

Nerve to popliteus muscle

Popliteus muscle

Interosseous nerve of leg

Soleus muscle (*cut and
partly retracted*)

Flexor digitorum
longus muscle

Tibialis posterior muscle

Flexor hallucis
longus muscle

Sural nerve (*cut*)

Lateral calcaneal branch

Medial
calcaneal branch

Flexor retinaculum (*cut*)

Lateral dorsal
cutaneous nerve

Common fibular (peroneal) nerve

Articular branch

Lateral sural cutaneous nerve (*cut*)

From
tibial nerve
{
Medial calcaneal
branches
(S1, 2)

Medial
plantar nerve
(L4, 5)

Lateral
plantar nerve
(S1, 2)
}

Saphenous nerve
(L3, 4)

Sural nerve
(S1, 2) via
lateral calcaneal
and lateral dorsal
cutaneous
branches

Cutaneous innervation of sole

Flexor
retinaculum
(*cut*)

**Tibial
nerve**

Medial
calcaneal
branch

**Medial plantar
nerve**

Flexor digitorum
brevis muscle
and nerve

Abductor hallucis
muscle and nerve

Flexor hallucis
brevis muscle
and nerve

1st lumbrical
muscle and
nerve

Common
plantar
digital
nerves

Proper
plantar
digital
nerves

Lateral calcaneal
branch of sural nerve

**Lateral plantar
nerve**

Nerve to abductor
digiti minimi muscle

Quadratus plantae
muscle and nerve

Abductor digiti
minimi muscle

Deep branch
to interosseous
muscles,
2nd, 3rd, and 4th
lumbrical muscles
and
Adductor hallucis
muscle

**Superficial
branch** to
4th interosseous
muscle
and
Flexor digiti minimi
brevis muscle

Common and
Proper plantar
digital nerves

Note: Articular branches not shown

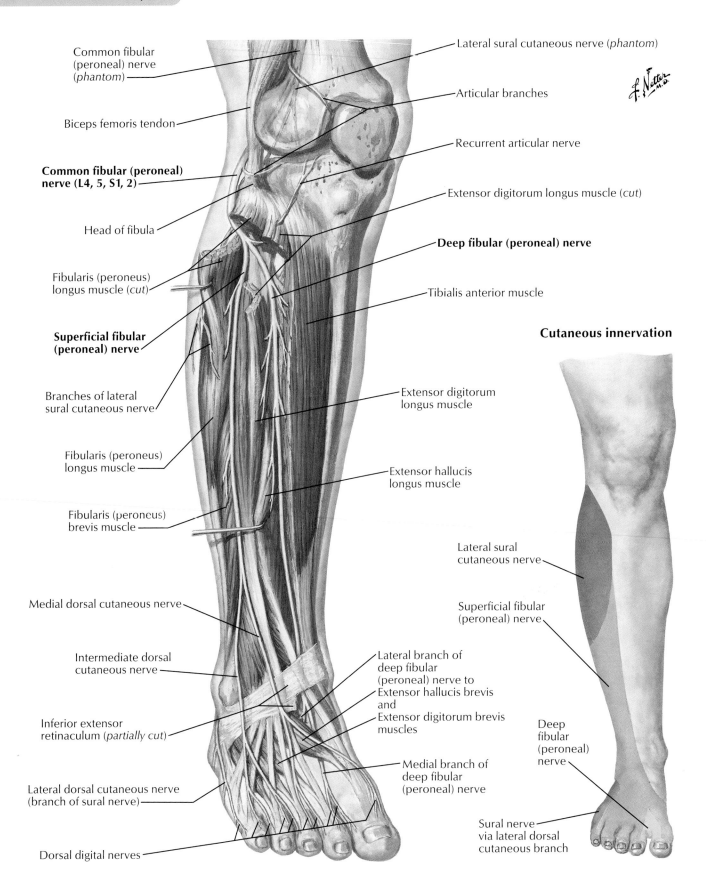

Common fibular (peroneal) nerve (*phantom*)

Lateral sural cutaneous nerve (*phantom*)

Biceps femoris tendon

Articular branches

Recurrent articular nerve

Common fibular (peroneal) nerve (L4, 5, S1, 2)

Extensor digitorum longus muscle (*cut*)

Head of fibula

Deep fibular (peroneal) nerve

Fibularis (peroneus) longus muscle (*cut*)

Tibialis anterior muscle

Superficial fibular (peroneal) nerve

Cutaneous innervation

Branches of lateral sural cutaneous nerve

Extensor digitorum longus muscle

Fibularis (peroneus) longus muscle

Extensor hallucis longus muscle

Fibularis (peroneus) brevis muscle

Medial dorsal cutaneous nerve

Lateral sural cutaneous nerve

Intermediate dorsal cutaneous nerve

Superficial fibular (peroneal) nerve

Lateral branch of deep fibular (peroneal) nerve to Extensor hallucis brevis and Extensor digitorum brevis muscles

Inferior extensor retinaculum (*partially cut*)

Deep fibular (peroneal) nerve

Medial branch of deep fibular (peroneal) nerve

Lateral dorsal cutaneous nerve (branch of sural nerve)

Sural nerve via lateral dorsal cutaneous branch

Dorsal digital nerves

Plate 542

Neurovasculature

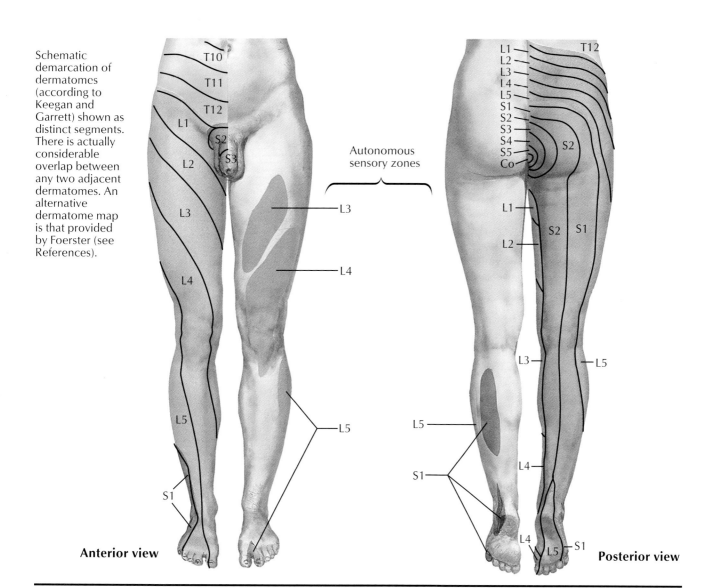

Schematic demarcation of dermatomes (according to Keegan and Garrett) shown as distinct segments. There is actually considerable overlap between any two adjacent dermatomes. An alternative dermatome map is that provided by Foerster (see References).

T10
T11
T12
L1
S2
L2
S3
L3
L4
L5
S1

Autonomous sensory zones

L3
L4
L5

Anterior view

L1
L2
L3
I4
L5
S1
S2
S3
S4
S5
Co
T12
S2

L1
S2   S1
L2
L3   L5
L5
S1
L4
L4   S1
L5

Posterior view

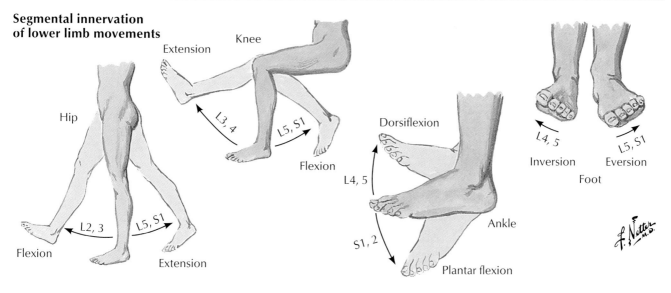

Segmental innervation of lower limb movements

Hip

Flexion
L2, 3   L5, S1
Extension

Extension
Knee
L3, 4   L5, S1
Flexion

Dorsiflexion
L4, 5
S1, 2
Ankle
Plantar flexion

Inversion   Eversion
L4, 5   L5, S1
Foot

F. Netter, M.D.

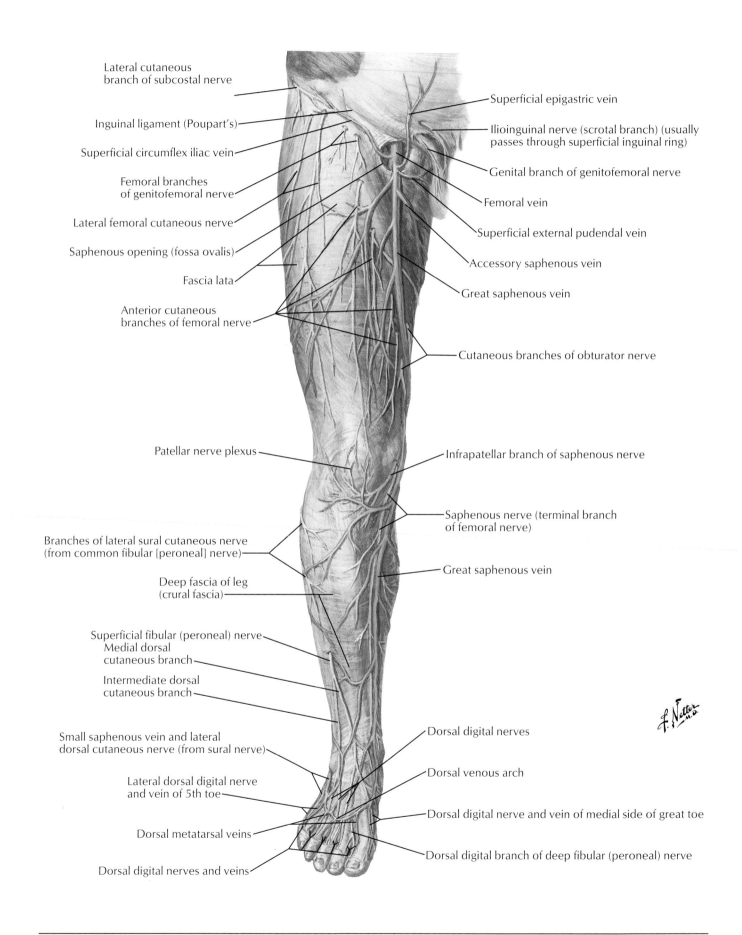

Lateral cutaneous branch of subcostal nerve

Inguinal ligament (Poupart's)

Superficial circumflex iliac vein

Femoral branches of genitofemoral nerve

Lateral femoral cutaneous nerve

Saphenous opening (fossa ovalis)

Fascia lata

Anterior cutaneous branches of femoral nerve

Patellar nerve plexus

Branches of lateral sural cutaneous nerve (from common fibular [peroneal] nerve)

Deep fascia of leg (crural fascia)

Superficial fibular (peroneal) nerve
Medial dorsal cutaneous branch

Intermediate dorsal cutaneous branch

Small saphenous vein and lateral dorsal cutaneous nerve (from sural nerve)

Lateral dorsal digital nerve and vein of 5th toe

Dorsal metatarsal veins

Dorsal digital nerves and veins

Superficial epigastric vein

Ilioinguinal nerve (scrotal branch) (usually passes through superficial inguinal ring)

Genital branch of genitofemoral nerve

Femoral vein

Superficial external pudendal vein

Accessory saphenous vein

Great saphenous vein

Cutaneous branches of obturator nerve

Infrapatellar branch of saphenous nerve

Saphenous nerve (terminal branch of femoral nerve)

Great saphenous vein

Dorsal digital nerves

Dorsal venous arch

Dorsal digital nerve and vein of medial side of great toe

Dorsal digital branch of deep fibular (peroneal) nerve

Plate 544   **Neurovasculature**

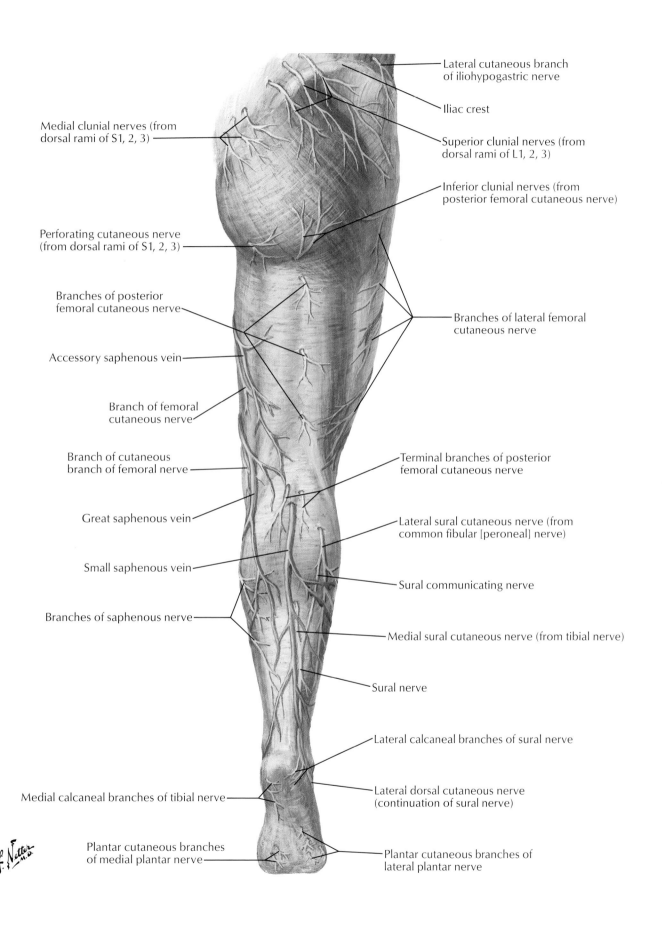

Lateral cutaneous branch of iliohypogastric nerve

Iliac crest

Medial clunial nerves (from dorsal rami of S1, 2, 3)

Superior clunial nerves (from dorsal rami of L1, 2, 3)

Inferior clunial nerves (from posterior femoral cutaneous nerve)

Perforating cutaneous nerve (from dorsal rami of S1, 2, 3)

Branches of posterior femoral cutaneous nerve

Branches of lateral femoral cutaneous nerve

Accessory saphenous vein

Branch of femoral cutaneous nerve

Branch of cutaneous branch of femoral nerve

Terminal branches of posterior femoral cutaneous nerve

Great saphenous vein

Lateral sural cutaneous nerve (from common fibular [peroneal] nerve)

Small saphenous vein

Sural communicating nerve

Branches of saphenous nerve

Medial sural cutaneous nerve (from tibial nerve)

Sural nerve

Lateral calcaneal branches of sural nerve

Medial calcaneal branches of tibial nerve

Lateral dorsal cutaneous nerve (continuation of sural nerve)

Plantar cutaneous branches of medial plantar nerve

Plantar cutaneous branches of lateral plantar nerve

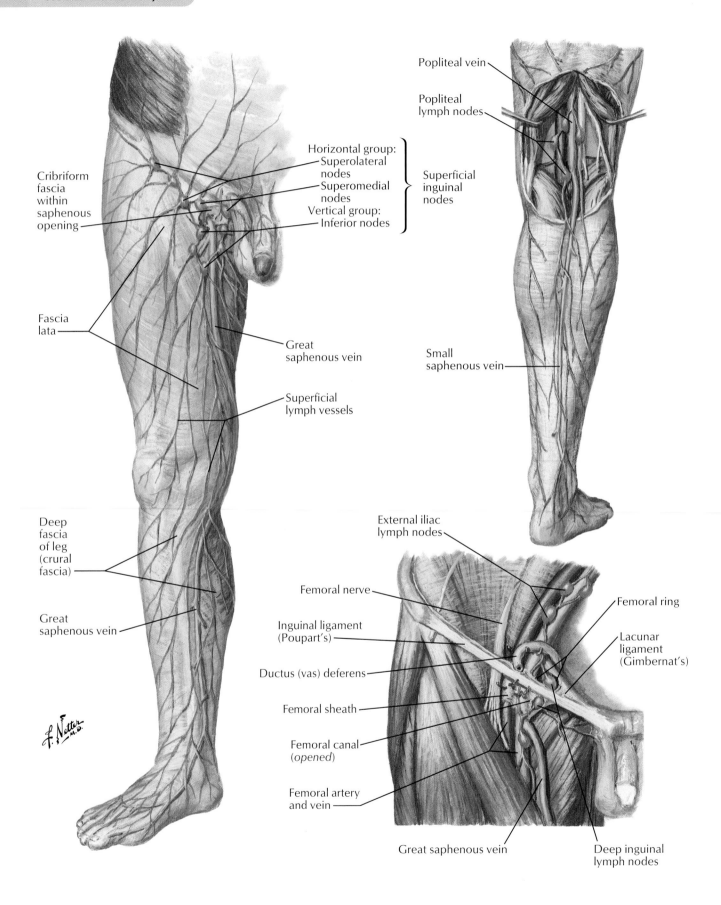

Cribriform fascia within saphenous opening

Horizontal group:
Superolateral nodes
Superomedial nodes
Vertical group:
Inferior nodes

Superficial inguinal nodes

Fascia lata

Great saphenous vein

Superficial lymph vessels

Deep fascia of leg (crural fascia)

Great saphenous vein

Popliteal vein

Popliteal lymph nodes

Small saphenous vein

External iliac lymph nodes

Femoral nerve

Inguinal ligament (Poupart's)

Ductus (vas) deferens

Femoral sheath

Femoral canal (opened)

Femoral artery and vein

Femoral ring

Lacunar ligament (Gimbernat's)

Great saphenous vein

Deep inguinal lymph nodes

Plate 546

Neurovasculature

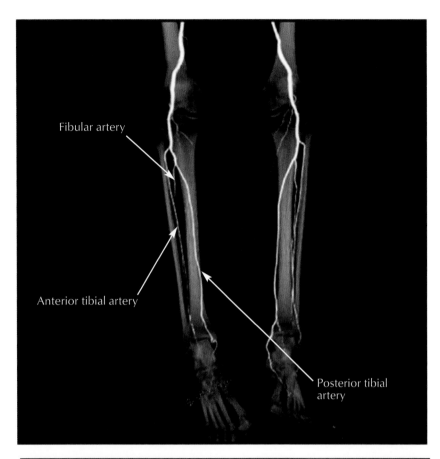

Fibular artery

Anterior tibial artery

Posterior tibial artery

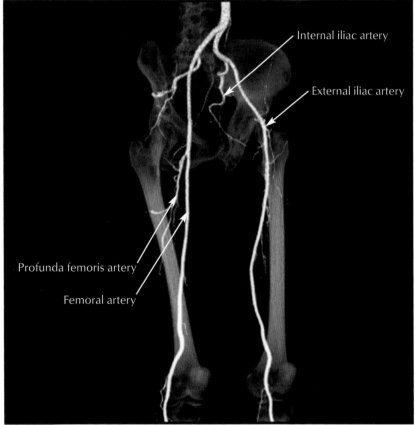

Internal iliac artery

External iliac artery

Profunda femoris artery

Femoral artery

Section 8 **Cross-Sectional Anatomy**

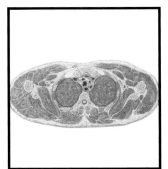
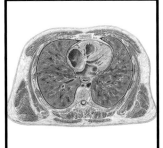

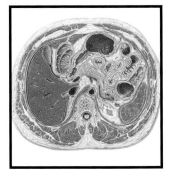
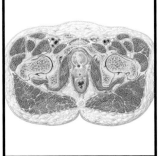

Plate 548

548 Key Figure for Cross Sections

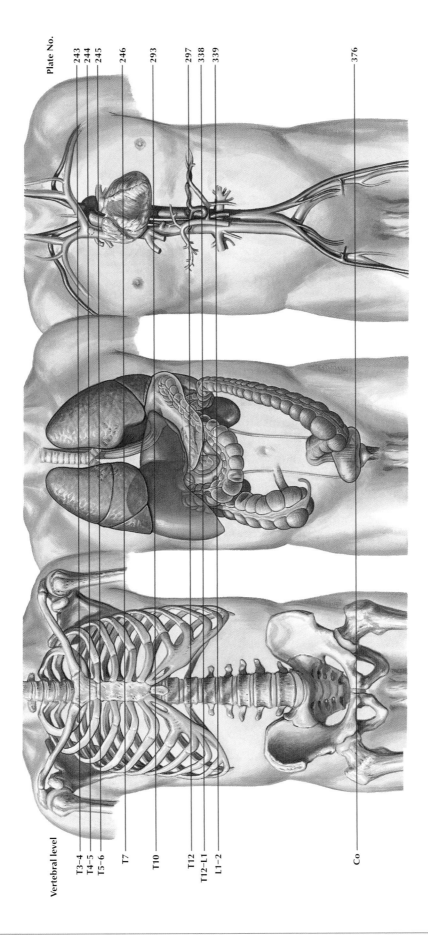

Plate No.

243
244
245
246
293
297
338
339
376

C. Machado M.D.

Vertebral level

T3–4
T4–5
T5–6
T7
T10
T12
T12–L1
L1–2
Co

References

Plate 58
Braus H. Anatomie des Menschen. Berlin, Verlag von Julius Springer, 1924.

Plate 89
Nishida S. The Structure of the Eye. New York, Elsevier North-Holland, 1982.

Plates 116, 117, 127
Lachman N, Acland RD, Rosse C. Anatomical evidence for the absence of morphologically distinct cranial root of the accessory nerve in man. Clin Anat 2002; 15:4.

Plates 164, 482, 525, 543
Foerster O. The dermatomes in man. Brain 1933; 56:1.

Garrett FD. The segmental distribution of the cutaneous nerves in the limbs of man. Anat Rec 1948; 102:409.

Keegan JJ. Dermatome hypalgesia with posterolateral herniation of lower cervical intervertebral disc. J Neurosurg 1947; 4:115.

Plate 172
Turnball IM. Bloody supply of the spinal cord. In Vinken PJ, Bruyn GW (eds): Handbook of Clinical Neurology, XII. Amsterdam, North-Holland, 1972, pp 478–491.

Plates 200, 201
Jackson CL, Huber JF. Correlated applied anatomy of the bronchial tree and lungs with a system of nomenclature. Dis Chest 1943; 9:319.

Plate 203
Ikeda S, Ono Y, Miyazawa S, et al. Flexible broncho-fiberscope. Otolaryngology (Tokyo) 1970; 42:855.

Plate 225
James TN. The internodal pathways of the human heart. Prog Cardiovas Dis 2001; 43:495.

Plates 253, 366, 370, 383
Myers RP, King BF, Cahill DR. Deep perineal "space" as defined by magnetic resonance imaging. Presented at 14th Annual Scientific Session of the American Association of Clinical Anatomists, Honolulu, HI, 1997. [Abstract: Clin Anat 1998;11].

Plate 282
DiDio LJA. Anatomo-Fisiologia do Piloro ileo-ceco-colica no homen. Actas das Primeiras Jornadas Interuniversitarías Argentinas de Gastroenterologia, Rosario, 1954.

_____. Dados anatomicos sobre o "piloro" ileo-ceco-colico. (Com observacao direta in vivo de "papila" ileo-ceco-colico.) [English summary]. Thesis, Fac Med, Univ de São Paulo, 1952.

Plate 290
Healey JE Jr, Schroy PC. Anatomy of the biliary duct within the human liver: analysis of the prevailing pattern of branchings and the major variations of the biliary ducts. Arch Surg 1953; 66:599.

Healey JE Jr, Schroy PC, Sörensen RJ. The intrahepatic distribution of the hepatic artery in man. J Int Coll Surg 1953; 20:133.

Plates 291, 292
Elias H. Liver morphology. Biol Rev 1955; 30:263.

_____. Origin and early development of the liver in various vertebrates. Act Hepat 1955;3:1.

_____. Morphology of the liver. In Liver Injury, Trans 11th Conference. New York, Macy Foundation, 1953.

_____. A re-examination of the structure of the mammalian liver: the hepatic lobule and its relation to the vascular and biliary system. Am J Anat 1949; 85:379.

_____. A re-examination of the structure of the mammalian liver: parenchymal architecture. Am J Anat 1949; 84:311.

Plates 305, 308
Michels NA. Blood Supply and Anatomy of the Upper Abdominal Organs, With a Descriptive Atlas. Philadelphia, JB Lippincott, 1955.

Plate 326
Thomas MD. In The Ciba Collection of Medical Illustrations, Vol 3, Part II. Summit, NJ, CIBA, p 78.

Plates 348, 361, 384, 396, 414
Stormont TJ, Cahill DR, King BF, Myers RP. Fascias of the male external genitalia and perineum. Clin Anat 1994; 7:115.

Plates 356, 360, 365, 370, 378, 379
Oelrich TM. The striated urogenital sphincter muscle in the female. Anat Rec 1983; 205:223.

Plates 359, 361
Myers RP, Goellner JR, Cahill DR. Prostate shape, external striated urethral sphincter and radical prostatectomy: the apical dissection. J Urol 1987; 138:543.

Plates 359, 361, 383, 384
Oelrich TM. The urethral sphincter muscle in the male. Am J Anat 1980; 158:229.

Plate 403
Flocks RH, Kerr HD, Elkins HB, et al. Treatment of carcinoma of the prostate by interstitial radiation with radio-active gold (Au 198): a preliminary report. J Urol 1952; 68(2):510.

Plate 482
Keegan JJ, Garrett FD. The segmental distribution of the cutaneous nerves in the limbs of man. Anat Rec 1948; 102:409.

Plate 543
Keegan JJ. Neurological interpretation of dermatome hypalgesia with herniation of the lumbar intervertebral disc. J Bone Joint Surg 1944; 26:238.

Last RJ. Innervation of the limbs. J Bone Joint Surg 1949; 31(B):452.

Index

Alveolar artery
anterior superior, 40
inferior, 40, 53, 60
lingual branch of, 69
mental branch of, 40, 69
middle superior, 40
posterior superior, 40, 69
Alveolar duct, 204
opening of, 204
Alveolar nerve, 53, 55, 122, 131, 134
anterior superior, 45
nasal branch of, 42
inferior, 16, 40, 53, 55, 60, 131, 134
branch of, 40
entering mandibular foramen, 46
middle superior, 45
posterior superior, 44, 45
superior, 62, 71
Alveolar sac, 204
Alveolar vein
inferior, 60, 70
posterior superior, 60, 70
Alveolus, 204
capillary bed in, 205
Amacrine cells, 120
Ampulla
ear, 95, 96
semicircular, 92
of uterine tube, 372
Amygdaloid body, 110, 112, 119
thalamus and, 110
Anal canal, 393
anatomical, 393
arteries of, 398
beginning of, 376
beginning of, transverse section of, 357, 521
longitudinal muscle of, 356, 357
muscularis mucosae of, 393, 394
sagittal MR images of, 397
surgical, 393
veins of, 399
Anal columns, 393
Anal glands, 393
Anal nerve, inferior, 410, 411, 414, 496, 503
Anal pit, 388
Anal sinus, 393
Anal sphincter muscle
external, 356, 358, 360, 365
deep part of, 394, 395, 396
peripheral view of, 395
subcutaneous of, 391, 393, 395, 396
superficial part of, 391, 393, 394, 395
internal, 393, 394
Anal triangle, 380
Anal tubercle, 388
Anal valve, 393
Anal verge, 393
Anastomosis
around elbow, 434
around scapula, 427
carotid-vertebral, 138
gastro-omental arterial, 272
in incisive canal, 40
obturator-pubic arterial, 259
paravertebral, 172
patellar, 500, 512
portacaval, 312
right-left, 138

Anastomosis (Continued)
between septal sphenopalatine artery
and greater palatine artery, 41, 138
subclavian-carotid, 138
subclavian-vertebral, 138
Anastomotic branch, 301
Anastomotic loop
of ileal arteries, 280
of jejunal arteries, 280
of posterior spinal arteries, 171
of small intestinal veins, 310
of small intestine, 306
Anastomotic vein
inferior, 102, 145
superior, 102
Anatomical snuffbox, 444
radial artery to, 469, 470
Anconeus muscle, 432, 444, 445, 477
nerve to, 432
origin of, 421
Angular artery, 23, 36, 68, 85, 138
Angular gyrus, 105
cerebral artery to, 141
cerebral branches to, 141, 142
Angular vein, 23, 70, 85
Ankle
dorsiflexion and plantar flexion of, 543
lateral ligament of, 514
ligaments and tendons of, 514
ligaments of, 527
medial ligament of, 514
radiograph of, 526
tendons of, 527
Annular ligament
of radius, 438
of trachea, 202
Anococcygeal body, 380, 381, 395, 396
Anococcygeal nerve, 411, 412, 499
Anocutaneous line, 392, 393, 394
Anoderm, 393
Anorectal hiatus, 358
Anorectal junction, circular muscle layer of, 359
Anorectal line, 393
Anorectal musculature, 394
Ansa cervicalis, 31, 32, 128, 129
inferior root of, 32, 34, 71, 74, 128, 129
superior root of, 32, 34, 71, 74, 128, 129
ventral rami of, 128
Ansa of Galen, 80
Ansa subclavia, 130, 209, 226, 240
Anserine bursa, 506, 507
Antebrachial vein
intermediate, 418, 479
median, 449
Anterior chamber, 81, 87, 88, 89, 90
endothelium of, 88
Anterolateral central arteries, 140, 141
Anteromedial central arteries, 140
Antidromic conduction, 167
Antihelix, 1, 93
crura of, 1, 93
Antitragus, 1, 93
Anulus fibrosus, 19, 155
Anum, fibrous septum of, 394
Anus, 360, 377, 380, 382, 388, 395
fetal, 388
transverse fibrous septum of, 393

Aorta, 207, 263, 324, 330, 342
abdominal, 27, 179, 195, 207, 225, 232, 270, 273, 274, 278, 298, 300, 301, 324, 327, 329, 330, 331, 332, 339, 341, 342, 363, 369, 398, 400, 401, 403, 412
cross section of, 338
abdominal, 412
arch of, 237, 244
ascending, 138, 215, 220, 223, 224, 225, 242, 245
axial CT images of, 242, 350
descending, 237, 242, 245, 246
thoracic, 194, 242
prenatal, 229
thoracic, 172, 297
cross section of, 297
descending, 172, 231, 241
esophageal branches of, 237
ureteric branch from, 341
Aortic arch. See Arch of aorta
Aortic hiatus, 195
Aortic lymph node, lateral, 266, 343, 406
Aortic lymph nodes, 266
Aortic nerve, 228
Aorticorenal ganglion, 165, 167, 267, 318, 320, 321, 322, 324, 344, 345, 346, 409
celiac, 267
left, 318, 320, 323, 410, 415
right, 318, 320, 323
superior mesenteric, 267
Aortic plexus, 321, 322, 412
Aortic sinus, 223, 224
Aortic valve
anatomy of, 223
semilunar cusps of, 221, 222, 223, 224, 225
left, 224
Apical foramen, 53
Apical ligament, of dens, 63, 65
Appendicular artery, 281, 306, 307, 322, 323
Appendicular nodes, 317
Appendicular plexus, 322, 323
Appendicular vein, 311, 312
Appendix, 126
fibrous, 287
vermiform, 271, 281, 283, 284, 362, 363
aggregate lymphoid nodules of, 283
barium radiograph of, 283
circular muscle of, 283
fixed retrocecal, 283
orifice of, 282
serosa of, 283
submucosa of, 283
variations in position of, 283
Arachnoid, 102, 109
cerebral veins penetrating, 102
Arachnoid–dura interface, 102
Arachnoid granulation, 100, 102, 109
granular foveola for, 99
skull indentation for, 99
Arachnoid mater, 169
lumbar, 170
thoracic, 170
Arantius, body of, 223

Arch of aorta, 74, 75, 80, 138, 206, 210, 211, 212, 213, 214, 215, 221, 232, 233
  groove for, 199
  radiograph of, 213
Arcuate artery, 335, 337, 530, 531, 536
  afferent glomerular arteriole from, 337
  lymph vessels along, 343
Arcuate eminence, 9
Arcuate ligament
  dorsal radial metaphyseal, 455
  lateral, 195, 263
  medial, 195, 263
  median, 195, 263
Arcuate line, 248, 251, 255, 259, 279, 348, 352, 353, 356, 486
  section above, 252
  section below, 252
Arcuate nucleus, 147
Arcuate popliteal ligament, 508, 511
Arcuate vein, 337
Arcus tendineous fasciae pelvis, 372
Areola, 182
Areolar gland, 182
Areolar tissue, 179, 251, 361, 471
  in anterior closed space of finger, 471
Areolar venous plexus, 256
Arm. See also Forearm
  arteries of, 484
  cutaneous nerves of, 479, 481
    inferior lateral, 432, 477, 479, 481
    medial, 257, 429, 432, 435, 473, 474, 479
    posterior, 432, 477, 479, 481
    superior lateral, 432, 477, 478, 479, 481
  deep artery of, 429, 432, 433, 434, 435
    middle collateral branch of, 445
  muscles of, 432
    anterior views of, 430
    deep layer of, 430, 432
    posterior, 432
    posterior view of, 432
    superficial layer of, 430, 432
    superior lateral, 432
  neurovascular compartment of, 435
  radial nerve in, 477
  serial cross section of, 435
  superficial veins of, 480
Arrector muscle, hair follicle, 167
Arteriae rectae, 307
Arteriogram, celiac, 303
Arteriole
  intralobular, 291
  periportal, 291
  portal, 291
Artery(ies). See also specific arteries
  of anterior abdominal wall, 255
  of arm, 484
  to brain, 136–137, 138, 141, 142
    frontal view of, 141
    lateral and medial views of, 142
  colic, 308
  of duodenum and head of pancreas, 301, 304
  of esophagus, 237
  of face, 23
  of female pelvic organs, 400
  of female pelvis, 403
  of female perineum and uterus, 405
  of femoral head, 504

Artery(ies) (Continued)
  of femoral head and neck, 504
  of fingers, 471
  of foot, 536
  of foot, deep, 536
  of hand, palmar view of, 466
  of head, 23
  of hip and thigh, 500–502
  of hypothalamus and hypophysis, 148
  intrarenal, 335
  intrinsic distribution of, in spinal cord, 172
  of large intestine, 307
  of liver, 301
  of liver, pancreas, duodenum, and spleen, 301, 305
  of liver and gallbladder, variations in, 305
  of male pelvis, 403
  of male perineum, 405
  of mammary gland, 183
  to meninges, 136
  of nasal cavity, 41
  of neck, 504
  of oral and pharyngeal regions, 69
  of oral region, 69
  of pancreas, 301
  of posterior abdominal wall, 264
  of posterior cranial fossa, 142, 143
  of rectum and anal canal, 398
  renal, 335
  of scalp, 23
  of spinal cord, 171
  of spleen, 301
  of stomach, liver, and spleen, 300
  of testis, 401
  of thigh
    anterior view of, 501
    posterior view of, 502
  of upper limb, 473
    computed tomography of, 484
  at wrist, 461
Articular cavity, 471
  of finger, 471
Articular disc, 16, 243
Articularis genus muscle, 505, 507, 511, 538
  attachment of, 489
Articular nerve
  great, 32
  recurrent, 542
Articular process
  inferior, lumbar, 155
  superior, lumbar, 155
Articular tubercle, 55
Aryepiglottic fold, 66, 67, 78
Aryepiglottic muscle, 78, 80
Arytenoid muscle
  oblique, 67, 78, 79, 80, 235
  transverse, 63, 78, 79, 80, 235
    action of, 79
Atlantoaxial joint, 19
  lateral, 19
    capsule of, 21
  median, superior view of, 22
  radiograph of, 17
Atlantooccipital joint capsule, 21, 22
Atlas (C1), 13, 17, 19, 22, 153, 160
  anterior, 21
  anterior arch of, 5, 17, 19, 37, 62, 137
  anterior tubercle of, 19
  dens of, articular facet for, 17
  inferior view of, 17

Atlas (C1) (Continued)
  lateral mass of, 17
  occipital condyle of, 17
  posterior, 21
  posterior arch of, 17, 18, 178
  posterior tubercle of, 17, 175, 176
  spinous process of, 18
  superior articular facet for, 17
  superior view of, 17
  transverse foramen of, 17
  transverse process of, 17, 21, 30, 39, 176
Atrioventricular bundle, 225
Atrioventricular node, 22, 218, 225
Atrioventricular valve
  left. See Mitral valve
  right. See Tricuspid valve
Atrium, 224
  internodal conduction pathways of, 225
  left, 214, 215, 220, 221, 224, 246
    auricle of, 212
    oblique vein of, 214, 215, 216
    section through, 221
  right, 212, 213, 214, 215, 220, 223, 224, 241, 246
    opened, 220
    radiograph of, 213
Auditory ossicles, 93
Auditory (pharyngotympanic, Eustachian) tube, 92, 93, 96, 125, 126
  cartilage of, 47
  cartilaginous part of, 52, 55, 64, 65, 67
  groove for, 8
  opening of, 37
  pharyngeal opening of, 63, 64, 66, 125
Auerbach's plexus. See Myenteric (Auerbach's) plexus
Auricle, 92, 97
  concha of, 93
  left, 212, 213, 215, 216, 224, 225
  lobule of, 93
  posteromedial surface of, 24
  right, 93, 212, 214, 219, 220, 224
Auricular artery
  anterior, 23
  deep, 40
  posterior, 23, 34, 40, 100, 136, 138, 178
Auricularis anterior muscle, 26
Auricularis posterior muscle, 26
Auricularis superior muscle, 26
Auricular muscle, facial nerve branches to, 123
Auricular nerve, 122
  anterior, 122
  articular branch of, 122
  great, 21, 22, 24, 32, 129, 177, 178
  greater, 31
  posterior, 25, 123
    occipital branch of, 123
Auricular tubercle (of Darwin), 93
Auricular vein, posterior, 23, 70
Auriculotemporal nerve, 16, 24, 40, 55, 71, 122, 125, 134
Auscultation, triangle of, 152, 246, 424
  precordial area of, 213
Autonomic ganglion, abdominal, 318
Autonomic nerves
  of abdomen, 318
  in head, 131

Brain, 48
  arteries to, 136, 141, 142
    frontal views of, 141
    inferior views of, 139
    lateral and medial views of, 142
    schema of, 138
  coronal section of, 108
  deep veins of, 145
  sagittal section of, in situ, 106
  subependymal veins of, 146
  ventricles of, 108
Brainstem
  anterior view of, 114
  cranial nerve nuclei in, 116, 117
    medial dissection of, 117
    posterior phantom view of, 116
    schema of, 117
  sectioned, 107
Bregma, 7
Broad ligament, 389
  anterior lamina of, 372
  of female ureter, 340
  mesometrium of, 371
  mesosalpinx of, 369
  posterior lamina of, 372
  subdivisions and contents of, 372
  uterine, 360, 362
Bronchial artery, 204, 205, 207
  esophageal branch of, 207
  inferior left, 207
  left, 199, 231
    esophageal branch of, 237
    inferior, 237
    superior, 237
  right, 199, 207, 230, 237
  superior left, 207
  variations in, 207
Bronchial vein
  left, 207
  right, 207
Bronchiole
  respiratory, 204, 205
  terminal, 204, 205
Bronchomediastinal lymphatic trunk, 208
  left, 266
  right, 266
Bronchopulmonary lymph nodes, 199, 208, 230, 231
Bronchopulmonary segments, 200, 201
  anterior view of, 200
  lateral view of, 201
  medial view of, 201
  nomenclature for, 203
  posterior view of, 200
Bronchus, 167, 202, 204, 234
  anterior basal, 203
  anteromedial basal, 203
  apicoposterior, 203
  elastic fibers of, 204
  extrapulmonary, 202
  inferior lobar, 202
  intermediate, 202
  intrapulmonary, 202, 204
  lateral basal, 203
  left, 203
    axial CT images of, 242
  left main branches of, 199, 206, 232, 233, 241
  lingular, 202

Bronchus *(Continued)*
  major, 202
  medial basal, 203
  middle lobar, 202, 203
  nomenclature of, 203
  posterior basal, 203
  right
    axial CT images of, 242
  intermediate, 206
  right main branches of, 207, 230, 245
  smooth muscle of, 204
  superior lobar, 202, 203, 206
Brunner's gland. *See* Duodenal glands
Buccal artery, 40, 69
Buccal nerve, 24, 40, 46, 62, 71, 122
  branches of, 25
Buccinator crest, 68
Buccinator lymph node, 72
Buccinator muscle, 15, 26, 48, 52, 54, 55, 60, 65, 68, 123
Buccopharyngeal fascia, 60, 63, 65
Buck's fascia. *See* Deep (Buck's) fascia
Bulbar conjunctiva, 81, 87
Bulbospongiosus muscle, 358, 366, 370, 380, 381, 383, 404, 405, 417
bulb of vestibule of, 366
Bulbourethral (Cowper's) gland, 253, 361, 366, 383, 384, 389, 417
  duct of, 383
    opening of, 384, 385
  perineal membrane and, 348
  primordium of, 389
Bulging septum, 37
Bursa
  anserine, 506, 507
  fibular collateral, 507
  of hand, 462
  iliopectineal, 496
  infrapatellar, 511
  patellar, 508
  radial, 460
  subdeltoid, 423
  ulnar, 460
Buttock, nerves of, 503

C

C1 spinal nerve, 127
  dorsal ramus of, 178
  dorsal roots of, 114
  exit of, 161
  ventral ramus of, 71
  ventral roots of, 114
C2 spinal nerve, 127
  dorsal ramus of, 177, 178
  ventral ramus of, 32, 71, 177
C3 spinal nerve, 19
  dorsal ramus of, 177
  ventral ramus of, 32, 71, 177
C4 spinal nerve, 127
C5 spinal nerve, ventral ramus of, 32
C8 spinal nerve, 160
  exit of, 161
C6 transverse process, 136
C1 vertebra. *See* Atlas (C1)
C2 vertebra. *See* Axis (C2)
C3 vertebra, 13
  inferior articular facet for, 19

C3 vertebra *(Continued)*
  tubercles of transverse process of
    anterior, 26
    posterior, 26
C4 vertebra
  anterior tubercle of, 18
  body of, 18
  lamina of, 18
  posterior tubercle of, 18
  posterosuperior view of, 17
C7 vertebra, 13, 153, 160
  posterior tubercle of transverse process of, 30
  spinous process of, 18, 152, 174, 175, 176, 424
  superior view of, 18
Calcaneal artery
  lateral, 534, 535
  medial, 534, 535
Calcaneal nerve
  lateral, 534, 535
  medial, 534, 535
Calcaneal (Achilles) tendon, 485, 515, 516, 517, 518, 521, 527
  soleus muscle insertion in, 515, 517
Calcaneocuboid ligament, 527, 536
  dorsal, 527
  plantar, 528
Calcaneofibular ligament, 514, 525, 527
Calcaneometatarsal ligament, 532
Calcaneonavicular ligament, 527
  plantar, 527, 528, 536
Calcaneus, 524, 527, 528
  anterior talar articular surface of, 525
  body of, 523, 524, 525
  dorsal view of, 523
  fibular, 524
  fibular trochlea of, 523
  functional relations of, 525
  groove for tendon of flexor hallucis longus, 523
  lateral process, 523, 533
  lateral view of, 525
  medial process, 523
  medial view of, 525
  middle talar articular surface of, 525
  plantar view of, 523
  posterior talar articular surface of, 525
  posterior view of, 525
  radiograph of, 54
  superior view of, 525
  sustentaculum tali of, 523
  trochlea of, 524
  tuberosity of, 485, 488, 516, 517, 523, 533, 534, 535
    radiograph of, 54
Calcar, 489
Calcar avis, 111, 112
Calcarine artery, 142, 143
Calcarine sulcus, 105, 106, 107, 111, 120
Callosomarginal artery, 141, 142
Calot, cystic node of, 315
Calot, triangle of, 301
Calvaria, 102
  inferior view of, 7
  superior view of, 7
Calyx, major, 339
Camper chiasm, 461
Camper's fascia, 348

Costal pleural, 231, 232
Costocervical trunk, 33, 69, 136, 137, 138
Costochondral joint, 186
Costoclavicular ligament, 186, 419
  attachment of, 419
Costocoracoid ligament, 188, 428
Costocoracoid membrane, 428
Costodiaphragmatic recess, 198, 230, 231, 293, 330, 332, 342, 349
  right, 206
Costomediastinal space, 331
  lateral, 198
  superior, 198
Costovertebral joint, 243
  left lateral view of, 187
  right posterolateral view of, 187
  transverse section of, 187
Cough receptor, 210
Cowper's gland. See Bulbourethral
  (Cowper's) gland
Coxal bone. See Hip bone
Cranial base
  bones of, 9
  foramina of, 10, 11
    inferior view of, 10
  inferior view of, 8
Cranial fossa
  anterior, 9
  middle, 9
  posterior, 9
    arteries of, 142, 143
    veins of, 144
  posterior veins of, 144
Cranial mesonephric (Gartner's) duct, 389
Cranial mesonephric tubule, 389
Cranial nerve, 116, 130–133, 134–135
  in carotid sheath, 60
  communicating branch of, 45
  motor and sensory distribution of, 118
  nuclei of
    medial dissection of, 117
    posterior phantom view of, 116
    schema of, 116
  palsy of, 101
Cranial nuclei, in brainstem, schema of, 117
Craniocervical ligaments
  external
    anterior view of, 21
    posterior view of, 21
    right lateral view of, 21
  internal, 22
Cremaster fascia, 250
Cremasteric artery, 255
Cremasteric muscle, 250, 251, 259, 261
  lateral origin of, 259
  medial origin of, 259
Cremasteric vessels, 260, 401
Cremaster muscle, 390
  lateral origin of, 259
  medial origin of, 259
Cribriform fascia, 546
Cribriform plate, 6, 9, 37, 39, 119
  foramina of, 11
Cricoarytenoid muscle
  lateral, 78, 80
    action of, 78, 79

Cricoarytenoid muscle (Continued)
  posterior, 78, 80, 235
    action of, 79
Cricopharyngeus muscle, 75, 76, 80, 233, 234, 235
Cricothyroid artery, 69
Cricothyroid joint, 77
  pivot point of, 79
Cricothyroid ligament
  lateral, 77
  median, 74, 77, 202
Cricothyroid muscle, 126
  action of, 79
  oblique part of, 79
  straight part of, 79
Crista galli, 3, 6, 9, 39
  coronal CT images of, 151
Crista terminalis, 220, 225
Cross section
  of abdomen
    at L1–2, 339, 349
    at L3, 349
    at L3, 4, 349
    at T10, 293
    at T12, 297, 331, 338
  of descending duodenum, 179
  forearm, serial, 449
  of gallbladder, 297
  of scrotum, 390
  of testis, 390
Cruciate ligament, 22, 507, 509
  anterior, 508, 509, 514
    attachment of, 508
    origin of, 514
  inferior longitudinal band of, 22
  posterior, 514
    attachment of, 514
  superior longitudinal band of, 22
  transverse, 22
C3 spinal nerve, 19, 127
  dorsal ramus of, 178
  ventral ramus of, 32, 71, 178
C2 spinal nerve, 133
  dorsal ramus of, 177, 178
  ventral ramus of, 32, 71, 177
Cubital fossa, 418
Cubital lymph nodes, 483, 484
Cubital node, 483
Cubital vein
  intermediate, 480
  median, 418, 479, 483, 484
Cuboid bone, 523, 524, 527, 536, 537
  articular surface for, 525
  base of, 523
  dorsal view of, 523
  groove for fibularis longus tendon insertion, 523
  plantar view of, 523
  radiograph of, 54
  shaft of, 523
  tuberosity of, 523, 524, 528, 536
Cuboideonavicular ligament, plantar, 528
Culmen, 113, 115, 144
Cuneate fasciculus, 114
Cuneate tubercle, 114
Cuneiform bone
  intermediate, 523, 536
  lateral, 523, 536
    radiograph of, 54

Cuneiform bone (Continued)
  medial, 523, 524, 527, 536
  plantar view of, 523
Cuneiform tubercle, 66, 67, 78
Cuneocuboid ligament, dorsal, 527
Cuneonavicular ligament
  dorsal, 527
  plantar, 528
Cuneus, 106
  apex of, 107
Cuspid teeth. See Teeth, canine
Cutaneous nerve(s)
  antebrachial lateral, 469
  dorsal, lower limb
    intermediate, 540, 541, 542
    lateral, 542, 545
    medial, 541, 542
  femoral
    lateral, 409
    posterior, 411
  of forearm, medial, 469
  of head, 24
  lateral antebrachial, 447
  lateral dorsal, 544
  lateral femoral, 329, 499, 538, 539
  medial antebrachial, 429, 432, 469
  of neck, 24, 31
  perforating, 411, 499
  posterior antebrachial, 469
  superior lateral brachial, 177
Cuticle, 471
C1 vertebra. See Atlas (C1)
C2 vertebra. See Axis (C2)
C3 vertebra, 13
  inferior articular facet for, 19
  tubercles of transverse process of
    anterior, 30
    posterior, 30
C4 vertebra
  anterior tubercle of, 18
  body of, 18
  lamina of, 18
  posterior tubercle of, 18
  posterosuperior view of, 18
  superior articular process of, 19
C7 vertebra, 13, 153, 160
  posterior tubercle of transverse process of, 30
  spinous process of, 18, 152, 174, 175, 176, 424
  superior view of, 18
Cymba, 93
Cystic artery, 294, 300, 301, 305
Cystic duct, 331
  smooth part of, 294
  spiral fold of, 294
  variations in, 296
Cystic node (of Calot), 315
Cystic vein, typical arrangement of, 313
Cystohepatic triangle, 301
Cystourethrograms, male and female, 368

D

Declive, 113
Deep (Buck's) fascia, 249, 250, 348, 361, 380, 381, 382, 383, 396, 401, 403, 405
  intercavernous septum of, 382, 385

Deep palmar arch, 465
Deltoid muscle, 152, 174, 177, 188, 189, 243, 244, 245, 423, 428, 429
  attachments of, 420
  insertion of, 420, 421
  origin of, 419, 420
Deltoid tuberosity, 420
Deltopectoral lymph node, 483, 484
Deltopectoral node, 483
Deltopectoral triangle, 247, 424
Denonvilliers' fascia. *See* Rectoprostatic (Denonvilliers') fascia
Dens, 137
  apical ligament of, 63, 65
  of axis, 19, 37
  posterior auricular facet of, 22
Dental plexus
  inferior, 122
  superior, 122
Dental pulp, 57
Dentate gyrus, 106, 108, 111, 112, 119
Dentate nucleus, 108, 112, 119
Denticulate ligament, 169, 170
Dentinal tubules, 57
Dentine, 57
Depressor anguli oris muscle, 54
Depressor labii inferioris muscle, 26, 54, 123
Depressor septi nasi muscle, 36, 123
Dermatomes
  anterior, 482
  levels of, 164
  of lower limb, 543
  posterior, 482
  schematic demarcation of, 164
  of upper limb
    anterior and posterior views of, 482
Descemet's membrane. *See* Posterior limiting lamina (Descemet's membrane)
Diaphragm, 198, 206, 211, 215, 230, 233, 236, 237, 272, 273, 275, 286, 327, 329, 331, 342, 498
  abdominal surface of, 195
  area for, 330
  caval opening for, 195, 263, 267
  central tendon of, 263
    right leaflet of, 194
  costal part of, 195, 258
  cross section of, 338
  crura of, 179, 293, 338, 342
    left, 263, 270, 297, 339
    right, 263, 270, 293, 297, 331, 339
  domes of, 213
    left, 196, 197
    right, 196, 197
  lateral view of, 233
  lumbar part of, 195
  pelvic, 361
    fascia of, 364
    female, 356, 357
    inferior and superior fascia of, 392
    male, 358–359
    superior fascia of, 360, 364, 365, 369, 394
  phrenic nerves to, 193
  slip of origin of, 349
  sternal part of, 195
  thoracic surface of, 193
Diaphragmatic constriction, 233

Diaphragmatic ligament, 389
Digastric fossa, 15
Digastric muscle, 29, 123
  anterior belly of, 27, 28, 29, 31, 32, 34, 46, 53, 61, 68
  intermediate tendon of, 59
    fibrous loop for, 59
  phantom, 34
  posterior belly of, 27, 28, 29, 32, 34, 40, 59, 73
  nerve to, 25
Digastric tendon, intermediate, 60
  fibrous loop for, 28, 29, 53
Digital artery
  common, computed tomography of, 484
  common palmar, 465
  common plantar, 536
  dorsal, 469, 471, 530, 536
  nutrient branches of, 471
  palmar
    common, 460
    proper, 460
  proper palmar, 460, 471
    dorsal branches of, 471
  proper plantar, 533, 535, 536
    dorsal branches of, 530
Digital creases, 418
Digital nerves
  common palmar, 476
  common plantar, 476, 541
  dorsal, 468, 471, 475, 542, 544
  lateral dorsal, 544
  palmar
    to fourth and fifth fingers, 460
    proper, 476
  proper palmar, 460, 471, 476
    dorsal branches of, 468
    to thumb, 460
  proper plantar, 535, 541
Digital vein
  dorsal, 468, 480, 544
Dilator pupillae muscle, 88, 121
Diploë, 7
Diploic vein, 102
  anterior temporal, 99
  coronal dissection of, 99
  frontal, 99
  occipital, 99
  posterior temporal, 99
Direct vein, lateral, 145, 146
Distal interphalangeal (DIP) joint, site of, 418
Distal medial striate artery (recurrent artery of Heubner), 140, 141, 142
Dorsalis pedis artery, 520, 530, 536
Dorsal ramus, spinal, 170, 258, 430
  medial clunial nerves from, 545
  perforating cutaneous nerves from, 545
Dorsal tubercle of radius (Lister's), 452
Dorsal venous arch, foot, 544
Dorsomedial nucleus, 147
Dorsum sellae, 9
Douglas, cul-de-sac of. *See* Rectouterine pouch (of Douglas)
Ductus arteriosus
  obliterated, 229
  prenatal, 229
Ductus choledochus. *See* Bile duct, common

Ductus (vas) deferens, 259, 261, 340, 389, 390, 409, 546
  ampulla of, 384
  artery to, 255, 264, 340, 398, 401, 403
Ductus deferens plexus, 409, 415
Ductus plexus, 409
Ductus reuniens, 96
Ductus venosus
  obliterated, 229
  prenatal, 229
Duodenal cap, 279
Duodenal flexure
  inferior, 279
  superior, 279
Duodenal fold
  inferior, 278
  superior, 270
Duodenal fossa
  inferior, 270
  superior, 270
Duodenal glands, 279
Duodenal impression, 287
Duodenal papilla
  major, 279, 294, 295
  minor, 279
Duodenal wall
  circular muscle layer of, 279
  longitudinal muscle layer of, 279
  submucosa of, 279
Duodenojejunal flexure, 270, 279, 342
Duodenojejunal junction, 179
Duodenum, 126, 248, 273, 275, 278, 288, 329, 340, 342
  arteries of, 301, 304
  ascending, 270, 278, 279
  barium radiograph of, 279
  circular muscle of, 277, 295
  descending, 272, 279, 294
    cross section of, 179
  descending part of, 270
  inferior part of, 270
  in situ, 278
  innervation of, 321
  junction with common bile duct, 295
  longitudinal fold of, 279
  longitudinal muscle of, 277
  mesentery root of, 278
  mucosa of, 279
  musculature of, 279
  nerves of, 319, 320, 321
  second-third parts of, 338
    junction of, 339
  submucosa of, 279
  superior, 276, 278
    cross section of, 297
  superior part of, 294
  superior (1st) part of, 297
  suspensory ligament of, 270
  suspensory muscle of, 270
  veins of, 309
Dural sac
  in lumbar puncture, 162
  sagittal MR images of, 397
  termination of, 160, 161
Dural venous sinuses, 104
  coronal section through, 104
  sagittal section of, 103
  superior view of, 104

Dura mater, 39, 91, 93, 96, 99, 100, 102, 109, 119, 137, 169
around bony and membranous labyrinths, 96
cerebral veins penetrating, 102
lumbar, 170
periosteal and meningeal layers of, 99
spinal, 160, 179
spinal arteries to, 172
of thoracic spine, 170
Dura–skull interface, 102

E

Ear, 93
bony and membranous labyrinths of, 95
external
coronal oblique section of, 93
superolateral view of, 93
lobule of, 1
middle coronal oblique section of, 93
surface anatomy of, 1
Edinger-Westphal nucleus, 116, 117, 132
Efferent ductule, 389, 390
Efferent fiber, to olfactory bulb, 119
Ejaculatory duct, 376
beginning of, 384
openings of, 316, 384, 385
Elbow
anastomoses around, 434
bones of, 436
ligaments of, 438
muscles of, 447–448
attachments of, 450, 451
radiographs of
anteroposterior, 437
lateral, 437
Emissary vein, 99, 102
communicating with cavernous sinus, 70
condylar, 137
coronal dissection of, 99, 102
mastoid, 23, 99, 137
occipital, 99
parietal, 23, 94, 99
parietal foramen for, 7
of skull, 99
to superior sagittal sinus, 7
Endolymphatic duct, 11, 95
opening for, 97
in vestibular aqueduct, 96
Endolymphatic sac, 96
Endometrium, 371
Endopelvic fascia, 364
Ependyma, 108
Epicolic nodes, 317
Epicondyles
lateral, 438, 440, 441, 442, 443, 489
radiograph of, 510
medial, 437, 440, 441, 442, 443, 447, 476, 489
Epicranial aponeurosis, 26, 178
Epicranius muscle
frontal belly of, 26
occipital belly of, 26
Epididymal duct, 390
Epididymis, 390
appendix of, 389
body of, 390
head of, 390

Epididymis *(Continued)*
sinus of, 390
tail of, 390
Epidural anesthesia, for lumbar puncture, 162
Epidural hematoma, 101
Epidural space
fat in, 170
in lumbar puncture, 162
Epigastric artery
superficial, 211, 511
superior, 188, 189, 192
Epigastric lymph nodes, inferior, 266
Epigastric region, 268
Epigastric vein
inferior, 251, 256, 265, 400
superficial, 247, 256, 265, 544
superior, 189, 256
Epigastric vessels
inferior, 251, 259, 261, 349, 362, 363, 401, 403
superficial, 249, 500
superior, 331, 500
Epiglottis, 13, 58, 63, 66, 67, 76, 77, 78, 135, 233, 235
Epiphyseal plate, 504
Epiphysis, 471
nutrient arterial branch to, 471
Epiploic appendices. *See* Omental appendices
Epiploic foramen, 331
Epiploic foramen. *See* Omental foramen
Episcleral artery, 90
Episcleral space, 83, 87
Episcleral vein, 90, 91
segment of, 91
Epithelial cell, stomach surface, 276
Epithelial tag, 388
Epitympanic recess, 92, 93
Eponychium, 471
Epoöphoron, 343
Epoöphoron canal, 389
Erector spinae muscle, 152, 174, 175, 179, 180, 192, 243, 258, 293, 330, 331
Esophageal artery, 207
Esophageal hiatus, 195
Esophageal impression, 287
Esophageal junction, 236
Esophageal muscle, 202
circular, 75, 235, 236
longitudinal, 75, 235, 236
cricoesophageal tendon of, 235
Esophageal plexus, 126, 165, 166, 206, 209, 230, 231, 232, 241, 321
anterior, 240
posterior portion of, 240
sympathetic branches to, 209, 240
Esophageal prominence, pericardial, 215
Esophageal vein, 312, 313
Esophagogastric junction, 236
transverse section of, 293
Esophagus, 63, 68, 76, 126, 194, 204, 206, 207, 230, 231, 233, 240, 241, 243, 244, 245, 246, 263, 264, 270, 274, 323, 329, 332, 348
abdominal part of, 233, 237, 275
anterior view of, 240

Esophagus *(Continued)*
arteries of, 237
common variations in, 237
bare area on ventral surface, 234
cervical part of, 237
circular muscle layer of, 234, 277
gradual slight muscular thickening of, 232
greater curvature of, 277
groove for, 199
in situ, 232
lateral view of, 233
longitudinal muscle layer of, 234, 277
lateral mass of, 234
mucosa of, 235, 236
junction with gastric mucosa, 276
musculature of, 239
nerves of, 240
opened posterior view of, 66
posterior view of, 240
pyloric part of, 277
recurrent arterial branch to, 195, 264
submucosa of, 235, 236
thoracic part of, 232, 237
topography and constrictions of, 233
zone of sparse muscles of, 234, 235
Ethmoidal artery
anterior, 11, 85
meningeal branch of, 100
septal and meningeal branches of, 41
posterior, 11, 85, 100
septal and meningeal branches of, 41
Ethmoidal bulla, 37, 38
Ethmoidal cells, 48, 49, 83
anterior, 50
opening of, 37, 38
semilunar hiatus of, 37
middle, 50
opening of, 37, 38
posterior, 37, 38
opening of, 38
Ethmoidal foramen
anterior, 2, 11, 12
posterior, 2, 11
Ethmoidal nerve
anterior, 11, 43, 86, 121, 122
external nasal branches to, 24, 122
lateral internal nasal branches to, 42, 43
medial internal nasal branches to, 42
posterior, 11, 45, 86, 121, 122
Ethmoidal vein
anterior, 122
posterior, 122
Ethmoid bone, 4, 6, 9, 38
anterior ethmoidal foramen of, 12
cribriform plate of, 37, 38, 39, 119
crista galli of, 39
middle nasal concha of, 2
nasal concha of, 38
orbital plate of, 2, 4, 12
perpendicular plate of, 2, 6, 39
uncinate process of, 38
Ethmoid sinus
axial MR image of, 150
coronal CT images of, 151
Eustachian tube. *See* Auditory (pharyngotympanic, Eustachian) tube

Genicular artery
descending, 512
articular branch of, 500, 512
saphenous branch of, 500, 512
inferior lateral, 512, 517, 518, 519, 520
inferior medial, 500, 512
middle, 512
superior lateral, 502, 512, 516, 517, 519, 520, 521
superior medial, 51, 500, 501, 502, 512, 516, 518, 519, 520
Geniculate body
lateral, 107, 110, 111, 114, 116, 120, 132, 143, 144, 145
of left thalamus, 143
medial, 107, 108, 110, 111, 114, 115, 139, 143, 144, 145
Geniculate nucleus
left dorsal lateral, 120
right dorsal lateral, 120
Geniculum (geniculate ganglion), 116, 131, 135
of facial nerve, 97, 116, 125
site of, 124
Genioglossus muscle, 29, 32, 59, 60, 128, 129
superior mental spine for origin of, 52
Geniohyoid muscle, 29, 53, 59, 128, 129
Genital cord, 389
Genitalia, 388
external, 167
female, 377, 388
homologues of, 388
innervation of, 168
male, 388
internal
female, 389
homologues of, 389
male, 389
lymph nodes and vessels of, 406, 407, 408
undifferentiated, 388
Genital tubercle
epithelial tag of, 388
glans area of, 388
lateral part of, 388
Genitofemoral nerve, 329, 340, 496, 498, 539, 409
femoral branch of, 267, 409, 498, 544
genital branch of, 259, 261, 267, 409, 544
testicular vessels and genital branch of, 259, 261
Genu, of corpus callosum, 146
Gerdy's tubercle, 494, 513
Gerota's fascia. See Renal fascia, Gerota's
Gimbernat's ligament. See Lacunar ligament (Gimbernat's)
Gingiva
epithelium of, 57
lamina propria of, 57
Gingival groove, 57
Glenohumeral joint, 423
Glenohumeral ligament
inferior, 423
superior, 423
Glenoid cavity, 185, 423
Glenoid labrum, 423

Glisson's capsule. See Perivascular fibrous (Glisson's) capsule
Globus pallidus, 108, 110, 539
Glomerular arteriole
afferent, 336
efferent, 336
Glomerulus, 119, 136
Glossoepiglottic fold
lateral, 58
median, 58
Glossopharyngeal nerve, 34, 114, 116, 117, 118, 123, 125, 126, 130, 131, 133, 135, 166
branch of, 168
carotid branch of, 34, 125, 126, 130, 131
inferior ganglion of, 125, 135
pharyngeal, tonsillar and lingual branches, 125
schema of, 118, 125, 134
tympanic branch of, 10
Gluteal aponeurosis, 330, 494, 495
over gluteus medius muscle, 174
Gluteal artery
inferior, 341, 499
superior, 499
Gluteal fold, 152
Gluteal line
anterior, 352, 486
right inferior, 352, 486
superior, 265, 311
Gluteal nerve
inferior, 160, 499, 503
superior, 160, 499, 503
Gluteal tuberosity, 489
Gluteal vein
inferior, 311
superior, 311
Gluteus maximus muscle, 152, 174, 177, 254, 330, 376, 381, 382, 395, 396, 410, 411, 413, 485, 494, 495, 502, 503, 504
attachments of, 491
Gluteus medius muscle, 152, 376, 492, 496, 500, 501, 502, 503
attachments of, 491
gluteal aponeurosis over, 330, 494, 495
Gluteus minimus muscle, 489, 495, 496, 500, 501, 502, 503
attachments of, 489, 491
tendon of, 376
Gonads, 389
male, descent of, 386
Gracile fasciculus, 114, 115
Gracile tubercle, 114, 115
Gracilis muscle, 489, 492, 493, 495, 500, 501, 502, 505, 506, 516
attachments of, 489, 515
innervation of, 540
Gracilis tendon, 485, 492, 493, 506, 507
Granular foveola, 99, 102
Granule cells, 119
Gray matter, 169
interomediolateral nucleus of, 44, 132, 134
lateral horn of, 170, 325, 346
spinal, 169
sympathetic preganglionic cell bodies in, 132
Great cerebral artery, quadrigeminal cistern of, 109

Great cerebral vein (of Galen), 103, 104, 106, 144, 145, 146
Groin
left, 268
right, 268
Gubernaculum, 389, 415
Gum, 57
Gut. See also Viscera
enteric plexus of, 325
prenatal, 229

H

Habenula, 110
Habenular commissure, 106, 111, 115
Habenular trigone, 111, 115
Hair cells (cochlear)
inner, 96
outer, 96
Hamate, 452, 455, 456, 474
anterior (palmar) view of, 452
coronal section of, 455
hook of, 442, 452, 454, 456
radiograph of, 457
posterior (dorsal) view of, 452
radiograph of, 457
Hamulus, 8, 14, 38, 52
of spiral lamina, 95
Hand
in abduction, 453
in adduction, 453
in anatomical position, 453
anterior (palmar) view of, 459, 465, 472
anterior view of, 460
arteries and nerves of, palmar view of, 466, 484
bones of, 456
bursae of, 462
cutaneous innervation of, 472, 476
deep digital crease of, 418
deep dorsal dissection of, 469
deeper palmar dissection of, 460
dorsal fascia of, 462
dorsal venous network of, 468, 483
dorsum of, 483
lymph vessels passing to, 483
in extension, 453
in flexion, 453
lymphatic pathway of, 468
lymph vessels passing to
around web in, 483
dorsum of, 483
middle digital crease of, 418
muscles of, 465
intrinsic, 465
nerves of, palmar view of, 466
palmar dissection of
deeper, 460
superficial, 459–460
palm of, 453
posterior (dorsal) view of, 465, 472
proximal digital crease of, 418
proximal palmar crease of, 418
radial dissection of, superficial, 467
radial longitudinal crease of, 418
radiograph of, anteroposterior, 457
septa between spaces of, 462
spaces and sheaths of, 462
spaces of, 462
superficial dorsal dissection of, 468

Hand *(Continued)*
  surface anatomy of, 418
  tendon sheaths of, 462
Hartmann's pouch. *See* Infundibulum
      (Hartmann's pouch)
Haustra, 284
Head. *See also* Brain; Skull; *specific parts
      of head*
  arteries of, 40–41
  autonomic nerves in, 131
  axial CT image of, 150
  axial MR image of, 150
  bones and ligaments of, 4–16
  coronal CT images of, 151
  cutaneous nerves of, 24
  fauces of, 64
  lymph vessels and nodes of, 72–73
  mastication muscles of, 54–55
  muscles of, 26
  nasal region of, 36–37, 46–47, 48–49
  nerves of, 24
  oral region of, 50–61
  sagittal MR image of, 149
  surface anatomy of, 1
Heart, 126, 233
  anterior exposure of, 212
  apex of, 212, 213, 214, 246
  atria, ventricles, and interventricular sep-
      tum of, 224
  base of
      posterior view of, 214
      surface of, 214
  conducting system of, 225
  diaphragmatic surface of, 214
  in diastole, 222
  fibrous skeleton of, 222
  inferior border of, 212
  in situ, 211
  innervation of, 227
  innervation of, schema of, 227
  left border of, 196
  left side of, 225
  membranous septum of, 221, 222
  nerves of, 226
  pericardial sac and, 282
  right border of, 196
  right side of, 225
  in systole, 222
  valves of, 222
Heiss, loops of, 367
Helicotrema, 92, 95, 96
Helix, 93
  crus of, 93
Helvetius, collar of, 236, 277
Hemiazygos vein, 236, 245
  accessory, 194, 207
**Hemothorax, chest drainage tube
      placement in,** 190
Henle's loop, 337
  ascending limb of, 336
  descending limb of, 336
  proximal segment of, 336
  thin segment of, 336
Hepatic artery, 297, 337
  branches of, 290, 291, 292
  common, 237, 264, 272, 279, 294, 300,
      301, 305, 306, 318, 321, 327, 331,
      349
      arteriogram of, 303
  cross section of, 297
  effects of obstruction on, 305

Hepatic artery *(Continued)*
  intermediate, 301
  left, 294, 300, 301, 305
  middle, 305
  origin of, 302
  proper, 273, 278, 279, 288, 290, 294,
      298, 301, 321, 330
      arteriogram of, 303
      bifurcation of, 331
      to lesser omentum, 348
  right, 294, 300, 301, 305
      accessory, 302
      origin of, 302
Hepatic duct, 290
  aberrant, 294, 296
  accessory, 296
  common, 287, 289, 290, 294, 301, 331
  left, 294
  right, 294
  variations in, 294, 296
Hepatic flexure. *See* Colic flexure, right
Hepatic lymph nodes, 314, 315
Hepatic nerve plexus, 349
Hepatic plexus, 126, 319, 320, 322
  anterior, 327
  branches from, 319
      to cardia, 320
      pyloric, 126
      vagal, 319
  common, 318
  posterior, 327
  pyloric branch from, 126
  vagal branch to, 319
Hepatic portal vein, 273, 278, 279,
      288, 294, 298, 300, 301, 311, 312,
      315, 331, 349
  to lesser omentum, 348
  prenatal, 229
  tributaries of, 312
  typical arrangement of, 313
  variations of, 313
Hepatic vein, 194, 232, 265, 274, 287,
      290, 309
  prenatal, 229
Hepatoduodenal ligament, 272, 275,
      278, 297
Hepatogastric ligament, 275, 288
Hepatogastric trunk, 302
Hepatomesenteric trunk, 302
Hepatopancreatic ampulla, 294
  sphincter of, 295, 327
**Hepatorenal recess (Morison's
      pouch),** 331
Hering, canal of, 291, 292
Hering-Breuer reflex, receptors for,
      210
Hernia
  inguinal
      indirect, 261
      site of, 261
  sliding, 236
Hernial sac, 261
  neck of, 261
Herniated disc. *See* Lumbar disc
      herniation
Hesselbach, triangle of. *See* Inguinal
      (Hesselbach's) triangle
Heubner, recurrent artery of. *See*
      Distal medial striate artery (recur-
      rent artery of Heubner)
High intestinal vein, 313

Hip
  anteroposterior radiograph of, 488
  arteries of, 500–502
  bony attachments of
      anterior view of, 490
      posterior view of, 491
  flexion and extension of, 543
  muscles of, 496
      lateral view of, 494
      posterior view of, 495
  nerves of, 503
Hip bone
  auricular cartilage of, 487
  lateral view of, 486
  medial view of, 486
Hip joint
  anteroposterior radiograph of, 488
  anterior view of, 487
  capsule of, 504
  iliofemoral ligament of, 496
  lateral view of, 487
  ligaments of, 492
  posterior view of, 487
Hippocampal fimbria, 119
Hippocampal sulcus, 112
Hippocampus, 110, 111, 112
  alveus of, 112
  fimbria of, 106, 108, 111, 112
  superior dissection of, 112
His, bundle of, 225
Horizontal cells, 120
Houston, valves of, 393
Humeral artery, circumflex
  anterior, 427, 429, 433, 434
  posterior, 427, 429, 432, 433, 434
Humeral ligament, transverse, 423
Humeral vein, circumflex, 479
Humeroulnar head, 447
Humerus, 433, 436, 438
  anatomical neck of, 420, 421
      anteroposterior radiograph of, 422
  anterior view of, 420
  anteroposterior radiograph of, 422
  capitulum of, 420, 436
  common extension tendon of, 421
  common flexor tendon of, 421
  condyles of, 420, 436
  coronoid fossa of, 420
  greater tubercle of, 420, 421, 423, 432
      crest of, 420
  head of, 420
      anteroposterior radiograph of, 422
  infraglenoid tubercle of, 421
  intertubercular sulcus of, 420
  intertubercular tubercle of, 420
  lateral epicondyle of, 420, 421, 436, 437,
      438, 441, 442, 444, 448
  lateral supracondylar ridge on, 420
  lesser tubercle of, 420, 423
  medial epicondyle of, 420, 421, 432,
      433, 437, 440, 442, 444, 445, 446,
      447, 476, 477
  medial supracondylar ridge on, 420
  olecranon fossa of, 421, 436, 437
  olecranon of, 437
  posterior view of, 421
  radial fossa of, 420
  radial groove of, 421
  radiographs of, 437
  right
      surgical neck of, 243

Humerus (Continued)
  shaft of, 244, 245
  surgical neck of, 420
    anteroposterior radiograph of, 422
  trochlea of, 420, 437
  ulnar nerve groove of, 421
Hyaloid canal, 87
Hydatid of Morgagni. *See* Vesicular
    appendix (hydatid of Morgagni)
Hymen
  annular, 377
  cribriform, 377
  septate, 377
Hymenal caruncle, 370, 377
Hyoepiglottic ligament, 63, 77
Hyoglossus muscle, 34, 60
Hyoid bone, 27, 28, 29, 34, 59, 60, 61,
    63, 65, 68, 74, 76, 77
  body of, 13, 53
  greater horn of, 13, 53, 75
  lesser horn of, 13, 53
  tip of greater horn of, 67, 75
Hyothenar muscle, 444, 476
Hypochondrium
  left, 268
  right, 268
Hypogastric nerve, 165, 218, 324, 344,
    345, 409, 410, 414, 415, 416
  inferior, 324
  left, 318, 323, 412
  pelvic, 414
  right, 318, 323, 412
  superior, 345, 415
Hypogastric plexus
  inferior, 165, 166, 168, 323, 324, 344,
    345, 409, 412, 499
  parasympathetic branch from, 165
  with periureteric loops, 344
  right, 323
  superior, 165, 318, 323, 324, 345, 409,
    412
Hypogastric sheath, 364
Hypoglossal canal, 8, 10, 11
Hypoglossal nerve, 10, 32, 34, 114,
    117, 129, 344
  distribution of, 118
  meningeal branch of, 128
  schema of, 118, 128
  vena comitans of, 59, 60, 70
Hypoglossal nucleus, 116, 128
  Hypoglossal trigone, 115
Hypoglossus muscle, 27, 53, 74, 77,
    128
  dorsal lingual vein medial to, 70
Hypophyseal artery
  inferior, 140, 148
  superior, 140, 148
Hypophyseal fossa, 5, 9
  at birth, 50
Hypophyseal portal system
  primary plexus of, 148
  secondary plexus of, 148
Hypophyseal portal vein
  long, 140, 148
  short, 148
Hypophyseal vein, efferent, 140
  to cavernous sinus, 148
Hypophysis, 106, 107, 147. *See also*
    Pituitary gland
  arteries and veins of, 148
Hypothalamic area, lateral, 135

Hypothalamic artery, 140
Hypothalamic sulcus, 106, 147
Hypothalamic vessels, 148
Hypothalamohypophyseal tract, 147
Hypothalamus, 108, 147, 324
  arteries of, 148
  nuclei of
    arcuate, 147
    dorsomedial, 147
    paraventricular, 147
    posterior, 147
    supraoptic, 147
    ventromedial, 147
  parasympathetic, 324
  sympathetic, 324
Hypothenar eminence, 418
Hypothenar muscle, 446, 462, 476
Hysterosalpingogram, uterus, 373

I

Ileal artery, 306, 307
  anastomotic loops of, 280
Ileal fold, 311, 313
Ileal orifice, 284
  muscles fibers of, 282
  papillary, 282
Ileal papilla, 282
Ileocecal fold, 281
**Ileocecal junction, muscle fibers
    around,** 282
Ileocecal lips, 282
Ileocecal recess
  inferior, 281
  superior, 281
Ileocecal region, 281, 282
Ileocolic artery, 281, 307, 322, 323,
    340
  colic branch of, 281, 306, 307
  ileal branch of, 281, 306, 307
Ileocolic lymph nodes, 317
Ileocolic plexus, 322, 323
Ileocolic vein, 311, 312, 313
Ileum, 269, 282, 284, 339, 349
  barium radiograph of, 280
  circular muscle layer of, 280, 282
  longitudinal muscle layer of, 280, 282
  lymphoid nodules of, 280
  mucosa of, 280
  muscle fibers to, 282
  musculature of, 280
  serosa of, 280
  submucosa of, 280
  terminal, 271, 281, 282, 362, 363
Iliac artery
  circumflex
    ascending branch of, 255, 264
    deep, 501, 512
    superficial, 247, 512
  common, 264, 274, 340, 341, 398, 400,
    412
    left, 318
      axial CT images of, 350
    right, 329
      axial CT images of, 350
    ureteric branch from, 341
  external, 264, 274, 318, 329, 340, 398,
    400, 402, 412, 501, 512
    right, 329

Iliac artery (Continued)
  internal, 264, 307, 318, 329, 340, 341,
    370, 398, 412
    anterior division of, 400
    posterior and anterior divisions of, 402
  right, 323, 329
Iliac crest, 152, 174, 175, 176, 177, 247,
    248, 254, 329, 330, 342, 351, 485,
    486, 494, 495, 496, 502, 503, 545
  inner lip of, 248, 352, 353
  intermediate zone of, 248, 352, 353, 486
  in lumbar puncture, 162
  outer lip of, 248, 352, 353, 486
  tuberculum of, 248, 352, 353, 486
  upper lip of, 486
Iliac fossa, 352, 353, 363, 486
Iliac lymph nodes
  common, 266, 317, 343, 408
  external, 266, 317, 343, 408, 546
    lymphatic pathways to, 408
  internal, 266, 317, 343, 408
  lateral, 406
  medial external, 406
Iliac plexus
  common, 412
  external, 318, 412
  internal, 318, 412
  left common, 317
  right internal, 323
Iliac spine
  anterior, 247, 248, 250, 486, 487, 492
  anterior superior, 248, 249, 259, 263,
    486, 487, 492, 493, 496, 500
  posterior inferior, 486
  posterior superior, 152, 352, 353, 486
Iliac tubercle, 353
Iliac tuberosity, 248
Iliacus muscle, 263, 329, 376, 490,
    496, 498, 499, 538
  attachment of, 490
  muscular branch of, 498
Iliacus wing, male, 354
  Iliac vein, superficial circumflex, 544
Iliac vessels
  circumflex
    deep, 364, 403
    superficial, 249, 500
  common, 271, 401, 412
  external, 259, 260, 281, 311, 360, 361,
    362, 364, 372, 392, 401, 403
  internal, 311
  superficial circumflex, 249
Iliococcygeus muscle, 356, 357, 358,
    359, 395
Iliocostalis cervicis muscle, 175
Iliocostalis lumborum muscle, 175
Iliocostalis muscle, 175, 331
Iliocostalis thoracis muscle, 175
Iliofemoral ligament, 487, 496
Iliohypogastric nerve, 160, 177, 267,
    329, 409, 496, 498, 539
  anterior branch of, 257
  anterior cutaneous branch of, 257, 267,
    410
  genital branch of, 409
  lateral cutaneous branch of, 545
  schema of, 498

Ilioinguinal nerve, 160, 257, 260, 267, 329, 330, 340, 409, 414, 496, 498, 539, 540, 544
anterior labial branch of, 413
anterior scrotal branches of, 267, 409
schema of, 498
scrotal branches of, 267, 409, 544
Iliolumbar artery, 264, 341, 402
Iliolumbar ligament, 330, 353
Iliolumbar vein, 330, 353
Iliopectineal bursa, 496
Iliopectineal line, 353, 392
iliac part of, 358
pubic part of, 358
Iliopsoas muscle, 259, 376, 489, 492, 493, 500
attachments of, 489, 491, 496
Iliopsoas tendon, 504
Iliopubic eminence, 248, 352, 486, 487
female, 354
Iliopubic tract, 259, 362, 363, 364
Iliotibial tract, 485, 492, 494, 495, 502, 506, 507, 514, 515, 519, 520
bursa deep to, 506, 507
insertions of, 515
lateral patellar retinaculum and capsule and, 508
Ilium
arcuate line of, 356
articular surface of, 486
axial CT images of, 350
body of, 352, 486
gluteal surface of, 352
radiograph of, 355
anteroposterior radiograph of, 488
wing of, 248, 352, 358, 486
Incisive canal, 37, 38, 39, 43, 63
anastomosis in, 40
posterior septal branch of sphenopalatine and greater palatine arteries in, 41
Incisive fossa, 10, 14, 52, 56
Incisive papilla, 52
Incisor teeth, 56, 233
Incus, 89, 93, 96, 124
articular surface for, 93
body of, 93
lateral view of, 93
long limb of, 93
posterior ligament of, 94
short limb of, 93
superior ligament of, 94
Infant, mandible of, 15
Inferior anastomotic vein (of Labbé), 102, 145
Infraglenoid tubercle, 420, 421
Infrahyoid muscle, 29
action of, 29
fascia of, 28, 428
Infraorbital artery, 23, 36, 40, 81, 85
Infraorbital canal, 45
Infraorbital foramen, 12, 36
Infraorbital groove, 2
Infraorbital margin, 1
Infraorbital nerve (V₂), 24, 36, 44, 81, 83, 121, 122
entering infraorbital canal, 45
internal nasal branches of, 122
superior alveolar branches of, 122
Infraorbital vein, 23, 70

Infrapatellar bursa
deep, 511
subcutaneous, 511
Infrapatellar synovial fold, 507, 508
Infraspinatus fascia, 174, 177
Infraspinatus muscle, 152, 180, 244, 245, 424, 425, 427, 428, 432
fascia over, 174
insertion of, 421
origin of, 421
Infraspinatus tendon, 423, 425
Infratemporal fossa, 4, 13
Infratrochlear nerve, 24, 36, 56, 81, 86, 122
from nasociliary nerve, 45
Infundibular nucleus, 147
Infundibular process, 147
capillary plexus of, 148
Infundibular recess, 108
Infundibular stem, 147
Infundibulum (Hartmann's pouch), 114, 140, 147, 294
body of, 114
fundus of, 114
neck of, 114
of uterine tube, 372
Inguinal canal, 260, 262
Inguinal falx, 250
conjoint tendon of, 250, 253, 259, 263
Inguinal fold, 389
Inguinal hernia
indirect, 261
site of, 261
Inguinal ligament (Poupart's), 247, 249, 250, 259, 263, 351, 356, 378, 380, 381, 407, 485, 492, 498, 500, 501, 544, 546
reflected, 250, 251, 259
Inguinal lymph nodes
deep, 266, 406, 407, 408, 546
highest deep, 266, 408
horizontal, 266
inferior, 266
superficial, 266, 317, 406, 407, 408, 546
superficial inferior, 407
superolateral, 407
superomedial, 407
Inguinal region, 259
anterior view of, 259
posterior view of, 259
Inguinal ring
deep, 251, 259, 261, 362, 363, 369, 386
site of, 274
superficial, 249, 259, 261, 386, 544
lateral and medial crus of, 259
Inguinal (Hesselbach's) triangle, 259
Insula, 105, 110, 141
central and circular sulci of, 105
limen of, 105, 141
short and long gyri of, 105
Interalveolar septa, 15
Interarticular ligament, 187
Interarytenoid notch, 66
Interatrial septum, 220, 246
Intercalated lymph node, 73
Intercapitular vein, 468, 480
Intercarpal ligament, 455
Intercavenous sinus
anterior, 103
superior, 103

Intercavernous septum, 382, 385
of deep fascia, 381
Interchondral joints, 186
Interclavicular ligament, 186, 419
Intercondylar area
anterior, 513
posterior, 513
Intercondylar condyle, radiograph of, 510
Intercondylar eminence, 514
anteroposterior radiograph of, 510
Intercostal artery, 183, 192, 305
anterior, 192
first posterior, 33
lower, anastomosis with, 255
posterior, 171, 172, 188, 189, 230, 231
dorsal branch of, 172
lateral mammary and cutaneous branches of, 183, 192
second, 33
third right, 207, 237
supreme, 33, 136, 138
Intercostal lymph nodes, 266
Intercostal membrane
external, 180, 189, 192, 258
internal, 180, 192, 230, 258
Intercostal muscle, 198, 243, 244, 245, 331
anterior cutaneous branch of, 180
external, 176, 188, 189, 192, 250, 258
external intercostal membranes anterior to, 189
innermost, 180, 192, 258
internal, 189, 192, 230, 231, 255, 258
lateral branch of, 188
medial branch of, 188
Intercostal nerve, 160, 170, 180, 189, 192, 331
abdominal portions of, 188
anterior, 258
anterior cutaneous branches of, 177, 188, 192, 257
collateral branch rejoining, 258
eighth, 209
first, 227, 430
lateral cutaneous branches of, 177, 188, 189, 192
lateral cutaneous branches to, 177, 188, 189, 257
posterior, 192, 230
seventh right, 321
sixth, 165, 209
third, 240
ventral ramus of, 180
Intercostal vein
anterior, 256
left superior, 231
posterior, 230, 231
right superior, 230
Intercostal vessels, 331
Intercostobrachial muscle, 189
Intercostobrachial nerve, 189, 257, 429, 474, 479, 481
Intercrural fibers, 249, 259
Intercuneiform ligament, dorsal, 527
Interglobular space, 57
Intergluteal cleft, 152
Interlobar artery, 335, 337
lymph vessels along, 343
Interlobar lymph vessels, 208

Interlumborum cervicis muscle, 176
Intermaxillary suture, 36
Intermediate nerve, 104, 114, 118, 123, 124, 133, 135
Intermediolateral cell column, 346
Intermediolateral nucleus, 133, 134
Intermediolateral nucleus, preganglionic sympathetic cell bodies in, 132
Intermesenteric plexus, 267, 318, 322, 323, 324, 344, 345, 412
   renal and upper ureteric branches from, 344
Intermetacarpal joint, 455
Intermuscular septum
  anterior, 522
  anteromedial, 492, 500, 501
  lateral, 430, 432, 435, 445, 448
   of arm, 477
  medial, 430, 432, 433, 445, 446, 447, 448
  posterior, 522
  transverse, 522
Intermuscular stroma, 326
Internal capsule, 108, 141
  cleft for, 110
  genu of, 110
  retrolenticular part of, 110
Interosseous artery
  anterior, 434, 447
   computed tomography of, 484
  common, 434, 447, 448, 449
  posterior, 434, 445, 448, 449
  recurrent, 434, 445
  termination of, 445
Interosseous intercarpal ligament, 455
Interosseous ligament, intercarpal, 455
Interosseous membrane, 439, 441, 443, 444, 454, 455, 511, 512, 517, 518, 520, 522, 525
Interosseous muscle, 528
  deep tibial nerve to, 541
  dorsal, 462, 465, 470, 476, 531, 536, 537
   first, 445, 460, 465, 530
  of foot, 536, 537
   dorsal, 536
  palmar, 465, 476
  plantar, 535
  plantar dorsal, 536
  superficial tibial nerve branch to, 541
Interosseous nerve
  anterior, 448, 449, 475
  of leg, 541
  plantar, 537
  posterior, 445, 449
Interosseous talocalcaneal ligament, 527
Interpectoral (Rotter's) lymph nodes, 184
Interpeduncular cistern, 109
Interphalangeal joint, 418
  capsules and ligaments of, 528
Interphalangeal ligaments, 458
Intersigmoid recess, 271, 340
Intersphincteric groove, 392, 393, 394
Interspinalis cervicis muscle, 176

Interspinous ligament
  lumbar, 176
  lumbosacral, 177
Interspinous plane, 268
Intertendinous connection, hand, 470
Interthalamic adhesion, 106, 108, 110, 111, 146
Intertragic notch, 93
Intertransversarius muscle, lateral, 176
Intertransverse ligament, 187
Intertrochanteric crest, 487, 503
  anteroposterior radiograph of, 488
Intertrochanteric line, 487, 489
Intertubercular plane, 268
Intertubercular tendon sheath, 423
Interureteric crest, 366
Interventricular foramen (of Monro), 106, 109, 111, 115, 145, 146
  left, 108
Interventricular septum, 216, 220
  muscular part of, 220, 223, 224, 225
Interventricular sulcus
  anterior, 246
  posterior, 214, 215
Intervertebral disc, 19, 155.
Intervertebral disc, 19, 155. *See also specific vertebrae*
  anulus fibrosis of, 155
  lumbar, 157, 339
  lumbosacral, 352
  nucleus pulposus of, 155
  sternal angle of, 245
Intervertebral disc space, 156
Intervertebral foramen, 19, 180
  lower margin of, 154
  lumbar, 155
   radiograph of, 156
Intervertebral joint, 18
Intervertebral vein, 137, 173
Intestinal glands, 326
Intestinal lymphatic trunk, 316
Intestinal trunk, 266
Intestine, 167. *See also* Colon; Duodenum; Jejunum; Mesocolon
  circular muscle of, 326
  intrinsic autonomic plexuses of, 326
  large
   arteries of, 307
   innervation of, 324
   lymph nodes vessels and nodes of, 317
   mucosa and musculature of, 284
   nerves of, 323, 324
    schema of, 324
   veins of, 311
  longitudinal muscle of, 326
  lumen of, 326
  mesenteric relations of, 270, 271
  mucosa of, 326
  small, 126, 269, 322
   area for, 329
   arteries of, 306
   innervation of, 324
   lymph nodes of, 316
   lymph vessels of, 316
   mesentery of, 348
   mucosa and musculature of, 280
   nerves of, 322
    schema of, 324

Intestine *(Continued)*
  small *(Continued)*
   veins of, 310
   submucosa of, 326
Intraarticular ligament, 187
Intraculminate vein, 144
Intrahepatic biliary system, schema of, 292
Intralaminar nuclei, 111
Intraparietal sulcus, 105
Intrapulmonary airway
  schema of, 204
Intrapulmonary blood circulation, 205
Intraspinatus tendon, 423
Intrinsic artery, of eye, 90
Intrinsic muscle
  action of, 79
  of larynx, 78
  of tongue, 128
Intrinsic nerve, pancreatic, 328
Intrinsic vein, of eye, 90
Iridocorneal angle, 87, 88, 90
  trabecular meshwork and spaces of, 88
Iris, 81, 87, 89, 90
  arteries of, 91
  folds of, 88
  major arterial circle of, 88, 90, 91
  minor arterial circle of, 88, 90, 91
  veins of, 91
Irritant receptors, 210
Ischial spine, 248, 263, 411, 486, 487, 503
  female, 354
  radiograph of, 355
Ischial tuberosity, 248, 352, 353, 359, 378, 379, 381, 390, 395, 398, 486, 487, 502, 503
  anteroposterior radiograph of, 488
  female, 354
  male, 354
  radiograph of, 355
Ischioanal fossa, 366, 392
  anterior recess of, 366, 370, 396
  fat body of, 376, 380, 392
  posterior communication between right and left, 396
  posterior recess of, 396
  preanal communication between right and left, 396
  pus in, 396
  roof of, 405
  transverse fibrous septum of, 392, 394, 395
Ischiocavernous muscle, 360, 361, 370, 378, 379, 381, 382, 383, 391, 395, 404, 405
  crus of, 366
Ischiococcygeus muscle, 263, 356, 357, 398, 402, 411, 412, 499
  nerve to, 499
Ischiocondylar muscle, 540
Ischiofemoral ligament, 487
Ischiopubic ramus, 359, 361, 378, 379, 380, 382, 383, 384, 395
Ischium
  anteroposterior radiograph of, 488
  body of, 486
  radiograph of, 355
  ramus of, 486

J

Jaw. *See also* Mandible; Maxilla
  angle of, 1
  closed, 16
  slightly opened, 16
  widely opened, 16
Jejunal artery, 306, 307
  anastomotic loop of, 280
  first, 302
  plexus on, 3190
Jejunal vein, 311, 313
Jejunum, 269, 270, 271, 278, 279, 297, 298
  barium radiograph of, 279, 280
  circular muscle layer of, 280
  cross section of, 297, 338
  longitudinal muscle layer of, 280
  lymphoid nodule of, 280
  mucosa of, 280
  musculature of, 280
  submucosa of, 280
Jugular foramen, 103, 125, 126, 127
Jugular fossa, 8, 11
Jugular lymphatic trunk, 208
Jugular nerve, internal, 1, 10
Jugular notch, 28, 181, 196
Jugular trunk, 72
    left, 266
    right, 266
Jugular vein
  anterior, 30, 74, 256
    communication to, 70
    termination of, 70
  external, 23, 31, 74, 198, 206, 211, 256
  internal, 23, 28, 29, 30, 31, 32, 34, 59, 74, 75, 76, 97, 128, 189, 198, 206, 211, 232, 256
    inferior bulb of, 75
    left, 137
    right, 137
Jugulodigastric muscle, 73
Juguloomohyoid node, 73
Jugum, 9

K

Kerckring, valves of, 279, 280
Kidneys, 167, 179, 272, 278, 338
  anterior surface of, 335
  base pyramid of, 334
  blood vessels in parenchyma of, 334, 337
  blood vessels of, 332, 333, 347
  cortex of, 334, 336, 337
  cortical radiate arteries of, 335
  fibrous capsule of, 334
  hilum of, 334
  inferior pole of, 334
  in situ
    anterior views of, 329
    posterior, 330
  innervation of, 345
  inner zone of, 336
  interlobar arteries of, 335
  lateral border of, 334
  left, 98, 197, 273, 299, 329, 331, 340, 347
  axial CT images of, 350
  frontal section of, 329
  superior pole of, 297

Kidneys *(Continued)*
  lymph vessels and nodes of, 343
  major calices of, 334
  medial border of, 334
  medulla of, 334
  minor calices of, 334
  nerves of, 334
  outer zone of, 336, 345
  perforating radiate artery of, 335
  posterior surface of, 335
  prenatal, 229
  renal column of, 334
  renal cortex of, 338
  renal papilla of, 334
  retroperitoneal, 288
  right, 197, 275, 298, 329, 330, 340, 342, 347
  subscapular zone of, 336, 337
  superior pole of, 272, 334
    cross section of, 338
Knee
  anterior views of, 507, 508
  anteroposterior radiograph of, 510
  arteries of, 507
  articular cavity of, 511
  attachment of, 511
  collateral ligaments of, 509
  cruciate ligaments of, 509
  in extension of, 507
  in flexion, 509, 543
  interior of, 508
  joint capsule of, 506, 508, 519
  lateral view of, 506
  ligaments of, 508, 509
  medial view of, 506
  posterior view of, 511
  right
    in extension, 507, 509
    in flexion, 509
  sagittal view of, 511
  slightly in flexion, 507
Kohn, pores of, 204

L

L4–5 disc herniation, 162
L5–S1 disc herniation, 162
L2 ganglion, 412
L1 spinal nerve, 160
  ventral ramus of, 177
L1–3 spinal nerves, dorsal rami of, 254
L5 spinal nerve, 160, 412
  anterior ramus of, 410
L1 vertebra, 153, 160
  body of, 273
  inferior articular process of, 156
  spinous process of, 179
  superior articular process of, 156
  transverse process of, 338
L2 vertebra
  body of, 179
  superior view of, 155
L3 vertebra
  body of, 156, 336, 337
  pedicle of, 156
  posterior view of, 155
  spinous process of, 156
  transverse process of, 156

L4 vertebra
  body of, 352
  inferior vertebral notch of, 156
  lamina of, 156
  posterior view of, 155
  spinous process of, 156
L5 vertebra, 153, 160
  body of, 352
  superior vertebral notch of, 156
Labbé vein. *See* Inferior anastomotic vein (of Labbé)
Labial artery
  inferior, 69
  posterior, 404
  superior, 69
Labial nerve, posterior, 413, 414
Labial vein
  inferior, 70
  superior, 70
Labioscrotal swelling, 388
Labium majus, 360, 365, 388
Labium minus, 360, 365, 388
Labyrinth
  bony, 95, 96
    common limbs of, 95
    right, 95
    schema of, 96
    superior projection of, right, 97
  common membranous limb of, 95
  membranous, 95, 96
    right, 95
    schema of, 96
  orientation of in skull, 97
Labyrinthine artery, 140, 141, 143
  internal, 143
  left, 136
Lacrimal apparatus, 82
Lacrimal artery, 85
  recurrent meningeal branch of, 100
Lacrimal bone, 2, 4, 6, 12, 38
  at birth, 46
Lacrimal canaliculi, 82
Lacrimal caruncle, 81, 82
Lacrimal gland, 83, 85, 86, 133, 166, 167, 168
  excretory ducts of, 82
  orbital part of, 82
  palpebral part of, 82
Lacrimal lake, 81, 82
Lacrimal nerve, 83, 86, 121, 122, 131
  cutaneous branch of, 45
  palpebral branch of, 82
Lacrimal papilla
  inferior, 81, 82
  superior, 81, 82
Lacrimal sac, 81, 82
  fossa for, 2, 4
Lactiferous duct, 182
Lactiferous sinus, 182
Lacuna
  lateral (venous), 99, 100
  magna, 385
Lacunar ligament (Gimbernat's), 250, 251, 259, 263, 546
Laimer, area of. *See* V-shaped area (of Laimer), 234, 235
Lambda, 7
Lamina, lumbar, 155
Lamina affixa, 111
Lamina cribrosa, 87
Lamina terminalis, 106, 107, 147

Liver (Continued)
duct distribution in, 289
falciform ligament of, 255
fibrous appendix of, 287
functional surgical segments of, 289
interior border of, 268, 275
in situ, 288
inlet venula of, 291
innervation of, 168, 326
intrahepatic vascular and duct systems
of, 290
intralobular arteriole of, 291
left lobe of, 269, 275, 288
left triangular ligament of, 274
ligaments of, 287, 312
lobes of, 289
low-power section of, 292
lymph pathways to, 184
normal lobular pattern of, 290
papillary process of, 287
parietal surface of, 289
periportal arteriole of, 291
perivascular fibrous capsule of, 290
portal arteriole of, 291
posterior lateral segment of, 289
posterior view of, 287
prenatal, 229
quadrate lobe of, 275
right lobe of, 269, 275, 288
axial CT images of, 350
round ligament of, 229, 256, 275, 349
segments of, 289
structure of, 29
sublobular lobes of, 290
surfaces of, 287
topography of, 286
variations in form of, 288
vascular system of, 290
veins of, 291
visceral peritoneum of, 331
visceral surface of, 287, 289
Liver plate cells, 290
Lobule (ear), 1
Locus ceruleus, 115
Longissimus capitis muscle, 175, 178
Longissimus cervicis muscle, 175
Longissimus erector spinae
muscle, 349
Longissimus muscle, 175, 331
Longissimus thoracic muscle, 175
Longitudinal esophageal muscle,
cricoid attachment of, 65, 67
Longitudinal intramuscular plexus,
326
Longitudinal ligament
anterior, 63, 65, 179, 187, 263, 331, 348,
349, 353, 362, 363
posterior, 22
Longitudinal muscle
conjoined, 392, 394
conjoined rectal, 393
of intestine, 326
rectal, 393
of tongue
inferior, 60
superior, 60
Longus capitis muscle, 27, 30
nerves to, 129
Longus colli muscle, 30
Loops of Heiss, 367

Lower limb. *See also* Leg
arteries of, 500–502, 504
cutaneous innervation of, 487–489
dermatomes of, 543
lymph nodes and vessels of, 546
muscles of, 490–503
neurovasculature of, 538–546
segmental innervation of movements of,
543
superficial nerves and veins of, 544
anterior view of, 545
posterior view of, 545
surface anatomy of, 485
Lumbar artery, 171
fifth, 264
lower, anastomosis with, 255
right, 264
Lumbar curvature, 153
Lumbar disc herniation, 162
characteristic posture in, 161
clinical manifestations of, 161
left-sided lower, 161
level of and clinical features of, 161
surgical exposure of, 161
Lumbar disc protrusion, 161
Lumbar enlargement, 161
Lumbar ganglion, 167, 318
Lumbar lymphatic trunk
to cisterna chyli and thoracic duct, 343
right and left, 316
Lumbar lymphatic trunk ganglion
lower, 228
upper, 228
Lumbar lymph nodes, 266
Lumbar nerve, 161
Lumbar nucleus pulposus,
herniated, 161
Lumbar plexus, 160, 496, 498, 538, 539
muscular branches from, 267
Lumbar puncture, 162
Lumbar region, 268
Lumbar spinal nerve, 161, 179
dorsal and ventral roots of, 170
dorsal rami of, 177
origin of, 170
Lumbar triangle (of Petit), 152, 254
internal oblique muscle in, 174
Lumbar trunk
ascending, 195, 263, 265, 332
left, 266
right, 266
Lumbar vein, ascending, 332
Lumbar vertebra
anterior view of, 171
arteries of, 171
assembled, 153
body of, 153
cross section through, 170
dura mater of, 162
foramen of, 155
inferior articular process of, 155
inferior vertebral notch of, 155
intervertebral disc of, 155
lamina disc of, 155
left lateral view of, 155
mammillary process of, 155
muscles of, 179
pedicle, sectioned of, 179
posterior view of, 153
radiographs of, 156
spinous process of, 155

Lumbar vertebra (Continued)
superior articular process of, 155
superior vertebral notch of, 155
superior view of, 155
transverse processes of, 248
transverse process of, 248
Lumbocostal ligament, 330
Lumbocostal triangle, 195
Lumborum muscle, interspinalis,
176
Lumbosacral articular surface, 157
Lumbosacral fascial sheath, 462
Lumbosacral trunk, 267, 496, 498,
499, 538, 539
Lumbosacral vertebrae
inferior articular process of, 159
invertebral foramen of, 159
lamina of, 159
ligaments of, 159
ligamentum flavum of, 159
pedicle of, 159
spinous process of, 159
superior articular process of, 159
transverse process of, 159
Lumbrical fascial sheath, 460
Lumbrical muscle, 465, 533, 534, 536
deep tibial nerve branch to, 541
in fascial sheaths, 460
first, 541
fourth, 460
in fascial sheath, 460
innervation of, 465, 541
schema of, 463
second, 460, 541
in fascial sheath, 460
tendons of, 535
third, 460
in fascial sheath, 460
third and fourth, 476, 541
Lumen, 326
Lunate, 376, 456, 487
anterior (palmar) view of, 452
area for, 439
coronal section of, 455
posterior (dorsal) view of, 452
radiograph of, 457
Lunate sulcus, 105
Lungs, 167, 168, 170, 342
anterior border of, 196
anterior view of, 200
apex of, 196, 197
area for esophagus in, 196
area for trachea in, 196
bronchopulmonary segments of, 200,
201
cardiac impression of, 196
cardiac notch of, 196, 198
diaphragmatic surface of, 196
great vessels of, 206
groove for esophagus in, 196
hilum of, 196
horizontal fissure of, 196, 197, 198
inferior border of, 196
inferior lobe of, 198, 200
medial view of, 199
in situ, anterior view of, 198
left, 197, 211, 215, 243, 245
bronchopulmonary segments of, 200,
201
inferior lobe of, 201, 293
medial view of, 199

Manubriosternal synchondrosis, 419
Manubrium, 186, 198, 243, 244, 419
Marginal artery, 307, 323
  of large intestine, 307
  left, 216
Marginal plexus, 323
Marginal sulcus, 106
Marshall, ligament of, 221
Masseteric artery, 40, 54, 55
Masseter nerve, 40, 54, 55, 122
Masseter muscle, 25, 27, 28, 47, 60, 61
  axial CT image of, 150
  axial MR image of, 150
  deep part of, 54
  insertion of, 54
  superficial part of, 54
Mastication, muscles of, 54, 55
Mastoid angle, 9
Mastoid antrum, 94
Mastoid canaliculus, 10
Mastoid cells, 94
Mastoid emissary vein, 10, 137
Mastoid foramen, 10
Mastoid process, 14, 25, 27, 28, 29,
    30, 34, 53, 59, 176
Maxilla, 2, 6, 38
  alveolar process of, 2, 4, 6, 13, 38, 48
  anterior nasal spine of, 2, 4, 6, 36, 38
  at birth, 50
  frontal process of, 2, 4, 36, 38, 81
  incisive canal of, 6, 38, 40
  incisive fossa of, 8
  infraorbital foramen of, 2, 4, 12
  infratemporal surface of, 4
  maxillary sinus in, 50
  medial palatine suture of, 8
  nasal spine of, anterior, 36
  nasal surface of, 6
  orbital surface of, 2
  palatine process of, 5, 6, 8, 14, 37, 38,
    52, 56
  tuberosity of, 4, 14
  zygomatic process of, 2, 8
Maxillary artery, 16, 34, 40, 54, 71,
    100, 131, 134
  branches of, 40
Maxillary bone, 47
Maxillary nerve (V₂), 45, 86, 121, 122,
    131, 133, 134, 135
  dental and gingival branches of, 45
  meningeal branch of, 86, 122
  nasal branch of, 122
  pharyngeal branch of, 122
  posterior superior lateral nasal branch of,
    42, 43
Maxillary plexus, 131
Maxillary sinus, 3, 5, 44, 47, 48, 49
  alveolar recess of, 48
  axial MR image of, 150
  coronal CT images of, 151
  growth of, 50
  infraorbital recess of, 48
  mucous membrane of, 45
  with opening into semilunar hiatus, 50
  openings of, 37, 38, 48, 49, 50
  postganglionic fibers to vessels and
    glands of, 44
  sagittal MR image of, 149
  zygomatic recess of, 48
Maxillary vein, 85
McBurney's point, 283

Medial rectus muscle, 83
Median aperture (foramen of
    Magendie), 109
Median nerve, 429, 433, 446, 447, 454,
    460, 465, 474, 475
  anterior interosseous part of, 476
  anterior view of, 475
  articular branch of, 475
  branches to thenar and lumbrical mus-
    cles, 465
  in carpal tunnel, 461
  common palmar digital branches of, 460
  communicating branch with ulnar nerve,
    476
  communicating with ulnar nerve, 475
  to cutaneous innervation, 475
  palmar branch of, 446, 447, 475, 481
  palmar digital branches of, 473, 481
  palmar view of, 475
  posterior view of, 475
  proper palmar digital branches of, 469
  recurrent branch of, 474
    to thenar muscles, 460
Median sulcus, dorsal, 115
Mediastinal lymph nodes, 184
  anterior, pathway to, 184
  posterior, 266
Mediastinum
  anterior lung area for, 194
  cross section of, 241
  fat pad in, 231
  left lateral view of, 231
  right lateral view of, 230
  superior, great vessels of, 206
Medulla oblongata, 11, 106, 124, 134,
    135, 168, 324, 345
  axial MR image of, 150
  cross section of, 124
  lower part of, 135
  nuclear layer of, 113
  sagittal MR image of, 149
Medullary artery
  anterior segmental, 171, 172
  posterior segmental, 171
Medullary lamina
  external, 111
  internal, 111
Medullary (renal) lymph vessels,
    343
Medullary vein
  anteromedian, 144
  anterior segmental, 173
  anteromedian, 144
  posterior, 173
Medullary velum
  inferior, 106, 113
  superior, 106, 113, 114, 115
Meibomian glands, 81
Meissner's plexus. See Submucous
    (Meissner's) plexus
Membranous ampulla
  anterior, 95
  lateral, 95
  posterior, 95
Membranous septum
  atrioventricular part of, 222, 223, 225
  interventricular part of, 223, 225
Meningeal artery, 99, 100
  accessory, 11, 40, 100
  anterior, 85
  left middle, 136

Meningeal artery *(Continued)*
  middle, 40, 55, 99, 100, 102, 131, 138
  posterior, 11
Meningeal nerve, 45
Meningeal plexus, middle, 131
Meningeal vein, middle, 102
Meningeal vessel grooves
  anterior, 9
  middle, 6, 7, 9
  posterior, 9
Meningeal vessels, middle, 10
Meninges, 10,136
  arteries of, 99, 136
  innervation of, 325
  spinal, 102, 324, 325
  superficial veins of, 102
  veins of, 99
Meningohypophyseal trunk, 100
Meniscofemoral ligament,
    posterior, 508, 509
Meniscus, 455
  lateral, 507, 508, 509, 511
    horns of, 508
  medial, 507, 508, 509
    horns of, 508
Mental foramen, 15
Mentalis muscle, 26, 54, 123
Mental nerve, 24, 46, 71, 122
Mental protuberance, 1
Mesencephalic vein
  lateral, 144
  posterior, 144, 146
Mesenteric artery
  inferior, 270, 278, 307, 308, 318, 323,
    329, 332, 340, 341
  superior, 179, 270, 281, 298, 301, 305,
    306, 307, 308, 319, 321, 322, 328,
    332, 339, 340, 342
  common origin of, 302
  relations of, 310
  in root of mesentery, 270
Mesenteric ganglion, 126
  inferior, 165, 167, 318, 323, 409
  superior, 165, 167, 168, 267, 298, 318,
    320, 322, 323, 324, 325, 328, 344,
    345, 346, 409
Mesenteric lymph nodes, 315
  inferior, 266, 317
  superior, 266, 314, 317, 321
Mesentericoparietal recess, 179,
    270, 271
Mesenteric plexus
  inferior, 165, 318, 323
  superior, 165, 166, 318, 319, 320, 322,
    328
Mesenteric vein
  inferior, 270, 298, 311, 312, 313, 315
  superior, 179, 279, 306, 311, 312, 313,
    338, 339, 342
  cross section of, 338
  relations of, 310
Mesenteric vessels, superior, 278,
    349
Mesentery
  of ileum, 280
  of jejunum, 280
  peritoneal layers of, 326
  root of, 270, 274, 278, 296, 298, 310,
    340, 362, 363
    superior mesenteric vein and, 310
  of small intestine, 349

Mesoappendix, 281, 283, 322
Mesocolic taenia, 281, 282, 284
Mesocolon
sigmoid, 271, 284, 307, 329, 340
attachment of, 274
transverse, 269, 270, 271, 272, 273, 278, 284, 307
attachment of, 298, 299
Mesometrium, 371
Mesonephric (wolffian) duct, 389
Mesonephric tubule
vestigial, 390
Mesosalpinx, 369
laminae of, 372
Mesothelial septum, 169
Mesovarium, 370
laminae of, 372
Metacarpal artery
dorsal, 469, 530
palmar, 465
Metacarpal bone, 456
anterior (palmar) view of, 452
base of, 456
fifth, 444
base of, radiograph of, 457
head of, 456
posterior (dorsal) view of, 452
second, 445
shaft of, 456
third, 456
Metacarpal ligament
deep transverse, 465
dorsal, 455
palmar, 465
superficial transverse, 480
Metacarpal vein, dorsal, 468
Metacarpophalangeal (MP) joint, 458
Metacarpophalangeal (MP) ligament, 458
Metaphyseal arcuate ligament, 455
Metaphysis, nutrient arterial branch to, 471
Metatarsal artery
dorsal, 530, 535, 536
anterior perforating branches of, 535
posterior perforating branches of, 535
plantar, 535, 536
anterior perforating branches of, 535
Metatarsal bone, 523, 524, 536
base of, 523
fifth, 523
tuberosity of, 523, 530, 535, 536, 537
first, 523, 524, 537
fourth, 523
head of, 523
plantar view of, 523
second, 523
shaft of, 523
third, 523
tuberosity of, 523, 524, 537
Metatarsal ligament
deep transverse, 536
dorsal, 536
plantar, 528, 536
superficial transverse, 532
Metatarsal vein, dorsal, 544
Midbrain
axial MR image of, 150
sagittal MR image of, 149

Midclavicular line
left, 268
right, 268
Midline groove, 58
Midpalmar space, 460, 462
Minute arteries, of finger, 471
Mitral cell, 119
Mitral valve, 213, 225
anatomy of, 223
anterior cusp of, 222, 223, 224
commissural cusps of, 222
fibrous ring of, 222
leaflet of, 246
left fibrous ring of, 222
posterior cusp of, 222, 223, 224
Molar teeth
first, 56
growth of, 50
second, 56
third, 56
Monro, foramen of. See Interventricular foramen (of Monro)
Morgagni, hydatid of. See Vesicular appendix (hydalid of Margagni)
Morison's pouch. See Hepatorenal recess (Morison's pouch)
Mouth
afferent innervation of, 62
floor of, 53
nerves of, 62
roof of, 52
anterior view of, 52
posterior view of, 52
Mucosa, intestinal, 279, 280
Mucous cell, stomach, 276
Müllerian duct. See Paramesonephric (müllerian) duct
Multifidus muscle, 176
Muscles. See also specific muscles
anorectal, 394
of arm
anterior view of, 430
posterior view of, 432
of back, 174, 175, 176
deep layers of, 176
intermediate layers of, 175
superficial layers of, 174
of dorsum of foot, 530
of duodenum, 279
of esophagus, 234
extrinsic eye, 84
of face, 123
of facial expression, 26, 60
of foot, 536
of forearm, 440, 441, 446, 447, 448
of hand, 465
of hip and thigh, 492–493
lateral view of, 494
posterior view of, 495
innervated by femoral nerve, 538
innervated by obturator nerve, 540
of large intestine, 284
of larynx, 78
of leg
anterior view of, 520
attachments of, 515
deep dissection of, 516, 520
posterior view of, 518
intermediate dissection of, 517
lateral view of, 521
posterior view of, 517

Muscles (Continued)
superficial dissection of
anterior view of, 518, 519
posterior view of, 516
of lower limb, 485
of mastication, 54, 55
of neck
anterior view of, 28
lateral view of, 27
of pharynx, 65, 67, 68
lateral view of, 68
of rotator cuff, 425
of shoulder, 424
of small intestine, 280
of sole of foot
first muscle layer of, 533
second muscle layer of, 534
third muscle layer of, 535
of stomach, 277
of thigh, 492–495
of tongue, 59, 60
of vermiform appendix, 283
Muscular artery, 90, 91
Muscularis mucosae, 276
of anal canal and rectum, 394
Muscular vein, 90
Musculocutaneous nerve, 429, 430, 433, 435, 447, 449, 474, 475, 480
terminal part of, 446, 469, 479, 482
Musculophrenic artery, 189, 198, 211, 215
Musculophrenic vein, 189, 256
Myelencephalon, 423. See also Medulla oblongata
Myenteric (Auerbach's) plexus, 326
Mylohyoid groove, 15
Mylohyoid line, 15
Mylohyoid muscle, 27, 28, 29, 31, 32, 34, 53, 59, 60
median raphe between, 53
nerve to, 55, 60
Mylohyoid nerve, 16, 40, 46, 53, 122
Myometrium, 371

N

Nail bed, 471
Nail matrix, 471
Nail root, 471
Nares
anterior, 1
posterior, 14
Nasal artery
dorsal, 23, 36, 40, 81, 85
external, 36
lateral, 36
Nasal bone, 1, 2, 4, 6, 12, 36, 38, 39
at birth, 50
Nasal cavity, 82, 83
arteries of, 41
autonomic innervation of, 44
bones of, at birth, 50
floor of, 37
growth of, 50
lateral wall of, 37, 38
medial wall of, 39
nerves of, 42–44
postganglionic fibers to vessels and glands of, 44
speculum view of, 37
Nasal cleft. See Intergluteal cleft

Nasal concha
axial MR image of, 150
highest, 38
inferior, 37, 38, 82
coronal CT images of, 151
othmoidal process of, 30
growth of, 50
sagittal MR image of, 149
middle, 2, 6, 37, 38, 48, 50, 82
growth of, 50
superior, 6, 37, 38
lower border of, 50
Nasalis muscle, 123
alar part of, 26, 76
transverse part of, 26, 36
Nasal meatus
atrium of middle, 37
inferior, 37, 82
opening into, 50
middle, 37
atrium of, 37
opening into, 49
superior, 37, 50
Nasal nerve
external, 36
inferior lateral, 131
posterior, 131, 133
posterior superior, 131
Nasal retinal arteriole
inferior, 90
superior, 90
Nasal retinal venule
inferior, 90
superior, 90
Nasal septum, 39, 41, 42, 47, 48, 63, 66
axial MR image of, 150
cartilage of, lateral process of, 38
coronal CT images of, 151
growth of, 48
Nasal slit, 11
Nasal spine
anterior, 39
posterior, 39
Nasal vein
dorsal, 23
external, 70
Nasal vestibule, 37, 39
Nasociliary nerve (V₁), 83, 86, 121,
122, 131, 132
infratrochlear nerve from, 45
Nasofrontal vein, 23, 85
Nasolabial lymph node, 72
Nasolabial sulcus, 1
Nasolacrimal canal, opening of, 38
Nasolacrimal duct, 82
in nasooptic furrow, 50
opening of, 37, 82
Nasolacrimal foramen, at birth, 50
Nasooptic furrow, 50
Nasopalatine nerve (V₂), 10, 42, 43,
44, 62
communicating with greater palatine
nerve, 42
passing to septum, 43
Nasopharynx, 92
airway to, 37
sagittal MR image of, 149
Navicular bone, 536, 537
plantar view of, 523
tuberosity of, 523, 524, 536
Navicular fossa, 361, 385

Neck
arteries of, 504
autonomic nerves in, 130
bony framework of, 185
cervical plexus in, 32
cutaneous nerves of, 24
fascial layers of, 28
lymph nodes and vessels of, 72
muscles of, 27
anterior view of, 28
posterior view of, 27
nerves of, 24
posterior triangle of, 174, 188
superficial veins and cutaneous nerves
of, 31
surface anatomy of, 1
Nephron
Henle's loop of, 337
schema of, 336
Nerves. *See also specific nerves*
abdominal, 258
of abdominal wall, 267
of back, 177
to blood vessels, 228
cochlear fibers of, 96
cutaneous
of arm and shoulder, 479
of forearm, 480
of head and neck, 224
of upper limb, 479, 481
of wrist and hand, 473
of esophagus, 240
of external genitalia, 409
of female pelvic viscera, 412
of female perineum and external
genitalia, 413
of female reproductive organs, 415
of fingers, 471
of forearm, 480
of hand, 472
palmar view of, 466
of heart, 226, 227
of hip and buttock, 503
of kidneys and ureters, 344, 345
of large intestine, 323, 324
of larynx, 80
of liver and biliary tract, 327
of lower limb, 544, 545
of male external genitalia, 409
of male pelvic viscera, 410
of male perineum, 411
of mouth, 62
of nasal cavity, 42–44
of neck, 130
of pancreas, 328
of shoulder, 477
of small intestine, 322, 324
of spinal cord and vertebral column, 173
of stomach and duodenum, 319, 320
of suprarenal glands, 345, 346
of thigh, 500, 501, 540
of tracheobronchial tree, 210
of upper limb, 473
of urinary bladder, 344
of wrist, 461, 472
Neuroendocrine G cell, 276
Neurohypophysis, 140, 147, 148
Neuropathways, in parturition, 415
Neurovasculature
of arm, 435
of lower limb, 538–546

Newborn, skull of, 12
Nipple, 181, 182
left, 196
right, 196
Nodose ganglion, 135
Nodule
cerebellar, 144
inferior vermis, 113
Nose. *See also* Nasal cavity
ala of, 1
anterolateral view of, 36
cross section of, 47
inferior view of, 36
lateral crus of, 36
medial crus of, 36
surface anatomy of, 1
Nostril, 1
Nuchal line
inferior, 14
of skull, 174, 175, 176
Nucleus ambiguus, 117, 126
Nucleus pulposus, 155, 162
lumbar, 19
Nutrient artery, femoral, 504, 513
Nutrient foramen, 489, 513

O

Obex, 115
Oblique aponeurosis, 261
external, 250, 251, 260, 261, 349
internal, 253, 257
Oblique cord, 438, 439
Oblique fissure, 198
external, 188, 331
internal, 188, 189
of left lung, 244
Oblique muscle
external, 174, 175, 177, 179, 182, 192,
247, 249, 250, 259, 263, 330, 424,
494
aponeurosis of, 250, 252, 259, 349
aponeurotic part of, 249
cross section of, 338
digitations of, 254
muscular part of, 249
inferior, 121
internal, 175, 179, 250, 259, 261, 263,
330
aponeurosis of, 252, 349
in lumbar triangle, 174
tendon of origin of, 179
superior, 83, 84, 86, 118, 121
Oblique popliteal ligament, 508
Oblique vein, left atrial, 214, 215, 221
Obliquus capitis inferior muscle,
175, 176, 178
Obliquus capitis superior muscle,
175, 176, 178
Obturator anastomotic vein, 265
Obturator anastomotic vessels,
262, 363
Obturator artery, 259, 264, 340, 369,
376, 398, 400, 402, 403, 410, 504,
512
acetabular branch of, 487
anterior branch of, 487
posterior branch of, 487
Obturator canal, 352, 358, 364, 365,
369, 402, 501
Obturator crest, 352, 486, 487

Obturator externus muscle, 489, 493, 539
  attachments of, 489, 491
Obturator foramen, 248
  anteroposterior radiograph of, 488
  radiograph of, 355
Obturator groove, 486
Obturator internus muscle, 263, 376, 398, 411, 495, 499, 503
  attachments of, 489, 491
  nerve to, 499, 503
  obturator fascia of, 364, 392, 402, 411
Obturator internus tendon, 359
Obturator lymph node, 406
Obturator membrane, 263, 352, 370, 487
Obturator nerve, 267, 340, 376, 498, 499, 538, 539, 540
  accessory, 267, 498
  articular branch of, 539
  cutaneous branches of, 501, 544, 545
  cutaneous branch of, 539
  to knee joint, 539
  posterior branch of, 539
Obturator-pubic arterial anastomosis, 259
Obturator vein, 311, 376
Obturator vessels, 259
  right, 403
Occipital artery, 23, 34, 100, 178
  descending branch of, 34
  mastoid branch of, 100
  medial, 142
  meningeal branch of, 23
  occasional branch of, 11
  sternocleidomastoid branch of, 34
Occipital bone, 4, 7, 8, 9, 12
  basilar part of, 6, 8, 9, 22, 30, 37, 38, 39, 52, 65, 66, 67
  clivus of, 22
  condylar canal and fossa of, 8
  condyle of, 9, 30, 128
  external occipital crest of, 8
  external occipital protuberance of, 4, 6, 8
  foramen magnum of, 6
  hypoglossal canal of, 6
  inferior nuchal line of, 8
  inferior petrosal sinus groove of, 6
  internal occipital crest of, 9
  internal occipital protuberance of, 9
  jugular foramen of, 6
  jugular process of, 30
  pharyngeal tubercle of, 8, 63
  superior nuchal line of, 83
  transverse sinus groove of, 6
Occipital condyle, 9, 30, 128
Occipital crest, external, 14
Occipital lobe, 105
  projection on, 120
Occipital lymph node, 72
Occipital nerve
  greater, 24, 177, 178
    from C2 dorsal ramus, 129
  lesser, 32, 129, 177, 178
  third, 24, 177, 178
Occipital pole, 105
  sagittal MR image of, 149
Occipital protuberance
  external, 14, 152
  internal, 9

Occipital sinus, 103, 144
  groove for, 9
Occipital sulcus, transverse, 105
Occipital vein, 23
  internal, 146
Occipitofrontalis muscle
  frontal belly of, 123
  occipital belly of, 123, 178
Occipitotemporal artery, 142
Occipitotemporal gyrus
  lateral, 106, 107
  medial, 106, 107
Occipitotemporal sulcus, 106, 107
Oculomotor nerve (III), 84, 86, 101, 114, 116, 117, 166
  branch of, 168
  distribution of, 118
  inferior branch of, 83, 86
  inferior division of, 118, 121
  schema of, 118
  superior branch of, 83, 86
  superior division of, 118, 121
Oculomotor nucleus, 116, 117, 121, 437, 438, 441, 444
  accessory, 132
Odontoblast layer, 57
Olecranon, 436
Olfactory bulb, 107
  cells of, 119
  contralateral, 119
Olfactory cells, 119
Olfactory mucosa, 119
Olfactory nerve (I), 119
  bundles of, 11
  distribution of, 118
  fibers of, 118, 119
  schema of, 118, 119
Olfactory nucleus, anterior, 119
Olfactory stria
  lateral, 119
  medial, 119
Olfactory sulcus, 107
Olfactory tract, 106, 107, 114
  lateral nucleus of, 119
Olfactory trigone, 119
Olfactory tubercle, 119
Olive, 114, 117
Omental appendices, 272, 284
Omental arterial arch, 305
Omental artery, 305
Omental bursa, 272, 331
  cross section of, 273
  lesser sac of, 273
  posterior wall of, 349
  posterior wall of, parietal peritoneum on, 331
  stomach reflected in, 272
  superior recess of, 272, 274, 287
Omental foramen (of Winslow), 272, 273, 275, 288, 331
  probe in, 272
Omental taenia, 281, 284
Omentum
  greater, 269, 271, 273, 284, 288, 339
    anterior layers of, 294, 319
    attachment of gastro-omental vessels to, 274
    posterior layers of, 319
  lesser, 273, 275, 288
    anterior layer of, 319
    attachment of gastric artery, 274

Omentum *(Continued)*
  blood vessels to right margin of, 348
  posterior layer of, 319
  right free margin of, 278, 279, 298
Omohyoid muscle, 29, 31, 34, 53, 189, 198, 420, 424, 428, 429
  inferior belly of, 1, 27, 29, 31, 32, 128, 129, 427
  invested by cervical fascia, 188
  invested by fascia of infrahyoid muscle, 428
  nerve to, 32, 71 31
  origin of, 420
  superior belly of, 27, 28, 29, 31, 32, 128, 129
Ophthalmic artery, 11, 23, 40, 83, 86, 132, 140, 143
  continuation of, 85
  muscular branch off, 85
  supraorbital branch from, 69
  supratrochlear branch from, 69
Ophthalmic nerve (V₁), 24, 45, 121, 122, 132, 133, 134, 135
  external nasal branches of, 122
  internal nasal branches of, 122
  lacrimal, frontal, and nasociliary branches of, 11
  tentorial branch of, 86, 122
Ophthalmic vein
  inferior, 85, 91
  superior, 83, 85, 91
Opponens digiti minimi muscle, 465, 476
Opponens pollicis muscle, 461, 465, 475
Optic canal, 2, 6, 11, 83
Optic chiasm, 48, 104, 106, 107, 114, 140, 141, 145, 146, 147
Optic disc, 90
Optic nerve (II), 83, 86, 87, 90, 106, 107, 113, 132, 143, 144
  coronal CT images of, 151
  distribution of, 118
  external sheath of, 91
  internal sheath of, 91
  vessels of, 91
  outer sheath of, 32, 83, 87
  sagittal MR image of, 149
  in visual pathway, 120
Optic radiation, 120
Optic tract, 107, 108, 112, 114, 144
Oral cavity, 39, 48, 52-53, 63. *See also* Lip; Mouth; Teeth; *specific parts of oral cavity*
  coronal CT images of, 151
  inspection of, 51
Oral region
  arteries of, 69
  nerves of, 71
  veins of, 70
Ora serrata, 87, 89, 90
Orbicularis ciliaris, 89
Orbicularis oculi muscle, 123
  orbital part of, 26
  palpebral part of, 26
Orbicularis oris muscle, 26, 36, 54, 81, 123
Orbiculus ciliaris, 89
Orbit
  arteries and veins of, 85
  fascia of, 85

Pancreaticoduodenal artery
(Continued)
inferior *(Continued)*
posterior, 306
posterior inferior, 320, 321
posterior superior, 305, 306, 320, 321
superior, 321
plexus on, 319
Pancreaticoduodenal lymph nodes,
315
Pancreaticoduodenal plexus,
inferior, 322, 323
Pancreaticoduodenal vein
anterior, 312
anterior inferior, 311
anterior superior, 311
inferior, 313
posterior, 312, 313
posterior inferior, 311
superior, 312
Pancreaticoduodenal artery
anterior superior, 301
inferior
anterior branch of, 301
posterior branch of, 301
phantom, 301
posterior superior, 301
Pancreatic vein, 311, 313
dorsal or superior, 313
great, 313
Papilla
muscle fibers to, 282
of teeth, 57
Papillary duct, 336
Papillary muscle
anterior, 220, 223, 224, 225
left anterior, 224
left posterior, 224
posterior, 220, 223, 225
right anterior, 224
right posterior, 224
septal, 220, 223, 224
Paracentral artery, 141, 142
Paracentral lobule, 106
Paracentral sulcus, 106
Paracolic gutter
left, 271, 362, 363
right, 271, 281, 362, 363
Paracolic lymph nodes, 317
Paradidymus, 389
Paraduodenal fossa, 270
Parahippocampal gyrus, 106, 107,
108, 119
Paramedian artery, 140
Paramesonephric (müllerian) duct,
389
Paramesonephric tubule, 389
Paranasal sinus
age-related changes in, 50
bones of, at birth, 50
coronal section of, 48
cross section of, 47
horizontal section of, 48
lateral dissection of, 49
sagittal section of, 49
Pararectal fossa, 362, 363, 369
floor of, 392
Pararenal fat, 179
Parasternal lymph nodes, 184
Parasympathetic fibers
postganglionic, 44
preganglionic, 44

Parasympathetic nerve, in tracheo-
bronchial tree, 210
Parasympathetic nervous system
schema of, 168
topography of, 166
Parathyroid gland, 76
inferior, 75, 76
right lateral view of, 75, 76
superior, 75, 76
superior view of, 75, 76
Paratracheal lymph nodes
left, 208
right, 208
Paraumbilical vein, 312
to round ligament of liver, 256
tributaries of, 256
Paraurethral (Skene's) glands, 389
primordium of, 389
Paraventricular nucleus, 147
Paravertebral anastomosis, 172
Paravesical fossa, 369
Parenchyma, blood vessels in, 337
Parietal artery, 141
anterior, 141, 142
anterior parietal, 142
posterior, 141, 142
Parietal bone, 2, 4, 6, 8, 9
tuber eminence of, 12
Parietal cells, 9, 276
Parietal emissary vein, 23
Parietal foramen, 7
Parietal limb, 220
Parietal lobe, 105
Parietal lobule
inferior, 105
superior, 105
Parietal operculum, 105
Parietal pleura
cervical, 196, 197, 230
costal, 194, 198, 206, 211, 230
left border of, 197
right border of, 197
diaphragmatic part of, 193, 194, 198,
206, 211
mediastinal part of, 193, 194, 198, 206,
211, 215, 230
Parietooccipital artery, 142, 143
Parietooccipital sulcus, 105, 106,
143
Parolfactory area, 106
Parotid duct, 25, 54
Parotid gland, 25, 26, 27, 28, 31, 32,
55, 125, 134, 166, 167
accessory, 61
cholinergic and adrenergic synapses to
serous, 61
horizontal section of, 25
Parotid lymph nodes
deep, 72
superficial, 72
Parotid papilla, 51
Parotid space, 34
Pars distalis, 147
Pars flaccida, 93
Pars interarticularis, 155
Pars intermedia, 147
Pars tensa, 93
Pars tuberalis, 147
Parturition, neuropathways in, 414

Passavant's ridge. *See*
Palatopharyngeal sphincter
(Passavant's ridge)
Patella, 485, 492, 493, 494, 501, 507,
511, 519, 521
anteroposterior radiograph of, 510
radiograph of, 510
Patellar anastomosis, 500, 512
Patellar bursa, 508
Patellar capsule, iliotibial tract
blended into, 508
Patellar ligament, 485, 489, 492, 493,
494, 508, 511, 514, 520, 521
Patellar nerve plexus, 544
Patellar retinaculum
iliotibial tract blended into, 508
lateral, 492, 493, 507, 508, 519, 520
medial, 492, 493, 501, 506, 508, 519, 520
Pecten, 393
Pecten pubis, 248, 486
Pectinate ligament, 88
Pectinate line, 393
Pectinate muscle, 220
Pectineal ligament (Cooper's), 188,
250, 251, 259, 262, 263
Pectineal line, 248, 263, 352, 353, 486,
489, 505, 538
Pectineus muscle, 376, 489, 492, 493,
500, 538
attachments of, 489, 491
Pectoralis major muscle, 27, 28, 181,
182, 188, 192, 198, 243, 244, 245,
246, 247, 249, 250, 418, 419, 428
abdominal part of, 424
clavicular head of, 181
deep to pectoral fascia, 182
fascia of, 26, 428
insertion of, 420
origin of, 419
sternocostal head of, 424
tendon of, 433
Pectoralis minor muscle, 198, 243,
244, 245, 420, 428, 433
fascia of, 428
insertion of, 420
invested by clavicopectoral fascia, 188
Pectoralis minor tendon, 429, 430
Pectoralis muscle, 189
Pectoral nerve
lateral, 188, 428, 430
medial, 188, 428, 429, 430
median, 428
Pedicle, lumbar, 155
Pelvic brim, 370
sacral part of, 157
Pelvic floor
contents of, 354–366
female, 356
Pelvic foramina, radiograph of, 355
Pelvic inlet
diameters of, 354
female, 354
male, 354
radiograph of, 355
Pelvic ligaments, 372
Pelvic organs, female, arteries and
veins of, 400
Pelvic outlet
anteroposterior diameter of, 354
female, 354
transverse diameter of, 354

Pneumothorax, chest drainage tube placement in, 190
Pons, 106, 114, 134, 135
  axial MR image of, 150
  sagittal MR image of, 149
Pontine artery, 140, 141, 143
Pontine taste area, 135
Pontine vein
  lateral, 144
  transverse, 144
Pontomesencephalic vein, anterior, 144
Popliteal artery, 512
Popliteal fossa, 485
Popliteal ligament, arcuate, 511
Popliteal ligament, oblique, 511
Popliteal lymph nodes, 546
Popliteal surface, 489
Popliteal vein, 546
Popliteal vessels, 495
Popliteus muscle, 491, 511, 515, 541
  attachments of 515, 541
  nerve to, 541
Popliteus tendon, 508, 510
origin of, 507
Pores of Kohn, 204
Portacaval anastomosis, 312
Porta hepatis, 287
Portal space, limiting plate of, 291, 292
Portal triad, 273, 278, 290, 297, 298
  cross section of, 273
Portal vein, 297
  branch of, 291, 292
  cross section of, 297, 338
Postanal space
  deep, 396
  superficial, 396
Postcaval lymph nodes, lateral, 343
Postcentral gyrus, 105
Postcentral sulcus, 105
Posterior chamber, 81, 87, 88, 90
Posterior limiting lamina (Descemet's membrane), 88
Posteromedial central artery, 140
Postganglionic sympathetic fibers, 346
  ciliary ganglion, 132
  female reproductive organ innervation, 415
  male reproductive organ innervation, 416
  urinary bladder and lower ureter innervation, 417
Postlunate fissure, 113
Poupart's ligament. See Inguinal ligament (Poupart's)
Preaortic lymph nodes, 317, 408
Precaval lymph nodes, lateral, 343
Prececal lymph nodes, 317
Precentral gyrus, 105
Precentral sulcus, 105
Prechiasmatic groove, 9
Preculminate vein, 144
Precuneal artery, 142
Precuneus, 106
Prefrontal artery, 141
Preganglionic sympathetic cell body, 44, 132

Preganglionic sympathetic fibers, 346
  ciliary ganglion, 132
  female reproductive organ innervation, 415
  male reproductive organ innervation, 416
  urinary bladder and lower ureter innervation, 417
Premolars, 56, 57
Preoccipital notch, 105
Prepatellar bursa, subcutaneous, 511
Prepontine cistern, 109
Prepuce, 388
  of clitoris, 388
  of penis, 361
  site of, 388
  site of future origin of, 388
Preputial gland, opening of, 382
Prepyloric vein, 311
Prerectal muscle fibers (of Luschka), 359
Presacral space, 364, 396
Presymphyseal node, 408
Pretracheal lymph node, 74
Prevertebral anastomosis, 172
Prevertebral muscle, 30
Prevesical lymph node, lateral, 343
Prevesical lymph plexus, 408
Prevesical plexus, 408
Princeps pollicis artery, computed tomography of, 484
Procerus muscle, 26, 36, 123
Profunda brachii artery, 429
Profundus flexor tendon, in common flexor sheath, 460
Promontorial lymph nodes, 343, 408
Promontory, 92, 93
Pronator quadratus muscle, 440, 448, 449, 450, 465, 475
Pronator teres muscle, 420, 433, 440, 446, 447
  humeral head of, 420, 447, 450, 474, 475
    origin of, 420
  ulnar head of, 350, 420, 447, 448, 475
    origin of, 420
Prostate gland, 167, 384
  arterial supply of, 403
  capsule of, 361, 366, 384
  fibromuscular stroma of, 384
  hyperplastic lateral lobe of, 403
  hyperplastic middle lobe of, 403
  inferolateral lobe of, 384
  inferoposterior lobe of, 384
  innervation of, 168
  isthmus lobe of, 384
  lymphatic drainage from, 408
  median lobe of, 384
  primordium of, 389
  with prostatic urethra, 376
  sagittal MR images of, 397
  skeletal muscle band of, 384
  sphincter urethrae muscle ascending anterior aspect of, 359
Prostatic duct, openings of, 384, 385
Prostatic plexus, 165, 344, 416
Prostatic sinus, 384, 385
Prostatic urticle, 389
Prostatic vein, right, 311
Prostatic venous plexus, 403

Proximal interphalangeal (PIP) joint, 418
Psoas major fascia, 342
Psoas major muscle, 179, 267, 278, 329, 339, 342, 492, 496, 498, 499
  area for, 330
  articular branch of, 538
  fascia of, 179, 342
  lower part of, 538
  origin of, 489, 496
Psoas minor muscle, 263, 496
  origin of, 496
Psoas muscle, 376, 496
  axial CT images of, 350
  muscular branch of, 498
Psoas tendon, 376
Pterion, 4
Pterygoid artery
  lateral, 40
  medial, 40
Pterygoid canal
  artery of, 40
  nerve of, 122, 123, 125, 131, 133, 135
Pterygoid fossa, posterior view of, 14
Pterygoid fovea, 15
Pterygoid hamulus, 4, 38, 46, 52, 55, 64, 65, 68
  at birth, 50
Pterygoid muscle
  lateral, 40, 54, 55
    axial MR image of, 150
  medial, 15, 25, 40, 52, 55
    nerve to, 71
Pterygoid nerve
  lateral, 46, 122
  medial, 46, 122
Pterygoid plate
  lateral, 13, 47, 55, 68
  medial, 52, 55, 64, 65
    hamulus of, 13
Pterygoid plexus, 70, 85
  deep facial nerve from, 23
Pterygoid process, 6, 8
  hamulus of, 12, 13, 14
  lateral plate of, 4, 12, 13, 14, 38, 39, 50
  medial plate of, 12, 13, 14, 38, 39, 50
  of palatine bone, 13
  plates of, 6
Pterygomandibular raphe, 15, 40, 52, 55, 65, 68
Pterygomaxillary fissure, 4
Pterygopalatine fossa, 4, 13, 14, 40, 44, 49
Pterygopalatine ganglion, 122, 123, 125, 131, 133, 135, 166, 168
  ganglionic branches of, 45
  in pterygopalatine fossa, 44
  schema of, 133
Pubic arch, 248
  female, 354
  male, 354
Pubic bone, 348, 357, 383
Pubic crest, 259, 376
Pubic hypogastric region, 268
Pubic ligament, inferior, 248, 356, 359, 360, 364, 365, 378, 383
Pubic ramus
  inferior, 248, 486
  superior, 248, 486, 496, 499

Pubic symphysis, 247, 259, 263
  female, 354
  male, 354
  radiograph of, 355
  sagittal MR images of, 397
  superior portion of, 376
Pubic tubercle, 247, 250, 263, 486,
    492, 493
Pubic vein, 265
Pubis
  anteroposterior radiograph of, 488
  body of, 376
  radiograph of, 355
  superior ramus of, 488, 493
  symphyseal surface of, 412
Pubocervical fascia, 372
Pubococcygeus muscle, 357, 358,
    359, 360
Pubofemoral ligament, 487
Puboprostatic ligament, lateral, 366
Puborectalis muscle, 356, 357, 358,
    359, 376, 398
  left, 356
Pubovesical ligament
  lateral, 364, 365
  medial, 364, 365
Pudendal artery
  deep external, 512
  internal, 341, 376, 499
  superficial external, 512
Pudendal canal (Alcock's), 392, 411
  internal pudendal artery in, 402, 404
  internal pudendal vein in, 399
  pudendal nerve in, 413
Pudendal canal, left internal
    pudendal vein in, 311
Pudendal cleft, 377
Pudendal nerve, 160, 267, 410, 411,
    412, 415, 416, 417, 499, 500, 503
  block of, 413
  internal, 392
Pudendal vein
  external, 256, 265
  internal, 376
  left internal, 311
  right internal, 311
  superficial external, 544
Pudendal vessels
  deep external, 401
  internal, 392
  superficial, 500
  superficial external, 401
Pudendal vessels, superficial, 249
Pudendum, 377
Pulmonary artery, 213
  axial CT images of, 242
  left, 206, 213, 214, 231, 245
    prenatal, 229
    radiograph of, 213
  right, 205, 206, 210, 214, 220, 230, 245
    prenatal, 229
Pulmonary ligament, 199, 208, 230,
    231
Pulmonary lymph nodes, 208
Pulmonary plexus, 126, 165, 166, 168,
    210
  anterior, 209
  posterior, 209

Pulmonary trunk, 206, 212, 215, 220,
    224, 225
  bifurcation of, 215
  outflow to, 224
  prenatal, 229
Pulmonary valve, 213, 220, 222, 225
  semilunar cusps of, 220, 222
Pulmonary vein
  left, 205, 206, 215, 221, 224, 231
    inferior, 214, 241
    prenatal, 229
    superior, 214
  right, 206, 215, 225, 230
    inferior, 214, 220, 246
    prenatal, 229
    superior, 212, 214, 220, 224
Pulvinar, 110, 111, 143, 144, 145
  left, 144
  right, 144
  of thalamus, 114
Pupil, 81
  dilator muscle of, 88, 121, 132
  muscles of, 132
  sphincter muscle of, 88, 121, 132
Pupillae muscle
  dilator, 121
  sphincter, 121
Purkinje fibers, 225
  subendocardial branches of, 225
Putamen, 108
Pyloric antrum, 275
  barium radiograph of, 279
Pyloric canal, 297
  cross section of, 297
Pyloric gland, 276
Pyloric lymph nodes, 315
Pyloric orifice, 276, 279
Pylorus, 275, 276, 278, 297
  barium radiograph of, 279
  cross section of, 297
Pyramid, 114, 144
  decussation of, 114
  inferior vermis, 113
  of vermis of cerebellum, 115
Pyramidalis muscle, 250, 260
Pyramidal process, 8, 12

Q

Quadrangular lobule, 113
Quadrangular space, posterior
    circumflex humeral artery
    in, 427
Quadratus femoris muscle, 492, 493,
    495, 503, 511, 538
  attachments of, 489, 491, 515
  nerve to, 499, 503
Quadratus lumborum muscle, 176,
    179, 263, 267, 329, 342, 496, 498
  area for, 330
  fascia of, 179
Quadratus plantae muscle, 534, 535,
    541
Quadratus plantae nerve, 541
Quadriceps femoris muscle, 538
  attachment of, 490
  patellar ligament of, 515
Quadriceps femoris tendon, 485,
    492, 501, 506, 511, 520, 521
Quadriceps tendon, 493

Quadrigeminal cistern, 109
Quadrigeminal plate, 115

R

Radial artery, 433, 445, 446, 447, 448,
    449, 454, 460, 461, 465, 474
  in anatomical snuffbox, 469, 470
  computed tomography of, 484
  palmar carpal branch of, 448, 465
  superficial palmar branch of, 454, 460,
    465
Radial bursa, 460, 462
Radial collateral artery, 434
Radial collateral ligament, 454, 455
Radial nerve, 429, 430, 432, 435, 447,
    448, 474, 475, 477
  in arm, 477
  branch of, 469
  communicating branch of, 468
  deep branch of, 445, 447, 449, 474
  dorsal digital branch of, 473, 481
  inferior lateral, 481
  posterior cutaneous, 469, 473, 481
  superficial branch of, 444, 447, 449, 468,
    469, 473, 474, 480, 481
    dorsal digital branch of, 469
Radial recurrent artery, 433, 434, 447
Radial styloid process, 452
Radiate artery, perforating, 335
Radiate capitate ligament, 454
Radiate ligament, 187
Radiate sternocostal ligament, 186
Radicular artery
  anterior, 172
  posterior, 172, 173
Radicular vein, 173
Radiocarpal joint, 453, 455
Radiocarpal ligament
  dorsal, 455
  palmar, 454
    radiocapitate part of, 454
    radioscapholunate part of, 454
Radiograph
  of ankle, 526
  barium
    of ileum, 279
    of jejunum, 279
    of long vermiform appendix, 283
    of stomach, duodenum, and proximal
      jejunum, 279
  of cervical vertebrae, 18
  of chest, 213
  of elbow, 437
  of female pelvis, 355
  of hand, 457
  of hip joint, 488
  of knee, 510
  lateral, of skull, 5
  of lumbar vertebrae
    anteroposterior, 156
    lateral, 156
  of male and female pelvis, 355
  of male pelvis, 355
  pelvic
    female, 355
    male, 355
  of shoulder, 422
  of wrist and hand, 457

Radiolunate ligament
long, 454
palmar, 454
short, 454
Radioscaphocapitate ligament, 454
Radioulnar joint, distal, 455
Radioulnar ligament
dorsal, 455
palmar, 454
Radius, 436, 438, 439, 440, 442, 443, 465
annular ligament of, 438
anterior branch of, 439
anterior (palmar) view of, 452
anterior surface of, 439
coronal section of, 439, 455
cross section of, 470
dorsal tubercle of, 452
head of, 439
right, 439
interosseous border of, 439
neck of, 437, 439
posterior cutaneous and inferior lateral cutaneous nerves of arm from, 479
posterior (dorsal) view of, 452
radiograph of, 437
rotators of, 440
tuberosity of, 437, 439
ulnar notch of, 439
Rami communicantes
gray, 130, 132, 133, 134, 165, 167, 169, 170, 180, 196, 209, 230, 240, 258, 267, 318, 324, 325, 327, 344, 412, 498, 499
white, 130, 132, 133, 134, 165, 167, 169, 180, 196, 209, 230, 240, 258, 267, 318, 321, 324, 325, 345, 398, 412, 499
Rathke's pouch, vestigial remnant of, 50
Rectal artery
inferior, 307, 398, 402, 403, 404, 405
middle, 264, 307, 323, 341, 364, 398, 400, 402, 403
superior, 264, 307, 318, 323, 324, 340, 364, 398, 400, 410
bifurcation of, 307
branch of, 307
Rectal lymph nodes, 317
middle, 317
superior, 317
Rectal nerve
inferior, 411, 503
superior, 503
Rectal plexus, 323, 344, 412
communication between internal and perimuscular, 399
middle, 323
superior, 318, 323
Rectal vein
inferior, 312
left, tributaries of, 311
left middle, 311
left superior, 312
middle, 312
right, tributaries of, 311
right inferior, 311
right middle, 311
right superior, 312
superior, 311
bifurcation of, 399

Rectal venous plexus
communication between internal and external, 399
external, 311, 393, 394, 399
internal, 393, 394, 399
perimuscular, 399
Rectal vessels, superior, 274
Rectineal ligament, 259
Rectocervical space, 369
Rectococcygeus muscle, 263
Rectoperinealis muscle, 262
Rectoprostatic (Denonvilliers') fascia, 348, 359, 361, 386, 391, 396
Rectosigmoid artery, 307, 323, 398
Rectosigmoid junction, 284, 391, 393, 394
Rectosigmoid plexus, 323
Rectosigmoid vein, 311, 312, 399
Rectourethralis superior muscle, 359
Rectouterine fold, 369
Rectouterine ligament, 369
Rectouterine pouch (of Douglas), 360, 362, 369, 371, 391
Rectovaginal space, 364, 369
Rectovesical pouch, 348, 361, 391
Rectovesical space
prerectal, 396
retroprostatic, 396
retrovesical, 396
Rectum, 263, 271, 284, 329, 356, 357, 361, 363, 364, 365, 378, 384, 391, 393, 400, 412
anal canal and, 393
arteries of, 398
circular muscle layer of, 393, 394
in situ, 391
female, 328, 396
male, 328, 396
innervation of, 168
ischioanal fossae of, 392
longitudinal muscle layer of, 393, 394
lymphatic pathway along, 408
marginal artery of, 398
muscularis mucosae of, 394
sagittal MR images of, 397
termination of, 376
transverse folds of, 393
veins of, 399
Rectus abdominis muscle, 189, 331
sagittal MR images of, 397
Rectus capitis anterior muscle, 73
Rectus capitis muscle. *See* Capitis muscle, rectus
Rectus capitis posterior major muscle, 175, 176, 178
Rectus capitis posterior minor, 175, 176, 178
Rectus femoralis tendon, 492
origin of, 492
Rectus femoris tendon, 485
Rectus muscle
inferior, 83, 84, 121, 151
lateral, 83, 84, 86, 121, 151
axial MR image of, 150
tendon of, 87
medial, axial MR image of, 150
superior, 83, 84, 86, 91, 121
tendon of, 91

Rectus sheath, 83, 189, 249, 250, 349
anterior layer of, 188, 250, 252, 259, 424
cross section of, 252
posterior layer of, 251, 252, 257, 259
Red nucleus, 107, 116, 117
Reil, island of. *See* Insula
Renal artery, 335, 341, 345
anterior branch of, 335
in situ, 332
left, 323, 329, 339, 347
posterior branch of, 335
right, 318, 321, 329
ureteric branch of, 335, 336
variations in, 333
Renal column (of Bertin), 337
Renal corpuscle
cortical, 336
juxtamedullary, 336
Renal cortex, 336, 337, 346
Renal ganglion, 344, 345
left, 346
right, 346
Renal fascia, 339, 342, 347
anterior layer of, 179
Gerota's, 342, 347
posterior layer of, 179, 342
sagittal section of, 342
transverse section of, 342
Renal medulla, 336, 337
preganglionic fibers and, 346
Renal papilla, 336
Renal parenchyma, 334
Renal plexus, 344, 345
left, 323, 346
right, 318, 346
Renal segment
arteries of, 335
vascular, 335
Renal sinus, 337
fat in, 334
perirenal fat of, 337
Renal vein, 341
in situ, 332
left, 329, 333
double, 333
entering inferior vena cava, 339
multiple, 333
right, 265, 329, 332, 339
Reproductive organs, male, innervation of, 415
Respiratory bronchiole, 204
Rete testis, area of, 390
Reticular nucleus, 111
Retina, 91
ciliary part of, 87, 88
iridial part of, 88
non-pigmented areas of, 91
optic part of, 87, 89
pigmented areas of, 91
projection on, 120
structure of, 120
Retinacular artery, 504
subsynovial, 504
Retinal artery, 90
central, 85, 87, 90, 91
Retinal vein, 90
central, 87, 91
Retinal vessels, right, 90
Retrobulbar fat, 83
Retrocecal recess, 271, 281

Subhiatal fat ring, 236
Sublingual artery, 59, 61
Sublingual caruncle, 51
  with openings of submandibular ducts, 51
Sublingual duct, 51
  openings of, 61
Sublingual fold, 51
  with openings of sublingual ducts, 51
Sublingual fossa, 15
Sublingual gland, 51, 53, 61, 123, 133,
    167
  mucous, 61
Sublingual nerve, 46
Sublobular vein, 290, 291
Submandibular duct, 51, 53, 59, 60
Submandibular fossa, 15
Submandibular ganglion, 59, 122,
    123, 131, 133, 166, 168
  schema for, 133
Submandibular gland, 27, 28, 31, 32,
    53, 123, 133, 166, 167
  mucous, 61
  serous, 61
Submandibular lymph nodes, 73
Submental artery, 40
Submental vein, 70
Submucosa
  of intestine, 326
  of stomach, 277
  of vermiform appendix, 283
Submucosal gland, 326
Submucosal plexus, 326
Submucous (Meissner's) plexus, 326
Submucous space, 392
  internal rectal venous plexus in, 393
  perianal, 396
Suboccipital nerve, 21, 178
Suboccipital triangle, 178
Subparotid node, 72
Subpleural capillary, 205
Subpleural lymphatic plexus, 208
Subpopliteal recess, 507, 508
Subpubic angle, radiograph of, 355
Subpyloric lymph nodes, 314
Subscapular artery, 427, 434
  computed tomography of, 484
Subscapular fossa, 185
Subscapularis muscle, 180, 192, 243,
    244, 245, 425, 428, 433
  insertion of, 420
  origin of, 420
  subtendinous bursa of, 423
Subscapularis tendinous muscle
  openings of, 423
  position of, 423
Subscapularis tendon, 423, 425
Subscapular nerve
  lower, 429, 430, 477
  upper, 429, 430
Subserous fascia, 412
Subserous plexus, 326
Substantia nigra, 107
Subtendinous bursa, 511
Subtrapezial plexus, 177
Subungual space, 471
Sulcal artery, 141
  central, 141, 142
  postcentral, 142
  precentral, 141
  prefrontal, 142

Sulcal vein
  anterior, 173
  posterior, 173
Sulcus
  dorsal median, mesothelial septum in,
    169
  hippocampal, 112
  hypothalamic, 147
  intraparietal, 105
  occipital transverse, 105
  occipitotemporal, 107
  olfactory, 107
Sulcus limitans, 115
Sulcus terminalis, 214
Superciliary arch, 1
Superficialis flexor tendon, in com-
    mon tendon sheath, 460
Superficial perineal (Colles') fascia,
    358, 361, 366, 370, 378, 380, 411
  attachment of, 380
Supinator artery, 447
Supinator muscle, 420, 440
  insertion of, 420
  origin of, 420
Supraclavicular nerve, 24, 31
  intermediate, 129, 479
  lateral, 129, 479
  medial, 129, 479
Supracondylar ridge, 436
Supraduodenal artery, 300, 301, 306
Supraglenoid tubercle, 420
Suprahyoid artery, 59
Suprahyoid muscle, action of, 29
Supramarginal gyrus, 105
Supraoptic nucleus, 147
Supraopticohypophyseal tract, 147
Supraoptic recess, 106, 108
Supraorbital artery, 23, 36, 40, 81, 85
Supraorbital nerve, 24, 36, 81, 122
  branches of, 86
  medial and lateral branches of, 86
Supraorbital notch, 1
  foramen, 2
Supraorbital vein, 23, 70, 85
Suprapatellar synovial bursa, 511
Suprapineal recess, 108
Suprapleural membrane, 230
  cervical, 231
Suprapyloric lymph nodes, 314
Suprarenal gland, 197, 278, 298, 299,
    329, 340, 342
  arteries and veins of, 332, 333
  cross section of, 347
  dissection of, 346
  in situ, 332
  left, 197, 272, 297, 329, 331, 338, 346
  nerves of, 344, 346
    dissection of, 346
  right, 197, 297, 329, 346
  schema of, 346
    dissection of, 346
Suprarenal impression, 287
Suprarenal-phrenic vein
    anastomosis, 265
Suprarenal plexus
  left, 323
  right, 318
Suprarenal vein, 333, 347
  inferior, 347
  middle, 347
  right, 332, 338

Suprascapular artery, 32, 74, 75, 76,
    427, 429
  infraspinous branch of, 427
Suprascapular nerve, 429
Suprascapular notch, 184, 185, 420,
    421, 423, 427
Suprascapular vein, 70
Supraspinatus ligament, 179
Supraspinatus muscle, 177, 423, 427
    428, 428
  insertion of, 420
  origin of, 420
Supraspinatus tendon, 423, 425
Suprasternal space, 28
Supratrochlear artery, 23, 40, 81, 85
Supratrochlear crest, 220, 224
Supratrochlear nerve, 81, 122
Supratrochlear vein, 23, 24, 85
Sural cutaneous nerve
  articular branches of, 541, 542
  communicating branch of, 540
  lateral, 540, 541, 542, 545
    branches of, 544
    communicating branch of, 545
  medial, 540, 541, 545
Sural nerve, 534, 540, 541, 545
  lateral calcaneal branch of, 541
  medial calcaneal branch of, 541
  via lateral calcaneal and lateral dorsal
    cutaneous branches, 541
Sustentaculum tali, 523, 524
Sweat gland, 9, 167
Sylvius, sulcus of, 141
Sympathetic ganglion, 409
  lumbar, 170
  superior cervical, 130, 132
  superior ganglion, 125, 128, 131, 133,
    134, 210, 226
  thoracic, 209
  thoracic, third, 240
Sympathetic nervous system
  general topography of, 165
  schema of, 167
Sympathetic trunk, 125, 133, 192,
    210, 230, 258, 263, 267, 290, 324,
    325, 327, 344, 409, 412, 499
  cervical, 165
  ganglia of, 321, 325, 344, 345
  ganglion of, first thoracic, 132
  left, 194, 318, 324, 346
  left lumbar, 323
  right, 194, 318, 328, 331, 346
  sacral, 323
    left, 412
    right, 412
  thoracic, 240
  thoracic ganglia of, 321
Synovial cavities, 22, 187
Synovial membrane, 423, 471
  attachment of to femur, 511
  of hip joint, 487

T

T1 spinal nerve, 132, 133, 134, 160
T2 spinal nerve, 133, 133
T7 spinal nerve, 414
  lateral cutaneous branch of, 254
  medial cutaneous branch of, 254

Ureter, 271, 334, 341, 362, 363, 364, 365, 366, 391, 400, 402, 403, 410, 412
  arteries of, 341
  diagonal course of, 340
  female, 340
  left, 340
  male, 340
  nerves of, 344, 345
  retroperitoneal, 340
  right, 318, 329, 340, 372
  upper, innervation of, 345
Ureteral plexus, right, 318
Ureteric fold, 362, 363, 369
Ureteric nerve, middle, 344
Ureteric orifice, 384
  left, 366
  right, 366
Ureteric plexus, 410
Ureteropelvic junction, 339
Urethra, 263, 367, 372, 389
  beginning of, 376
  cavernous, 368, 385
    bulbous portion of, 371
    pendulous portion of, 371
  in children, 368
  female, 356, 357, 360, 361, 389
    frontal section, anterior view of, 379
    schematic reconstruction of, 379
  male, 381, 383
    floor of, 385
    hiatus for, 358
    roof of, 385
  membranous, 368, 385, 408
    lymphatic pathway from, 408
  musculofascial extensions to, 357
  prostatic, 366, 368, 376, 384, 385
  spongy, bulbous portion of, 366
Urethral artery, 384, 405
Urethral crest, 384
Urethral fold, 388
  partly fused, 388
Urethral gland, 380, 385
  lacunae and openings of, 379
Urethral lacuna, 385
Urethral meatus, external, 361
Urethral orifice, 388
  external, 360, 377, 379, 382, 385, 388
  female external, 395
Urethral raphe, 388
Urethral sphincter, internal, 366, 367, 384, 385
Urethrovaginal sphincter, 367
Urinary bladder, 167, 269, 323, 329, 340, 367, 412
  apex of, 361, 365
  arteries of, 341
  body of, 361, 365, 366
  fascia of, 361, 364
  female, 366
  fundus of, 361, 365, 366
  innervation of, 168, 417
  interior of, 376
  lateral ligament of, 364
  lymph vessels and nodes of, 343
  male, 366
  mucosa of, 340
  neck of, 362, 365, 366
  nerves of, 344
  orientation and supports of, 365
  sagittal MR images of, 397
  trigone of, 361, 365, 366, 385

Urinary bladder *(Continued)*
  ureteric orifice of, 366
  uvula of, 366, 385
  voiding cystourethrography of, 368
Urogenital fold, 388
Urogenital groove, 388
Urogenital hiatus, 367
Urogenital sinus, 389
Urogenital triangle, 380
Urticle, 92, 95, 96, 124
Uterine artery, 340, 341, 372
  cardinal ligament with, 364
  vaginal branches of, 404
Uterine ostium, 371
Uterine (fallopian) tube, 360, 362, 369, 370, 389, 400, 412, 415
  abdominal ostium of, 371
  ampulla of, 371, 372
  fimbriae of, 371, 372
  folds of, 371
  infundibulum of, 371, 372
  isthmus of, 371
  uterine part of, 371
Uterine vein, 404
  superior, 399
Uterine venous plexus, 399
Uterine vessels, 360, 361, 371
  ovarian branches of, 372
Uterosacral fold, 362, 392
Uterosacral ligament, 360, 371, 372, 373
Uterovaginal venous plexus, 412
Uterovesical pouch, 372
Uterus, 370, 380, 388, 389, 400, 412
  age changes and muscle pattern of, 373
  anteflexion of, 377
  arteries and veins of, 404
  body of, 360, 371
  cervix of, 360, 364, 369, 370, 371
  degrees of retroversion of, 377
  external os of, 371
  frontal section of, 371
  fundus of, 360, 362, 365, 369, 371
  internal os of, 371
  retracted, 412
  round ligament of, 340, 389
  sagittal MR images of, 397
U-V junction, 372
Uvula, 51
  of urinary bladder, 366, 385
Uvular muscle, 52

V

Vagal cardiac nerve, 130
Vagal fibers, 126
Vagal nucleus, dorsal, 116
Vagal trunk, 263, 321, 322, 323, 328
  anterior, 126, 166, 209, 318, 319, 320, 321, 327, 344, 346
    anterior gastric branch of, 319
    celiac branches of, 216
    celiac branch of, 319, 320, 321, 322
    gastric branches of, 126
    hepatic branch of, 126, 319, 320, 323, 327
  celiac branches of, 320

Vagal trunk *(Continued)*
  posterior, 166, 318, 320, 321, 322, 323, 327, 328, 344, 346
    branch to celiac plexus, 240
    celiac branches of, 216, 319, 320, 321, 322
    posterior gastric branch of, 320, 328
Vagina, 367
  horizontal portion of, 372
  musculofascial extensions to, 356
  sagittal MR images of, 397
  supporting structures of, 370
  upper four-fifths of, 389
  vertical portion of, 372
  vestibule of, 370, 377
Vaginal artery, 340
Vaginal fornix, 371
  anterior part of, 360
  posterior part of, 360
Vaginal orifice, 388
Vaginal vein, 398
Vaginal venous plexus, 398
Vaginal vestibule, 389
  artery of bulb of, 370
  bulb of, 370, 404
  artery to, 404
Vaginal wall, 370, 373
Vagus nerve (X), 32, 34, 74, 75, 76, 114, 116, 117, 118, 125, 126, 127, 130, 131, 135, 206, 209, 210, 211, 325, 345
  auricular branch of, 10, 24, 126
  cardiac branch of, 209
  celiac branch of, 321
  cervical cardiac branch of
    inferior, 126
    superior, 126
  cholinergic, 210
  communicating branch of, 126
  communication to, 32
  distribution of, 118
  inferior ganglion of, 126, 127, 128, 135
  left, 243, 244
  meningeal branch of, 126
  nucleus of, 324
  pharyngeal branch of, 125, 126, 130
  posterior nucleus of, 116, 117, 126, 324, 345
  pulmonary plexus branch of, 209
  right, 75, 80, 193, 226, 230
  schema of, 118, 126
  superior cervical cardiac branch of, 130, 131
  superior ganglion of, 126, 127
  thoracic cardiac branch of, 126, 226
Vallate papillae, 58, 135
Vallecula, 58
Vane comitantes, 59, 60
Vasa rectae spuria, 337
Vasa rectae vera, 337
Vastus intermedius muscle, 489, 493, 507, 538
  attachments of, 489, 491
Vastus lateralis muscle, 485, 489, 491, 492, 493, 494, 500, 507, 538
  attachments of, 489, 491
Vastus medialis muscle, 485, 489, 492, 493, 500, 538
  attachments of, 489, 491, 538
  nerve to, 500

Visual fields, overlapping, 120
Visual pathway, 120
Vitreous body, 87
Vitreous chamber, 90
  coronal CT images of, 151
Vocalis muscle, 78, 80
  action of, 79
Vocal ligament, 77, 78
  abduction of, 79
  adduction of, 79
  lengthening of, 79
  shortening of, 79
Voiding cystourethrograms, male
  and female, 368
Vomer, 39
Vomerine groove, 39
Vorticose vein, 85, 90, 91
  anterior tributaries of, 91
  bulb of, 91
  posterior tributaries of, 91
  suprachoroidal tributaries of, 91
V-shaped area (of Laimer), 234, 235
Vulva, 377

W

White matter, spinal, 169
Willis, circle of. *See* Cerebral arterial
  circle (of Willis)
Winslow, foramen of. *See* Omental
  foramen (of Winslow)

Wolffian duct. *See* Mesonephric
  (wolffian) duct)
Wrist
  anterior (palmar) view of, 472
  anterior view of, 460
  arteries of, 461
  articular disc of, 455
  bones of, 456
  coronal section of, 455
  cross section, transverse, 461
  cutaneous innervation of, 472
  deep dorsal dissection of, 469
  deeper palmar dissection of, 460
  extensor muscles of, 441
  extensor tendons at, 470
  flexor muscles of, 442
  flexor tendons, arteries, and nerves at,
    461
  ligaments of, 454, 455
  movements of, 453
  nerves at, 461
  palmar dissection, deeper, 460
  posterior (dorsal) view of, 455, 470, 472
  radial dissection, superficial, 467
  radiograph of, anteroposterior, 457
  sagittal section of, 453
  superficial dorsal dissection of, 468
  superficial palmar dissection of, 459
  tendons of, 461

X

Xiphoid process, 185, 191, 196, 198,
  247, 248, 249, 285, 286, 293,
  297, 298
  cross section of, 297

Z

Zigzag (Z) line, 236
Zona orbicularis, 487
Zonular fibers, 87, 88, 89, 90
Zygapophyseal (facet) joint, 246
  C2–3, 19, 21, 22
    capsule of, 21, 22
  C3–4, 21
Zygomatic arch, 14, 54, 151
Zygomatic bone, 81
Zygomatic nerve, 121
Zygomaticofacial artery, 23
Zygomaticofacial nerve, 24, 122
Zygomaticofacial vein, 23
Zygomaticotemporal artery, 23
Zygomaticotemporal nerve, 24, 122
Zygomaticotemporal vein, 23
Zygomaticus major muscle, 26, 54,
  123
Zygomaticus minor muscle, 26, 54,
  123